Mitochondria in Health and Diseases

Mitochondria in Health and Diseases

Special Issue Editors

Sabzali Javadov
Andrey V. Kozlov
Amadou K.S. Camara

MDPI • Basel • Beijing • Wuhan • Barcelona • Belgrade

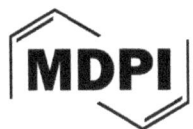

Special Issue Editors

Sabzali Javadov
Department of Physiology
School of Medicine
University of Puerto Rico
USA

Andrey V. Kozlov
Ludwig Boltzmann Institute
for Experimental and
Clinical Traumatology
Austria

Amadou K.S. Camara
Department of Anesthesiology
and Anesthesia Research,
Medical College of Wisconsin
USA

Editorial Office
MDPI
St. Alban-Anlage 66
4052 Basel, Switzerland

This is a reprint of articles from the Special Issue published online in the open access journal *Cells* (ISSN 2073-4409) from 2019 to 2020 (available at: https://www.mdpi.com/journal/cells/special_issues/Mitochondria_Health_Diseases).

For citation purposes, cite each article independently as indicated on the article page online and as indicated below:

LastName, A.A.; LastName, B.B.; LastName, C.C. Article Title. *Journal Name* **Year**, *Article Number*, *Page Range*.

ISBN 978-3-03936-384-1 (Hbk)
ISBN 978-3-03936-385-8 (PDF)

Cover image courtesy of Sabzali Javedov.

© 2020 by the authors. Articles in this book are Open Access and distributed under the Creative Commons Attribution (CC BY) license, which allows users to download, copy and build upon published articles, as long as the author and publisher are properly credited, which ensures maximum dissemination and a wider impact of our publications.

The book as a whole is distributed by MDPI under the terms and conditions of the Creative Commons license CC BY-NC-ND.

Contents

About the Special Issue Editors ix

Sabzali Javadov, Andrey V. Kozlov and Amadou K. S. Camara
Mitochondria in Health and Diseases
Reprinted from: *Cells* **2020**, *9*, 1177, doi:10.3390/cells9051177 1

Wonhee Hur, Byung Yoon Kang, Sung Min Kim, Gil Won Lee, Jung-Hee Kim, Min-Kyung Nam, Hyangshuk Rhim and Seung Kew Yoon
Serine Protease HtrA2/Omi Deficiency Impairs Mitochondrial Homeostasis and Promotes Hepatic Fibrogenesis via Activation of Hepatic Stellate Cells
Reprinted from: *Cells* **2019**, *8*, 1119, doi:10.3390/cells8101119 10

Jyotsna Mishra, Ariea J. Davani, Gayathri K. Natarajan, Wai-Meng Kwok, David F. Stowe and Amadou K.S. Camara
Cyclosporin A Increases Mitochondrial Buffering of Calcium: An Additional Mechanism in Delaying Mitochondrial Permeability Transition Pore Opening
Reprinted from: *Cells* **2019**, *8*, 1052, doi:10.3390/cells8091052 30

Adolfas Toleikis, Sonata Trumbeckaite, Julius Liobikas, Neringa Pauziene, Lolita Kursvietiene and Dalia M. Kopustinskiene
Fatty Acid Oxidation and Mitochondrial Morphology Changes as Key Modulators of the Affinity for ADP in Rat Heart Mitochondria
Reprinted from: *Cells* **2020**, *9*, 340, doi:10.3390/cells9020340 53

Rebecca M. Parodi-Rullán, Xavier Chapa-Dubocq, Roberto Guzmán-Hernández, Sehwan Jang, Carlos A. Torres-Ramos, Sylvette Ayala-Peña and Sabzali Javadov
The Role of Adenine Nucleotide Translocase in the Assembly of Respiratory Supercomplexes in Cardiac Cells
Reprinted from: *Cells* **2019**, *8*, 1247, doi:10.3390/cells8101247 73

Yang Ni, Muhammad A. Hagras, Vassiliki Konstantopoulou, Johannes A. Mayr, Alexei A. Stuchebrukhov and David Meierhofer
Mutations in *NDUFS1* Cause Metabolic Reprogramming and Disruption of the Electron Transfer
Reprinted from: *Cells* **2019**, *8*, 1149, doi:10.3390/cells8101149 86

Assunta Lombardi, Rosa Anna Busiello, Rita De Matteis, Lillà Lionetti, Sabrina Savarese, Maria Moreno, Alessandra Gentile, Elena Silvestri, Rosalba Senese, Pieter de Lange, Federica Cioffi, Antonia Lanni and Fernando Goglia
Absence of Uncoupling Protein-3 at Thermoneutrality Impacts Lipid Handling and Energy Homeostasis in Mice
Reprinted from: *Cells* **2019**, *8*, 916, doi:10.3390/cells8080916 108

Laura Poženel, Andrea Lindenmair, Katy Schmidt, Andrey V. Kozlov, Johannes Grillari, Susanne Wolbank, Asmita Banerjee and Adelheid Weidinger
Critical Impact of Human Amniotic Membrane Tension on Mitochondrial Function and Cell Viability In Vitro
Reprinted from: *Cells* **2019**, *8*, 1641, doi:10.3390/cells8121641 124

Denis Nalobin, Svetlana Alipkina, Anna Gaidamaka, Alexander Glukhov and Zaza Khuchua
Telomeres and Telomerase in Heart Ontogenesis, Aging and Regeneration
Reprinted from: *Cells* **2020**, *9*, 503, doi:10.3390/cells9020503 136

Anna Herminghaus, Eric Laser, Jan Schulz, Richard Truse, Christian Vollmer, Inge Bauer and Olaf Picker
Pravastatin and Gemfibrozil Modulate Differently Hepatic and Colonic Mitochondrial Respiration in Tissue Homogenates from Healthy Rats
Reprinted from: *Cells* **2019**, *8*, 983, doi:10.3390/cells8090983 148

Chupalav M. Eldarov, Irina M. Vangely, Valeriya B. Vays, Eugene V. Sheval, Susanne Holtze, Thomas B. Hildebrandt, Natalia G. Kolosova, Vasily A. Popkov, Egor Y. Plotnikov, Dmitry B. Zorov, Lora E. Bakeeva and Vladimir P. Skulachev
Mitochondria in the Nuclei of Rat Myocardial Cells
Reprinted from: *Cells* **2020**, *9*, 712, doi:10.3390/cells9030712 160

Andrey V. Kuznetsov, Sabzali Javadov, Michael Grimm, Raimund Margreiter, Michael J. Ausserlechner and Judith Hagenbuchner
Crosstalk between Mitochondria and Cytoskeleton in Cardiac Cells
Reprinted from: *Cells* **2020**, *9*, 222, doi:10.3390/cells9010222 174

Anna V. Kotrys and Roman J. Szczesny
Mitochondrial Gene Expression and Beyond—Novel Aspects of Cellular Physiology
Reprinted from: *Cells* **2020**, *9*, 17, doi:10.3390/cells9010017 198

Shubha Gururaja Rao, Piotr Bednarczyk, Atif Towheed, Kajol Shah, Priyanka Karekar, Devasena Ponnalagu, Haley N. Jensen, Sankar Addya, Beverly A.S. Reyes, Elisabeth J. Van Bockstaele, Adam Szewczyk, Douglas C. Wallace and Harpreet Singh
BK_{Ca} (*Slo*) Channel Regulates Mitochondrial Function and Lifespan in *Drosophila melanogaster*
Reprinted from: *Cells* **2019**, *8*, 945, doi:10.3390/cells8090945 223

Ji-Eun Kim, Hana Park, Seo-Hyeon Choi, Min-Jeong Kong and Tae-Cheon Kang
TRPC6-Mediated ERK1/2 Activation Increases Dentate Granule Cell Resistance to Status Epilepticus via Regulating Lon Protease-1 Expression and Mitochondrial Dynamics
Reprinted from: *Cells* **2019**, *8*, 1376, doi:10.3390/cells8111376 242

Ji-Eun Kim, Hana Park, Seo-Hyeon Choi, Min-Jeong Kong and Tae-Cheon Kang
CDDO-Me Selectively Attenuates CA1 Neuronal Death Induced by Status Epilepticus via Facilitating Mitochondrial Fission Independent of LONP1
Reprinted from: *Cells* **2019**, *8*, 833, doi:10.3390/cells8080833 258

A Ra Kho, Bo Young Choi, Song Hee Lee, Dae Ki Hong, Jeong Hyun Jeong, Beom Seok Kang, Dong Hyeon Kang, Kyoung-Ha Park, Jae Bong Park and Sang Won Suh
The Effects of Sodium Dichloroacetate on Mitochondrial Dysfunction and Neuronal Death Following Hypoglycemia-Induced Injury
Reprinted from: *Cells* **2019**, *8*, 405, doi:10.3390/cells8050405 276

Yanjie Tan, Yi Jin, Qian Wang, Jin Huang, Xiang Wu and Zhuqing Ren
Perilipin 5 Protects against Cellular Oxidative Stress by Enhancing Mitochondrial Function in HepG2 Cells
Reprinted from: *Cells* **2019**, *8*, 1241, doi:10.3390/cells8101241 296

René Günther Feichtinger, Daniel Neureiter, Ralf Kemmerling, Johannes Adalbert Mayr, Tobias Kiesslich and Barbara Kofler
Low VDAC1 Expression Is Associated with an Aggressive Phenotype and Reduced Overall Patient Survival in Cholangiocellular Carcinoma
Reprinted from: *Cells* **2019**, *8*, 539, doi:10.3390/cells8060539 320

Vincenzo Migliaccio, Ilaria Di Gregorio, Rosalba Putti and Lillà Lionetti
Mitochondrial Involvement in the Adaptive Response to Chronic Exposure to Environmental Pollutants and High-Fat Feeding in a Rat Liver and Testis
Reprinted from: *Cells* **2019**, *8*, 834, doi:10.3390/cells8080834 332

Anastasia Graf, Lidia Trofimova, Alexander Ksenofontov, Lyudmila Baratova and Victoria Bunik
Hypoxic Adaptation of Mitochondrial Metabolism in Rat Cerebellum Decreases in Pregnancy
Reprinted from: *Cells* **2020**, *9*, 139, doi:10.3390/cells9010139 349

Miroslav Ferko, Natália Andelová, Barbara Szeiffová Bačová and Magdaléna Jašová
Myocardial Adaptation in Pseudohypoxia: Signaling and Regulation of mPTP via Mitochondrial Connexin 43 and Cardiolipin
Reprinted from: *Cells* **2019**, *8*, 1449, doi:10.3390/cells8111449 365

Elena Starikovskaya, Sofia Shalaurova, Stanislav Dryomov, Azhar Nazhmidenova, Natalia Volodko, Igor Bychkov, Ilia Mazunin and Rem Sukernik
Mitochondrial DNA Variation of Leber's Hereditary Optic Neuropathy in Western Siberia
Reprinted from: *Cells* **2019**, *8*, 1574, doi:10.3390/cells8121574 383

Matthias L. Riess, Reem Elorbany, Dorothee Weihrauch, David F. Stowe and Amadou K.S. Camara
PPARγ-Independent Side Effects of Thiazolidinediones on Mitochondrial Redox State in Rat Isolated Hearts
Reprinted from: *Cells* **2020**, *9*, 252, doi:10.3390/cells9010252 396

Anna Picca, Robert T. Mankowski, George Kamenov, Stephen D. Anton, Todd M. Manini, Thomas W. Buford, Sunil K. Saini, Riccardo Calvani, Francesco Landi, Roberto Bernabei, Emanuele Marzetti and Christiaan Leeuwenburgh
Advanced Age Is Associated with Iron Dyshomeostasis and Mitochondrial DNA Damage in Human Skeletal Muscle
Reprinted from: *Cells* **2019**, *8*, 1525, doi:10.3390/cells8121525 408

About the Special Issue Editors

Sabzali Javadov M.D., Ph.D. completed his MD at the Russian Medical University, Moscow, in 1983, his PhD at the Russian Cardiology Center, Moscow, in 1986, and his DSc at the Moscow University, in 1992. He worked as a postdoctoral researcher and a visiting scientist at Magdeburg Medical University, Germany (1987), National Institute of Cardiology, Hungary (1991), University of Bristol, England (1997–2001), and Western University, Canada (2003–2008). Since 2009, he has been a professor at the Department of Physiology at the University of Puerto Rico School of Medicine, USA. Dr. Javadov has specific training and expertise in cardiac biochemistry and physiology, with a focus on the role of mitochondria in cardiac dysfunction induced by ischemia-reperfusion and heart failure. Currently, his laboratory elucidates the relationship between mitochondrial reactive oxygen species, permeability transition, and electron transport chain supercomplexes in myocardial infarction. Dr. Javadov has published over 100 papers in reputed journals and books and has served as an editorial board member for numerous biomedical journals. He has served as a review committee member for research foundations in the USA and Europe.

Andrey V. Kozlov M.D., Ph.D. completed his MD in 1980 and his PhD in 1986 for studies in medical biophysics from the Russian State Medical University (Moscow, Russia). In 2003, he received his habilitation (post-doctoral lecturing qualification) in pharmacology and toxicology at the University of Veterinary Medicine (Vienna, Austria). He worked as a postdoctoral researcher at the Institute of General Pathology, University of Modena (1993–1994, Modena, Italy), at the Department of Occupational and Environmental Health and Toxicology, University of Pittsburgh (1995, Pittsburgh, USA), and at the University of Veterinary Medicine (1996–2003, Vienna, Austria). Currently, he is the deputy director of, and principle investigator at, the Ludwig Boltzmann Institute for Experimental and Clinical Traumatology (Vienna, Austria). Dr. Kozlov's research has focused on metabolic disorders induced by hypoxia and inflammation occurring in shock, sepsis, ischemia-reperfusion, and more recently in neurotrauma. Particular attention is given to the function/dysfunction of subcellular organelles, mitochondria and endoplasmic reticulum, reactive oxygen and nitrogen species, free iron metabolism, oxidative stress reactions, and the pharmacology and toxicology of nitric oxide. He has published over 100 articles (original and review articles and book chapters), and serves on the editorial boards of several journals related to his research area.

Amadou K.S. Camara Ph.D. completed his PhD in renal and cardiovascular physiology at the Department of Physiology, Medical College of Wisconsin (MCW), in 1995. His dissertation focused on the brain renin angiotensin-aldosterone system, seeking to understand the mechanisms of renal neurogenic hypertension following a chronic NaCl diet in rats. From 1995–1999, he completed his postdoctoral training in cardiac electrophysiology at the Department of Anesthesiology, MCW. In 2000, he was elevated to the position of assistant professor in the department. In 2013, he was promoted to professor and was awarded a tenure in 2018. Dr. Camara's research has focused on cardiac physiology/pathophysiology, with an emphasis on ischemia reperfusion injury and cardioprotective strategies targeted to mitochondria. In particular, he studies mitochondrial Ca2+ regulation, with an emphasis on the molecular components responsible for Ca2+ efflux/influx (mitochondrial Ca2+ uniporter, Na+/Ca2+ exchanger, voltage-dependent anion channel), mitochondrial buffering capacity and the role of reactive oxygen species under normal and IR injury conditions. With his background in neuroscience, he has recently embarked on an investigation of the role of mitochondria in mild traumatic brain injury. He has published over 100 articles (original and review articles and book chapters) on IR and mitochondria-related studies. He has recently co-sponsored four Special Issues on mitochondria, served on numerous editorial boards, and been an ad hoc reviewer for more than two dozen journals. Dr. Camara has served on NIH study sections and has reviewed for numerous international grant organizations, including the Medical Research Council, England.

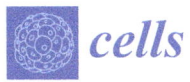

Editorial

Mitochondria in Health and Diseases

Sabzali Javadov [1,*], Andrey V. Kozlov [2,*] and Amadou K. S. Camara [3,4,5,*]

1. Department of Physiology, School of Medicine, University of Puerto Rico, San Juan, PR 00936-5067, USA
2. Ludwig Boltzmann Institute for Experimental and Clinical Traumatology, 1200 Vienna, Austria
3. Department of Anesthesiology, Medical College of Wisconsin, Milwaukee, WI 53226, USA
4. Department of Physiology, Medical College of Wisconsin, Milwaukee, WI 53226, USA
5. Cancer Center, Medical College of Wisconsin, Milwaukee, WI 53226, USA
* Correspondence: sabzali.javadov@upr.edu (S.J.); andrey.kozlov@trauma.lbg.ac.at (A.V.K.); aksc@mcw.edu (A.K.S.C.)

Received: 29 April 2020; Accepted: 6 May 2020; Published: 9 May 2020

Abstract: Mitochondria are subcellular organelles evolved by endosymbiosis of bacteria with eukaryotic cells characteristics. They are the main source of ATP in the cell and play a pivotal role in cell life and cell death. Mitochondria are engaged in the pathogenesis of human diseases and aging directly or indirectly through a broad range of signaling pathways. However, despite an increased interest in mitochondria over the past decades, the mechanisms of mitochondria-mediated cell/organ dysfunction in response to pathological stimuli remain unknown. The Special Issue, "Mitochondria in Health and Diseases," organized by *Cells* includes 24 review and original articles that highlight the latest achievements in elucidating the role of mitochondria under physiological (healthy) conditions and, in various cell/animal models of human diseases and, in patients. Altogether, the Special Issue summarizes and discusses different aspects of mitochondrial metabolism and function that open new avenues in understanding mitochondrial biology.

Keywords: mitochondria; energy metabolism; signaling pathways; ion homeostasis; human diseases

1. Introduction

Mitochondria have been recognized as the "power plants" that provide over 90% of ATP required for cell metabolism. Also, they are engaged in other aspects of cell metabolism and function and participate in the regulation of ion homeostasis, cell growth, redox status, cell signaling, and, thus, play a pivotal role in both cell survival and cell death mechanisms. Due to their central role in cell life and death, mitochondria are also involved in the pathogenesis and progression of numerous human diseases, including, among others, cancer, neurodegenerative and cardiovascular disorders, diabetes, traumatic brain injury, and inflammation (Figure 1). Mitochondria involvement in these diseases has been attributed to the pivotal role the organelle plays in the sequelae of events that culminate in cell death through various programmed (apoptosis, necroptosis, pyroptosis, ferroptosis, and autophagy) and non-programmed (necrosis) cell death mechanisms. A growing body of evidence on the important role of mitochondria under physiological conditions and human diseases is associated with increased number of biomedical studies in mitochondrial research. Since 2010, the number of mitochondria-related publications has exceeded other organelles including the nucleus, endo(sarco)plasmic reticulum, and the Golgi apparatus [1].

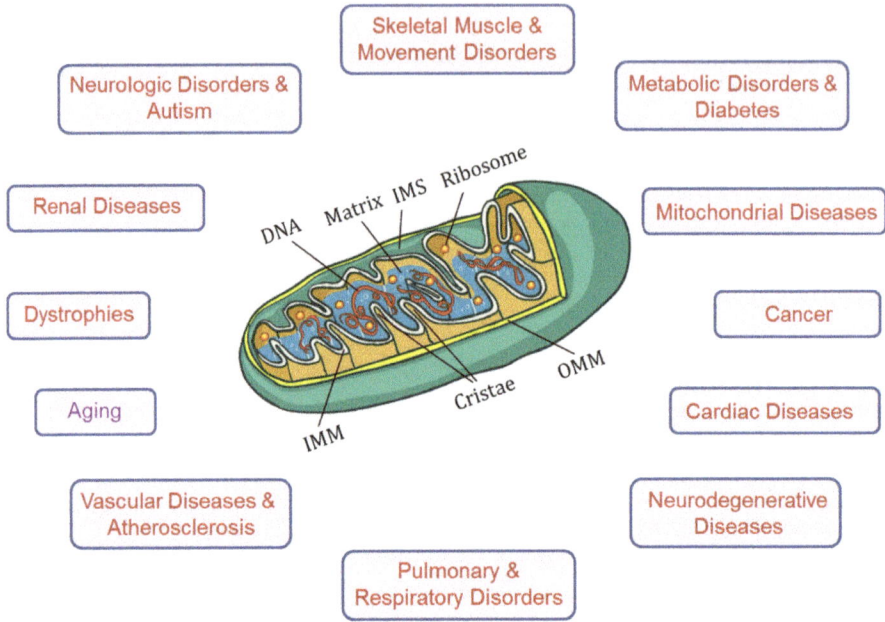

Figure 1. Mitochondria are involved in the pathogenesis of human diseases, and aging. IMM, inner mitochondrial membrane; IMS, intermembrane space; OMM, outer mitochondrial membrane.

Increased attention to mitochondria in recent decades stimulated preclinical studies on various cell and animal models to elucidate mitochondria as a therapeutic target for the treatment of a broad spectrum of human diseases. A large number of preclinical studies demonstrated beneficial effects of various pharmacological agents targeting mitochondrial ion channels, electron transfer chain (ETC), oxidative phosphorylation (OXPHOS), tricarboxylic acid (TCA) cycle, reactive oxygen species (ROS) production, permeability transition pore, DNA, membrane integrity, and apoptotic proteins, among others (Figure 2). However, despite an increased number of clinical trials conducted during recent decades, no single mitochondria-targeted compound has been approved by the U.S. FDA (Food and Drug Administration) so far that could be clinically applicable. Failure of the clinical trials can be explained by the fact that precise mechanisms whereby mitochondria are involved in the regulation of basic physiological functions, as well as their role in the cell under pathophysiological conditions, remain unknown. Furthemore, the mechanisms of interactions between mitochondria and other subcellular compartments and organelles such as endo(sarco)plasmic reticulum, nucleus, and lysosomes remain to be elucidated. Lack of in-depth knowledge of the regulatory mechanisms of mitochondrial metabolism and function as well as interplay between the factors that transform the organelle from the pro-suvival player to the pro-death contributor has hindered the development of new mitochondria-targeted pharmacological and conditional approaches for the treatment of human diseases.

To further improve our understanding of mitochondria, *Cells* organized the Special Issue entitled "Mitochondria in Health and Diseases" to highlight the latest achievements in elucidating mitochondrial metabolism and function under physiological and pathological conditions. The Special Issue published 24 articles consisting of 5 review articles and 19 original articles that cover a broad spectrum of mitochondrial research.

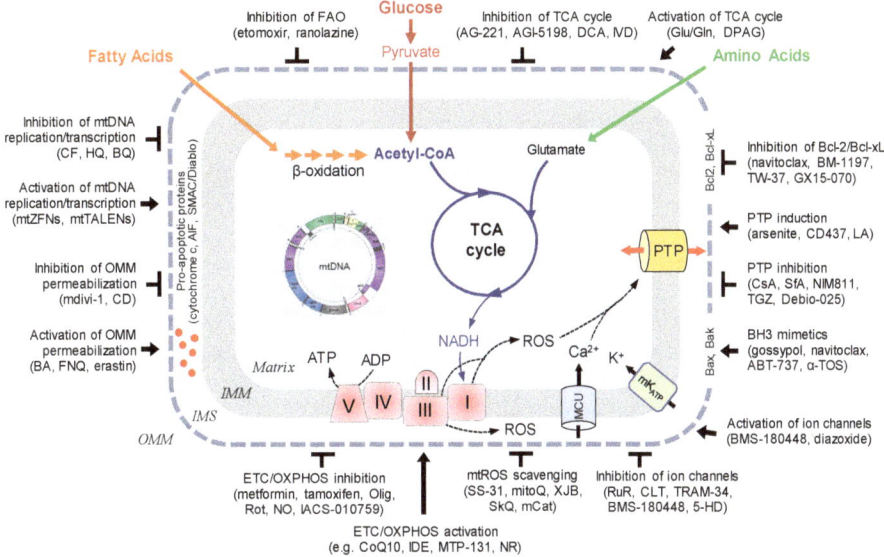

Figure 2. Mitochondria are promising therapeutic target for human diseases. *Abbreviations:* AIF, apoptosis-inducing factor; BA, betulinic acid; BQ, p-benzoquinone, mCAT, mitochondrial-targeted catalase; CD, chlorodiazepam; CF, ciprofloxacin; CLT, clotrimazole; CsA, cyclosporin A; DCA, dichloroacetate; DPAG, dipyruvyl-acetyl-glycerol; FAO, fatty acid oxidation; FNQ furanonaphthoquinone; 5-HD, 5-hydroxydecanoate; HQ, hydroquinone; Glu/Gln glutamate/glutamine; IDE, idebenone; IMM, inner mitochondrial membrane; IMS, intermembrane space; IVD, ivosidenib; mK_{ATP}, mitochondrial ATP-sensitive potassium channel; LA, lonidamine; MCU, mitochondrial calcium uniporter; NR, nicotinamide riboside; Olig, oligomycin, OMM, outer mitochondrial membrane; PTP, permeability transition pore; Rot, rotenone; RuR, ruthenium red; SfA, sanglifehrin A; mtTALENs, mitochondrially targeted transcription activator like effectors (TALE) fused with a Fok1 nuclease; α-TOS, α-tocopheryl succinate; TGZ, troglitazone; mtZFNs mitochondrially targeted zinc finger nucleases. *The names of representative compounds are shown in brackets.*

2. Mitochondria in Health

This section of the Editorial focuses on the role of mitochondria in maintaining normal and healthy physiology. In this endeavor, 13 articles (10 original research and 3 review articles) elucidating different aspects of mitochondria in maintaining health in the organism have been published. These studies can be grouped in the following four sections: (1) *Mitochondrial homeostasis*, (2) *Mitochondrial and cellular metabolism*, (3) *Crosstalk between mitochondria and other subcellular compartments*, and (4) *Mitochondrial ion channels*. The review articles highlight (a) the significance of mitochondria crosstalk with cytoskeletal proteins key in normal mitochondrial and cellular physiology, (b) mitochondrial gene regulation in different cellular contexts, and the importance of emerging aspects of mitochondrial transcripts and gene regulation in human health and disease, and (c) the role of telomeres and telomerase in cardiac aging. Altogether, these seminal articles provide a broad spectrum of new and unique perspectives in our understanding of the role of mitochondria in health and disease.

Mitochondrial homeostasis: To preserve themself and the host cell, mitochondria must maintain a balance between mitochondrial proliferation (biogenesis) and degradation (mitophagy). To mitigate degradation, mitochondria rely on intrinsic strategies to maintain quality. In this effort, Hur et al. [2] explored a novel role of HtrA2/OMI, a serine protease, in the regulation of mitochondrial homeostasis during hepatic fibrogenesis. The authors showed that overexpression of HtrA2/OMI led to antifibrotic effect due to CCl_4, by enhancing the antioxidant activity of mitochondria in hepatocytes.

In an unrelated study, but with a similar focus on mitochondria self-preservation during stress due to excess of Ca^{2+}, Mishra et al. [3] reported an intriguing observation that cyclosporin A bolsters mitochondrial Ca^{2+} buffering capacity in a phosphate-dependent manner in guinea pig cardiomyocytes isolated mitochondria. This novel observation indicates that cyclosporin A activates, yet determined, mitochondrial molecular mechanisms involved in Ca^{2+} sequestration. This additional insight into the action of cyclosporin A could potentially reveal different therapeutic approaches targeted at regulating mitochondria Ca^{2+} homeostasis and reduce cardiac injury in Ca^{2+} overload.

Mitochondrial and cellular metabolism: Normal mitochondrial and cellular metabolisms are tightly coupled. In healthy conditions, mitochondria account for the majority of the ATP produced in the cell via OXPHOS. In healthy cardiomyocytes, most of the acetyl CoA consumed by the heart is from fatty acids, with the remainder from pyruvate. In their study, Toleikis et al. [4], investigated the effects of fatty acid oxidation-induced changes in mitochondrial morphology and conformational changes in adenine nucleotide translocase (ANT) on the kinetics of the regulation of mitochondrial respiration in rat skinned cardiac fibers. Fatty acids alone or in combination with pyruvic acid was the substrate. The key message from this study is that fatty acids could regulate cellular energy metabolism by increasing the affinity of the ADP/ATP transporter for ADP, via conformational changes of the transporter. This study provides new understandings of the metabolic changes in altered age-related cardiovascular diseases.

In another study, Parodi-Rullán et al. [5] sought to elucidate whether ANT knockdown affects respiratory chain supercomplex formation in H9c2 cardiomyoblasts. This study is predicated on a previous observation by the same group that pharmacological inhibition of ANT disintegrated respirasome, the main respiratory chain supercomplex containing ETC complexes I, III, and IV, in cardiac mitochondria [6] suggesting an essential role of ANT in respirasome formation. ANT1 knockdown in the H9c2 cells reduced the $\Delta\Psi_m$ but increased total cellular ATP levels [5]. Furthermore, ANT1 downregulation did not alter the enzymatic activity of the ETC complexes I-IV but reduced the level of the respirasome. The results of this study not only confirm the previous observations of the role of ANT in respirasome formation, it also provides new convincing data, never reported previously with significant physiological implications for cellular metabolism. The reliance on electron transfer and the respirasome as key regulators of cellular metabolism was further reported by Ni et al. [7]. This study focused on the impact of specific mutations on two core subunits of complex I on metabolic reprogramming and disruption of electron transfer. The authors used an elaborate and integrative proteome and metabolome on human patient skin fibroblast (pluripotent cells). Mutations of the complex led to impaired integrity of the respirasome with increased ROS, increased $NADH/NAD^+$ ratio, and a switch towards glycolysis for cellular metabolism. These observations link the intactness of the respiratory complexes to the ability of mitochondria to execute OXPHOS and preserve normal cellular metabolism. The switch to anaerobic metabolism and ROS production is emblematic of the disruption of mitochondrial metabolism.

The prerequisite in bridging the gap between mitochondrial metabolism, thermal regulation, and body mass is mitochondrial uncoupling proteins (UCPs) and fatty acid oxidation. The physiological role of UCP3 in normal physiology, and its emerging role in pathophysiology, provide exciting potential for bridging this gap. Lombardi et al. [8] investigated the role of UCP3 in metabolic control in a situation where thermal stress was eliminated. There was no significant difference in weight gain and body composition between the two genotypes under low-fat diet; however, when animals were fed a high-fat diet, the UCP3 knockout animals showed enhanced energy efficiency and lean tissue mass. This novel observation indicates that temperature is the determinant factor for the outcome of metabolic effects elicited by UCP3.

Functional mitochondria are potentially key to tissue regeneration. Poženel et al. [9] looked at the potential contribution of mitochondrial metabolism in preserving the integrity of the human amniotic membrane (hAMs). The premise of this study is that in the common cell culture environment, the viability of amniotic cells decreases rapidly, but the underlying mechanisms of this phenomenon are unclear. Exposing hAM cells to tension or no tension, the study showed that tension applied to the cells in the culture environment displayed greater viability, in part, due to the preservation of mitochondrial bioenergetics and concomitantly reduced apoptotic events. These observations are a harbinger for improving stem cell maturation and tissue regeneration by using media conducive to mitochondrial preservation.

Cardiovascular diseases are associated with age and have a detrimental impact on the whole organism. Telomere length and telomerase activity play a role in cellular aging. In their review article Nalobin et al. [10] discussed the emerging role of telomere length and telomerase in cardiac development, aging, and regeneration. With the surge in interest in this topic and the contribution of mitochondria, the review is timely and highly appropriate. It postulates that the cumulative knowledge gained from the regenerative capacity of hearts will help in the formation of new approaches in the field of regenerative medicine for the treatment of diseases, for example, myocardial infarction and heart failure.

Altering mitochondrial metabolism is the hallmark of numerous pharmacological agents with significant clinical utility. Herminghaus et al. [11] explored the untoward effects of two clinically effective drugs in the management of hypertriglyceridemia. Utilizing hepatic and colonic tissue homogenates of healthy rats, the study showed that both drugs negatively impacted hepatic mitochondrial metabolism, as manifested in diminished mitochondrial respiration and OXPHOS. In contrast, in colonic mitochondria, the drugs either did not significantly impact mitochondrial metabolism or increased it in some cases. This carefully executed study reveals that the side effects of these drugs are organ-specific. A note of caution is that the studies were conducted in the in vitro condition, and some of the dosages used are out of the clinical range. So, extrapolation to human experience is tempered.

Crosstalk between mitochondria and other subcellular compartments: Mitochondria form an intricate network of connectivity with each other and with other cell structures, including the nucleus and the cytoskeleton. This dynamic interaction provides the framework for efficient mitochondrial function and cell survival. The anatomical and functional connection between mitochondria and the nucleus provides a coordinated cellular response to intracellular changes. The study by Eldarov et al. [12] explored the idea that mitochondria interaction with the nucleus is beyond intramembrane connection; it espouses the notion that a tiny fraction of the organelle could reside in the nucleus. This provocative concept has its genesis from earlier studies, but the results at the time generated skepticisms. Furthermore, other studies reported that mitochondria fragments found in the nucleus were indicative of pathology. With the advent of higher resolution technologies, this current study provided compelling new data obtained from healthy rat cardiomyocytes that support the localization of mitochondria in the nucleus.

Two review articles discussed the crosstalk between mitochondria and the cytosolic compartment. A review contribution by Kuznetsov et al. [13] provided a detailed and insightful summary of the physiological relevance of the crosstalk between mitochondria and cytoskeletal proteins. The review highlights the role of these proteins on mitochondrial intracellular organization and interaction with other organelles, the regulation of mitochondrial function, ATP production, and energy transfer. This anatomical and functional coupling is the hub for the integration of mitochondrial function with normal cell physiology and the preservation of life. In a different perspective on the interaction between mitochondria and cytosolic constituents, Kotrys and Szczesny [14] reviewed the impact of the mitochondrial genome on normal cell physiology and pathophysiology. The mitochondrial genome encodes for only 13 proteins involved in mitochondrial respiration; however, they also encode RNAs, which influence cell physiology when released into the cytosol. The review specifically focuses on the latest knowledge on mitochondrial transcripts, including mitochondrial long non-coding RNAs and novel functions of these transcripts. These novel mitochondrial gene regulation transcripts extend the repertoire of potential mechanisms by which mitochondria influence cell physiology.

Mitochondrial ion channels: In mammals, mitochondrial K_{Ca} channels have been reported to regulate mitochondrial function and to provide protection against cell injury. A study by Gururaja

Rao et al. [15] reported, for the first time, the presence of the BKCa (Slo) channel in mitochondria of the Drosophila (fruit fly). Mutation of the *slo* gene increased ROS generation, which could decrease survival and lifespan. The study is further bolstered by experiments that showed a reversal in mortality and improved lifespan following the overexpression of the human *slo* gene in the flies. The implications of the study are noteworthy; they provide new physiological understandings that may be relevant in our effort to decipher the underlying mechanisms of aging-related diseases.

3. Mitochondria in Diseases

Recently, different aspects of mitochondrial dysfunction have been associated with multiple human diseases, and hence, mitochondria are becoming a promising pharmacological target for the treatment of a broad range of diseases. This section of the Editorial comprising 11 articles focuses on the role of mitochondrial dysfunction in several pathological conditions. These studies can be grouped in the following four sections based on disease types: (1) *Neurological disorders*, (2) *Liver diseases*, (3) *Diseases associated with oxygen deficiency*, and (4) *Inborn and metabolic diseases*.

Neurological disorders: A study by Kim et al. [16] described a novel mechanism potentially regulating mitochondrial dynamics and seizure activity in the central nervous system. They provide novel evidence that transient receptor potential canonical channel-6 (TRPC6) regulates mitochondrial Lon protease 1 (LONP1) expression via the ERK1/2-mediated pathway. Activation of this pathway dramatically changes mitochondrial dynamics and assumed as an important therapeutic target for neuroprotection from various neurological diseases. In another study, the same group of authors [17] demonstrated that 2-cyano-3,12-dioxo-oleana-1,9(11)-dien-28-oic acid methyl ester (CDDO-Me), an analog of oleanolic acid exhibiting promising therapeutic effects in cancer, inflammatory, and neural diseases, irreversibly inhibits Lon protease-1 (LONP1) and activates ERK1/2 and c-Jun N-terminal kinase (JNK) pathways. They showed that CDDO-Me may selectively attenuate seizure activity in the cornu ammonis area 1 by rescuing the abnormal mitochondrial machinery, but in contrast to data reported above, this pathway was independent of LONP1 activity. Another report by Kho et al. [18] addressed the effect of glucose reperfusion after hypoglycemia on seizure, unconsciousness, and neuronal death. The data obtained by these authors suggest that abnormally elevated levels of pyruvate dehydrogenase kinase (PDK), and subsequent inhibition of pyruvate dehydrogenase play a critical role in this phenomenon. The authors found that sodium dichloroacetate, an inhibitor of PDK, can alleviate hippocampal neuronal death induced by hypoglycemia.

Liver diseases: A study by Tan et al. [19] investigated the impact of lipid droplet accumulation on cellular oxidative stress. They have shown that overexpression of Perilipin 5 (PLIN5), a key lipid droplet protein required for the formation of contacts between mitochondria and lipid droplets, reduces ROS levels and improves mitochondrial function in HepG2 cells. They assume that the upregulation of PLIN5 is a survival strategy of cells in response to stress. Feichtinger et al. [20] examined cholangiocellular carcinoma biopsies in order to better understand the impact of mitochondria. They have found that the expression of voltage-dependent anion-selective channel 1 (VDAC-1) in the outer mitochondrial membrane inversely correlates with UICC (Union Internationale Contre le Cancer) cancer stage classification. Also, significantly lower survival was observed for low/moderate VDAC1 expressors compared to high expressors. These data suggest that lower mitochondrial mass is associated with shorter survival of patients with cholangiocellular carcinoma. Also, one review contributed to this section. Migliaccio at al. [21] contributed a review article summarizing recent findings on mitochondrial adaptive response and oxidative stress induction in the liver, the main tissue involved in fat metabolism and pollutant detoxification, and in male gonads, the main targets of endocrine disruption induced by both high-fat feeding and environmental pollutants. This review provided novel insights into the mechanisms underlying cellular response to the exposure to stressful environmental stimuli and metabolic adaptation to promote cellular survival.

Diseases associated with oxygen deficiency: In a study by Graf et al. [22], they reported the changes in cerebellar amino acid metabolism in pregnancy with particular emphasis on the role of 2-oxoglutarate dehydrogenase complex. Hormonal changes occurring in pregnancy are known to coordinate a broad range of physiological adaptations, including changes in amino acid metabolism. The data obtained by this group suggest that these changes critically influence mitochondrial function and the resistance of pregnant rats to hypoxia. The authors suggest that specific patterns of amino acids and the activity of the α-ketoglutarate dehydrogenase complex in mitochondria can be used as sensitive markers for the adaptation to hypoxia. In a review article, Ferko et al. [23] summarized and discussed previous studies that evaluated the factors affecting the regulatory mechanisms in mitochondria at the level of mitochondrial permeability transition and its impact on comprehensive myocardial protection. The review put particular emphasis on signaling pathways leading to mitochondrial energy maintenance during partial oxygen deprivation.

Inborn and metabolic diseases: Leber's hereditary optic neuropathy (LHON), an inherited mitochondrial disease, was the focus of the study by Starikovskaja et al. [24]. The authors performed an entire mtDNA genome sequencing and provided genealogical and molecular genetic data on mutations and haplogroup background of LHON patients in Russia (Siberia) and Europe. The results indicate that haplogroup affiliation and the mutational spectrum of the Western Siberian LHON cohort substantially deviated from those of European populations. Another study by Riess et al. [25] was focused on the adverse effects of thiazolidinediones, a class of anti-diabetic drugs, which sometimes were associated with heart failure. The latter was not clear, because these drugs activate the peroxisome proliferator-activated receptor-gamma (PPARγ), which is believed to play a key role in cardioprotection. However, Riess and coauthors [25] showed that there is another PPARγ-independent mechanism of thiazolidinedione action based on a reversible increase in mitochondrial oxidation, causing an increase in ROS production and a decrease in membrane potential. Both mechanisms may cause damage to the myocardium and have to be considered in the treatment of diabetic patients. The study by Picca et al. [26] attempted to evaluate the impact of iron metabolism on the process of muscle aging with an emphasis on mitochondrial homeostasis. Their data show that the changes in iron metabolism are strongly associated with mtDNA content and damage. The authors assume that muscle iron homeostasis is altered in old age, which contributes to the loss of mtDNA stability and impairs muscle metabolism. Muscle iron metabolism may, therefore, represent a target for therapeutic interventions against muscle aging.

In conclusion, the Special Issue "Mitochondria in Health and Diseases" includes the most recent studies that elucidate the physiological role of mitochondria in cell life as well as the response of mitochondria to various pathological stimuli in cell/animal models of human diseases, and in patients. The articles in this Special Issue will further improve our understanding of mitochondrial biology under physiological and pathological conditions, and open new avenues for the development of new pharmacological compounds and conditional approaches for the treatment of human diseases through targeting mitochondria.

Author Contributions: Conceptualization: Validation: All authors; Formal analysis: All authors; Writing—original draft: All authors; Writing—review & editing: All authors. All authors have read and agreed to the published version of the manuscript.

Funding: This work was supported by the National Institute of General Medical Sciences (Grant SC1 GM128210 to S.J.) and the National Heart, Lung, and Blood Institute (Grant R01 HL-131673 to A.K.S.C.) of the National Institutes of Health, the Advancing A Healthier Wisconsin (AHW; Grant 5520444 to A.K.S.C.), and Austrian Research Promotion Agency (Grant FFG 854180 to A.V.K.).

Conflicts of Interest: The authors declare no conflict of interest.

References

1. Picard, M.; Wallace, D.C.; Burelle, Y. The rise of mitochondria in medicine. *Mitochondrion* 2016, *30*, 105–116. [CrossRef] [PubMed]
2. Hur, W.; Kang, B.Y.; Kim, S.M.; Lee, G.W.; Kim, J.H.; Nam, M.K.; Rhim, H.; Yoon, S.K. Serine Protease HtrA2/Omi Deficiency Impairs Mitochondrial Homeostasis and Promotes Hepatic Fibrogenesis via Activation of Hepatic Stellate Cells. *Cells* 2019, *8*, 1119. [CrossRef] [PubMed]
3. Mishra, J.; Davani, A.J.; Natarajan, G.K.; Kwok, W.M.; Stowe, D.F.; Camara, A.K.S. Cyclosporin A Increases Mitochondrial Buffering of Calcium: An Additional Mechanism in Delaying Mitochondrial Permeability Transition Pore Opening. *Cells* 2019, *8*, 1052. [CrossRef] [PubMed]
4. Toleikis, A.; Trumbeckaite, S.; Liobikas, J.; Pauziene, N.; Kursvietiene, L.; Kopustinskiene, D.M. Fatty Acid Oxidation and Mitochondrial Morphology Changes as Key Modulators of the Affinity for ADP in Rat Heart Mitochondria. *Cells* 2020, *9*, 340. [CrossRef] [PubMed]
5. Parodi-Rullán, R.M.; Chapa-Dubocq, X.; Guzman-Hernandez, R.; Jang, S.; Torres-Ramos, C.A.; Ayala-Pena, S.; Javadov, S. The Role of Adenine Nucleotide Translocase in the Assembly of Respiratory Supercomplexes in Cardiac Cells. *Cells* 2019, *8*, 1247. [CrossRef] [PubMed]
6. Jang, S.; Javadov, S. Elucidating the contribution of ETC complexes I and II to the respirasome formation in cardiac mitochondria. *Sci Rep* 2018, *8*, 17732. [CrossRef]
7. Ni, Y.; Hagras, M.A.; Konstantopoulou, V.; Mayr, J.A.; Stuchebrukhov, A.A.; Meierhofer, D. Mutations in NDUFS1 Cause Metabolic Reprogramming and Disruption of the Electron Transfer. *Cells* 2019, *8*, 1149. [CrossRef]
8. Lombardi, A.; Busiello, R.A.; De Matteis, R.; Lionetti, L.; Savarese, S.; Moreno, M.; Gentile, A.; Silvestri, E.; Senese, R.; de Lange, P.; et al. Absence of Uncoupling Protein-3 at Thermoneutrality Impacts Lipid Handling and Energy Homeostasis in Mice. *Cells* 2019, *8*, 916. [CrossRef]
9. Pozenel, L.; Lindenmair, A.; Schmidt, K.; Kozlov, A.V.; Grillari, J.; Wolbank, S.; Banerjee, A.; Weidinger, A. Critical Impact of Human Amniotic Membrane Tension on Mitochondrial Function and Cell Viability In Vitro. *Cells* 2019, *8*, 1641. [CrossRef]
10. Nalobin, D.; Alipkina, S.; Gaidamaka, A.; Glukhov, A.; Khuchua, Z. Telomeres and Telomerase in Heart Ontogenesis, Aging and Regeneration. *Cells* 2020, *9*, 503. [CrossRef]
11. Herminghaus, A.; Laser, E.; Schulz, J.; Truse, R.; Vollmer, C.; Bauer, I.; Picker, O. Pravastatin and Gemfibrozil Modulate Differently Hepatic and Colonic Mitochondrial Respiration in Tissue Homogenates from Healthy Rats. *Cells* 2019, *8*, 983. [CrossRef] [PubMed]
12. Eldarov, C.M.; Vangely, I.M.; Vays, V.B.; Sheval, E.V.; Holtze, S.; Hildebrandt, T.B.; Kolosova, N.G.; Popkov, V.A.; Plotnikov, E.Y.; Zorov, D.B.; et al. Mitochondria in the Nuclei of Rat Myocardial Cells. *Cells* 2020, *9*, 712. [CrossRef] [PubMed]
13. Kuznetsov, A.V.; Javadov, S.; Grimm, M.; Margreiter, R.; Ausserlechner, M.J.; Hagenbuchner, J. Crosstalk between Mitochondria and Cytoskeleton in Cardiac Cells. *Cells* 2020, *9*, 222. [CrossRef] [PubMed]
14. Kotrys, A.V.; Szczesny, R.J. Mitochondrial Gene Expression and Beyond-Novel Aspects of Cellular Physiology. *Cells* 2019, *9*, 17. [CrossRef]
15. Gururaja Rao, S.; Bednarczyk, P.; Towheed, A.; Shah, K.; Karekar, P.; Ponnalagu, D.; Jensen, H.N.; Addya, S.; Reyes, B.A.S.; Van Bockstaele, E.J.; et al. BKCa (Slo) Channel Regulates Mitochondrial Function and Lifespan in Drosophila melanogaster. *Cells* 2019, *8*, 45. [CrossRef]
16. Kim, J.E.; Park, H.; Choi, S.H.; Kong, M.J.; Kang, T.C. TRPC6-Mediated ERK1/2 Activation Increases Dentate Granule Cell Resistance to Status Epilepticus Via Regulating Lon Protease-1 Expression and Mitochondrial Dynamics. *Cells* 2019, *8*, 1376. [CrossRef]
17. Kim, J.E.; Park, H.; Choi, S.H.; Kong, M.J.; Kang, T.C. CDDO-Me Selectively Attenuates CA1 Neuronal Death Induced by Status Epilepticus via Facilitating Mitochondrial Fission Independent of LONP1. *Cells* 2019, *8*, 833. [CrossRef]
18. Kho, A.R.; Choi, B.Y.; Lee, S.H.; Hong, D.K.; Jeong, J.H.; Kang, B.S.; Kang, D.H.; Park, K.H.; Park, J.B.; Suh, S.W. The Effects of Sodium Dichloroacetate on Mitochondrial Dysfunction and Neuronal Death Following Hypoglycemia-Induced Injury. *Cells* 2019, *8*, 405. [CrossRef]
19. Tan, Y.; Jin, Y.; Wang, Q.; Huang, J.; Wu, X.; Ren, Z. Perilipin 5 Protects against Cellular Oxidative Stress by Enhancing Mitochondrial Function in HepG2 Cells. *Cells* 2019, *8*, 1241. [CrossRef]

20. Feichtinger, R.G.; Neureiter, D.; Kemmerling, R.; Mayr, J.A.; Kiesslich, T.; Kofler, B. Low VDAC1 Expression Is Associated with an Aggressive Phenotype and Reduced Overall Patient Survival in Cholangiocellular Carcinoma. *Cells* **2019**, *8*, 539. [CrossRef]
21. Migliaccio, V.; Gregorio, I.D.; Putti, R.; Lionetti, L. Mitochondrial Involvement in the Adaptive Response to Chronic Exposure to Environmental Pollutants and High-Fat Feeding in a Rat Liver and Testis. *Cells* **2019**, *8*, 834. [CrossRef] [PubMed]
22. Graf, A.; Trofimova, L.; Ksenofontov, A.; Baratova, L.; Bunik, V. Hypoxic Adaptation of Mitochondrial Metabolism in Rat Cerebellum Decreases in Pregnancy. *Cells* **2020**, *9*, 139. [CrossRef] [PubMed]
23. Ferko, M.; Andelova, N.; Szeiffova Bacova, B.; Jasova, M. Myocardial Adaptation in Pseudohypoxia: Signaling and Regulation of mPTP via Mitochondrial Connexin 43 and Cardiolipin. *Cells* **2019**, *8*, 1449. [CrossRef] [PubMed]
24. Starikovskaya, E.; Shalaurova, S.; Dryomov, S.; Nazhmidenova, A.; Volodko, N.; Bychkov, I.; Mazunin, I.; Sukernik, R. Mitochondrial DNA Variation of Leber's Hereditary Optic Neuropathy in Western Siberia. *Cells* **2019**, *8*, 1574. [CrossRef] [PubMed]
25. Riess, M.L.; Elorbany, R.; Weihrauch, D.; Stowe, D.F.; Camara, A.K.S. PPARgamma-Independent Side Effects of Thiazolidinediones on Mitochondrial Redox State in Rat Isolated Hearts. *Cells* **2020**, *9*, 252. [CrossRef] [PubMed]
26. Picca, A.; Mankowski, R.T.; Kamenov, G.; Anton, S.D.; Manini, T.M.; Buford, T.W.; Saini, S.K.; Calvani, R.; Landi, F.; Bernabei, R.; et al. Advanced Age Is Associated with Iron Dyshomeostasis and Mitochondrial DNA Damage in Human Skeletal Muscle. *Cells* **2019**, *8*, 1525. [CrossRef]

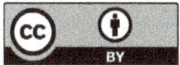 © 2020 by the authors. Licensee MDPI, Basel, Switzerland. This article is an open access article distributed under the terms and conditions of the Creative Commons Attribution (CC BY) license (http://creativecommons.org/licenses/by/4.0/).

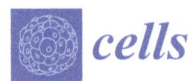

Article

Serine Protease HtrA2/Omi Deficiency Impairs Mitochondrial Homeostasis and Promotes Hepatic Fibrogenesis via Activation of Hepatic Stellate Cells

Wonhee Hur [1], Byung Yoon Kang [1], Sung Min Kim [1], Gil Won Lee [1], Jung-Hee Kim [1], Min-Kyung Nam [2], Hyangshuk Rhim [2] and Seung Kew Yoon [1],*

1. Catholic University Liver Research Center, College of Medicine, The Catholic University of Korea, Seoul 06591, Korea; wendyhur@catholic.ac.kr (W.H.); kby2132@catholic.ac.kr (B.Y.K.); ring704@nate.com (S.M.K.); lgw0429@catholic.ac.kr (G.W.L.); kim.jh@catholic.ac.kr (J.-H.K.)
2. Department of Biomedicine and Health Sciences, College of Medicine, The Catholic University of Korea, Seoul 06591, Korea; wangmouse@catholic.ac.kr (M.-K.N.); hrhim@catholic.ac.kr (H.R.)
* Correspondence: yoonsk@catholic.ac.kr; Tel.: +82-2-2258-7534; Fax: +82-2-536-9559

Received: 8 July 2019; Accepted: 19 September 2019; Published: 20 September 2019

Abstract: The loss of mitochondrial function impairs intracellular energy production and potentially results in chronic liver disease. Increasing evidence suggests that mitochondrial dysfunction in hepatocytes contributes to the activation of hepatic stellate cells (HSCs), thereby resulting in hepatic fibrogenesis. High-temperature requirement protein A2 (HtrA2/Omi), a mitochondrial serine protease with various functions, is responsible for quality control in mitochondrial homeostasis. However, little information is available regarding its role in mitochondrial damage during the development of liver fibrosis. This study examined whether HtrA2/Omi regulates mitochondrial homeostasis in hepatocyte during the development of hepatic fibrogenesis. In this study, we demonstrated that HtrA2/Omi expression considerably decreased in liver tissues from the CCl_4-induced liver fibrotic mice model and from patients with liver cirrhosis. Knockdown of HtrA2/Omi in hepatocytes induced the accumulation of damaged mitochondria and provoked mitochondrial reactive oxygen species (mtROS) stress. We further show that the damaged mtDNA isolated from HtrA2/Omi-deficient hepatocytes as a form of damage-associated molecular patterns can induce HSCs activation. Moreover, we found that motor neuron degeneration 2-mutant mice harboring the missense mutation Ser276Cys in the protease domain of HtrA2/Omi displayed altered mitochondrial morphology and function, which increased oxidative stress and promoted liver fibrosis. Conversely, the overexpression of HtrA2/Omi via hydrodynamics-based gene transfer led to the antifibrotic effects in CCl_4-induced liver fibrosis mice model through decreasing collagen accumulation and enhancing anti-oxidative activity by modulating mitochondrial homeostasis in the liver. These results suggest that suppressing HtrA2/Omi expression promotes hepatic fibrogenesis via modulating mtROS generation, and these novel mechanistic insights involving the regulation of mitochondrial homeostasis by HtrA2/Omi may be of importance for developing new therapeutic strategies for hepatic fibrosis.

Keywords: mitochondrial function; hepatic fibrogenesis; HtrA2/Omi; reactive oxygen species stress; mitochondrial homeostasis

1. Introduction

Hepatic fibrosis is a histological consequence of the wound-healing process resulting from chronic liver injuries induced by various causes. Advanced fibrosis progresses to liver cirrhosis leading to various life-threatening complications and hepatocellular carcinoma [1]. During long-standing liver injuries, the activation of hepatic stellate cells (HSCs) following hepatocyte damage and the recruitment of inflammatory mediators lead to the accumulation of extracellular matrix (ECM) [2]. At this time, reactive oxygen species (ROS) are primarily generated in the mitochondria and endoplasmic reticulum of hepatocytes, leading to further hepatocyte damage that results in HSC activation and enhanced ECM production [3]. These vicious pathogenic events of involving hepatocyte damage, inflammation, ROS production, and excessive ECM accumulation can accelerate hepatic fibrosis.

Mitochondria in hepatocytes serve as the primary source of energy; however, their dysfunction is commonly associated with increased ROS production. Moreover, along with being the source of ROS, mitochondria and mitochondrial DNA (mtDNA) can suffer damage by ROS. Thus, mitochondrial ROS homeostasis is critical for preventing oxidative injury in hepatocytes [4,5]. Once mtDNA is damaged by ROS produced in mitochondria, a cascade of events culminating in apoptosis or cell death proceeds. Studies have suggested that mitochondrial dysfunction in injured hepatocytes can initiate the apoptotic pathway, leading to increased collagen production via HSC stimulation [6–8]. Growing evidence supports a link between mitochondrial dysfunction and liver fibrogenesis, and mitochondrial quality control-based therapy has emerged as a new therapeutic strategy. However, it remains unknown whether mitochondrial dysfunction, specifically in hepatocytes, plays a role in the fibrogenesis, or whether mediators from hepatocyte mitochondrial damage promote liver fibrosis.

High-temperature requirement protein A2 (HtrA2, also known as Omi) is a nuclear encoded serine protease that localizes in the intermembrane space of mitochondria under normal conditions, and it is released into the cytosol upon apoptosis in response to various cellular stresses [9]. The pro-apoptotic function of HtrA2/Omi protease is at least partially mediated via the binding and proteolytic removal of inhibitor of apoptosis proteins. Recent studies illustrated that HtrA2/Omi inactivation does not cause early lethality in non-neuronal tissue, unlike its effects in neuronal tissue, but it leads to increased accumulation of mtDNA deletions and premature aging in mammals [10,11]. It has also been demonstrated that HtrA2/Omi deficiency causes mtDNA damage through ROS generation and DNA mutation, which can lead to the accumulation of unfolded proteins in the mitochondria, oxidative stress, and defective mitochondrial respiration, suggesting that HtrA2/Omi is important for mitochondrial homeostasis. Furthermore, our previous studies indicated that HtrA2/Omi deficiency or point mutations in its protease domain cause mtDNA conformational changes through ROS production in cultured cells [12]. The Ser276Cys (S276C) missense mutation in HtrA2/Omi was found to be the cause of symptoms such as muscle wasting, neurodegeneration, involution of the spleen and thymus, and death by 40 days of age in mnd2 (motor neuron degeneration 2) mutant mice. In these mice, the protease activity of HtrA2/Omi is greatly reduced.

Given that both ROS and mitochondrial dysfunction contribute to liver fibrogenesis and that hepatocyte mtDNA can exacerbate HSC activation, we hypothesized that HtrA2/Omi plays a pivotal role in liver fibrosis by modulating mitochondrial homeostasis.

In the present study, we demonstrated that the progression of fibrosis in both animal models and patients is associated with decreased expression of HtrA2/Omi, which modulates mitochondrial function and ROS generation. The modulation of HtrA2/Omi through mitochondrial homeostasis might be a promising anti-fibrotic therapeutic approach. These findings suggest the therapeutic value of HtrA2/Omi in the treatment of liver fibrosis.

2. Materials and Methods

2.1. Clinical Samples and Animal Studies

Five liver fibrosis tissues were obtained from patients with diagnosed chronic liver diseases who underwent liver transplantation (Seoul St. Mary's Hospital, Seoul, South Korea) prior to 2010 and stored in liquid nitrogen. None of them had history of any treatment. In addition, three liver tissues (as controls) were also obtained from patients without viral hepatitis during surgical procedures, and they were described in a previous report [13]. All patients provided written informed consent for the storage of liver tissue samples according to the ethical guidelines of Seoul St. Mary's Hospital in the Catholic University of Korea. Their personal information was restricted to analytical purposes. Such information is not available to the public.

All animal care and experimental protocols were conducted in accordance with the guidelines for the Care and Use of Laboratory Animals provided by the Research Supporting Center for Medical Science of the Catholic University of Korea (2016-0005-03). BALB/C and heterozygous *mnd2* (mnd2+/−) mice of the B6(Cg)-Htra2^{mnd2}/J strain were purchased from Orient Bio (Seongnam, Republic of Korea) and Jackson Laboratory (stock no. 004608). Mnd2/mnd2, mnd2/+, and WT mice were obtained by crossing mnd2 heterozygous (mnd2/+) mice. The genotypes of the mice were identified via PCR-AluI-RFLP genotype analysis as previously described [14]. Mice were used when 6–8 weeks old, excluding mnd2/mnd2 mice, which were used at 3 weeks of age, and housed in a standard laboratory animal facility.

To establish an animal model of liver fibrosis, male BALB/C or mnd2/+ mice (from five to seven mice per group) were treated via intraperitoneal injections of CCl_4 (Sigma, St. Louis, MO) as previously described [15]. Briefly, mice received CCl_4 dissolved in mineral oil (1/4 ratio) or mineral oil alone at a dose of 0.5 mL/kg body weight twice a week for 8 weeks to induce liver fibrosis. The control group received mineral oil alone at the same time. For the preventive study, liver-targeted hydrodynamic gene delivery to the mice was performed as previously described [16,17]. In brief, saline containing 30 μg of pFLAG-HtrA2/Omi plasmid, an expression vector containing the murine HtrA2/Omi open reading frame [18], or its control plasmid was hydrodynamically injected into the liver via a catheter with temporal blood flow occlusions. The injection volume and flow rate were fixed at 5% body weight and 1 mL/s, respectively. CCl_4 and the pFLAG-HtrA2/Omi plasmid were administered from five to seven mice in each group every 3 days for 8 weeks. The mice were sacrificed, and their livers were harvested.

2.2. Histological Analysis and Immunohistochemistry

Liver tissues were fixed in 3.7% buffered formalin, and then embedded in paraffin wax. The samples were cut into 3-μm sections and stained with hematoxylin & eosin (H&E) and Sirius Red (Direct Red 80, Aldrich, Milwaukee, WI) to detect collagen deposition. For immunohistochemistry, serial sections were deparaffinized and hydrated through a graded alcohol series. Antigen retrieval was performed by heating the sample in 0.01 M citrate buffer (pH 6.0) using a microwave vacuum histoprocessor (RHS-1, Milestone, Bergamo, Italy) at a controlled final temperature of 121 °C for 15 min. To block endogenous peroxide activity, the sections were quenched in 3% hydrogen peroxide in methanol and then blocked with 1% bovine serum albumin in PBS. Sections were incubated with primary antibodies against α-SMA and HtrA2/Omi diluted 1:500 in Antibody Diluent (Golden Bridge, Mukilteo, WA) at 4 °C. After washing, the peroxidase EnVision System (HRP rabbit/Mouse Envision System TM, Dakocytomation, Denmark) was applied at room temperature for 5–10 min. Peroxidase activity was detected with 3,3′-diaminobenzidine tetrachloride (DakoCytomation) and hematoxylin counterstain (DakoCytomation). The percent staining was calculated by the software of the Optimas 6.5 system.

2.3. TUNEL Assay

The TUNEL assay was performed using an in-situ cell death detection kit (Roche Diagnostics GmbH, Mannheim, Germany) following the manufacturer's protocol. After staining, the sections were mounted with mounting medium with 4, 6-diamidino-2-phenylindole (DAPI; Sigma). Apoptotic cells were quantified by counting TUNEL-positive nuclei. For each sample, the number of TUNEL-positive cells was observed under a fluorescent or confocal microscope (Zeiss, Jena, Germany) and counted under ×400 magnification. Six representative fields were evaluated for each mouse in all the experimental groups.

2.4. Isolation of Mouse Primary Hepatocytes and Cell Culture

Mice were intraperitoneally anesthetized with Rompun (10 mg/kg) and Zoletil (40 mg/kg). These mice were then exsanguinated. Livers were perfused in situ through portal vein with calcium- and magnesium-free Hanks' balanced salt solution (HBSS, Welgene, Daegu, Republic of Korea) until the firm texture was lost. After perfusion, soft liver tissue was removed and placed in a 1:1 mixture of Dulbecco's modified Eagle's medium and Ham's F-12 medium (DMEM/F12, Invitrogen, Carlsbad, CA). Subsequently, the liver suspension was poured through sterile 70-μm nylon mesh (BD Sciences, San Jose, CA) and then the homogenate was centrifuged at 50 × g for 2 min. The pellet containing parenchymal cells was washed twice with DMEM/F12 containing 10% fetal bovine serum (FBS, Invitrogen). Isolated primary hepatocytes were plated onto collagen coated plates and cultured in DMEM/F12 supplemented with 10% FBS. The non-tumorigenic mouse hepatocyte cell line FL83B cells was cultured in Ham's F-12K medium containing 10% FBS (Invitrogen), 100 μg/mL penicillin, and 0.25 μg/mL streptomycin. The LX-2 human hepatic stellate cell line (Merck Millipore, Billerica, MA; SCC064) with key features of hepatic stellate cytokine signaling and fibrogenesis was used as described previously [19]. LX-2 cells were cultured in DMEM supplemented with 10% FBS (Invitrogen), 100 μg/mL penicillin, and 0.25 μg/mL streptomycin. The cells were maintained in a humidified incubator at 37 °C with 5% CO_2.

2.5. Western Blot Analysis

Protein was extracted from cell lysates using RIPA lysis buffer (10 mM Tris-HCl, pH 7.5; 10 mM EDTA; 1% NP-40; 0.1% SDS; 150 nM NaCl; 0.5% sodium deoxychloride; protease inhibitors) for western blotting. Protein extracts were heated at 100 °C for 5 min before loading followed by separation on 10% or 12% SDS-polyacrylamide gels, transfer onto nitrocellulose membranes (Schleicher & Schuell, Dassel, Germany), and blocking for 1 h at room temperature in 5% skim milk. The membranes were incubated with primary antibodies overnight at 4 °C, followed by incubation (2 h at room temperature) with HRP-conjugated secondary antibodies (Amersham Biosciences, Cardiff, UK). Target proteins were detected using an enhanced chemiluminescence system (Amersham Pharmacia Biotech, Uppsala, Sweden) according to the manufacturer's instructions. The density of each band was analyzed using the Multi Gauge V3.0 program (Fujifilm, Tokyo, Japan).

2.6. Transmission Electron Microscopy (TEM)

Cells were collected and fixed with 4% paraformaldehyde and 2.5% glutaraldehyde in 0.1 M phosphate buffer, pH 7.2, at 4 °C overnight. After rinsing with 0.1 M phosphate buffer three times for 30 min each, the cells were treated with 1% osmium tetroxide in 0.1 M phosphate buffer for 1 h, dehydrated through a graded series of ethanol and acetone, embedded in Epon 812, and polymerized at 60 °C for 3 days. Ultrathin sections (60–70 nm) were prepared using an ultramicrotome (Leica Ultracut UCT; Leica Microsystems GmbH, Wetzlar, Germany). The sections on Formvar-coated slot grids were examined under a transmission electron microscope (JEM 1010; JEOL Ltd., Tokyo, Japan) operated at 60 kV. Images were recorded using a CCD digital camera (Orius SC1000; Gatan, Pleasanton, CA). All experiments were repeated three to five times to ensure reproducibility.

2.7. Immunofluorescence Staining

Cells were fixed with 4% paraformaldehyde for 20 min and permeabilized with 0.5% Triton X (Sigma). After washing three times each with PBS, the cells were blocked with 1% bovine serum albumin in PBS. Subsequently, the cells were incubated overnight at 4 °C with the primary antibodies. The cells were washed three times with PBS and incubated with Alexa Flour 488-labeled anti-rabbit IgG (Life Technologies, Carlsbad, CA). Nuclei were visualized by staining for 5 min with 1 μg/mL DAPI. After washing, the preparations were mounted using Kaiser's Glycerol gelatin (Merck, Darmstadt, Germany). The fluorescence intensity of the preparations was detected using a confocal microscopy (Zeiss). Fluorescence intensity in cells per sections was measured with microscope image-analysis software (ZEN blue software) by a single investigator who was blind to sample identity. In each of four replicate experiments, 20 images were recorded, and the fluorescent cells in each image were counted (every image contained approximately 20 cells). Finally, the cell concentration was calculated from the average number of cells per image.

2.8. Serum Aminotransferase Activity and Hydroxyproline Determination

Hepatotoxicity was assessed by quantifying the activities of serum alanine aminotransferase (ALT) using an ALT assay kit according to the manufacturer's protocol (Vettest 8008 Chemistry Analyzer; IDEXX Lab., UK). The accumulation of collagen in the liver tissue was determined by estimating the hydroxyproline content, an amino acid characteristic of collagen. Hydroxyproline levels in mouse livers were measured using a hydroxyproline assay kit (BioVision, Milpitas, CA) according to the manufacturer's instructions. The results are reported as milligrams of hydroxyproline per gram of wet liver tissue.

2.9. Lentiviral Vector Transduction

To establish a stable HtrA2/Omi-depleted cell line, FL83B cells were infected with a mouse HtrA2/Omi specific shRNA-encoded lentivirus (Sigma; SHCLNV-NM_019752). An shRNA negative control lentiviral particle (LV-Control) was used as a negative control. To generate a stable cell line, FL83B cells were plated at a density of 1×10^5 cells per 60-mm culture dish and infected overnight with five multiplicities of infection (MOI) lentiviral particles in the presence of 8 µg/mL hexadimethrine bromide (Sigma). After infection, the transduced cells were selected using 10 mg/mL puromycin (Sigma) for 2 weeks and incubated at 37 °C in a humidified incubator with 5% CO_2. Suppression of HtrA2/Omi expression in selected cells was confirmed by western blot analysis.

2.10. Quantitative Real Time-PCR-Based Gene Expression

Total RNA was extracted with TRIzol reagent (Invitrogen) and treated with DNase I (Invitrogen). For first-strand cDNA synthesis, 1.5 µg of total RNA were reverse-transcribed at 42 °C for 1 h using a random hexamer primer (Applied Biosystems) and Superscript II reverse transcriptase (Invitrogen). mRNA levels were measured using SYBR Premix Ex Taq (Takara, Japan). The relative mRNA levels were quantified using the comparative ΔCT method, normalized to β-actin. Primer sequences are listed in Supplementary Table S1.

2.11. Mitochondrial Fractionation and mtDNA Extraction

Following cell lysis, mitochondria were prepared using a mitochondria isolation kit (Pierce Biotechnology, Inc., Rockford, IL), according to the manufacturer's protocol. Isolation and DNase treatment of mitochondrial pellets were performed as described previously [20]. The DNase and RNase-treated mitochondrial pellet was resuspended in lysis buffer via gentle pipetting and the suspension was incubated at 37 °C for 1 h. A measure of 2 mg of proteinase K (Roche Diagnostics) was added and the lysate was incubated for 1 h at 37 °C. mtDNA was purified according to the genomic DNA extraction protocol using a DNeasy Blood & Tissue Kit (Qiagen, Santa Clarita, CA).

2.12. Genomic DNA Extraction and Quantitative PCR (qPCR)

Preparation of total genomic DNA from cell or liver tissue was performed using a DNeasy Blood & Tissue Kit (Qiagen, Santa Clarita, CA). Kits were used according to the manufacturer's instructions with the inclusion of RNAse A treatment to generate RNA-free genomic DNA, and genomic DNA was eluted using sterile deionized water. Quantitative PCR (qPCR) was conducted on genomic DNA using SYBR Premix Ex Taq in triplicate for each sample.

mtDNA damage was determined as a ratio of the copy number of short mtDNA-79 bp fragments (indicative of damaged mtDNA) to the copy number of long mtDNA-230 bp fragments (indicative of undamaged mtDNA) of the mitochondrial 16S-RNA gene as previously reported (Supplementary Table S1) [21]. In addition, the mtDNA copy number was compared to determine the relative mtDNA:nDNA ratio. Primers were designed within the mitochondria NADH dehydrogenase 1 (*mt-ND1*), and cytochrome oxidase 1 (*mt-COX1*) region of the mitochondrial genome (Supplementary Table S1). The nuclear NADH dehydrogenase flavoprotein 1 (*Ndufv1*) gene was used to standardize the mtDNA copy number to the diploid chromosomal DNA content [22]. Relative gene expression was normalized to that of the single-copy nuclear *Ndufv1* gene (ΔCT) in each sample.

2.13. Mitochondrial Membrane Potential and ROS Production

Cells were incubated with 2 uM CM-H_2DCFDA (Molecular Probes/Invitrogen) resuspended in warm HBSS or HBSS alone for unstained controls for exactly 15 min. The cells were analyzed on a FACSCalibur flow cytometer (BD). The cellular subset was identified according to size and granularity. We used a mitochondria-specific dye (MitoTracker Green FM) that binds the mitochondrial membrane independently of the membrane potential, and thus, the staining intensity is considered an index of mitochondrial mass. For MitoSOX Red-based flow cytometric detection of mitochondrial superoxide, cells were then incubated with MitoSOX Red superoxide indicator (Invitrogen) for 30 min, washed, and then analyzed on a FACSCalibur. The mean channel fluorescence was converted to absolute fluorescence using an inverse log transformation and normalized to that of untreated cells or WT hepatocytes.

2.14. Measurement of Mitochondrial Respiration

The OCR and extracellular acidification rate of cells were measured using a Seahorse XF24 extracellular flux analyzer (Seahorse Bioscience, Billerica, MA). In brief, hepatocytes were plated on Seahorse XF 24well plates at a density of 5×10^4 per well to achieve 80–90% confluency at the time of assay. Following the overnight attachment of cells, the medium was replaced with Seahorse XF medium, and the manufacturer's protocol for the Mitostress kit was followed (Seahorse Bioscience). In this analysis, sequential injections of 1 μM oligomycin, 1 μM FCCP, and 0.5 μM rotenone/antimycin A were added to the cells to define the basal OCR, ATP-linked OCR, proton leak, maximal respiratory capacity, reserve respiratory capacity, and non-mitochondrial oxygen consumption. Results for mitochondrial respiration were normalized to the total protein content.

2.15. Serine Protease Activity Assy

The protease activity of HtrA2/Omi in liver sections from WT and mnd2 heterozygous (mnd2/+) mice was assayed with the substrates β-casein. Liver lysates were immunoprecipitated (IP) with HtrA2/Omi-specific polyclonal antibody. The IP complexes were incubated for the indicated times at 37 °C with β-casein as a substrate. The reaction samples were resolved by 15% SDS-PAGE, and the processing pattern of β-casein was visualized by staining with Coomassie Brilliant Blue dye (CBB). The level of the HtrA2 was analyzed by western bolt with HtrA2/Omi Ab.

2.16. Statistical Analysis

All results are expressed as the mean ± SEM. Comparisons between two groups were performed using two-tailed Student's *t*-test. * $p < 0.05$, ** $P < 0.005$, *** $p < 0.001$.

Comparisons between multiple groups were performed via two-way analysis of variance (ANOVA). When ANOVA identified significant differences, individual means were compared using the post hoc Bonferroni test. Statistical analyses were performed using GraphPad Prism software 6.0.

3. Results

3.1. Mitochondrial Dysfunction Is Present in the CCl_4-Induced Mouse Model of Liver Fibrosis

As has been reported for liver fibrosis, most forms of chronic liver diseases are associated with the accumulation of damaged mitochondria, which are responsible for abnormal ROS formation and respiratory complex alterations [23]. To investigate whether alterations in mitochondrial structure or functions in hepatocyte were associated with the progression of liver fibrosis, we established a mouse model of CCl_4-induced liver fibrosis. As shown in Figure 1A, liver sections from the CCl_4 group displayed a distorted architecture with extensive collagen deposition upon staining with H&E and Sirius Red. Further examination via TEM revealed obvious swelling in mitochondria, and the cristae disappeared in mouse livers during the progression of hepatic fibrosis, suggesting that the mitochondrial structure was damaged along with these fibrotic changes (Figure 1A). Based on these findings, we hypothesized that the structural alterations of mitochondria were due to mitochondrial damage and that mtDNA damage, such as damage-associated molecular patterns (DAMPs), accumulated in necrotic hepatocytes. Therefore, we performed a quantitative evaluation of damaged mtDNA and mtDNA content in CCl_4-induced fibrotic livers. As in previous reports [21], we isolated genomic DNA, and then performed qPCR assay for two different mtDNA, namely 79 bp fragment (damaged), and 230 bp fragment (undamaged). The structurally damaged mitochondria in CCl_4-induced fibrotic model showed an increase in the damaged mtDNA at the ratios of the 79 bp fragment and 230 bp fragment (Figure 1B). In addition, we performed qPCR assay for two different mtDNA markers, namely mt-ND1 and mt-COX1. The levels of these mtDNA markers were normalized against NADH dehydrogenase flavoprotein 1 (Ndufv1) levels to examine the relative mtDNA to nuclear DNA ratios as described previously [24]. As shown in Figure 1C, the copy numbers of *mt-ND1* and *mt-COX1* per *Ndufv1* were significantly increased by 2.2- and 2.3-fold, respectively in CCl_4-induced fibrotic model. Based on these results, the increased damaged mtDNA and mtDNA content in CCl_4-induced fibrotic livers can result in malfunctioning proteins and altered mtDNA replication and/or transcription efficiency. Next, we examined the expression levels of mitochondrial respiratory and complex activity-encoded genes in mouse livers during the progression of hepatic fibrosis using qRT-PCR and western blot analysis. As shown in Figure 1D, the expression levels of nuclear-encoded subunit of complex IV *ATP5A* (Complex V) and *COX5B* (Complex IV) mRNA were decreased in CCl_4-induced fibrotic livers. Furthermore, immunoblots illustrated that the levels of subunits of ATP5A and MTCO1 (Complex IV) were significantly decreased in CCl_4-induced fibrotic livers, whereas those of the SDHB (Complex II) subunit were unchanged (Figure 1E). Therefore, these findings indicated that the pathogenesis of liver fibrosis is associated with mitochondrial damage or mitochondrial dysfunction.

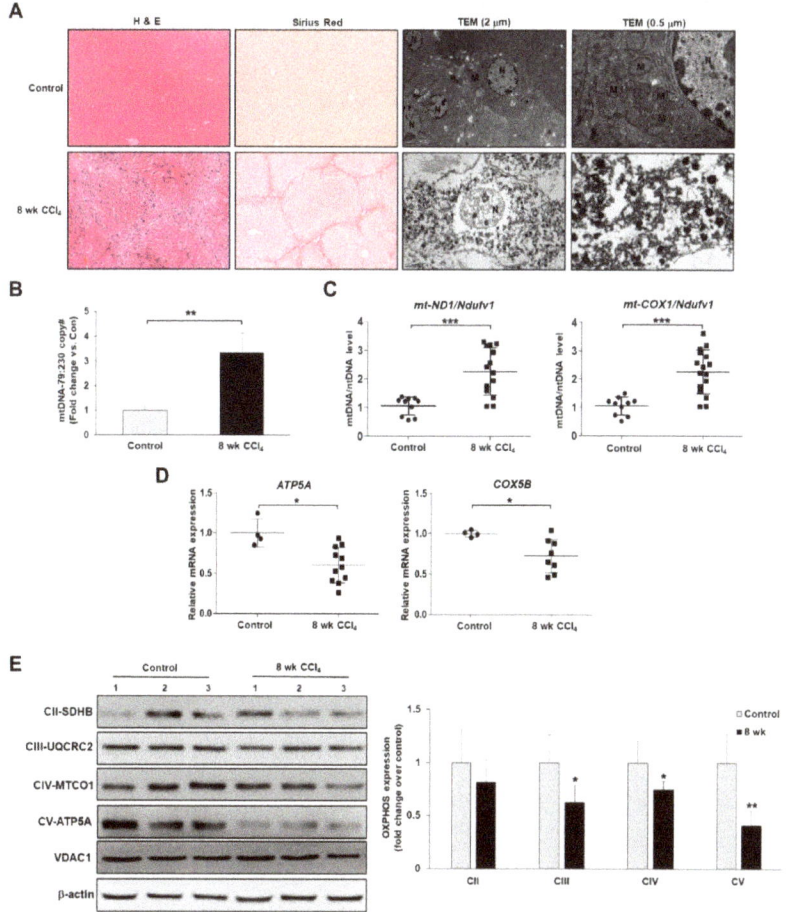

Figure 1. Morphological and functional abnormalities in mitochondrial are present in the mouse model of CCl_4-induced liver fibrosis. Male BALB/c mice were injected intraperitoneally with CCl_4 biweekly for 8 weeks to establish a hepatic fibrosis mouse model. (**A**) Representative images of H&E and Sirius red staining (original magnification, X200) of liver sections. TEM analysis of hepatocyte showing nucleus (N) and mitochondria (M) (scale bar = 2 & 0.5 μm). (**B**) Damaged mtDNA levels of the 79 bp fragment (damaged) and 230 bp fragment (undamaged) in gDNA isolated from livers of mice were assessed by qPCR. Bars represent mean copy number ratios of mtDNA-79:230, normalized to 18S levels. (**C**) Analysis of mtDNA content to obtain the mtDNA/nDNA ratio. gDNA isolated from livers of mice was analyzed by qPCR for the indicated genes. (**D**) Total RNA isolated from livers of mice was analyzed by qRT-PCR for the indicated genes. (**E**) Western blot analysis of representative subunits of OXPHOS complexes expression.

3.2. HtrA2/Omi Expression Is Decreased in CCl_4-Induced Fibrotic Mice and Patients with Liver Fibrosis

We attempted to identify and characterize the role of the mitochondrial serine protease HtrA2/Omi in improving mitochondrial damage during the progression of hepatic fibrosis. We first used fibrotic mouse models to validate the association of HtrA2/Omi expression with liver fibrosis. We found that HtrA2/Omi expression was downregulated in CCl_4-treated mouse livers via immunohistochemistry and western blotting. Staining assays revealed that HtrA2/Omi predominantly localized in the cytoplasm of hepatocytes and its levels were lower in fibrotic livers than in normal livers (Figure 2A).

Likewise, immunoblotting demonstrated that HtrA2/Omi expression was markedly decreased in mouse livers during the progression of hepatic fibrosis (Figure 2B). We detected α-smooth muscle actin (α-SMA) expression as a marker of HSC activation in fibrotic liver tissues. These findings were consistent with results obtained via western blotting using liver tissue samples from patients with fibrosis and healthy controls (Figure 2C). Immunohistochemistry of HtrA2/Omi in human fibrotic liver revealed that liver tissue from patients with late-stage fibrosis (grade 4) had lower HtrA2/Omi expression than that from patients with early-stage fibrosis (grades 1–2) (Figure 2D). These results suggest that HtrA2/Omi expression is downregulated in liver fibrosis with mtDNA alterations or mitochondrial dysfunction.

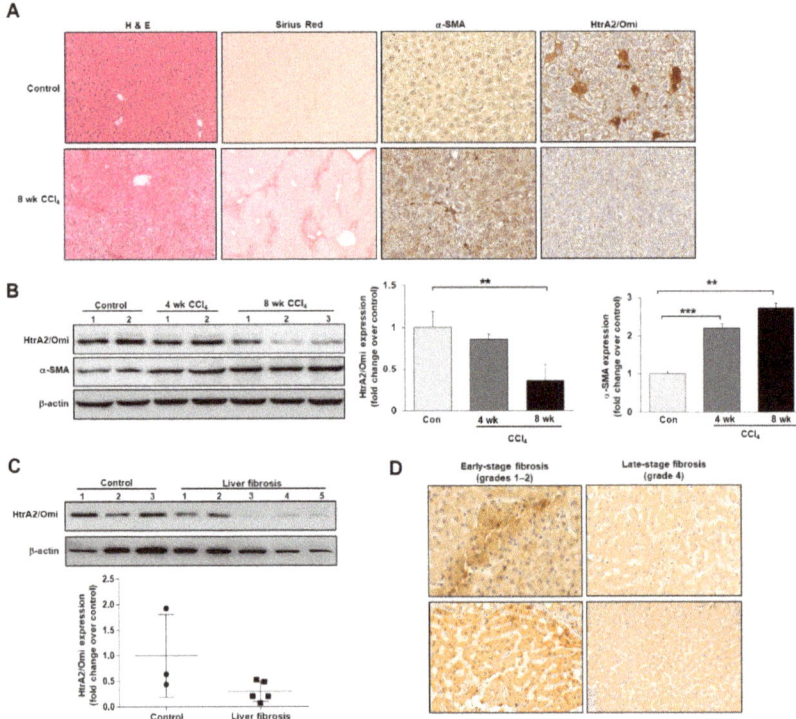

Figure 2. HtrA2/Omi expression is downregulated in CCl_4-induced liver fibrosis and human fibrotic livers. (**A**) Representative images of H&E, Sirius red (original magnification, X200) and immunohistochemistry staining (X400) of liver sections. (**B**) Western blot analysis of HtrA2/Omi, α-SMA and β-actin expression. (**C**) The protein levels of HtrA2/Omi in liver tissue from patients with fibrosis and healthy controls, as evaluated by western blotting. (**D**) Immunohistochemical staining of HtrA2/Omi in human fibrotic liver (X200).

3.3. HtrA2/Omi-Deficient Hepatocytes Cause Mitochondrial Accumulation and Structural Anomalies

To investigate the direct relationship between HtrA2/Omi downregulation and mitochondrial function in hepatocyte during liver fibrogenesis, we transfected a plasmid encoding shRNA targeting HtrA2/Omi into FL83B mouse hepatocytes, which were named lenti-shHtrA2 cells. As shown in Supplemental Figure S1A, HtrA2/Omi protein levels were significantly lower in lenti-shHtrA2 cells than in negative control lenti-shNC cells. We previously reported that HtrA2/Omi deficiency causes mtDNA damage through mutation and ROS generation, which can lead to mitochondrial dysfunction and consequent cell death [12]. Therefore, we examined the effect of HtrA2/Omi depletion on intracellular total ROS and mitochondria ROS (mtROS) levels in lenti-shHtrA2 hepatocytes using CM-H$_2$DCFDA and MitoSox. As shown in Figure 3A,B, lenti-shHtrA2 cells produced greater amounts of mtROS despite a decrease of total ROS than lenti-shNC cells. Recent reports suggested that mitochondria play a key role in regulating cell size by affecting the balance of cell growth and proliferation through metabolic activity [25]. Therefore, we measured the distributions of cell volume by analyzing forward (FSC) and side (SSC) light scatter as a cell-size and granularity index and then measured the mitochondrial mass via staining with a mitochondria-specific dye (MitoTracker FM) and intracellular voltage-dependent anion channel (VDAC) expression in HtrA2/Omi-depleted FL83B cells. In addition to the absence of changes in the cell-size and granularity index (Supplemental Figure S1C), the MitoTracker signal and VDAC expression revealed that the average mitochondrial mass was not changed in HtrA2/Omi-depleted hepatocytes (Supplemental Figure S1B). Next, the degree of mtDNA damage induced by mtROS was measured in HtrA2/Omi-depleted hepatocyte via qPCR assay. As shown in Figure 3C, the ratios of the 79 bp fragment and 230 bp fragment were significantly increased by 1.7-fold in HtrA2/Omi-depleted hepatocyte. Furthermore, an interesting observation was that *mt-ND1* mtDNA content per *Ndufv1* in HtrA2/Omi-depleted FL83B cells was significantly increased by approximately 6-fold compared with control levels, whereas *ND1* mRNA levels were significantly decreased (Figure 3D,E). These results are consistent with previous findings that MEF cells lacking HtrA2/Omi displayed increased mtDNA levels relative to paired control cell lines [12]. Mitochondrial oxidative stress-induced mtDNA damage was associated with a decrease in mitochondrial respiration [26]. Next, we examined the effect of HtrA2/Omi depletion on mitochondrial respiration by measuring the oxygen consumption rate (OCR) using an extracellular flux analyzer. Three basal OCRs were recorded, followed by the sequential injection of oligomycin, FCCP, and antimycin A. As shown in Figure 3F, HtrA2/Omi-depleted FL83B cells displayed impaired mitochondrial respiration either under basal or maximal oxygen consumption induced by FCCP treatment. Taken together, these results indicate that HtrA2/Omi-deficient hepatocytes exhibit mitochondrial dysfunction and a concomitant elevation of mtROS levels.

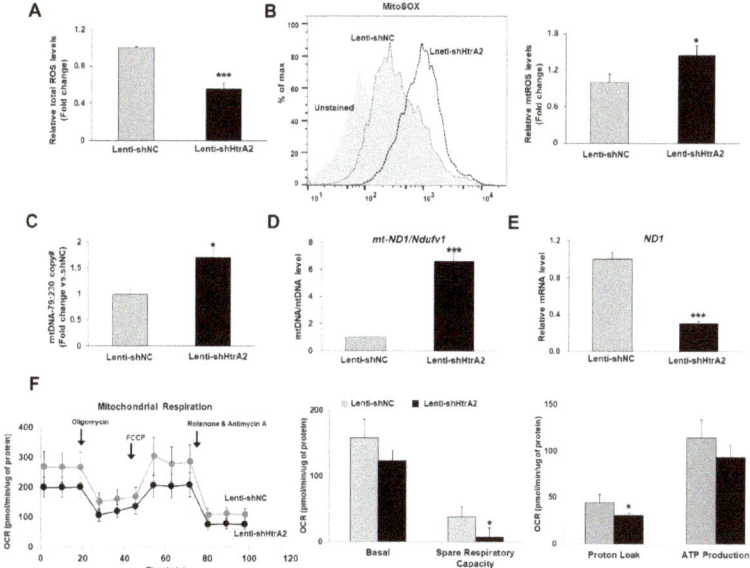

Figure 3. Lentivirus-mediated HtrA2/Omi depletion in hepatocyte lead to impaired mitochondrial function and metabolism.

(**A**) Intracellular ROS levels were measured by FACS-analysis using CM-H$_2$DCFDA staining. (**B**) Mitochondrial superoxide level was measured by FACS-analysis using MitoSOX red staining. The fluorescence mean intensity of MitoSOX red per cell was quantified. (**C**) Damaged mtDNA levels of the 79 bp fragment (damaged) and 230 bp fragment (undamaged) in gDNA isolated from cells were assessed by qPCR. Bars represent mean copy number ratios of mtDNA-79:230, normalized to 18S levels. (**D**) Real time qPCR analysis of *mt-ND1* DNA normalized to nuclear *Ndufv1* DNA. (**E**) *ND1* mRNA expression, as determined by qRT-PCR. (**F**) OCR measurements were obtained using an extracellular flux analyzer. Results for mitochondrial respiration were normalized to the total protein content.

3.4. Loss of HtrA2/Omi Protease Activity in Hepatocytes Results in the Accumulation of Dysfunctional Mitochondria and Oxidative Stress

We attempted to confirm the association of mitochondrial dysfunction with mtROS levels following the loss of HtrA2/Omi mitochondrial protease activity as well as HtrA2/Omi depletion in hepatocytes. Motor neuron degeneration 2 (mnd2)-mutant mice carry a single missense mutation (Ser276Cys) in the HtrA2/Omi gene that inactivates the protease activity of HtrA2/Omi [27]. Consistent with previous studies [28], mnd2-mutant mice exhibited striatal neuron loss; severe muscle wasting; weight loss; general decreases in the sizes of organs such as the liver, thymus, heart, and spleen; and death before 40 days of age (Supplemental Figure S2A). We next examined whether HtrA2/Omi mutation influences the quantity and function of mitochondria in hepatocytes as well as liver fibrogenesis. We observed mitochondrial morphology using TEM in liver tissue from wild-type (WT) or mnd2-mutant mice at postnatal day 32. Compared with the findings in WT mice, the liver tissue sections from mnd2-mutant mice appeared to have greater numbers of mitochondria and a slightly larger volume (Supplemental Figure S2B). In addition, the mitochondria in the liver tissue sections from mnd2-mutant mice were swollen compared with those in WT mice. These findings indicate that HtrA2/Omi mutation induces mitochondrial accumulation, mitochondrial swelling, and disruption of the cristae, and the results are similar for primary hepatocytes isolated from mnd2-mutant mouse livers (Supplemental Figure S2C).

Based on the abnormal mitochondrial morphology and biogenesis in the livers of mnd2-mutant mice, HtrA2/Omi mutation in hepatocytes is expected to lead to mitochondrial dysfunction. We hypothesized that pathologic changes in mitochondria caused by HtrA2/Omi mutation result from abnormalities of respiratory complex subunits. As mentioned previously, mnd2-mutant mice displayed decreases in liver size, and thus, we compared the cell-size and granularity index of primary hepatocytes isolated from WT and mnd2-mutant mouse livers at postnatal day 32 via FSC and SSC analysis (Figure 4A). FACS analysis illustrated that the cell-size and granularity index was lower for hepatocytes from mnd2 mutant mice. A previous study found that mitochondrial activity changes with cell size, resulting in allometric scaling of metabolism at the cellular level [25,29]. To determine whether HtrA2/Omi mutation in hepatocytes affects mitochondrial mass and mtROS, we assessed VDAC expression, MitoTracker Green, and MitoSOX staining in primary hepatocytes isolated from mnd2-mutant mouse livers via western blot, flow cytometry, and confocal microscopy. As shown in Figure 4B, mtROS levels to be higher in mnd2-mutant hepatocytes than in WT hepatocytes. However, no differences in mitochondrial mass by VDAC expression and MitoTracker staining were observed between hepatocytes isolated from mnd2-mutant and WT mouse livers. Furthermore, confocal microscopy revealed that mnd2-mutant hepatocytes had smaller mitochondrial areas, but higher mitochondrial fluorescence intensity for MitoSOX Red than WT hepatocytes (Figure 4C). We also measured intracellular ROS levels using the intensity of CM-H$_2$DCFDA fluorescence in H$_2$O$_2$-treated hepatocytes. As shown in Figure 4D, intracellular ROS levels were increased in mnd2-mutant mouse hepatocytes treated with 1.5 mM H$_2$O$_2$. ROS levels were higher in mnd2-mutant mouse hepatocytes, and mnd2-mutant mouse hepatocytes are more sensitive to H$_2$O$_2$-induced oxidative stress than in WT hepatocytes. These findings suggest that the number of mitochondria per cell was not changed by mnd2 mutation in primary hepatocytes, whereas mtROS and intracellular ROS levels were elevated.

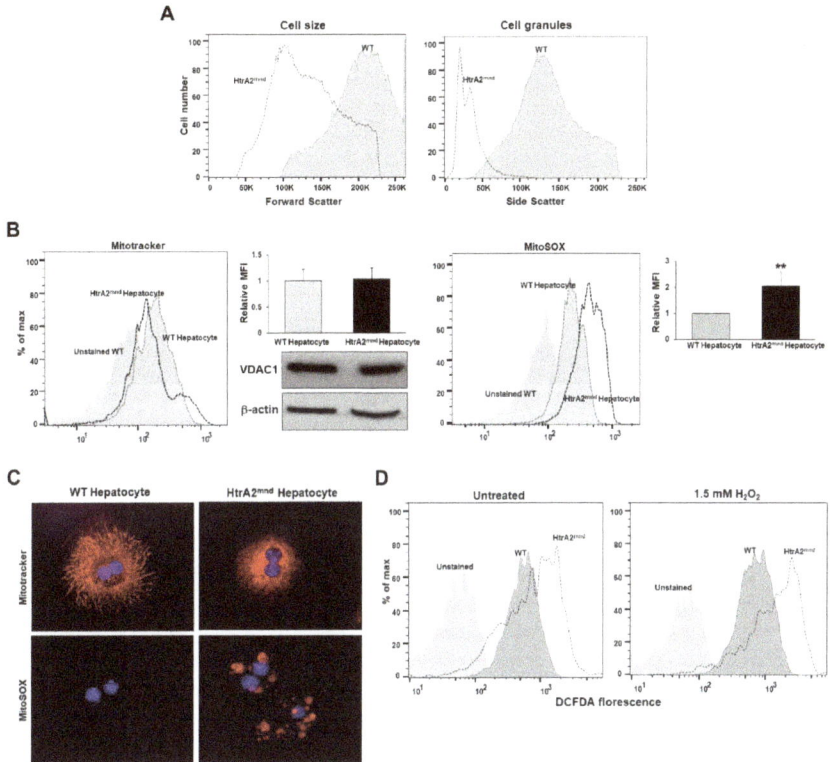

Figure 4. Loss of HtrA2/Omi in hepatocyte results in the accumulation of dysfunctional mitochondria and oxidative stress. (**A**) Exemplary flow cytometry plot and histogram of showing populations of primary hepatocyte in light scatters. (**B**) Mitochondrial morphology and superoxide levels in isolated hepatocyte were measured by FACS-analysis using MitoTracker green and MitoSOX red staining. The fluorescence mean intensity per cell was quantified. Western blotting for VDAC, mitochondrial mass proteins in WT and mnd2-mutant hepatocytes, with β-actin as a loading control. (**C**) Confocal microscopy of Mitotracker and MitoSOX red staining in primary hepatocyte. Nuclei were stained blue by DAPI. (**D**) Intracellular ROS levels in primary hepatocyte were measured by FACS-analysis using CM-H_2DCFDA staining.

To clarify whether increased mtROS levels are involved in mitochondrial dysfunction in primary hepatocytes isolated from mnd2-mutant mouse livers, we assessed damaged mtDNA and mtDNA content using real-time qPCR. As shown in Supplemental Figure S2D,E, *mt-ND1* and *mt-COX1* were detectable at higher levels in mnd2 hepatocyte, whereas their mRNA levels were significantly lower. In addition, the ratios of the 79 bp fragment and 230 bp fragment were significantly increased by 5.5-fold in mnd2 hepatocyte. These results are consistent with those in HtrA2/Omi-deficient hepatocytes and CCl_4-induced fibrotic livers. In addition, mitochondrial respiration (*ATP5A, COX5B*) and biogenesis (*ERRα*) genes were downregulated in mnd2-mutant hepatocytes compared with their levels in WT hepatocytes (Supplemental Figure S2F). These results reveal statistically significant associations between mtDNA damage and the concomitant elevation of mtROS levels in mnd2-mutant hepatocytes.

3.5. Loss of HtrA2/Omi Mitochondrial Protease Activity in mnd2-Mutant Mice Promotes Liver Fibrosis

The abnormal mitochondrial shape and mitochondrial dysfunction observed in HtrA2/Omi-deficient liver tissue might be closely linked to liver fibrogenesis. Next, we induced chronic liver injury in mnd2 heterozygous (mnd2/+) mice via repetitive CCl_4 injections to observe the development of extensive bridging fibrosis and substantial collagen deposits. As shown in Supplemental Figure S3A, we demonstrated that the heterozygous (mnd2/+) mice for this deletion showed a 50–70% reduction in mitochondrial protease activity. The mnd2/+ mice were used because mnd2 homozygous (mnd2/mnd2) mice die before 40 days of age. After 8 weeks of CCl_4 treatment, mnd2/+ mice displayed significant hepatic fibrosis, as demonstrated by quantification of Sirius-red positive area (Supplemental Figure S3B,C), compared with the findings in WT mice. Moreover, the concentration of hydroxyproline in mnd2/+ mouse livers was also increased after CCl_4 injection compared with the levels in WT mice (Supplemental Figure S3D). These results suggest that loss of HtrA2/Omi mitochondrial protease activity in mnd2-mutant mice promotes liver fibrosis by increasing mtDNA damage and mtROS levels.

3.6. HtrA2/Omi Deficient Hepatocyte Derived-mtDNA Induces Liver Fibrogenesis

Based on the aforementioned results, we demonstrated a direct link between increased mtDNA damage in HtrA2/Omi-deficient or HtrA2/Omi-mutated hepatocytes and liver fibrogenesis. HtrA2/Omi was predominantly expression in hepatocyte, but there is little information available regarding the effects of potential paracrine stimulation by hepatocyte-derived mtDNA or mtROS on HSC activation either in vivo or in culture. Therefore, we hypothesized that the accumulation of damaged mtDNA in hepatocyte may serve as DAMPs to link the HSC activation. We isolated damaged mtDNA from HtrA2/Omi-deficient or HtrA2/Omi-mutated hepatocytes and examined whether mtDNA can induce HSC activation as DAMP molecules. Forty-eight hours after adding the same concentration (500ng) of mtDNA extracted from HtrA2/Omi-deficient hepatocytes, upregulation of the mRNA transcripts for *collagen 1* and *α-SMA* was observed in inactivated LX-2 cells with serum-free medium (Figure 5A). Furthermore, LX-2 cells underwent morphological changes in response to damaged mtDNA treatment, as shown in stained images (Figure 5B). Consistent with the upregulation of *collagen 1* and *α-SMA* transcripts in LX-2 cell treated with mtDNA from HtrA2/Omi-mutated hepatocytes, *collagen 1* and *α-SMA* expression was upregulated in LX-2 cell treated with mtDNA from primary hepatocytes isolated from mnd2-mutant mice (Figure 5C,D). These results, together with the previously mentioned data, strongly suggested that the accumulation of damaged mtDNA due to a loss of HtrA2/Omi in hepatocyte is associated with liver fibrosis through crosstalk with the activation of HSC.

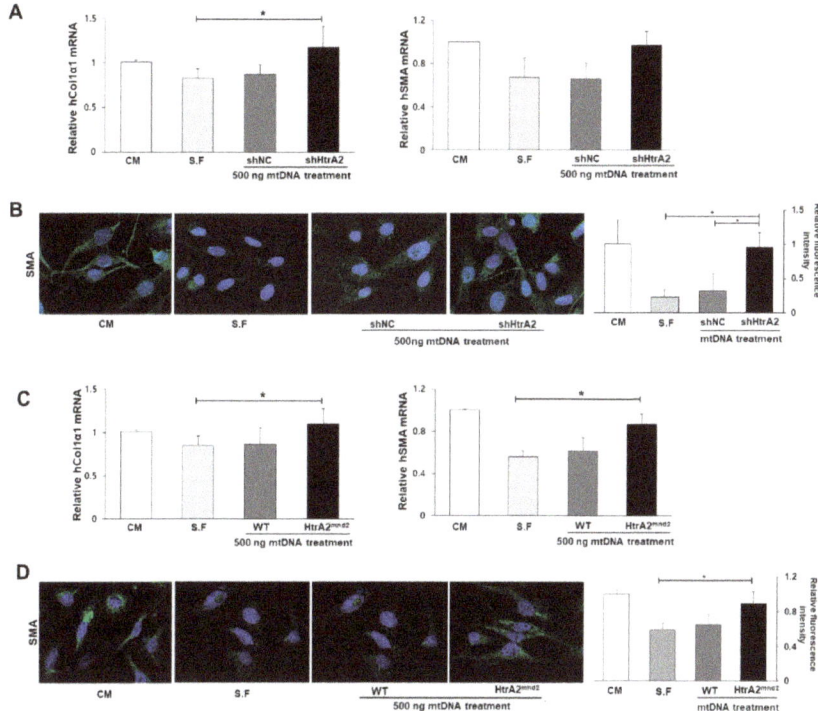

Figure 5. Loss of HtrA2/Omi mitochondrial protease activity promotes liver fibrosis. (**A,C**) Collagen 1 and α-SMA mRNA expression in LX-2 cell treated with the same concentration (500 ng) of hepatocyte derived-mtDNA, as determined by qRT-PCR. (**B,D**) Immunofluorescence staining for α-SMA (green) performed in LX-2 cell treated with hepatocyte derived-mtDNA. Nuclei were stained with DAPI (blue). The relative intensity measurement of immunofluorescence is shown as histogram for α-SMA. Original magnification, X400. CM: cultured LX-2 cells in completed media condition; S.F.: cultured LX-2 cells in serum free media condition.

3.7. Restoration of HtrA2/Omi Expression Rescues CCl_4-Induced Liver Fibrosis and Reverses Mitochondrial Dysfunction in Hepatocyte

Because HtrA2/Omi expression is downregulated during hepatic fibrogenesis, it was expected that HtrA2/Omi plays a protective role in our CCl_4-induced liver fibrosis model. To further confirm the protective role of HtrA2/Omi, we examined the effects of the hydrodynamic gene delivery of pFLAG-HtrA2/Omi in the CCl_4-induced liver fibrosis model. In a standard CCl_4-induced mouse model of liver fibrosis, serum ALT activity was significantly changed in mice treated with CCl_4 twice weekly for 8 weeks. The hydrodynamic injection of HtrA2/Omi attenuated the elevation of ALT activity in CCl_4-treated mice (Figure 6B). Subsequent experiments were performed to analyze liver histological alterations occurring in response to HtrA2/Omi injection in CCl_4-treated mouse livers. Semiquantitative IHC detection of HtrA2/Omi expression cells confirmed a transient increase in the HtrA2/Omi-injected liver than in control CCl_4- treated livers (Figure 6C). Intriguingly, pFLAG-HtrA2/Omi administration inhibited the development of hepatic fibrosis, as confirmed by H&E and Sirius red staining (Figure 6A). Quantification indicated that the Sirius red-positive area was smaller (by 5.8%) in fibrotic livers from mice injected with pFLAG-HtrA2/Omi plasmids than in livers from CCl_4-treated mice (Figure 6D). The hydroxyproline content was significantly lower in livers treated with pFLAG-HtrA2/Omi (1.1 μg/mg, $p < 0.01$) than in control CCl_4- treated livers (2.17 μg/mg) (Figure 6E). Hepatic HtrA2/Omi expression significantly decreased the hepatic hydroxyproline level. Immunohistochemical staining using α-SMA antibody illustrated that strong α-SMA expressions was limited to scarred areas in the CCl$_4$ treatment group, but pFLAG-HtrA2/Omi administration decreased α-SMA expression in fibrotic areas (Figure 6A). As previous studies reported that HtrA2/Omi directly contributes to apoptosis [9], we evaluated apoptosis using the terminal deoxynucleotidyl transferase dUTP nick-end labeling (TUNEL) assay in HtrA2/Omi-injected tissues. In the CCl$_4$-treated group, 76% of cells were TUNEL-positive, versus 67% of cells in the HtrA2/Omi-injected group (Supplemental Figure S4A,B). Consistent with the percent of TUNEL-positive apoptotic cells, we found that cleaved caspase 3 levels were reduced in the HtrA2/Omi-injected group compared with those in CCl$_4$-treated group (Supplemental Figure S4A,C). These results suggest that HtrA2/Omi expression appears to reverse, or at least prevent, further progression of liver fibrosis.

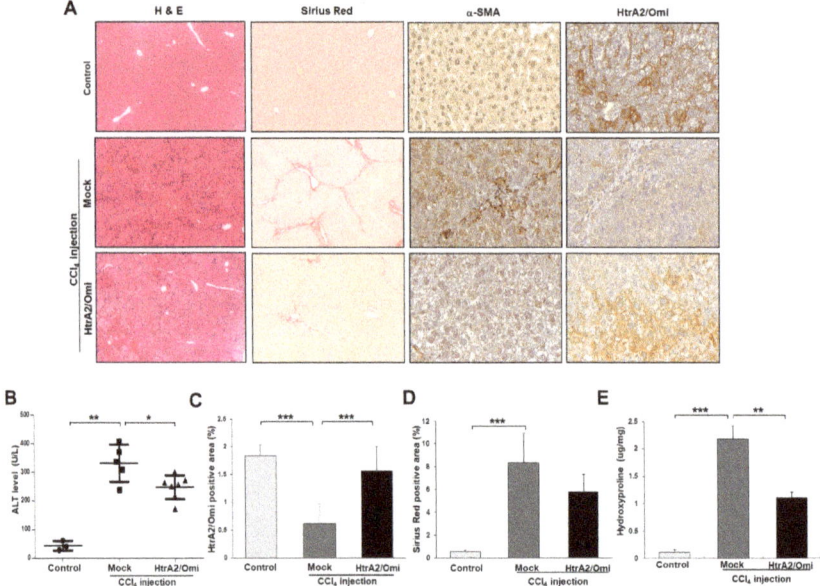

Figure 6. HtrA2/Omi expression in mouse model of CCl$_4$-induced liver fibrosis alleviates liver fibrosis by protecting hepatocytes damage. HtrA2/Omi expression in CCl$_4$-treated mice following the hydrodynamic tail vein injection of 30 μg HtrA2/Omi-encoding plasmid DNA ($n = 7$) compared with the mock control group ($n = 5$) over 8 weeks at 4-day intervals. Hepatic fibrosis was induced by injection of CCl$_4$ two times per week for 8 weeks. (**A**) Representative images of H&E, Sirius red (original magnification, X200) and immunohistochemistry staining (X400) of liver sections. (**B**) Effects of HtrA2/Omi expression on serum ALT. (**C**) IHC quantification of HtrA2/Omi positivity and (**D**) semi-quantitative analysis of Sirius red staining. (**E**) The hydroxyproline content in mouse livers.

Furthermore, to determine whether HtrA2/Omi expression could reverse mitochondrial dysfunction induced by CCl$_4$ in hepatocyte, we compared the mitochondrial ultrastructure and mtDNA content in the fibrotic livers of mice injected with pFLAG-HtrA2/Omi plasmids. Additional analyses revealed that mitochondria more frequently had a normal structure within hepatocyte from the HtrA2/Omi-injected group (Figure 7A). As shown in Figure 7B, the ratios of the 79 bp fragment and 230 bp fragment were decreased in the HtrA2/Omi-injected group than in the CCl$_4$-treated control group. The *mt-ND1* and *mt-COX1* mtDNA contents were significantly lower in the HtrA2/Omi-injected group than in the CCl$_4$-treated control group (Figure 7C). Conversely, there was no difference in *ATP5A* and *COX5B* mRNA levels between the HtrA2/Omi-injected and CCl$_4$-treated groups

(Supplemental Figure S4D), but MnSOD and CuZnSOD expression in antioxidant enzymes was restored by HtrA2/Omi treatment (Figure 7D). Taken together, these data suggested that HtrA2/Omi has an important role in maintaining mitochondrial homeostasis that might decrease vulnerability to liver injury and the development of liver fibrosis.

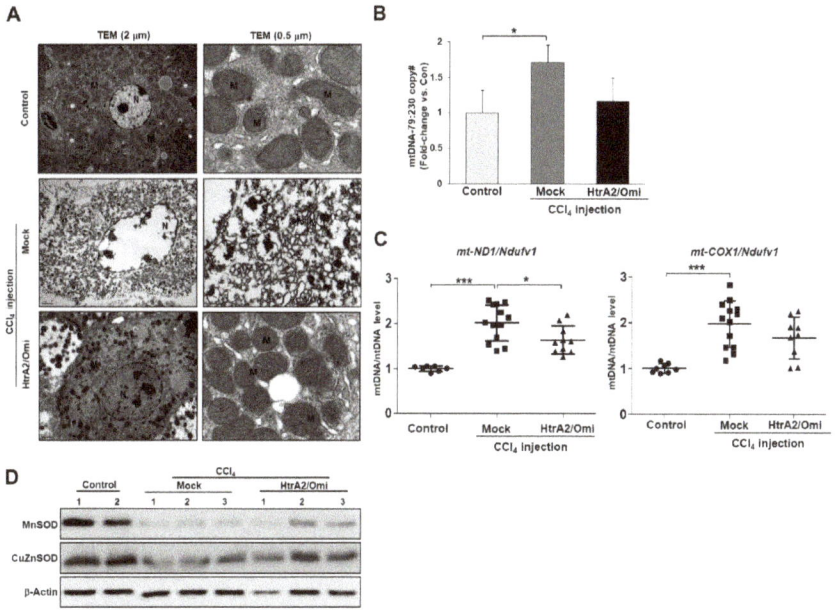

Figure 7. HtrA2/Omi expression in CCl_4-induced liver fibrosis protects mitochondrial damage of hepatocyte. (A) TEM analysis of hepatocyte showing nucleus (N) and mitochondria (M) (scale bar = 2 & 0.5 µm). (B) Damaged mtDNA levels of the 79 bp fragment (damaged) and 230 bp fragment (undamaged) in gDNA isolated from liver tissue were assessed by qPCR. Bars represent mean copy number ratios of mtDNA-79:230, normalized to 18S levels. (C) qPCR analysis of *mt-ND1* and *mt-COX1* DNA normalized to nuclear *Ndufv1* DNA. (D) Western blot analysis of MnSOD and CuZnSOD expression in liver tissue from pFLAG-HtrA2/Omi treated fibrotic mice compared to mock vector treated fibrotic mice.

4. Discussion

In this study, we demonstrated that mitochondrial dysfunction in hepatocytes is closely linked to hepatic fibrosis, and HtrA2/Omi might play a critical role in preventing of hepatic fibrogenesis through regulating mitochondrial homeostasis. Mitochondria are vital intracellular organelles that are altered in response to cellular stress and metabolic changes in hepatocytes. Oxidative stress is considered a key accelerator of liver fibrosis, and ROS produced by hepatocytes promote HSCs activation, resulting in excessive ECM deposition [30,31]. Furthermore, increased ROS production is associated with mitochondrial dysfunction in hepatocytes during liver damage [23,32], and subsequent mitochondrial dysfunction leads to oxidative stress and changes in mtDNA damage and calcium homeostasis, resulting in an energy crisis that can eventually lead to hepatocyte death. In the present study, we evaluated the alteration in the mitochondrial structure or function in a mouse model of CCl_4-induced liver fibrosis. In addition, we demonstrate that downregulation of HtrA2/Omi expression in CCl_4-induced liver fibrosis has a major role in modulating mitochondrial function and ROS generation in vivo and in vitro. Studies have shown that mitochondrial dysfunctions associated with HtrA2/Omi is a key causative factor inducing cell death in various chronic pathological conditions in numerous human diseases, such as neurodegeneration and cardiovascular diseases [33,34]. However, the relationship between mitochondrial dysfunction induced by HtrA2/Omi and chronic liver disease is unclear. Our analysis revealed that HtrA2/Omi-deficient and HtrA2/Omi-mutant hepatocytes have considerable reductions in mitochondrial electron transport chain activity and altered mitochondrial ultrastructural organization. However, we found that mitochondrial mass remained unchanged and the production of total ROS and mtROS increased in HtrA2/Omi deficient hepatocytes. These observations are consistent with previous studies demonstrating that HtrA2/Omi deficiency is involved in the accumulation of intracellular ROS [12,35,36], suggesting that mitochondrial damage in chronic liver injury leads to oxidative stress and changes in mtDNA damage that can eventually result in hepatocyte death. Although there was no change in the mitochondrial mass, the reason for the increased mtDNA contents in HtrA2/Omi deficient or mutation hepatocytes was that the destruction of mtDNA, which exists as a supercoiled form, caused morphological transfer to mtDNA of relaxed circular and linear forms. Accumulating evidence has demonstrated an association that the accumulation of relaxed and linearized mtDNA was used as a relatively good template for DNA amplification.

A number of recent studies reported correlations between elevated levels of intracellular or circulating mtDNA and various human diseases [37–39]. A study by Zhang et al. found that traumatic injury induces the release of mitochondrial DAMPs such as formyl peptides and mtDNA into the circulation, and these circulating mitochondrial DAMPs activate multiple inflammatory signal pathways through a specific receptor, toll-like receptor 9 (TLR9) [40]. TLR9 is in intracellular compartments and recognizes unmethylated cytosine phosphate guanine-containing DNA. Similarly, serum mtDNA levels are significantly higher in patients where acetaminophen-induced liver injury is significantly higher than in healthy controls, suggesting that the extent of mtDNA release into the circulation can be measured as a mechanistic biomarker of mitochondrial damage in patients with liver injury [41–43]. However, studies on how damaged mtDNA accumulated in hepatocytes or mtDNA released from hepatocytes affect non-parenchymal liver cells such as HSCs and cause liver fibrogenesis are still limited. Although we did not extract the damaged mtDNA released from HtrA2/Omi deficient and HtrA2/Omi mutated hepatocytes, it showed the possibility that the accumulation of damaged mtDNA in hepatocytes can induce HSC activation in the form of DAMP molecules. These results were the first to demonstrate that HtrA2/Omi expression regulates mtDNA damage and mitochondrial homeostasis in hepatocytes during liver fibrogenesis.

Initially, the roles of HtrA2/Omi in apoptosis, mitochondrial protein folding quality control, and cell survival were investigated [9]. A recent study reported that HtrA2/Omi regulates autophagy and inflammasome signaling by preventing prolonged accumulation of the inflammasome adaptor ASC [44]. In addition, Michell et al. found that expression of the pro-apoptotic protein Bcl-2 in the liver protected against CCl_4 induced-mitochondrial dysfunction and -oxidative stress in hepatocytes [8]. Therefore, we observed that, by protecting the mitochondria, HtrA2/Omi could restore mitochondrial structure and mitochondrial function, and subsequent play a pathophysiological role in the liver fibrogenesis in CCl_4-induced liver fibrosis model. By hydrodynamics-based gene transfer, the overexpression of HtrA2/Omi leads to antifibrotic effects in CCl_4-induced liver fibrosis mice model through decreasing collagen accumulation and enhancing anti-oxidative activity by modulating mitochondrial homeostasis in the liver. These results suggest that suppression of HtrA2/Omi expression promotes hepatic fibrogenesis by modulating mitochondrial ROS generation, and these novel mechanistic insights involving the regulation of mitochondrial homeostasis by HtrA2/Omi may be of importance for developing new therapeutic strategies for hepatic fibrosis.

Supplementary Materials: The following are available online at http://www.mdpi.com/2073-4409/8/10/1119/s1.
Figure S1. Lentivirus-mediated HtrA2/Omi depletion in hepatocyte lead to impaired mitochondrial function and metabolism. (**A**) HtrA2-shRNA encoding lentivirus were infected at MOI of 5 into FL83B cells. HtrA2/Omi protein levels were assayed using western blotting in lenti-shHtrA2 and lenti-shNC hepatocyte. (**B**) Mitochondrial morphology was measured by FACS-analysis using MitoTracker green staining. Western blotting for VDAC, mitochondrial mass proteins in lenti-shHtrA2 and lenti-shNC hepatocyte, with β-actin as a loading control. (**C**) Exemplary flow cytometry plot and histogram of showing populations of primary hepatocyte in light scatters;

FSC and SSC. The fluorescence mean intensity of FSC and SSC was quantified. **Figure S2.** Loss of HtrA2/Omi in hepatocyte results in the accumulation of dysfunctional mitochondria and oxidative stress. (**A**) Changes of mitochondrial ultrastructure in liver tissue from WT or mnd2-mutant mice at postnatal day 40. Appearance of normal (WT, left panel), mnd2-mutant (right panel) mice and liver. (**B**) H&E staining (original magnification, X200) and TEM images of liver sections. (**C**) Representative TEM images of hepatocytes isolated from WT and mnd2-mutant mice. (**D**) qRT-PCR analysis of mt-ND1 and mt-COX1 DNA normalized to nuclear Ndufv1 DNA in primary hepatocyte. (**E** & **G**) ND1, COX1, ATP5A, COX5B and ERRα mRNA expression in hepatocyte, as determined by qRT-PCR. (**F**) Damaged mtDNA levels of the 79 bp fragment (damaged) and 230 bp fragment (undamaged) in gDNA isolated from hepatocyte of mice were assessed by qPCR. Bars represent mean copy number ratios of mtDNA-79:230, normalized to 18S levels. **Figure S3.** Loss of HtrA2/Omi mitochondrial protease activity promotes liver fibrosis. (**A**) Loss of serine protease activity of HtrA2/Omi in liver sections from WT and mnd2 heterozygous (mnd2/+) mice. Liver lysates were immunoprecipitated (IP) with HtrA2/Omi-specific polyclonal antibody. The IP complexes were incubated for the indicated times at 37 °C with β-casein as a substrate. The reaction samples were resolved by 15% SDS-PAGE, and the processing pattern of β-casein was visualized by staining with Coomassie Brilliant Blue dye (CBB). The level of the HtrA2 was analyzed by IB with HtrA2/Omi Ab. (**B**) Representative images of H&E and Sirius red staining of liver sections from WT and mnd2 heterozygous (mnd2/+) mice via repetitive CCl_4 injections (original magnification, X200). (**C**) Semi-quantitative analysis of Sirius red staining in the fibrotic livers. (**D**). The hydroxyproline content. Figure S4. HtrA2/Omi expression in mouse model of CCl_4-induced liver fibrosis alleviates liver fibrosis by protecting hepatocytes damage. HtrA2/Omi expression in CCl_4-treated mice following the hydrodynamic tail vein injection of HtrA2/Omi-encoding plasmid DNA ($n = 7$) compared with the mock control group ($n = 5$) over 8 weeks. Hepatic fibrosis was induced by injection of CCl_4 two times per week for 8 weeks. (**A**&**B**) HtrA2/Omi expression alleviates CCl_4-induced hepatocyte death. Representative pictures of TUNEL and activated caspase 3 staining for apoptosis detection. Nuclei were stained with DAPI (blue). (**C**) The immunohistochemistry staining for cleaved caspase-3 was quantified by Image-Pro Plus 6 software. (**D**) ATP5A and COX5B mRNA expression in liver tissue, as determined by qRT-PCR.

Author Contributions: B.Y.K., S.M.K., and G.W.L. conducted experiments. W.H., J.-H.K., M.-K.N., and H.R. analyzed data and interpreted the results. W.H. and S.K.Y. designed the studies and wrote the manuscript. All coauthors reviewed the manuscript.

Funding: This research was supported by grants of the Basic Science Research Program through the National Research Foundation of Korea (NRF) funded by the Ministry of Education, Science, and Technology (2016R1D1A1B03931395 & 2017R1D1A1A09000911 & 2019R1I1A1A01056842) and the Korea Health Technology R&D Project through the Korea Health Industry Development Institute (KHIDI) funded by the Ministry of Health & Welfare (HI17C0509).

Conflicts of Interest: The authors declare no conflict of interest.

References

1. Friedman, S.L. Evolving challenges in hepatic fibrosis. *Nat. Rev. Gastroenterol. Hepatol.* **2010**, *7*, 425–436. [CrossRef] [PubMed]
2. Seki, E.; Schwabe, R.F. Hepatic inflammation and fibrosis: Functional links and key pathways. *Hepatology* **2015**, *61*, 1066–1079. [CrossRef] [PubMed]
3. Poelstra, K.; Schuppan, D. Targeted therapy of liver fibrosis/cirrhosis and its complications. *J. Hepatol.* **2011**, *55*, 726–728. [CrossRef] [PubMed]
4. Begriche, K.; Massart, J.; Robin, M.A.; Bonnet, F.; Fromenty, B. Mitochondrial adaptations and dysfunctions in nonalcoholic fatty liver disease. *Hepatology* **2013**, *58*, 1497–1507. [CrossRef] [PubMed]
5. Auger, C.; Alhasawi, A.; Contavadoo, M.; Appanna, V.D. Dysfunctional mitochondrial bioenergetics and the pathogenesis of hepatic disorders. *Front. Cell Dev. Biol.* **2015**, *3*, 40. [CrossRef] [PubMed]
6. Guimaraes, E.L.; Best, J.; Dolle, L.; Najimi, M.; Sokal, E.; van Grunsven, L.A. Mitochondrial uncouplers inhibit hepatic stellate cell activation. *Bmc Gastroenterol.* **2012**, *12*, 68. [CrossRef] [PubMed]
7. De Minicis, S.; Seki, E.; Oesterreicher, C.; Schnabl, B.; Schwabe, R.F.; Brenner, D.A. Reduced nicotinamide adenine dinucleotide phosphate oxidase mediates fibrotic and inflammatory effects of leptin on hepatic stellate cells. *Hepatology* **2008**, *48*, 2016–2026. [CrossRef]
8. Mitchell, C.; Robin, M.A.; Mayeuf, A.; Mahrouf-Yorgov, M.; Mansouri, A.; Hamard, M.; Couton, D.; Fromenty, B.; Gilgenkrantz, H. Protection against hepatocyte mitochondrial dysfunction delays fibrosis progression in mice. *Am. J. Pathol.* **2009**, *175*, 1929–1937. [CrossRef]
9. Vande Walle, L.; Lamkanfi, M.; Vandenabeele, P. The mitochondrial serine protease HtrA2/Omi: An overview. *Cell Death Differ.* **2008**, *15*, 453–460. [CrossRef]

10. Kang, S.; Louboutin, J.P.; Datta, P.; Landel, C.P.; Martinez, D.; Zervos, A.S.; Strayer, D.S.; Fernandes-Alnemri, T.; Alnemri, E.S. Loss of HtrA2/Omi activity in non-neuronal tissues of adult mice causes premature aging. *Cell Death Differ.* **2013**, *20*, 259–269. [CrossRef]
11. Kang, S.; Fernandes-Alnemri, T.; Alnemri, E.S. A novel role for the mitochondrial HTRA2/OMI protease in aging. *Autophagy* **2013**, *9*, 420–421. [CrossRef] [PubMed]
12. Goo, H.G.; Jung, M.K.; Han, S.S.; Rhim, H.; Kang, S. HtrA2/Omi deficiency causes damage and mutation of mitochondrial DNA. *Biochim. Biophys. Acta* **2013**, *1833*, 1866–1875. [CrossRef] [PubMed]
13. Kim, J.H.; Sung, P.S.; Lee, E.B.; Hur, W.; Park, D.J.; Shin, E.C.; Windisch, M.P.; Yoon, S.K. GRIM-19 Restricts HCV Replication by Attenuating Intracellular Lipid Accumulation. *Front. Microbiol.* **2017**, *8*, 576. [CrossRef] [PubMed]
14. Shin, H.A.; Kim, G.Y.; Nam, M.K.; Goo, H.G.; Kang, S.; Rhim, H. A Simple and Accurate Genotype Analysis of the motor neuron degeneration 2 (mnd2) Mice: An Easy-to-Follow Guideline and Standard Protocol Applicable to Mutant Mouse Model. *Interdiscip. Bio Cent.* **2012**, *4*, 1–7. [CrossRef]
15. Kim, S.M.; Choi, J.E.; Hur, W.; Kim, J.H.; Hong, S.W.; Lee, E.B.; Lee, J.H.; Li, T.Z.; Sung, P.S.; Yoon, S.K. RAR-Related Orphan Receptor Gamma (ROR-gamma) Mediates Epithelial-Mesenchymal Transition Of Hepatocytes During Hepatic Fibrosis. *J. Cell Biochem.* **2017**, *118*, 2026–2036. [CrossRef] [PubMed]
16. Liu, F.; Song, Y.; Liu, D. Hydrodynamics-based transfection in animals by systemic administration of plasmid DNA. *Gene* **1999**, *6*, 1258–1266. [CrossRef] [PubMed]
17. Huang, M.; Sun, R.; Huang, Q.; Tian, Z. Technical Improvement and Application of Hydrodynamic Gene Delivery in Study of Liver Diseases. *Front. Pharm.* **2017**, *8*, 591. [CrossRef] [PubMed]
18. Nam, M.K.; Seong, Y.M.; Park, H.J.; Choi, J.Y.; Kang, S.; Rhim, H. The homotrimeric structure of HtrA2 is indispensable for executing its serine protease activity. *Exp. Mol. Med.* **2006**, *38*, 36–43. [CrossRef]
19. Xu, L.; Hui, A.Y.; Albanis, E.; Arthur, M.J.; O'Byrne, S.M.; Blaner, W.S.; Mukherjee, P.; Friedman, S.L.; Eng, F.J. Human hepatic stellate cell lines, LX-1 and LX-2: New tools for analysis of hepatic fibrosis. *Gut* **2005**, *54*, 142–151. [CrossRef]
20. Higuchi, Y.; Linn, S. Purification of all forms of HeLa cell mitochondrial DNA and assessment of damage to it caused by hydrogen peroxide treatment of mitochondria or cells. *J. Biol. Chem.* **1995**, *270*, 7950–7956. [CrossRef]
21. Sadikot, R.T.; Bedi, B.; Li, J.; Yeligar, S.M. Alcohol-induced mitochondrial DNA damage promotes injurious crosstalk between alveolar epithelial cells and alveolar macrophages. *Alcohol* **2018**. pii: S0741–8329, 30181–30188. [CrossRef]
22. Haemmerle, G.; Moustafa, T.; Woelkart, G.; Buttner, S.; Schmidt, A.; van de Weijer, T.; Hesselink, M.; Jaeger, D.; Kienesberger, P.C.; Zierler, K.; et al. ATGL-mediated fat catabolism regulates cardiac mitochondrial function via PPAR-alpha and PGC-1. *Nat. Med.* **2011**, *17*, 1076–1085. [CrossRef]
23. Mansouri, A.; Gattolliat, C.H.; Asselah, T. Mitochondrial Dysfunction and Signaling in Chronic Liver Diseases. *Gastroenterology* **2018**, *155*, 629–647. [CrossRef]
24. Moiseeva, O.; Bourdeau, V.; Roux, A.; Deschenes-Simard, X.; Ferbeyre, G. Mitochondrial dysfunction contributes to oncogene-induced senescence. *Mol. Cell Biol.* **2009**, *29*, 4495–4507. [CrossRef]
25. Miettinen, T.P.; Bjorklund, M. Mitochondrial Function and Cell Size: An Allometric Relationship. *Trends Cell Biol.* **2017**, *27*, 393–402. [CrossRef]
26. Mikhed, Y.; Daiber, A.; Steven, S. Mitochondrial Oxidative Stress, Mitochondrial DNA Damage and Their Role in Age-Related Vascular Dysfunction. *Int. J. Mol. Sci.* **2015**, *16*, 15918–15953. [CrossRef]
27. Jones, J.M.; Datta, P.; Srinivasula, S.M.; Ji, W.; Gupta, S.; Zhang, Z.; Davies, E.; Hajnoczky, G.; Saunders, T.L.; Van Keuren, M.L.; et al. Loss of Omi mitochondrial protease activity causes the neuromuscular disorder of mnd2 mutant mice. *Nature* **2003**, *425*, 721–727. [CrossRef]
28. Martins, L.M.; Morrison, A.; Klupsch, K.; Fedele, V.; Moisoi, N.; Teismann, P.; Abuin, A.; Grau, E.; Geppert, M.; Livi, G.P.; et al. Neuroprotective role of the Reaper-related serine protease HtrA2/Omi revealed by targeted deletion in mice. *Mol. Cell Biol.* **2004**, *24*, 9848–9862. [CrossRef]
29. Miettinen, T.P.; Pessa, H.K.; Caldez, M.J.; Fuhrer, T.; Diril, M.K.; Sauer, U.; Kaldis, P.; Bjorklund, M. Identification of transcriptional and metabolic programs related to mammalian cell size. *Curr. Biol.* **2014**, *24*, 598–608. [CrossRef]
30. Gandhi, C.R. Oxidative Stress and Hepatic Stellate Cells: A PARADOXICAL RELATIONSHIP. *Trends Cell Mol. Biol.* **2012**, *7*, 1–10.

31. Gandhi, C.R. Hepatic stellate cell activation and pro-fibrogenic signals. *J. Hepatol.* **2017**, *67*, 1104–1105. [CrossRef]
32. Shinde, A.B.; Baboota, R.K.; Denis, S.; Loizides-Mangold, U.; Peeters, A.; Espeel, M.; Malheiro, A.R.; Riezman, H.; Vinckier, S.; Vaz, F.M.; et al. Mitochondrial disruption in peroxisome deficient cells is hepatocyte selective but is not mediated by common hepatic peroxisomal metabolites. *Mitochondrion* **2018**, *39*, 51–59. [CrossRef]
33. Satapati, S.; Kucejova, B.; Duarte, J.A.; Fletcher, J.A.; Reynolds, L.; Sunny, N.E.; He, T.; Nair, L.A.; Livingston, K.A.; Fu, X.; et al. Mitochondrial metabolism mediates oxidative stress and inflammation in fatty liver. *J. Clin. Invest.* **2015**, *125*, 4447–4462. [CrossRef]
34. Khacho, M.; Clark, A.; Svoboda, D.S.; MacLaurin, J.G.; Lagace, D.C.; Park, D.S.; Slack, R.S. Mitochondrial dysfunction underlies cognitive defects as a result of neural stem cell depletion and impaired neurogenesis. *Hum. Mol. Genet.* **2017**, *26*, 3327–3341. [CrossRef]
35. Krick, S.; Shi, S.; Ju, W.; Faul, C.; Tsai, S.Y.; Mundel, P.; Bottinger, E.P. Mpv17l protects against mitochondrial oxidative stress and apoptosis by activation of Omi/HtrA2 protease. *Proc. Natl. Acad. Sci. USA* **2008**, *105*, 14106–14111. [CrossRef]
36. Wan, J.; Cui, J.; Wang, L.; Wu, K.; Hong, X.; Zou, Y.; Zhao, S.; Ke, H. Excessive mitochondrial fragmentation triggered by erlotinib promotes pancreatic cancer PANC-1 cell apoptosis via activating the mROS-HtrA2/Omi pathways. *Cancer Cell Int.* **2018**, *18*, 165. [CrossRef]
37. Okochi, O.; Hibi, K.; Uemura, T.; Inoue, S.; Takeda, S.; Kaneko, T.; Nakao, A. Detection of mitochondrial DNA alterations in the serum of hepatocellular carcinoma patients. *Clin. Cancer Res.* **2002**, *8*, 2875–2878.
38. Yu, M. Circulating cell-free mitochondrial DNA as a novel cancer biomarker: Opportunities and challenges. *Mitochondrial Dna* **2012**, *23*, 329–332. [CrossRef]
39. Boyapati, R.K.; Tamborska, A.; Dorward, D.A.; Ho, G.T. Advances in the understanding of mitochondrial DNA as a pathogenic factor in inflammatory diseases. *F1000Res* **2017**, *6*, 169. [CrossRef]
40. Zhang, Q.; Raoof, M.; Chen, Y.; Sumi, Y.; Sursal, T.; Junger, W.; Brohi, K.; Itagaki, K.; Hauser, C.J. Circulating mitochondrial DAMPs cause inflammatory responses to injury. *Nature* **2010**, *464*, 104–107. [CrossRef]
41. McGill, M.R.; Staggs, V.S.; Sharpe, M.R.; Lee, W.M.; Jaeschke, H.; Acute Liver Failure Study, G. Serum mitochondrial biomarkers and damage-associated molecular patterns are higher in acetaminophen overdose patients with poor outcome. *Hepatology* **2014**, *60*, 1336–1345. [CrossRef]
42. Marques, P.E.; Amaral, S.S.; Pires, D.A.; Nogueira, L.L.; Soriani, F.M.; Lima, B.H.; Lopes, G.A.; Russo, R.C.; Avila, T.V.; Melgaco, J.G.; et al. Chemokines and mitochondrial products activate neutrophils to amplify organ injury during mouse acute liver failure. *Hepatology* **2012**, *56*, 1971–1982. [CrossRef]
43. McGill, M.R.; Sharpe, M.R.; Williams, C.D.; Taha, M.; Curry, S.C.; Jaeschke, H. The mechanism underlying acetaminophen-induced hepatotoxicity in humans and mice involves mitochondrial damage and nuclear DNA fragmentation. *J. Clin. Invest.* **2012**, *122*, 1574–1583. [CrossRef]
44. Rodrigue-Gervais, I.G.; Doiron, K.; Champagne, C.; Mayes, L.; Leiva-Torres, G.A.; Vanie, P., Jr.; Douglas, T.; Vidal, S.M.; Alnemri, E.S.; Saleh, M. The mitochondrial protease HtrA2 restricts the NLRP3 and AIM2 inflammasomes. *Sci. Rep.* **2018**, *8*, 8446. [CrossRef]

© 2019 by the authors. Licensee MDPI, Basel, Switzerland. This article is an open access article distributed under the terms and conditions of the Creative Commons Attribution (CC BY) license (http://creativecommons.org/licenses/by/4.0/).

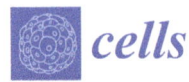

Article

Cyclosporin A Increases Mitochondrial Buffering of Calcium: An Additional Mechanism in Delaying Mitochondrial Permeability Transition Pore Opening

Jyotsna Mishra [1], Ariea J. Davani [1], Gayathri K. Natarajan [1], Wai-Meng Kwok [1,2,3,4], David F. Stowe [1,2,5,6] and Amadou K.S. Camara [1,2,4,6,*]

1. Department of Anesthesiology, Medical College of Wisconsin, Milwaukee, WI 53226, USA
2. Cardiovascular Center, Medical College of Wisconsin, Milwaukee, WI 53226, USA
3. Department of Pharmacology and Toxicology, Medical College of Wisconsin, Milwaukee, WI 53226, USA
4. Cancer Center, Medical College of Wisconsin, Milwaukee, WI 53226, USA
5. Research Service, Zablocki VA Medical Center, Milwaukee, WI 53295, USA
6. Department of Physiology, Medical College of Wisconsin, Milwaukee, WI 53226, USA
* Correspondence: aksc@mcw.edu; Tel.: +1-(414)-955-5624

Received: 6 July 2019; Accepted: 3 September 2019; Published: 7 September 2019

Abstract: Regulation of mitochondrial free Ca^{2+} is critically important for cellular homeostasis. An increase in mitochondrial matrix free Ca^{2+} concentration ($[Ca^{2+}]_m$) predisposes mitochondria to opening of the permeability transition pore (mPTP). Opening of the pore can be delayed by cyclosporin A (CsA), possibly by inhibiting cyclophilin D (Cyp D), a key regulator of mPTP. Here, we report on a novel mechanism by which CsA delays mPTP opening by enhanced sequestration of matrix free Ca^{2+}. Cardiac-isolated mitochondria were challenged with repetitive $CaCl_2$ boluses under Na^+-free buffer conditions with and without CsA. CsA significantly delayed mPTP opening primarily by promoting matrix Ca^{2+} sequestration, leading to sustained basal $[Ca^{2+}]_m$ levels for an extended period. The preservation of basal $[Ca^{2+}]_m$ during the $CaCl_2$ pulse challenge was associated with normalized NADH, matrix pH (pH_m), and mitochondrial membrane potential ($\Delta\Psi_m$). Notably, we found that in PO_4^{3-} (P_i)-free buffer condition, the CsA-mediated buffering of $[Ca^{2+}]_m$ was abrogated, and mitochondrial bioenergetics variables were concurrently compromised. In the presence of CsA, addition of P_i just before pore opening in the P_i-depleted condition reinstated the Ca^{2+} buffering system and rescued mitochondria from mPTP opening. This study shows that CsA promotes P_i-dependent mitochondrial Ca^{2+} sequestration to delay mPTP opening and, concomitantly, maintains mitochondrial function.

Keywords: cyclosporin A; mitochondria calcium buffering; mitochondria bioenergetics; mitochondria permeability transition pore; inorganic phosphate

1. Introduction

Regulation of intra-mitochondrial free calcium ($[Ca^{2+}]_m$) is critical in cardiac physiology and pathophysiology. Under physiological conditions, a moderate increase in $[Ca^{2+}]_m$ is believed to stimulate key enzymes of the Krebs cycle and oxidative phosphorylation and to drive mitochondrial ATP production to match cellular energy demand [1,2]. In contrast, a pathological increase in $[Ca^{2+}]_m$ causes opening of the mitochondrial permeability transition pore (mPTP), a key factor in initiation of cell death [3,4]. Pathophysiological dysregulation of $[Ca^{2+}]_m$ is a primary mediator in cardiac ischemia and reperfusion (IR) injury, as Ca^{2+} overloading can lead to apoptosis [5–7].

$[Ca^{2+}]_m$ is regulated by a dynamic balance between mitochondrial Ca^{2+} uptake, intra-mitochondrial Ca^{2+} buffering, and mitochondrial Ca^{2+} release. Mitochondrial Ca^{2+} uptake is mediated primarily through the mitochondrial Ca^{2+} uniporter (MCU) [8–10], and is controlled by the large membrane potential ($\Delta\Psi_m$: −180 to −200 mV) across the inner mitochondrial membrane (IMM). The $\Delta\Psi_m$ in turn is generated by the flow of electrons and proton pumping along the respiratory chain complexes [11]. When [Ca^{2+}]$_m$ increases, this depolarizes $\Delta\Psi_m$, which is compensated by enhanced H$^+$ pumping/extrusion to alkalinize the matrix. Therefore, powerful, dynamic buffering of matrix pH (pH$_m$) and Ca^{2+} are required to enable sufficient recovery of $\Delta\Psi_m$ and to avoid overloading the matrix with a high [Ca^{2+}]. Inorganic phosphate (P$_i$) has been recognized as a major player in maintaining the trans-matrix pH gradient when accompanied by the effective cotransport of H$^+$ [12] and buffering of matrix Ca^{2+} through the formation of amorphous calcium phosphate (Ca–P$_i$) granules [13–15]. The Ca–P$_i$ buffer system sets the free Ca^{2+} at a steady-state level, enabling greater mitochondrial Ca^{2+} loading without impeding the Ca^{2+} uptake and affecting the efflux system [16–18]. The efflux systems that regulate [Ca^{2+}]$_m$ are the Na$^+$/Ca^{2+} exchanger (NCLX) [17], and the putative Na$^+$-independent Ca^{2+} exchanger/Ca^{2+}-hydrogen exchanger (CHE) [19]. Any disruption in the uptake, and or impairment in the buffering or efflux of Ca^{2+} would disrupt the delicate balance of the [Ca^{2+}]$_m$ and lead to impaired bioenergetics and to opening of the mPTP [3,4].

The opening of the high conductance mPTP channel is associated with a high degree of mitochondrial swelling, dissipation of $\Delta\Psi_m$, uncoupling of oxidative phosphorylation, membrane rupture and release of sequestered Ca^{2+}, metabolites, and apoptotic signaling molecules [20–23]. Although the molecular components of the mPTP and its regulation remain largely unclear, cyclophilin D (Cyp D) is the only unambiguously recognized regulatory component of the mPTP. Cyp D is a mitochondrial matrix peptidyl-prolyl cis-trans isomerase (PPIase) that is translocated to the IMM during high matrix Ca^{2+} conditions; Cyp D is proposed to facilitate conformational changes in the putative mPTP core proteins thereby regulating pore opening [24–26].

Adenine nucleotides (AdN: ATP and ADP) have been implicated in the inhibition of Ca^{2+}-dependent mPTP opening [27,28]. A previous study from our laboratory suggested that matrix AdN modulate [Ca^{2+}]$_m$, potentially by increased buffering of [Ca^{2+}]$_m$ [29]. Oligomycin (OMN), an F$_0$F$_1$-ATP synthase inhibitor, influences the AdN (ATP/ADP) pool, and has been shown to modulate mPTP opening [30]. Cyclosporin A (CsA), a potent mPTP inhibitor is also believed to suppress pore opening by inhibiting matrix Cyp D, thereby preventing the Cyp D-induced conformational changes in mPTP core proteins [31,32]. CsA has long been known to desensitize mPTP from early opening during Ca^{2+} challenges by impeding Ca^{2+} interaction with Cyp D; however, the direct effects of CsA on the [Ca^{2+}]$_m$ buffering system have not been investigated systematically. It is worth noting that in a previous study from Chalmers and Nicholls [14], it was proposed that CsA enhances the Ca^{2+} loading capacity of mitochondria without changing the relationship between free [Ca^{2+}]$_m$ and total [Ca^{2+}]$_m$ during continuous Ca^{2+} infusion in isolated rat liver and brain mitochondria. Altschuld et al. [33] proposed that CsA increases mitochondrial Ca^{2+} influx and reduces its efflux. Later, Wei et al. [34] demonstrated that although CsA had no effect on MCU activity, it inhibited NCLX activity at higher concentrations. Altogether, these findings raise important questions about how CsA delays Ca^{2+}-induced mPTP opening while increasing net [Ca^{2+}]$_m$ accumulation. Our study sought to answer these questions by (i) examining the effect of CsA during repeated CaCl$_2$ challenges over an extended time-period on mitochondrial Ca^{2+} buffering, and (ii) by examining the underlying changes in bioenergetics during excessive Ca^{2+} overload.

To address our objective, we investigated systematically the effect of CsA on mitochondrial Ca^{2+} buffering and compared its effect with a known matrix buffering component, the AdN pool (OMN+ADP), by monitoring [Ca^{2+}]$_e$, [Ca^{2+}]$_m$, and key mitochondrial bioenergetics variables, $\Delta\Psi_m$, pH$_m$, and NADH (redox state), under conditions of repeated Ca^{2+} loading. Furthermore, we determined the effect of CsA on the rescue of buffering capability and bioenergetics of failing mitochondria just before mPTP opening. We found that CsA enhanced the sequestration of mitochondrial Ca^{2+}, maintained [Ca^{2+}]$_m$ at a steady-state level, and markedly delayed mPTP opening. In addition, CsA preserved $\Delta\Psi_m$, NADH, and pH$_m$ during CaCl$_2$ bolus challenges. However, in the absence of P$_i$, this

CsA-induced matrix Ca^{2+} sequestration was abrogated, and in turn led to the early mPTP opening. The results described herein reveal a novel way by which CsA modulates matrix Ca^{2+} sequestration to maintain $[Ca^{2+}]_m$, despite increased Ca^{2+} loading. CsA-mediated Ca^{2+} sequestration is likely achieved via a P_i-dependent $[Ca^{2+}]_m$ buffering system that delays Ca^{2+}-induced mPTP opening.

2. Materials and Methods

2.1. Materials

All chemical reagents were purchased from Sigma-Aldrich (St. Louis, MO, USA), unless stated otherwise. Fluorescent probes Fura-4F, Fura-4F^{AM}, tetramethylrhodamine methyl ester perchlorate (TMRM) and 2′,7′-Bis-(2-Carboxyethyl)-5-(and-6)-carboxyfluorescein, acetoxymethyl ester (BCECF^{AM}) were purchased from Life Technologies (Eugene, OR, USA).

2.2. Animals

Albino Hartley guinea pigs of both sexes weighing between 250 to 350 g were procured from Kuiper Rabbit Farm (Gary, IN, USA). All procedures were carried out in accordance with the National Institutes of Health (NIH) Guide for the Care and Use of Laboratory Animals (NIH Publication No. 85-23, revised 1996) and were approved by the Institutional Animal Care and Use Committee of the Medical College of Wisconsin.

2.3. Mitochondria Isolation

Mitochondria were isolated from guinea pig hearts as described previously [29,35,36]. Briefly, the guinea pig was anesthetized with an intraperitoneal injection of 30 mg ketamine plus 700 units of heparin, for anticoagulation, and the heart was rapidly excised and minced in ice-cold isolation buffer containing 200 mM mannitol, 50 mM sucrose, 5 mM KH_2PO_4, 5 mM MOPS, 1 mM EGTA, and 0.1% bovine serum albumin (BSA) at pH 7.15 (adjusted with KOH). The suspension was homogenized at low speed for 20 s in ice-cold isolation buffer containing 5 U/mL protease (from *Bacillus licheniformis*) and the homogenate was centrifuged at 8000× *g* for 10 min. The supernatant was discarded, and the pellet was suspended in 25 mL isolation buffer, and centrifuged at 850× *g* for 10 min. The supernatant was centrifuged further at 8000× *g* to yield the final mitochondrial pellet, which was suspended in isolation buffer and kept on ice until experimentation. All isolation procedures were performed at 4 °C and all experiments were conducted at room temperature. Protein concentration was determined by the Bradford method and the final mitochondrial suspension was adjusted to 12.5 mg protein/mL with isolation buffer.

The functional integrity of mitochondria was determined by the respiratory control index (RCI) as described before [29,37]. Mitochondria were energized with pyruvic acid (PA, 0.5 mM; pH 7.15, adjusted with KOH) followed by ADP (250 µM) addition. RCI was defined as the ratio of state 3 (after added ADP) to state 4 respiration (after complete phosphorylation of the added ADP). Only mitochondrial preparations with RCIs ≥ 10 were used to conduct further experiments.

2.4. Experimental Groups and Protocols

Two protocols (Protocol A and Protocol B) were used to assess the effect of CsA and AdN on mitochondrial Ca^{2+} handling and bioenergetics in normal and Ca^{2+}-overloaded mitochondria, as shown in Figure 1. Protocol A investigated the ability of CsA and AdN to modulate mitochondrial Ca^{2+} handling and delay mPTP opening. To further substantiate CsA-mediated buffering of matrix Ca^{2+}, Protocol B was designed to test the effectiveness of CsA and AdN on rescuing a failing mitochondrial Ca^{2+} buffering system from imminent mPTP opening. There were five experimental groups: vehicle (DMSO), CsA, ADP, OMN, and OMN+ADP. Experiments were also conducted in the presence of deionized H_2O as another vehicle (not shown). Each group was subjected to two different experimental protocols (Protocol A and Protocol B) that differed in the order of treatment and addition of $CaCl_2$ boluses to the mitochondrial suspension in experimental buffer.

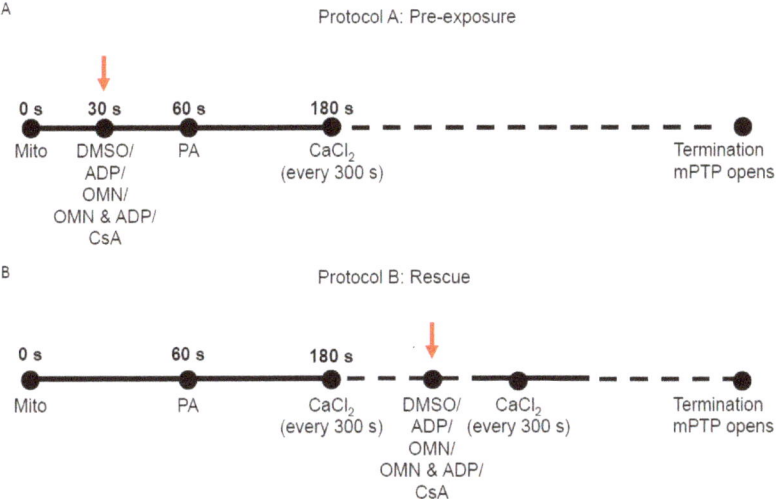

Figure 1. Schema of experimental timeline used to study the effect of Cyclosporin A (CsA) and adenine nucleotide (AdN) on mitochondrial Ca^{2+} handling and bioenergetics during repeated $CaCl_2$ pulses. (**A**) In Protocol A, at t = 0 s, mitochondria (mito, 0.5 mg) were added to the Na^+-free experimental buffer solution. The mitochondrial suspension was exposed to 0.5 µM CsA, 250 µM ADP, 10 µM oligomycin (OMN), or a combination of OMN+ADP at t = 30 s. Pyruvic acid (PA, 0.5 mM), was added at t = 60 s to energize mitochondria (state 2). At t = 180 s, 20 µM of $CaCl_2$ was added, followed by sequential additions of 20 µM $CaCl_2$ at every 300 s intervals until mPTP (mitochondrial permeability transition pore) opened or no further Ca^{2+} uptake was observed. (**B**) In Protocol B, the mitochondrial suspension was exposed to similar treatments as in Protocol A, but given after the last consecutive $CaCl_2$ bolus preceding the imminent onset of mPTP opening.

Delayed opening of mPTP (Protocol A): At t = 0 s, the experiment was initiated by suspending 0.5 mg of isolated mitochondria into the experimental buffer containing 130 mM KCl, 5 mM K_2HPO_4, 20 mM MOPS, 1 mM EGTA, 0.1% BSA, and EGTA ~0.036–0.040 µM at pH 7.15 (adjusted with KOH). At t = 30 s, mitochondria were treated with DMSO (1 µM), ADP (250 µM), OMN (10 µM), OMN+ADP or CsA (0.5 µM); at t = 60 s, mitochondria were energized with PA (0.5 mM). At t = 180 s, $CaCl_2$ bolus (20 µM final concentration) was added and subsequent $CaCl_2$ boluses added at 5 min intervals until pore opening (Figure 1A). Note that all experiments were conducted under state 2 conditions, except in the ADP-and OMN+ADP-treated groups.

Rescue of mitochondria from mPTP opening (Protocol B): The mitochondrial suspension was exposed to repetitive boluses of $CaCl_2$ (20 µM) as described in Protocol A; rescue of mitochondria from mPTP opening with the different treatments was carried out at 1 min of the last $CaCl_2$ bolus in which mitochondria Ca^{2+} uptake was observed before pore opening (Figure 1B). The onset of mPTP opening was predicted based on calcium retention capacity (CRC) of the DMSO (control)-treated group for each day's experiment. The pulse preceding mPTP opening observed in the control was the pulse chosen for targeted intervention in all subsequent experiments. In all experiments, extrusion of Ca^{2+} via the Na^+/Ca^{2+} exchanger (NCLX) was prevented by conducting all the experiments in Na^+-free conditions. That is, the respiration buffer, mitochondrial substrates, and all reagents/drugs were Na^+-free to prevent activation of the NCLX. Some experiments were conducted in the presence of 10 µM CGP 37157 (Tocris Bioscience), an NCLX inhibitor, which ascertained there was no potential Na^+ contamination in the respiration buffer from other sources [35,38,39].

2.5. Mitochondrial Function Measurements

Fluorescence spectrophotometry (Qm-8, Photon Technology International, Horiba, Birmingham, NJ, USA) was used to measure mitochondrial function, including mitochondria extra- and intra-matrix free [Ca^{2+}] ([Ca^{2+}]$_e$ and [Ca^{2+}]$_m$, respectively), $\Delta\Psi_m$, redox state (NADH), and pH$_m$. Fura-4F penta-potassium salt (1 µM, Invitrogen™, Eugene, OR) was used to measure [Ca^{2+}]$_e$. For [Ca^{2+}]$_m$ measurements, mitochondria were incubated with Fura-4F AM (5 µM, Invitrogen™, Eugene, OR) for 30 min at room temperature (25 °C) followed by a final spin and resuspension to remove any residual dye. $\Delta\Psi_m$ was assessed using the cationic lipophilic dye TMRM (1 µM, Invitrogen™, Eugene, OR, USA) in a ratiometric excitation approach [40]. NADH was measured by tissue autofluorescence, and matrix pH (pH$_m$) was assessed by incubating mitochondria in 5 µM BCECF^{AM} (Invitrogen, Carlsbad, CA, USA) for 30 min at room temperature (25 °C) followed by a final spin and resuspension [29,35,38,39].

2.6. Measurements of Free Ca^{2+}

Quantification of [Ca^{2+}]$_e$ and [Ca^{2+}]$_m$ were made using the fluorescent Ca^{2+} indicator probe Fura-4F with dual-excitation wavelengths (λ_{ex}) at 340/380 nm and a single emission wavelength (λ_{em}) at 510 nm. Ca^{2+} fluorescent intensities with Fura-4F are not influenced by background noise (e.g., NADH autofluorescence), so a background subtraction was unnecessary [38]. Fura-4F fluorescence ratios (F_{340}/F_{380}) were used to calculate [Ca^{2+}] using the equation described by Grynkiewicz: [41].

$$[Ca^{2+}] = K_d \frac{S_{f2}}{S_{b2}} \frac{(R - R_{min})}{(R_{max} - R)}. \quad (1)$$

The K_d value for Fura-4F binding to Ca^{2+} is 890 nM, which was described by us previously [38]. R is the ratio of the fluorescence intensities at λ_{ex} 340 and 380 nm, S_{f2}/S_{b2} is the ratio of fluorescence intensities measured at λ_{ex} 380 nm in Ca^{2+}-free (f)/Ca^{2+}-saturated (Ca^{2+}-bound, b) conditions. R_{min} (Ca^{2+}-free) and R_{max} (Ca^{2+}-saturated) are R values for Fura 4F, carried out after mPTP opening, adding 1 mM CaCl$_2$, followed by 10 mM EGTA, pH 7.1. The free [Ca^{2+}] in the buffer was calculated using an online version of MaxChelator program (http://www.stanford.edu/~{}cpatton/maxc.html) and accordingly, a standard curve was generated for the Fura-4F signal to the free [Ca^{2+}] in the experimental solution by fitting to the Grynkiewicz equation, as described above in Equation 1 [41].

2.7. Calculation of Mitochondrial Ca^{2+} Buffering Capacity

The ability of mitochondria to sequester Ca^{2+} is an index of its Ca^{2+} loading capacity, without altering mitochondrial function. Here we calculated mitochondrial Ca^{2+} buffering capacity (mβ_{Ca}) using the model described by Bazil et al. [42]. Briefly, experimental data for extra-and intra-matrix Ca^{2+} were fit with smooth trend curves satisfying the equation:

$$y(t) = p_1 + p_2 e^{\frac{(t-p_3)}{p_4}} + p_5 t, \quad (2)$$

where y(t) was either [Ca^{2+}]$_e$ or [Ca^{2+}]$_m$ at any given time, t. Global trend-fits were performed in MATLAB (Mathworks, Inc., MA) and parameters p_1 (offset value), p_2 (pre = exponential constant), p_3 (time lag), p_4 (decay time constant), and p_5 (steady-state slope) were estimated and optimized using the lsqnonlin and fmincon functions.

Mitochondrial Ca^{2+} buffering capacity for the second Ca^{2+} pulse (a cumulative of 40 µM added Ca^{2+}) was then calculated [42] as:

$$m\beta_{Ca} = -\beta_{Ca,e} V_r \frac{d[Ca^{2+}]_e}{dt} \bigg/ \frac{d[Ca^{2+}]_m}{dt}, \quad (3)$$

where, mβ_{Ca}, is the intra-mitochondrial Ca^{2+} buffering power, $\beta_{Ca,e}$ is the extra-mitochondrial Ca^{2+} buffering power determined by:

$$\beta_{Ca,e} = 1 + \frac{\partial [CaEGTA]_e}{\partial [Ca^{2+}]_e}. \qquad (4)$$

Vr is the volume ratio of the extra-mitochondrial space and matrix space (~2000), $d[Ca^{2+}]_e/dt$ and $d[Ca^{2+}]_m/dt$ are the rates of change of extra-and intra-mitochondrial free $[Ca^{2+}]$, respectively. $d[Ca^{2+}]_e/dt$ and $d[Ca^{2+}]_m/dt$ were estimated by evaluating the analytical derivative of Equation (2) using parameter estimates obtained from the trend fits [42].

Trend fits for data in Figure S4 were performed in Origin 2017 (OriginLab Corporation, Northampton, MA, USA).

2.8. Measurement of $\Delta\Psi_m$, Redox State (NADH) and Matrix pH

Membrane potential was assessed by the dual-excitation ratiometric approach using the fluorescent dye, TMRM, as described by Scaduto and Grotyohann [40] and in our published work [35,38,39]. Fluorescence changes were determined by two excitations, λ_{ex} 546 and 573 nm, and a single emission λ_{em} 590 nm. The calculated ratio of λex 573/546 is proportional to $\Delta\Psi_m$ and has the advantage of a broader dynamic range when compared to a single wavelength technique. Changes in mitochondrial redox state (NADH) were determined by autofluorescence (i.e., by exciting the energized mitochondria at λ_{ex} 350 nm and collecting data at λ_{em} 456 nm). An increase in the signal reflects an increase in the redox ratio of NADH to NAD^+ (i.e., a shift to a more reduced state). Matrix pH was assessed using BCECF^{AM} (5 µM) at λ_{ex} 504 nm and λ_{em} 530 nm. This fluorescent probe emits less fluorescence in an acidic environment, thus a decrease in signal indicates matrix acidification and an increase in signal indicates matrix alkalization [29].

2.9. Depletion of Endogenous Mitochondrial Phosphate

Given the important role of P_i in the mitochondrial Ca^{2+} buffering system [14,29], we tested the effect of P_i in CsA-induced mitochondrial Ca^{2+} buffering. Isolated cardiac mitochondria were depleted of endogenous P_i by pre-incubating mitochondria for 10 min at room temperature with 0.75 units/mL hexokinase, 1 mM glucose, 0.5 mM ADP, 1 mM $MgCl_2$, and 5 mM PA, as previously described [14,43,44].

2.10. Statistical Analyses

Data were transferred from PTI FelixGX (Version 3) into Microsoft® Excel® (2007). An unpaired Student's t-test was used to evaluate significant differences between means of CsA-treated versus DMSO- and AdN-treated groups on specific variables ($[Ca^{2+}]_m$, $[Ca^{2+}]_e$, $\Delta\Psi_m$, NADH, or pH_m) in both Protocols A and B. The final data of a specific variable were expressed as mean ± standard error (SE) over at least 4 replicates of the same variable ($n = 4$). Comparisons within and between groups were performed by one-way ANOVA (analysis of variance) with Tukey's post-hoc test to examine differences among individual groups. $p < 0.05$ (two-tailed) was considered significant. See Figure legends for statistical notations.

3. Results

3.1. Effect of CsA on Extra-Matrix Free $[Ca^{2+}]$

To determine the effect of CsA on matrix Ca^{2+} uptake, we measured $[Ca^{2+}]_e$ during repetitive additions of 20 µM $CaCl_2$ boluses at 5 min (300 s) intervals to allow characterization of the detailed kinetics of steady-state Ca^{2+} dynamics (influx and buffering). Figure 2 shows the dynamics of $[Ca^{2+}]_e$ during $CaCl_2$ pulse challenges, with different treatments. Panels A, B, C and panels D, E, F depict the Ca^{2+} dynamics profile using Protocols A and B, respectively. Each panel consists of five traces representing different treatment groups (DMSO, ADP, OMN, OMN+ADP, and CsA) in the presence of approximately 40 µM EGTA (carried over from the isolation buffer). In response to each $CaCl_2$ pulse, an increase in Fura-4F fluorescence intensity was observed, which then returned to a baseline; the steady-state (ss) level is marked by the flat response as mitochondria take up and sequester the added Ca^{2+}. The opening of mPTP is evident by cessation of mitochondrial Ca^{2+} uptake and a sharp rise in the extra-matrix dye fluorescent intensity. Ca^{2+} concentrations were determined from the fluorescence ratios using Equation (1).

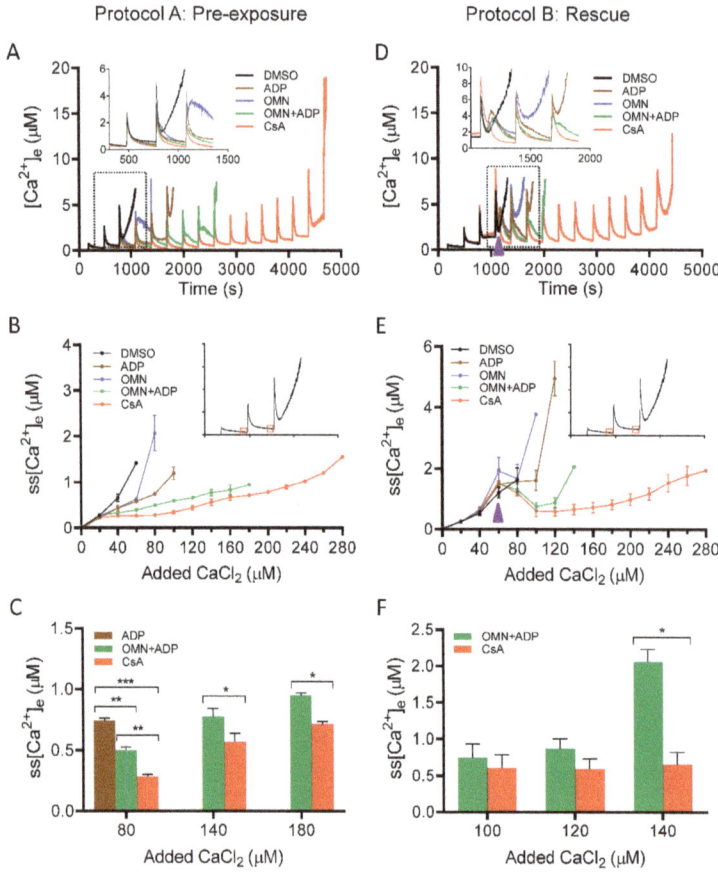

Figure 2. Effect of CsA and AdN on extra-mitochondrial calcium ($[Ca^{2+}]_e$) dynamics. Mitochondrial Ca^{2+} uptake and buffering for each of the treatment groups: DMSO (control; black trace), CsA (red trace), ADP (brown trace), OMN (blue trace), or OMN+ADP (green trace) are shown using the protocols depicted in Figure 1. Mitochondrial suspension was exposed to 0.5 µM CsA, 250 µM ADP, 10 µM OMN, or OMN+ADP before adding boluses of 20 µM $CaCl_2$ (Protocol A; left column). Mitochondrial suspension was exposed to added boluses of $CaCl_2$ (20 µM) and rescued mitochondria from mPTP opening (Protocol B; right column) with similar treatments as in Protocol A, at a time point at which it would initiate pore opening. Representative traces show change in extra-matrix free Ca^{2+} ($[Ca^{2+}]_e$) over time (**A**), and rescue of mitochondria from mPTP opening (**D**). Insets (**A**,**D**) show Ca^{2+} uptake kinetics in detail. Steady-state $[Ca^{2+}]_e$ (ss$[Ca^{2+}]_e$), 270 s after initiation of Ca^{2+} uptake, plotted as function of added Ca^{2+} (20 µM) every 300 s, in delay of mPTP opening (**B**), and rescue of mitochondria from mPTP opening (**E**). Insets (**B**,**E**) indicate the time points at which ss$[Ca^{2+}]_e$ was calculated. Quantification of steady-state $[Ca^{2+}]_e$ after a cumulative of 80, 140, and 180 µM $CaCl_2$ during delay of pore opening (**C**) and cumulative of 100, 120, and 140 µM $CaCl_2$ during rescue of mitochondria from mPTP opening (**F**). Error bars represent mean ± SEM (* $p < 0.05$; ** $p < 0.01$; *** $p < 0.005$). Arrowhead indicates time of addition of DMSO, ADP, OMN, OMN+ADP, or CsA during Protocol B.

We plotted steady-state $[Ca^{2+}]_e$ ($ss[Ca^{2+}]_e$) as a function of cumulative added $CaCl_2$ at each pulse (Figure 2B). The detailed dynamics of $ss[Ca^{2+}]_e$ for the initial four $CaCl_2$ pulses, in each group, are illustrated in the enlarged scale inset (Figure 2A). The exposure of mitochondria to DMSO and OMN, followed by repeated boluses of $CaCl_2$, resulted in a gradual increase in $ss[Ca^{2+}]_e$ with less mitochondrial Ca^{2+} uptake and rapid Ca^{2+} release by the third or fourth $CaCl_2$ pulse. The total CRC for the DMSO and OMN were comparable (i.e., 133.3 ± 13.3 nmol Ca^{2+}/mg protein and 146.6 ± 13.3 nmol Ca^{2+}/mg protein, respectively) (Figure S1). In the presence of ADP, mitochondria took up more Ca^{2+} before pore opening and the CRC was further augmented with OMN+ADP; the CRC value increased from 213.3 ± 13.3 nmol Ca^{2+}/mg protein for ADP alone to 373.3 ± 35.3 nmol Ca^{2+}/mg protein for OMN+ADP (Figure S1). Mitochondria treated with CsA before the addition of $CaCl_2$ boluses displayed a more robust Ca^{2+} uptake, with a significantly higher CRC value, 573.3 ± 26.6 nmol Ca^{2+}/mg protein, compared with all other groups (Figure 2A and Figure S1). Importantly, in CsA-treated mitochondria, the addition of $CaCl_2$ pulses (20 µM) did not significantly increase the $ss[Ca^{2+}]_e$ until the sixth to seventh pulse (Figure 2B), suggesting enhanced Ca^{2+} uptake. Figure 2C, summarizes the effects of the different treatments on the $ss[Ca^{2+}]_e$ for cumulative additions of 80, 140, and 180 µM of Ca^{2+}, which corresponds to the fourth, seventh, and ninth $CaCl_2$ pulses, respectively. The addition of CsA strongly blunted the Ca^{2+}-induced increase in $ss[Ca^{2+}]_e$ by stimulating faster and more Ca^{2+} uptake. We observed that the $ss[Ca^{2+}]_e$ was significantly lower for the CsA-treated mitochondria than for OMN+ADP-treated mitochondria after the cumulative addition of $CaCl_2$ of 80 µM (0.28 ± 0.0 µM vs. 0.50 ± 0.02 µM), 140 µM (0.57 ± 0.06 µM vs. 0.77 ± 0.06 µM), and 180 µM (0.71 ± 0.02 µM vs. 0.95 ± 0.1 µM) $CaCl_2$, respectively (Figure 2B,C). The sustained low $ss[Ca^{2+}]_e$ for an extended period of $CaCl_2$ additions in the CsA-treated group indicates a maintained $\Delta\Psi_m$ for Ca^{2+} uptake, resulting in enhanced Ca^{2+} loading capacity because of improved buffering.

We next examined $[Ca^{2+}]_e$ dynamics in the situation in which mitochondrial matrix Ca^{2+} nearly reached threshold, as determined by the predicted opening of mPTP; in this case we added CsA just before the anticipated mPTP opening. Using Protocol B (Figure 1), $[Ca^{2+}]_e$ was measured and the kinetics were compared in response to adding either DMSO, ADP, OMN, OMN+ADP, or CsA just before the onset of the mPTP opening (Figure 2D). The dynamic changes in $ss[Ca^{2+}]_e$ during the addition of different treatments are illustrated in more detail in the inset of Figure 2D. In the DMSO-treated mitochondria, three to four Ca^{2+} pulses (cumulative addition of 68 ± 4.9 µM $CaCl_2$) were sufficient to induce the release of matrix Ca^{2+}. Addition of ADP or OMN reversed the initial pore opening and delayed matrix Ca^{2+} release by one to two pulses compared to DMSO. Addition of OMN+ADP also showed a significant reversal of Ca^{2+} release with reduction in the $ss[Ca^{2+}]_e$ (0.74 ± 0.18 µM). Thus, there was a considerable increase in the CRC by OMN+ADP compared to DMSO (Figure 2D and Figure S1) and a further delay in mPTP opening by one additional $CaCl_2$ bolus compared to OMN or ADP alone. More impressively, the addition of CsA not only reversed the increasing trend of $ss[Ca^{2+}]_e$ to the baseline levels (0.42 ± 0.06 µM) (Figure 2D,E), it further maintained the $ss[Ca^{2+}]_e$ at a constant low value for an additional twelve to thirteen Ca^{2+} pulses. This resulted in a four-fold and a two-fold increase in the CRC, compared to DMSO and OMN+ADP, respectively (Figure 2E,F and Figure S1).

Altogether, these results demonstrate that CsA enhances mitochondrial Ca^{2+} uptake, thereby inhibiting a consequent increase in free $[Ca^{2+}]_e$ during $CaCl_2$ pulse challenges, leading to an increase in the CRC of the mitochondria. This sustained low $ss[Ca^{2+}]_e$ and concomitant increase in Ca^{2+} uptake are likely explained by enhanced $[Ca^{2+}]_m$ buffering to maintain basal $[Ca^{2+}]_m$, which results in a preserved $\Delta\Psi_m$ for Ca^{2+} uptake and greater CRC. To investigate further the potential for CsA on mediating Ca^{2+} buffering, it was necessary to examine the effects of CsA on matrix $[Ca^{2+}]_m$ dynamics in the next set of experiments.

3.2. Effect of CsA on Matrix Free [Ca^{2+}] Handling

Matrix Ca^{2+} was assessed with Fura-4 AM as described in Materials and Methods. We explored the effect of CsA on $[Ca^{2+}]_m$, under identical conditions and protocols as shown in Figure 1 (Protocols A,B). Mitochondrial Ca^{2+} buffering was measured as a function of a decrease in Ca^{2+} fluorescence, reaching a steady-state at approximately 270 s after each bolus of CaCl$_2$ added. The magnitude of mitochondrial Ca^{2+} uptake for the first CaCl$_2$ pulse (20 µM) was similar in all groups; however, on subsequent additions of CaCl$_2$, the ADP- and/or OMN-treated groups showed faster declines in [Ca^{2+}]$_m$ with lower mitochondrial steady-state [Ca^{2+}]$_m$ (ss[Ca^{2+}]$_m$) and delayed mPTP opening compared to DMSO (Figure 3A,B). Interestingly, the CsA-treated group showed a small increase in ss[Ca^{2+}]$_m$ with each CaCl$_2$ pulse, but a gradual decline in ss[Ca^{2+}]$_m$ was observed after [Ca^{2+}]$_m$ exceeded 3 ± 0.10 µM with the cumulative addition of 100–150 µM CaCl$_2$ (Figure 3A,B) and a significant increase in CRC up to fifteen to sixteen pulses. This suggested that the buffering effect of CsA on matrix Ca^{2+} is triggered when [Ca^{2+}]$_m$ reaches a certain value.

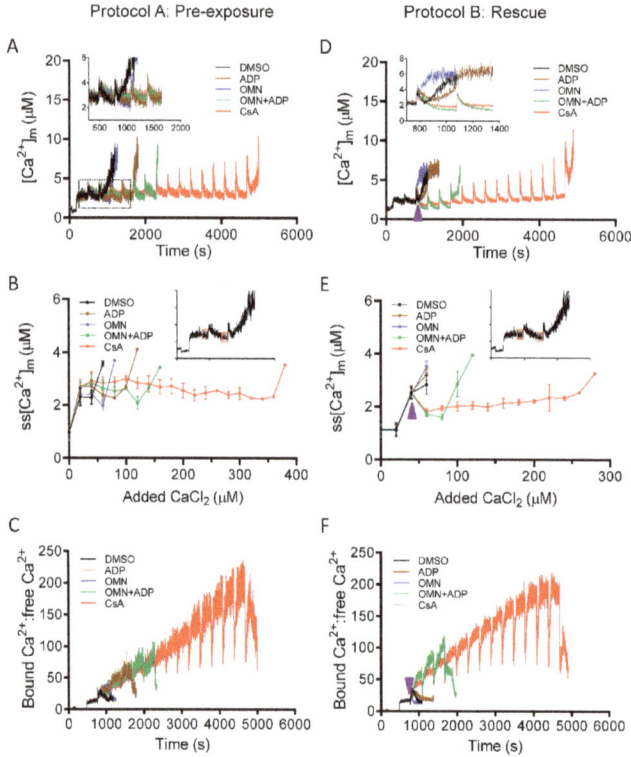

Figure 3. Effect of CsA and AdN on intra-matrix free Ca^{2+} ([Ca^{2+}]$_m$) dynamics. Mitochondrial Ca^{2+} uptake and buffering for each treatment groups, DMSO (control; black trace), CsA (red trace), ADP (brown trace), oligomycin (OMN, blue trace), or combination of OMN+ADP (green trace) are shown using the protocols depicted in Figure 1. Mitochondrial suspension was exposed to 0.5 µM CsA, 250 µM ADP, 10 µM OMN, or OMN+ADP before adding boluses of 20 µM CaCl$_2$ (Protocol A; left column). Mitochondrial suspension was exposed to added boluses of CaCl$_2$ (20 µM) and rescued from mPTP opening (Protocol B; right column) with similar interventions as in Protocol A, at a time point at which it would initiate mPTP opening. Representative traces show changes in [Ca^{2+}]$_m$ over time in delay of mPTP opening (**A**) and rescue of mitochondria from mPTP opening (**D**). Insets (**A**,**D**) show Ca^{2+} uptake kinetics in detail. Steady-state [Ca^{2+}]$_m$ (ss[Ca^{2+}]$_m$), 270 s after initiation of Ca^{2+} uptake, plotted as function of added Ca^{2+} (20 µM) every 300 s in delay of mPTP opening (**B**) and rescue of mitochondria from mPTP from opening (**E**). Insets (**B**,**E**) indicate the time points at which ss[Ca^{2+}]$_m$ was calculated. Change in matrix-bound Ca^{2+}:free Ca^{2+} over time in delay of mPTP opening (**C**) and rescue of mitochondria from mPTP opening (**F**). Arrowhead indicates time of addition of DMSO, ADP, OMN, OMN+ADP, or CsA during Protocol B.

To estimate the mitochondrial Ca^{2+} buffering capacity, the ratio of bound Ca^{2+}:free Ca^{2+} was calculated from the change in $[Ca^{2+}]_m$ (Figure 3A) to the total amount of Ca^{2+} taken up from the extra-matrix medium (ΣCa^{2+}_{uptake}): (ΣCa^{2+}_{uptake}-$[Ca^{2+}]_m$)/$[Ca^{2+}]_m$, as described previously [45]. Although the extent of bound Ca^{2+}:free Ca^{2+} at each Ca^{2+} pulse was comparable in all the treated groups (Figure 3C), the addition of CsA maintained the buffering capacity, with a gradual increase in the capacity to bind Ca^{2+} up to fifteen or sixteen Ca^{2+} pulses (Figure 3C).

Greater uptake of Ca^{2+} from the extra-matrix space (indicated by lower $ss[Ca^{2+}]_e$), combined with lower $ss[Ca^{2+}]_m$, indicated a greater Ca^{2+} buffering capacity of mitochondria in the presence of CsA. Consistent with this notion, the calculated matrix Ca^{2+} buffering capacity ($m\beta_{Ca}$) in CsA-treated mitochondria was about ten-fold higher compared to DMSO and two-fold higher than with OMN+ADP (Figure 4). This CsA-mediated increase in $m\beta_{Ca}$ is possibly due to an effect of CsA in triggering the matrix physiological buffers to enhance sequestration of Ca^{2+}.

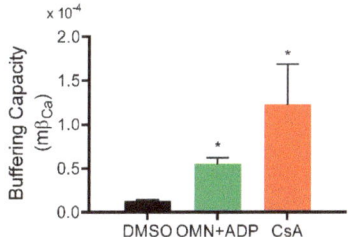

Figure 4. Effect of CsA and AdN on mitochondrial Ca^{2+} buffering capacity. Mitochondrial Ca^{2+} buffering capacity calculated from trend fits of $[Ca^{2+}]_e$ and $[Ca^{2+}]_m$ for DMSO-(control), CsA-, and OMN+ADP-treated mitochondria as described by Equations (2)–(4) in Materials and Methods. Buffering capacity for each treatment was calculated from three-five experiments each for $[Ca^{2+}]_e$ and $[Ca^{2+}]_m$ and averaged. Error bars represent mean ± SEM (* $p < 0.01$ compared with DMSO).

After observing the high buffering capacity of mitochondria pre-treated with CsA before the $CaCl_2$ bolus challenges, we next examined the effect of CsA on the rescue of mitochondria from Ca^{2+} release when the matrix Ca^{2+} buffering system (MCBS) becomes overwhelmed by the added boluses of $CaCl_2$ (Figure 1B). As shown in Figure 3D,E, OMN and ADP, each failed to reverse the mitochondrial Ca^{2+} efflux with added boluses; however, adding CsA or OMN+ADP at similar time points significantly reduced $ss[Ca^{2+}]_m$ by reinstating Ca^{2+} sequestration. This reversal was more effective and sustained in the presence of CsA than with OMN+ADP. This observation is consistent with the calculated values of bound Ca^{2+}: free Ca^{2+}, which increased two-fold for CsA compared to OMN+ADP (Figure 3F). Taken together, these data demonstrate that CsA increases the mitochondrial Ca^{2+} threshold for mPTP opening by activating $[Ca^{2+}]_m$ buffering that results in maintenance of a low $ss[Ca^{2+}]_m$.

3.3. Effect of CsA on Ca^{2+}-Mediated Changes in $\Delta\Psi_m$, NADH, and Matrix pH

A major driving force for Ca^{2+} uptake, in addition to the chemical gradient, is a high IMM potential gradient ($\Delta\Psi_m$); but increased Ca^{2+} uptake without efflux or sequestration can decrease $\Delta\Psi_m$ by flooding the matrix with positive charges. To strengthen the thesis that CsA increases the capacity of mitochondria to sequester Ca^{2+}, we next investigated the effect of CsA on mitochondrial bioenergetics. $\Delta\Psi_m$, NADH, and pH_m were assessed using the same protocols as described in Figure 1 for CRC to correlate changes in $[Ca^{2+}]_m$ to changes in bioenergetics over time. mPTP opening was marked by a sudden rise in the TMRM signal, indicating maximal depolarization of Ψ_m. Correspondingly, the oxidation of NADH was marked by a decrease in matrix NADH signal intensity when mPTP opens. Figure 5 shows representative traces of $\Delta\Psi_m$, NADH, and pH_m for each experimental condition. The rate of $\Delta\Psi_m$ depolarization and NADH oxidation correlated well with the induction of mPTP, as seen in the CRC data. The loss of CRC coincided with total $\Delta\Psi_m$

dissipation and NADH oxidation. DMSO-treated mitochondria (control) exhibited rapid Ca^{2+}-induced $\Delta\Psi_m$ depolarization and NADH oxidation (black trace) after only a few $CaCl_2$ pulses. Addition of OMN+ADP significantly delayed the Ca^{2+} induced $\Delta\Psi_m$ depolarization and NADH oxidation when compared to DMSO, with 533.3 ± 26.7 nmol Ca^{2+}/mg protein vs. 200 ± 23 nmol Ca^{2+}/mg protein and 546.7 ± 18.9 nmol Ca^{2+}/mg protein vs.173.3 ± 13.3 nmol Ca^{2+}/mg protein Ca^{2+} capacity, respectively (Figure 5A,B). Mitochondria treated with CsA maintained $\Delta\Psi_m$ and NADH for a higher number of $CaCl_2$ pulses than with OMN+ADP (666.7 ± 13.3 nmol Ca^{2+}/mg protein, and 626.6 ± 13.3 nmol Ca^{2+}/mg protein, respectively) (Figure 5A,B). Mitochondrial matrix pH (pH_m) is known to modulate mitochondrial P_i concentration and thus influence the matrix Ca^{2+} buffering [14]. The presence of CsA maintained pH_m at a basal level until mPTP opened (Figure 5C).

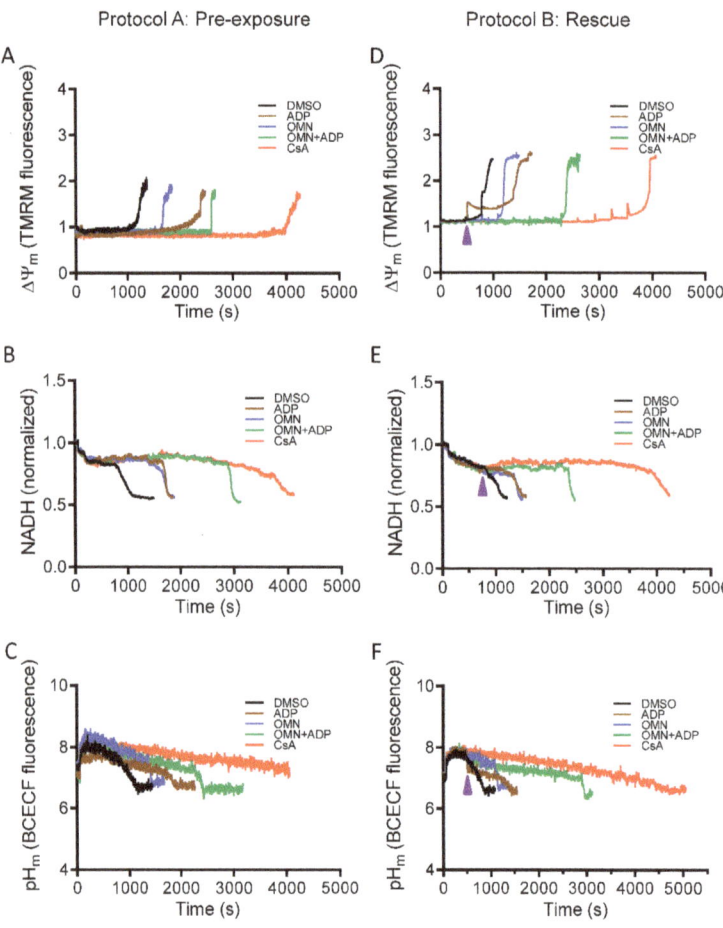

Figure 5. Effect of CsA and AdN on mitochondrial bioenergetics. The bioenergetic responses during Protocols A (left column) and B (right column) were monitored using the $\Delta\Psi_m$ sensitive dye TMRM (tetramethylrhodamine methyl ester perchlorate) (**A,D**), NADH autofluorescence (**B,E**), and pH_m-sensitive dye BCECF[AM] (2′,7′-Bis-(2-Carboxyethyl)-5-(and-6)-carboxyfluorescein, acetoxymethyl ester AM) (**C,F**). Purple arrowhead indicates time of addition of DMSO (1 μM), ADP (250 μM), OMN (10 μM), OMN+ADP, or CsA (0.5 μM) during Protocol B.

In Protocol B, intervention with OMN + ADP or CsA maintained $\Delta\Psi_m$, mitochondrial NADH, and pH_m (Figure 5D–F), and contributed to the improved capacity of mitochondria to take up and sequester additional Ca^{2+} after $CaCl_2$ pulses. However, OMN+ADP was less effective in preserving $\Delta\Psi_m$, NADH, and pH_m compared to CsA. This incapacity to sustain the bioenergetic status in the OMN+ADP- vs. CsA-treated mitochondria during $CaCl_2$ challenges reflects a lower capacity to sequester Ca^{2+} in the matrix for a protracted time.

In summary, maintenance of $\Delta\Psi_m$, NADH, and pH_m in the presence of CsA is consistent with changes in $[Ca^{2+}]_e$ and $[Ca^{2+}]_m$ that reflect greater Ca^{2+} sequestration (Figure S2) and uptake. Collectively, these results indicate that CsA reduced the accumulation of $[Ca^{2+}]_m$, by potentiating matrix Ca^{2+} buffering, which in turn, maintained $\Delta\Psi_m$, NADH, and pH_m necessary for normal mitochondrial function. Together, these mitochondrial variables preserve mitochondria and protect against mPTP opening.

3.4. Time Dependent Effect of CsA Addition on Rescue of Mitochondria from Imminent Ca^{2+}-Induced mPTP Opening

After demonstrating that CsA can reverse the induction of mPTP opening (Figures 2, 3 and 5), we next investigated the dynamics of $[Ca^{2+}]_e$, $[Ca^{2+}]_m$ and $\Delta\Psi_m$, by adding CsA at three different time points, before the onset of mPTP opening. This approach allowed us to determine the threshold at which CsA can effectively restore the mitochondrial sequestration system that will protect mitochondria from Ca^{2+} overload-mediated pore opening. Figure 6, panels A-C, show changes in $[Ca^{2+}]_e$, $[Ca^{2+}]_m$, and $\Delta\Psi_m$ depolarization, induced by adding CsA at 1, 2, and 3 min after the last $CaCl_2$ bolus in which mitochondrial Ca^{2+} uptake was observed before pore opened. Right panels D-F show detailed (close up) comparison of kinetics of $[Ca^{2+}]_e$, $[Ca^{2+}]_m$, and $\Delta\Psi_m$ after adding CsA at different time points. Adding CsA at all three tested time points, markedly delayed the large increase in $[Ca^{2+}]_e$ due to mitochondrial Ca^{2+} release. However, the effect of CsA to prolong Ca^{2+} uptake, which eventually maintains $ss[Ca^{2+}]_e$ at baseline, diminished as the interval before CsA addition and $[Ca^{2+}]_e$ accumulation was lengthened (Figure 6A). Adding CsA at 1 min caused a decline in $[Ca^{2+}]_e$, with a marked decrease in $ss[Ca^{2+}]_e$ (0.39 ± 0.07 µM) of the succeeding Ca^{2+} pulses, compared to adding CsA at 2 min (0.67 ± 0.03 µM) and 3 min (0.84 ± 0.05 µM) (Figure 6D; inset). In addition, we examined for changes in kinetics of $[Ca^{2+}]_m$ with CsA added at the same time points (Figure 6B). The rate of maximal Ca^{2+} buffering (i.e., the time to reach steady-state $[Ca^{2+}]_m$) and the Ca^{2+} threshold for pore opening was significantly higher when CsA was added at the early time points (i.e., 1 and 2 min) compared to the late time point of 3 min (Figure 6E, inset).

Next, in a parallel study, we monitored the corresponding changes in $\Delta\Psi_m$ profile at the same rescue time points (1, 2, or 3 min). Adding CsA reversed the Ca^{2+}-induced $\Delta\Psi_m$ depolarization even after a large depolarization (i.e., at 3 min; Figure 6C,F). Similar to its effect on $[Ca^{2+}]_e$ and $[Ca^{2+}]_m$, CsA restored and maintained $\Delta\Psi_m$ for a longer period at rescue points of 1 min vs. 2 and 3 min. Thus, at these points of intervention, CsA suppressed mPTP opening by increasing matrix Ca^{2+} buffering capacity, which maintained $\Delta\Psi_m$ and the driving force for further Ca^{2+} uptake (Figure 6C). Together, these results demonstrate that the magnitude of CsA-mediated increase in Ca^{2+} threshold for mPTP opening and maintenance of mitochondrial integrity is dependent on the $[Ca^{2+}]_m$ level before CsA intervention.

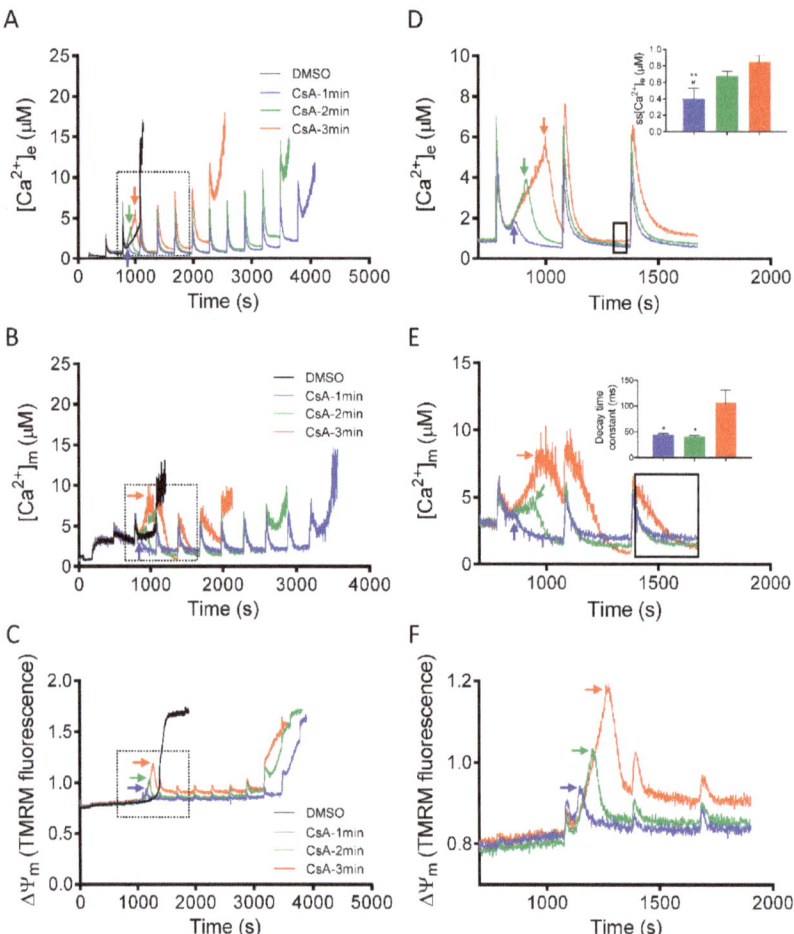

Figure 6. Time-dependent effects of CsA on mitochondrial Ca^{2+} dynamics and bioenergetics during rescue of mitochondria from mPTP opening. Changes in (**A**) extra-matrix free Ca^{2+} ($[Ca^{2+}]_e$), (**B**) intra-matrix free Ca^{2+} ($[Ca^{2+}]_m$) and (**C**) $\Delta\Psi_m$, when CsA was added at 1 min (blue trace), 2 min (green trace), and 3 min (red trace) after the last Ca^{2+} bolus before another Ca^{2+} bolus would have caused mPTP opening. Right panels show the effect of CsA on (**D**) $[Ca^{2+}]_e$, (**E**) $[Ca^{2+}]_m$, and (**F**) $\Delta\Psi_m$ dynamics during rescue of mitochondria from mPTP opening in greater detail. Insets (**D**,**E**) show relative $ss[Ca^{2+}]_e$ and decay time constant (ms) at specified time points (black dotted box), respectively. Arrows indicate time of addition of CsA (0.5 µM). Error bars represent mean ± SEM (* $p < 0.05$, ** $p < 0.01$ vs. 3 min and # $p < 0.05$ vs. 2 min).

3.5. Role of Inorganic Phosphate in CsA-Induced $[Ca^{2+}]_m$ Regulation.

Inorganic phosphate (P_i) is a required component for mitochondrial matrix Ca^{2+} buffering [14,29]. To gain insight into the mechanism that underlies CsA-mediated activation of the MCBS, we monitored mitochondrial Ca^{2+} handling and $\Delta\Psi_m$ during repeated boluses of 20 µM $CaCl_2$ every 5 min, as described in Materials and Methods, but now in the absence of P_i. With mitochondria depleted of P_i, and in P_i-free media, the CRC of mitochondria treated with CsA before the $CaCl_2$ pulses was not different from DMSO (control). In addition, these mitochondria showed a gradual increase in $ss[Ca^{2+}]_e$ and interestingly, after cumulative additions of $CaCl_2$ to 80 ± 15 µM, there was a significant decrease in mitochondrial Ca^{2+} uptake during additional CaCl$_2$ pulses (Figure 7A). These results implicated a P$_i$-dependent mechanism in the CsA-mediated delay in mPTP opening. In contrast, ADP and OMN+ADP, but not OMN alone, caused a significant delay in mPTP opening (Figure 7A) in the absence of P$_i$.

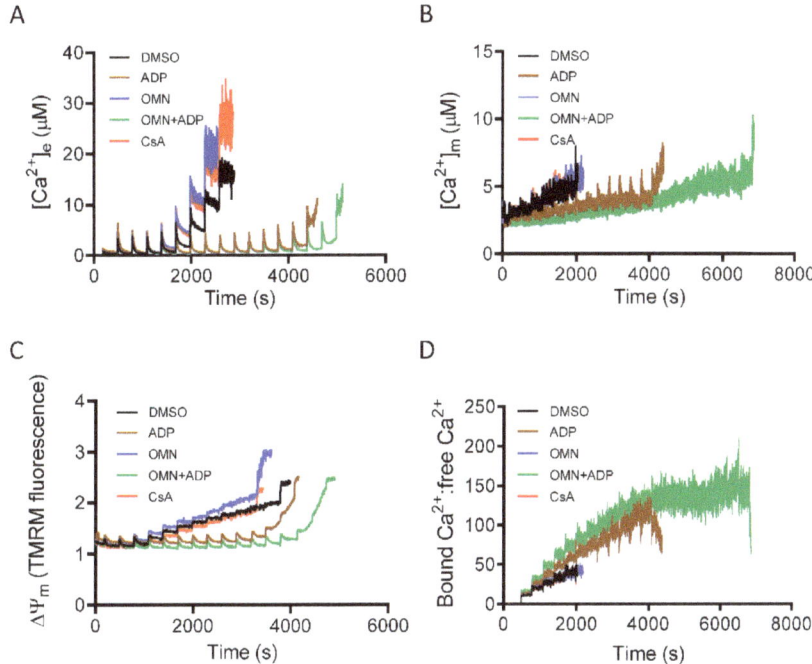

Figure 7. Effect of P$_i$ on CsA-induced mitochondrial Ca^{2+} handling and bioenergetics. Time course of [Ca^{2+}]$_e$ (**A**), [Ca^{2+}]$_m$ (**B**), $\Delta\Psi_m$ (**C**), and matrix-bound Ca^{2+}:free Ca^{2+} (**D**) during consecutive additions of 20 µM CaCl$_2$ to a suspension of P$_i$-depleted mitochondria, pre-exposed to DMSO (control), CsA, ADP, OMN, or OMN+ADP.

Along with observing the P$_i$-mediated effect of CsA on [Ca^{2+}]$_e$ dynamics, we also measured [Ca^{2+}]$_m$ under identical conditions. In the absence of P$_i$, mitochondria showed a gradual increase in ss[Ca^{2+}]$_m$; matrix Ca^{2+} sequestration was strongly blunted in both DMSO-and CsA-treated groups. This reflected diminished buffering capacity with the increase in [Ca^{2+}]$_m$ (Figure 7B). However, in the presence of ADP and OMN+ADP in the P$_i$-depleted condition, mitochondria displayed robust CRC and enhanced Ca^{2+} buffering and thus decreased [Ca^{2+}]$_m$ (Figure 7B). Intriguingly, this effect was stronger than in the P$_i$ replete condition (Figure 3). Mitochondria also showed an increased ratio of bound Ca^{2+}:free Ca^{2+} in the OMN+ADP-treated group, but not in the DMSO and CsA groups (Figure 7D). These data further support the premise that P$_i$ is crucial in CsA-induced matrix Ca^{2+} buffering and P$_i$ is a requisite component of matrix calcium sequestration.

Since we observed significant attenuation of Ca^{2+} uptake and buffering by CsA in the absence of P$_i$, we addressed how the altered mitochondrial Ca^{2+} dynamics impacted $\Delta\Psi_m$. Analysis of $\Delta\Psi_m$ in mitochondria depleted of P$_i$ during CaCl$_2$ bolus challenges revealed a gradual depolarization with each Ca^{2+} pulse over time in the DMSO-, OMN-, and CsA-treated groups (Figure 7C); this was consistent with the low CRC in these three groups due to the poor buffering after additional CaCl$_2$ pulses. In contrast, mitochondria exposed to ADP or OMN+ADP in the P$_i$-depleted state exhibited restored and sustained $\Delta\Psi_m$, which supported a robust CRC (Figure 7C).

To further confirm the requisite role of P_i in mediating CsA-induced activation of the MCBS, a rescue experiment with 5 mM P_i was performed with DMSO-and CsA-treated groups in P_i-depleted condition. With addition of deionized H_2O (vehicle), pore opening was not prevented in either group (data not shown). The addition of exogenous P_i to the buffer triggered a rapid reversal of Ca^{2+} release (decrease in ([Ca^{2+}]$_e$) in parallel with complete restoration of $\Delta\Psi_m$ (Figure 8). In contrast, additional Ca^{2+} pulses in the P_i free DMSO-treated group failed to maintain ss[Ca^{2+}]$_e$ and basal Ψ_m, and induced rapid Ca^{2+} efflux (Figure 8). However, the CsA-treated mitochondria showed a robust uptake of [Ca^{2+}]$_e$ with low ss[Ca^{2+}]$_e$ and sustained $\Delta\Psi_m$ maintenance with additional $CaCl_2$ boluses (Figure 8). Taken together, these results establish that P_i is required for CsA-mediated mitochondrial Ca^{2+} buffering that maintains low [Ca^{2+}]$_m$ and preserves $\Delta\Psi_m$; this in turn contributes to the capacity for more Ca^{2+} uptake and thus increases the Ca^{2+} threshold for mPTP opening.

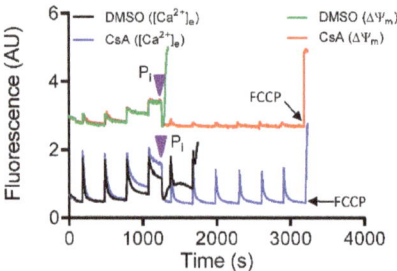

Figure 8. Mitochondrial Ca^{2+} modulation by CsA is phosphate (P_i)-dependent. Representative traces show change in extra-matrix Ca^{2+} fluorescence (Fura-4F Ŕatio) and $\Delta\Psi_m$ during consecutive 20 µM $CaCl_2$ boluses to induce mPTP opening in P_i-depleted mitochondria. P_i was added (purple arrowhead) at threshold point when mitochondria exhibited limited uptake of Ca^{2+} from the buffer.

4. Discussion

Matrix free [Ca^{2+}] ([Ca^{2+}]$_m$) plays two important roles: (i) Activation of Ca^{2+}-dependent dehydrogenases for oxidative phosphorylation at low concentrations [46]; and (ii) regulation of cytosolic Ca^{2+} by sequestration of excess Ca^{2+} at high concentrations [47]. Excessive accumulation of free [Ca^{2+}]$_m$ is a leading factor in inducing mPTP opening. It is well established that repetitive mitochondrial Ca^{2+} loading triggers a gradual increase in [Ca^{2+}]$_m$, leading to a loss of IMM integrity that results in dissipation of $\Delta\Psi_m$ and release of Ca^{2+}. CsA is known to delay pore opening, in part, by inhibiting the PPIase activity of Cyp-D [31]. Whether CsA-mediated delay in mPTP opening involves regulation of [Ca^{2+}]$_m$ by P_i-induced matrix Ca^{2+} buffering has not been addressed before. In this study, we investigated the effects of CsA on [Ca^{2+}]$_m$ regulation during repeated Ca^{2+} loading and its functional significance in mPTP opening. Additionally, we determined if changes in [Ca^{2+}]$_m$ induced by CsA correlated with changes in mitochondrial bioenergetics under identical experimental conditions and if matrix P_i was required for the observed CsA effects.

Since the key postulate was that CsA contributes to mitochondrial Ca^{2+} buffering, all experiments were performed in Na^+-free condition to completely block NCLX as a route for efflux of excess matrix Ca^{2+}. This allowed us to directly assess mitochondrial Ca^{2+} buffering capacity under different treatments. Our major findings during repetitive $CaCl_2$ bolus challenges are: (i) CsA maintained basal ss[Ca^{2+}]$_m$ owing to increased mitochondrial Ca^{2+} buffering capacity; (ii) the effectiveness of CsA to maintain basal ss[Ca^{2+}]$_m$ correlates well with preserved mitochondrial bioenergetics; (iii) the buffering effect of CsA in a P_i-replete buffer was more pronounced than the known buffering effect of OMN+ADP; (iv) CsA-induced buffering was abolished in P_i-depleted mitochondria and P_i-free experimental medium. We conclude that the CsA-mediated delay in mPTP opening could, in large part, be attributed to CsA-induced activation of a P_i-dependent mitochondrial Ca^{2+} buffering system (MCBS), which maintains a low free [Ca^{2+}]$_m$ and preserves mitochondrial bioenergetics.

4.1. CsA-Mediated Inhibition of mPTP Opening Relates to the ss[Ca^{2+}]$_m$

Using the two protocols (Figure 1A,B), we examined the changes in [Ca^{2+}]$_e$ and [Ca^{2+}]$_m$ in response to boluses of $CaCl_2$ in the presence of vehicle (DMSO), CsA, ADP, OMN, or OMN+ADP over time. Our experimental approaches allowed us to define the contribution of CsA in the regulation of [Ca^{2+}]$_m$ when CsA was given before the $CaCl_2$ boluses (Protocol A) and at the threshold for pore opening under condition of increased free [Ca^{2+}]$_m$ accumulation (Protocol B). Our results clearly indicate that the effect of CsA on delaying mPTP opening is due largely to its efficacy in maintaining free ss[Ca^{2+}]$_m$ by activating the MCBS in a P_i-dependent manner, and thereby preclude early mitochondrial Ca^{2+} overload and delay induction of mPTP opening. Sustained low ss[Ca^{2+}]$_e$ in the CsA-treated group indicated increasing mitochondrial Ca^{2+} uptake driven by the enhanced sequestration of free [Ca^{2+}]$_m$ to maintain a transmembrane Ca^{2+} gradient and a charged $\Delta\Psi_m$ that facilitated additional Ca^{2+} uptake (Figure 2). Unlike previous studies [14,33,34], NCLX was blocked under our experimental conditions, to prevent Ca^{2+} efflux during the repetitive $CaCl_2$ additions; therefore, the net free ss[Ca^{2+}]$_m$ in our study was determined by the balance between Ca^{2+} uptake and Ca^{2+} sequestration.

Notably, the CsA-induced buffering of mitochondrial Ca^{2+} resulted in greater Ca^{2+} uptake to attain a steady-state, as shown by the gradual decrease in ss[Ca^{2+}]$_m$ with each added $CaCl_2$ pulse (Figure 3). Insofar as Ca^{2+}–P_i precipitation is a major mechanism for mitochondrial Ca^{2+} buffering, the sustained ss[Ca^{2+}]$_m$ after each $CaCl_2$ bolus indicated matrix Ca^{2+} storage, likely in the form of various inorganic Ca–P_i complexes [14]. The low and maintained ss[Ca^{2+}]$_m$ during continuous matrix Ca^{2+} uptake is consistent with formation of these complexes. Although our study did not provide direct experimental evidence for CsA-induced matrix Ca–P_i complex formation, the continuous rise in estimated bound Ca^{2+}:free Ca^{2+} ratio with each $CaCl_2$ bolus as well as the ten-fold increase in mβ_{Ca} clearly reflects a CsA effect on [Ca^{2+}]$_m$ buffering capacity (Figure 3).

The protective effect of CsA in delaying mPTP opening has long been reported [28,31,32]. Our findings; however, provide the first direct evidence for a novel effect of CsA to enhance the capacity of mitochondria to sequester Ca^{2+} by which it obviates Ca^{2+}-induced mPTP formation. Moreover, the effect of CsA in mediating greater matrix Ca^{2+} buffering explains the sustained free [Ca^{2+}]$_m$ reported by Chalmers and Nicholls [14] and the CsA-induced inhibition of mitochondrial Ca^{2+} efflux observed in other prior studies [33,34].

4.2. Underlying Mechanism of the CsA-Mediated [Ca^{2+}]$_m$ Regulation

It is well established that mitochondria are able to sequester large amounts of Ca^{2+}, while maintaining free [Ca^{2+}]$_m$ over a range of 0.1 and 10 μM depending on the Ca^{2+} load [14]; however, the mechanism and kinetics for this are unclear. Matrix Ca^{2+} buffering capacity is determined by: i) The quantity of Ca^{2+} that can be retained, and ii) the Ca^{2+} threshold level for release when Ca^{2+} exchangers are blocked or maximally operated [48]. The role of P_i as a physiological buffer in regulation of [Ca^{2+}]$_m$ has been extensively studied [14,44,45,49]. The major mechanism of P_i-mediated Ca^{2+} sequestration in mitochondria is believed to be achieved by formation of amorphous Ca^{2+}–P_i complexes in the matrix [48,50,51], which in turn maintain the free [Ca^{2+}]$_m$ at a low level. Hence, sustained [Ca^{2+}]$_m$ cyclically promotes more Ca^{2+} uptake via the MCU due to better preservation of both the Ca^{2+} gradient and $\Delta\Psi_m$.

Though P_i plays an essential role in matrix Ca^{2+} buffering, P_i has also been suggested to induce mPTP opening [52]. A recent study associated Ca^{2+}–P_i precipitation with complex I inhibition and reduced ATP synthase rate during Ca^{2+} overload [53]. Another report demonstrated that increasing [P_i] decreased the mitochondrial Ca^{2+} loading capacity [14]. It was suggested that the mPTP-sensitizing effects of P_i was likely due to its effect in decreasing matrix-free Mg^{2+}, an mPTP inhibitor [20]. In addition, formation of polyphosphate, a known inducer of mPTP, could be a factor in regulating the Ca^{2+} threshold for mPTP activation [54,55]. Interestingly, two prior studies [56,57] indicated that P_i is necessary for the inhibitory effect of CsA on mPTP opening. However, two other studies reported that CsA inhibits mPTP opening even in the absence of P_i [58,59]. Conversely, in our study, the CsA-induced enhancement of matrix Ca^{2+} buffering was completely annulled when both mitochondria and the experimental medium were depleted of P_i (Figure 7). This loss of Ca^{2+} sequestration by CsA was reinstated when exogenous P_i was added just before activation of the mPTP (Figure 8). These observations provide the essential explanation for the requirement of P_i in the CsA-mediated MCBS and delay in mPTP opening.

The importance of mitochondrial matrix Ca^{2+} buffering via P_i is underscored by the studies of Wei et al. [44,45]. They reported that P_i modulates the total amount of Ca^{2+} uptake with smaller $CaCl_2$ boluses, whereas P_i modulates Ca^{2+} buffering capacity with larger $CaCl_2$ boluses. Since we had P_i in our experimental medium and the mitochondria were replete with exogenous P_i, the observation that CsA induced low $ss[Ca^{2+}]_e$ and $ss[Ca^{2+}]_m$ could be explained by the following: (i) CsA activates P_i-dependent matrix Ca^{2+} buffering potentially by maintaining the rate of Ca^{2+}–P_i complex formation; and (ii) CsA may activate P_i transport processes (via H^+/P_i transporter and/or phosphate carrier) that help to maintain both the IMM pH_m and $\Delta\Psi_m$ gradients. These processes would limit the increase in free $[Ca^{2+}]_m$, which in turn would contribute to more Ca^{2+} uptake and retention by increasing the electrochemical driving force for Ca^{2+} influx.

4.3. CsA vs. ADP; As a Regulator of $[Ca^{2+}]_m$

AdN are implicated as one of the multiple matrix factors responsible for sequestering Ca^{2+} by mitochondria [29,60–62]. AdN can potentiate mitochondrial Ca^{2+} buffering by maintaining high matrix P_i concentrations that can facilitate precipitation of AdN-Ca–P_i complexes, including, ATP-Mg^{2-}/P_i^{2-} and HADP$^{2-}/P_i^{2-}$, and thereby increase the Ca^{2+} threshold for mPTP opening [60,63]. In a study by Carafoli et al. [60], it was reported that mitochondrial Ca^{2+}-buffering is proportional to mitochondrial ADP uptake. In our P_i-replete study, OMN+ADP had a relatively small effect on Ca^{2+} buffering compared to CsA, but it had a significantly larger effect than ADP or OMN alone (Figures 2, 3 and 5). A reasonable explanation could be that OMN, an ATP synthase (Complex V) inhibitor [64], could contribute towards augmenting the AdN pool and thus enhance matrix Ca^{2+} buffering. Consistent with our findings, a previous study also showed a greater CRC with a low-concentration of ADP with OMN compared to 10-fold larger concentration of ADP alone [30]. Thus, in agreement with Sokolova et al. [30], the observed high buffering capacity and expanded CRC with OMN+ADP is largely attributed to the ADP component of the matrix AdN pool. However, a previous study [62] reported that AdN also prevent mitochondrial Ca^{2+} influx by directly chelating Ca^{2+} by a Ca–ATP complexation [61]. Contrary to this observation, in our study, the direct effect of ADP on binding free Ca^{2+} was negligible, as assessed by adding ADP and $CaCl_2$ together in mitochondria-free experimental buffer (Figure S4). Additionally, carboxyatractyloside-mediated inhibition of ADP uptake via adenine nucleotide translocase precluded matrix Ca^{2+} buffering and blunted the CRC by OMN+ADP or ADP alone (Figure S5). In this case, the extra-matrix ADP that accumulated did not chelate the Ca^{2+} added to the buffer. Altogether, these observations indicate that a direct sequestration of Ca^{2+} outside the mitochondria does not explain the effect of ADP alone or OMN+ADP on the enhanced CRC in our study.

A previous study [42] from our group proposed that the MCBS relies on at least two classes of Ca^{2+} buffers. The first class could represent classical Ca^{2+} buffers, including mostly metabolites (ATP, ADP, and P_i) and mobile proteins that bind a single Ca^{2+} ion at a single binding site. A second class of buffers could be associated with the formation of amorphous Ca^{2+} phosphates, which may be capable of binding multiple Ca^{2+} ions at a single site in a cooperative fashion [35,38,39,42]. Genge et al. [65] showed, in an in vitro study, that annexins, a diverse class of proteins, are required for Ca^{2+}-phosphate nucleation. Additionally, many studies have suggested an AdN-dependent Ca^{2+}-binding property of annexins [66]. Interestingly, mitochondria exposed to ADP alone or OMN+ADP retained their ability to maintain low $ss[Ca^{2+}]_e$ and $ss[Ca^{2+}]_m$ for an extended period of cumulative $CaCl_2$ additions, and showed a higher Ca^{2+} threshold for mPTP opening without P_i compared to with P_i (Figure 7). This extended delay in mPTP opening in the P_i-depleted state compared to the P_i-replete state reflects the ability of P_i to induce early mPTP opening under certain conditions [52]. In this case, the presence of P_i appears to counteract the ADP delay effect and induce a much earlier pore opening compared to the P_i-depleted state. The mechanisms for this AdN-mediated massive matrix Ca^{2+} loading capacity in the absence of exogenous P_i is unclear and needs to be further investigated. A plausible hypothesis could be that, in the absence of P_i, a significant Ca^{2+} loading capacity of AdN might be mediated via direct interaction with annexins. CsA, on the other hand, might function as a mediator that activates a P_i-dependent Ca^{2+} buffering system. Another possibility is that Cyp D, as a PPIase, reduces free phosphate levels in the matrix or blocks the Ca^{2+} binding property of annexins; this then would be relieved by CsA's effect to block Cyp D.

4.4. Implication of CsA-Mediated Ca^{2+} Buffering on Mitochondrial Bioenergetics

Elevated $[Ca^{2+}]_m$ over the nanomolar range is reported to increase NADH generation in part by stimulating Ca^{2+}-sensitive dehydrogenases of the TCA cycle [67,68] and activating the F_0F_1-ATP synthase [69], thereby accelerating oxidative phosphorylation (OXPHOS). However, excess mitochondrial free Ca^{2+} can dissipate $\Delta\Psi_m$ and impede OXPHOS. The IMM $\Delta\Psi_m$ is the key factor in generating the proton motive force across the IMM; it is also one of the primary driving forces for Ca^{2+} uptake via the MCU [70] and triggers Ca^{2+} efflux via the NCLX [71,72]. Therefore, if mitochondria continue to take up Ca^{2+} under increased extra-matrix Ca^{2+} exposure, the Ca^{2+} would have to be buffered or ejected to prevent excess free $[Ca^{2+}]_m$ accumulation that could dissipate $\Delta\Psi_m$ and increase oxidation of NADH.

The stability of Ca^{2+}–P_i precipitates inside the mitochondrial matrix largely depends on pH_m [50]. It is also proposed that the matrix $[P_i]$ depends on the pH gradient (e.g., a change in pH from 7 to 8 has been estimated to increase $[P_i]$ by a factor of 1000 [14,50]). Thus, matrix alkaline conditions could facilitate Ca^{2+}–P_i precipitation, whereas matrix acidification could lead to a destabilization of the Ca^{2+}–P_i precipitate and so enhance matrix free Ca^{2+} levels [14]. Consequently, we correlated the changes in $[Ca^{2+}]_m$ with indices of mitochondrial bioenergetics ($\Delta\Psi_m$, NADH, and pH) (Figure 5) to have a better understanding of the CsA-mediated MCBS. Mitochondria exposed to CsA before the repetitive $CaCl_2$ boluses, exhibited robust mitochondrial Ca^{2+} uptake and rapid $[Ca^{2+}]_m$ buffering while maintaining basal $\Delta\Psi_m$, NADH, and an alkalinized pH_m until mPTP opened (Figure 5). Maintaining $\Delta\Psi_m$ during excess Ca^{2+} uptake in the absence of functioning NCLX suggests a strong matrix buffering effect that is induced by CsA.

In Protocol B, when CsA was added just before the onset of pore opening, NADH and $\Delta\Psi_m$ levels transiently increased but immediately returned to baseline with each added $CaCl_2$ bolus. This transient depolarization and NADH oxidation with each addition of $CaCl_2$ was not observed in Protocol A. The reason for this is unclear. Nonetheless, the observed transient oxidation of NADH helped to restore $\Delta\Psi_m$ after Ca^{2+} induced transient depolarization before the next $CaCl_2$ bolus (Figure 5D,E). The transient redox oxidation and $\Delta\Psi_m$ depolarization suggest that the CsA added at the point just before mPTP opening activated MCBS more slowly compared to Protocol A. In addition, CsA maintained the pH_m gradient during prolonged Ca^{2+} pulse challenges (Figure 5C). This finding also likely excludes a contribution of the mitochondrial calcium–hydrogen exchange (mCHE) to the Ca^{2+} extrusion in the absence of NaCl. We have recently reported that CsA obviates mCHE activity at low extra-matrix pH [19]. However, based on our current results, it is likely that CsA triggered an enhancement of mitochondrial Ca^{2+} buffering so that the resulting low $[Ca^{2+}]_m$ and maintained $\Delta\Psi_m$ and pH_m accounted for the inactivity of mCHE.

5. Conclusions

The salient observation of this study is that CsA mitigated mPTP opening by promoting the maintenance of a low $[Ca^{2+}]_m$, by stimulating and/or potentiating MCBS. Specifically, we showed that the presence of CsA, (i) significantly delayed the mPTP opening when compared to ADP or

OMN+ADP (Protocol A); (ii) overturned the high amplitude increase in $[Ca^{2+}]_m$ (Protocol B); (iii) maintained pH_m, redox state (NADH) and basal $\Delta\Psi_m$, which maintains the driving force for more Ca^{2+} uptake and sequestration; and (iv) activates P_i-dependent mitochondrial Ca^{2+} sequestration to delay mPTP opening.

Our study provides a novel insight into how CsA-mediates a delay in mPTP opening by activating the MCBS, which lowers $ss[Ca^{2+}]_m$ below the threshold for mPTP activation. This concept is shown in the scheme presented in Figure 9. Our finding supports the notion that CsA facilitates P_i-dependent matrix Ca^{2+} buffering, which maintains matrix free Ca^{2+} and enables massive Ca^{2+} loading capacity, without diminishing the driving force for Ca^{2+} influx by maintaining $\Delta\Psi_m$. CsA may delay mPTP opening by enhancing P_i-dependent matrix Ca^{2+} buffering and by inhibiting Cyp D [31,32]. The culmination of these two mechanisms, and possibly others not yet identified, might be responsible for CsA protection against mitochondrial Ca^{2+} overload. Together, these findings add to our understanding of the mechanism of CsA-mediated modulation of mPTP. Importantly, we believe that therapeutic approaches targeted at regulating $[Ca^{2+}]_m$ homeostasis represent a promising strategy to reduce cardiac injury due to Ca^{2+} overload by delaying mPTP opening and preventing induction of apoptosis.

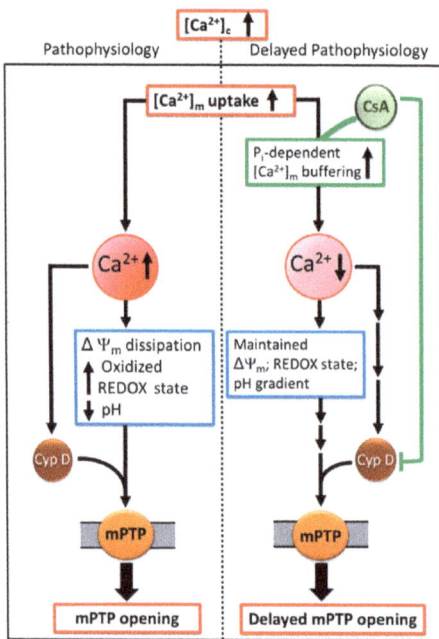

Figure 9. Schema of the potential mechanism by which CsA mediates delay in Ca^{2+}-induced mPTP opening. Pathological conditions, like cardiac ischemia-reperfusion injury, leads to an increase in cytosolic Ca^{2+} ($[Ca^{2+}]_c$). This in turn increases $[Ca^{2+}]_m$ and generation of reactive oxygen species (ROS), impairs respiration and substrate utilization, and leads to uncoupling of oxidative phosphorylation. Lower $\Delta\Psi_m$, oxidized redox state, and dissipation of the pH_m gradient, together induces mPTP opening which triggers apoptosis. These detrimental consequences that underlie IR injury could be mollified by CsA, which allows the mitochondria to maintain their basal $[Ca^{2+}]_m$ via enhanced P_i-dependent matrix Ca^{2+} buffering, in addition to, or through, Cyp D inhibition. Sustained low $[Ca^{2+}]_m$ maintains mitochondrial integrity and function and delays mPTP opening.

Supplementary Materials: The following are available online at http://www.mdpi.com/2073-4409/8/9/1052/s1. Figure S1: Quantification of calcium retention capacity (CRC) for each treatment, DMSO (control), ADP, oligomycin (OMN), OMN+ADP, and CsA during Protocol A (A) and Protocol B (B). Figure S2: Average Ca^{2+} added before mPTP opening, $\Delta\Psi_m$ collapse, NADH oxidation, and matrix acidification. Figure S3: Trend-fits for calculation of buffering rate. Figure S4: Fura-4F ratio representing the change in $[Ca^{2+}]_e$ before and after adding a 20 μM $CaCl_2$ bolus in the absence or presence of 250 μM ADP in the mitochondria-free experimental buffer. Figure S5: Representative raw traces of extra-matrix Ca^{2+} fluorescence (Fura-4F ratio) and Ca^{2+} uptake in mitochondria pretreated with 0.5% DMSO (control), OMN+ADP, and CATR (carboxyatractyloside)+OMN+ADP prior to mPTP opening.

Author Contributions: J.M. and A.K.S.C., conceptualized and designed the experiments; J.M. and A.J.D., performed experiments; J.M., A.J.D. and G.K.N., analyzed data; J.M., W.-M.K., D.F.S. and A.K.S.C., interpreted results; J.M. and A.K.S.C., drafted the manuscript and figures; J.M., G.K.N., W.-M.K., D.F.S. and A.K.S.C., critically read/edited the manuscript. All authors have read and approved the manuscript.

Funding: This project was supported by the Veterans Administration (Merit Review BX-002539-01).

Acknowledgments: The authors are thankful to James S. Heisner for technical assistance.

Conflicts of Interest: The authors declare no conflicts of interest.

References

1. Denton, R.M.; McCormack, J.G. The calcium sensitive dehydrogenases of vertebrate mitochondria. *Cell Calcium* **1986**, *7*, 377–386. [CrossRef]
2. Jouaville, L.S.; Pinton, P.; Bastianutto, C.; Rutter, G.A.; Rizzuto, R. Regulation of mitochondrial ATP synthesis by calcium: Evidence for a long-term metabolic priming. *Proc. Natl. Acad. Sci. USA* **1999**, *96*, 13807–13812. [CrossRef] [PubMed]
3. Bernardi, P. Mitochondrial transport of cations: Channels, exchangers, and permeability transition. *Physiol. Rev.* **1999**, *79*, 1127–1155. [CrossRef] [PubMed]
4. Hajnoczky, G.; Csordas, G.; Das, S.; Garcia-Perez, C.; Saotome, M.; Sinha Roy, S.; Yi, M. Mitochondrial calcium signalling and cell death: Approaches for assessing the role of mitochondrial Ca2+ uptake in apoptosis. *Cell Calcium* **2006**, *40*, 553–560. [CrossRef] [PubMed]
5. Brookes, P.S.; Yoon, Y.; Robotham, J.L.; Anders, M.W.; Sheu, S.S. Calcium, ATP, and ROS: A mitochondrial love-hate triangle. *Am. J. Physiol. Cell Physiol.* **2004**, *287*, C817–C833. [CrossRef] [PubMed]
6. O'Rourke, B.; Cortassa, S.; Aon, M.A. Mitochondrial ion channels: Gatekeepers of life and death. *Physiology (Bethesda)* **2005**, *20*, 303–315. [CrossRef]
7. Camara, A.K.; Lesnefsky, E.J.; Stowe, D.F. Potential therapeutic benefits of strategies directed to mitochondria. *Antioxid. Redox Signal.* **2010**, *13*, 279–347. [CrossRef]
8. Gunter, T.E.; Buntinas, L.; Sparagna, G.; Eliseev, R.; Gunter, K. Mitochondrial calcium transport: Mechanisms and functions. *Cell Calcium* **2000**, *28*, 285–296. [CrossRef]
9. Baughman, J.M.; Perocchi, F.; Girgis, H.S.; Plovanich, M.; Belcher-Timme, C.A.; Sancak, Y.; Bao, X.R.; Strittmatter, L.; Goldberger, O.; Bogorad, R.L.; et al. Integrative genomics identifies MCU as an essential component of the mitochondrial calcium uniporter. *Nature* **2011**, *476*, 341–345. [CrossRef]
10. De Stefani, D.; Raffaello, A.; Teardo, E.; Szabo, I.; Rizzuto, R. A forty-kilodalton protein of the inner membrane is the mitochondrial calcium uniporter. *Nature* **2011**, *476*, 336–340. [CrossRef]
11. Mitchell, P. Coupling of phosphorylation to electron and hydrogen transfer by a chemi-osmotic type of mechanism. *Nature* **1961**, *191*, 144–148. [CrossRef] [PubMed]
12. Mitchell, P. Keilin's respiratory chain concept and its chemiosmotic consequences. *Science* **1979**, *206*, 1148–1159. [CrossRef] [PubMed]
13. Greenawalt, J.W.; Rossi, C.S.; Lehninger, A.L. Effect of Active Accumulation of Calcium and Phosphate Ions on the Structure of Rat Liver Mitochondria. *J. Cell Biol.* **1964**, *23*, 21–38. [CrossRef] [PubMed]
14. Chalmers, S.; Nicholls, D.G. The relationship between free and total calcium concentrations in the matrix of liver and brain mitochondria. *J. Biol. Chem.* **2003**, *278*, 19062–19070. [CrossRef] [PubMed]
15. Starkov, A.A. The molecular identity of the mitochondrial Ca2+ sequestration system. *FEBS J.* **2010**, *277*, 3652–3663. [CrossRef]
16. Carafoli, E.; Tiozzo, R.; Lugli, G.; Crovetti, F.; Kratzing, C. The release of calcium from heart mitochondria by sodium. *J. Mol. Cell. Cardiol.* **1974**, *6*, 361–371. [CrossRef]

17. Palty, R.; Silverman, W.F.; Hershfinkel, M.; Caporale, T.; Sensi, S.L.; Parnis, J.; Nolte, C.; Fishman, D.; Shoshan-Barmatz, V.; Herrmann, S.; et al. NCLX is an essential component of mitochondrial Na+/Ca2+ exchange. *Proc. Natl. Acad. Sci. USA* **2010**, *107*, 436–441. [CrossRef]
18. Boyman, L.; Williams, G.S.; Khananshvili, D.; Sekler, I.; Lederer, W.J. NCLX: The mitochondrial sodium calcium exchanger. *J. Mol. Cell. Cardiol.* **2013**, *59*, 205–213. [CrossRef]
19. Haumann, J.; Camara, A.K.S.; Gadicherla, A.K.; Navarro, C.D.; Boelens, A.D.; Blomeyer, C.A.; Dash, R.K.; Boswell, M.R.; Kwok, W.M.; Stowe, D.F. Slow Ca(2+) Efflux by Ca(2+)/H(+) Exchange in Cardiac Mitochondria Is Modulated by Ca(2+) Re-uptake via MCU, Extra-Mitochondrial pH, and H(+) Pumping by FOF1-ATPase. *Front. Physiol.* **2018**, *9*, 1914. [CrossRef]
20. Bernardi, P.; Vassanelli, S.; Veronese, P.; Colonna, R.; Szabo, I.; Zoratti, M. Modulation of the mitochondrial permeability transition pore. Effect of protons and divalent cations. *J. Biol. Chem.* **1992**, *267*, 2934–2939.
21. Szabo, I.; Zoratti, M. The mitochondrial megachannel is the permeability transition pore. *J. Bioenerg. Biomembr.* **1992**, *24*, 111–117. [CrossRef] [PubMed]
22. Crompton, M. The mitochondrial permeability transition pore and its role in cell death. *Biochem. J.* **1999**, *341 Pt 2*, 233–249. [CrossRef] [PubMed]
23. Kim, J.S.; He, L.; Lemasters, J.J. Mitochondrial permeability transition: A common pathway to necrosis and apoptosis. *Biochem. Biophys. Res. Commun.* **2003**, *304*, 463–470. [CrossRef]
24. Nakagawa, T.; Shimizu, S.; Watanabe, T.; Yamaguchi, O.; Otsu, K.; Yamagata, H.; Inohara, H.; Kubo, T.; Tsujimoto, Y. Cyclophilin D-dependent mitochondrial permeability transition regulates some necrotic but not apoptotic cell death. *Nature* **2005**, *434*, 652–658. [CrossRef] [PubMed]
25. Basso, E.; Fante, L.; Fowlkes, J.; Petronilli, V.; Forte, M.A.; Bernardi, P. Properties of the permeability transition pore in mitochondria devoid of Cyclophilin, D. *J. Biol. Chem.* **2005**, *280*, 18558–18561. [CrossRef] [PubMed]
26. Baines, C.P.; Kaiser, R.A.; Purcell, N.H.; Blair, N.S.; Osinska, H.; Hambleton, M.A.; Brunskill, E.W.; Sayen, M.R.; Gottlieb, R.A.; Dorn, G.W.; et al. Loss of cyclophilin D reveals a critical role for mitochondrial permeability transition in cell death. *Nature* **2005**, *434*, 658–662. [CrossRef]
27. Hunter, D.R.; Haworth, R.A. The Ca2+-induced membrane transition in mitochondria. I. The protective mechanisms. *Arch. Biochem. Biophys.* **1979**, *195*, 453–459. [CrossRef]
28. Halestrap, A.P.; Connern, C.P.; Griffiths, E.J.; Kerr, P.M. Cyclosporin A binding to mitochondrial cyclophilin inhibits the permeability transition pore and protects hearts from ischaemia/reperfusion injury. *Mol. Cell. Biochem.* **1997**, *174*, 167–172. [CrossRef]
29. Haumann, J.; Dash, R.K.; Stowe, D.F.; Boelens, A.D.; Beard, D.A.; Camara, A.K. Mitochondrial free [Ca2+] increases during ATP/ADP antiport and ADP phosphorylation: Exploration of mechanisms. *Biophys. J.* **2010**, *99*, 997–1006. [CrossRef]
30. Sokolova, N.; Pan, S.; Provazza, S.; Beutner, G.; Vendelin, M.; Birkedal, R.; Sheu, S.S. ADP protects cardiac mitochondria under severe oxidative stress. *PLoS ONE* **2013**, *8*, e83214. [CrossRef]
31. Griffiths, E.J.; Halestrap, A.P. Further evidence that cyclosporin A protects mitochondria from calcium overload by inhibiting a matrix peptidyl-prolyl cis-trans isomerase. Implications for the immunosuppressive and toxic effects of cyclosporin. *Biochem. J.* **1991**, *274 Pt 2*, 611–614. [CrossRef] [PubMed]
32. Waldmeier, P.C.; Feldtrauer, J.J.; Qian, T.; Lemasters, J.J. Inhibition of the mitochondrial permeability transition by the nonimmunosuppressive cyclosporin derivative NIM811. *Mol. Pharmacol.* **2002**, *62*, 22–29. [CrossRef]
33. Altschuld, R.A.; Hohl, C.M.; Castillo, L.C.; Garleb, A.A.; Starling, R.C.; Brierley, G.P. Cyclosporin inhibits mitochondrial calcium efflux in isolated adult rat ventricular cardiomyocytes. *Am. J. Physiol.* **1992**, *262*, H1699–H1704. [CrossRef]
34. Wei, A.C.; Liu, T.; Cortassa, S.; Winslow, R.L.; O'Rourke, B. Mitochondrial Ca2+ influx and efflux rates in guinea pig cardiac mitochondria: Low and high affinity effects of cyclosporine A. *Biochim. Biophys. Acta* **2011**, *1813*, 1373–1381. [CrossRef] [PubMed]
35. Blomeyer, C.A.; Bazil, J.N.; Stowe, D.F.; Pradhan, R.K.; Dash, R.K.; Camara, A.K. Dynamic buffering of mitochondrial Ca2+ during Ca2+ uptake and Na+-induced Ca2+ release. *J. Bioenerg. Biomembr.* **2013**, *45*, 189–202. [CrossRef] [PubMed]
36. Aldakkak, M.; Stowe, D.F.; Dash, R.K.; Camara, A.K. Mitochondrial handling of excess Ca2+ is substrate-dependent with implications for reactive oxygen species generation. *Free Radic. Biol. Med.* **2013**, *56*, 193–203. [CrossRef] [PubMed]

37. Agarwal, B.; Dash, R.K.; Stowe, D.F.; Bosnjak, Z.J.; Camara, A.K. Isoflurane modulates cardiac mitochondrial bioenergetics by selectively attenuating respiratory complexes. *Biochim. Biophys. Acta* **2014**, *1837*, 354–365. [CrossRef] [PubMed]
38. Blomeyer, C.A.; Bazil, J.N.; Stowe, D.F.; Dash, R.K.; Camara, A.K. Mg(2+) differentially regulates two modes of mitochondrial Ca(2+) uptake in isolated cardiac mitochondria: Implications for mitochondrial Ca(2+) sequestration. *J. Bioenerg. Biomembr.* **2016**, *48*, 175–188. [CrossRef]
39. Boelens, A.D.; Pradhan, R.K.; Blomeyer, C.A.; Camara, A.K.; Dash, R.K.; Stowe, D.F. Extra-matrix Mg2+ limits Ca2+ uptake and modulates Ca2+ uptake-independent respiration and redox state in cardiac isolated mitochondria. *J. Bioenerg. Biomembr.* **2013**, *45*, 203–218. [CrossRef]
40. Scaduto, R.C., Jr.; Grotyohann, L.W. Measurement of mitochondrial membrane potential using fluorescent rhodamine derivatives. *Biophys. J.* **1999**, *76*, 469–477. [CrossRef]
41. Grynkiewicz, G.; Poenie, M.; Tsien, R.Y. A new generation of Ca2+ indicators with greatly improved fluorescence properties. *J. Biol. Chem.* **1985**, *260*, 3440–3450. [PubMed]
42. Bazil, J.N.; Blomeyer, C.A.; Pradhan, R.K.; Camara, A.K.; Dash, R.K. Modeling the calcium sequestration system in isolated guinea pig cardiac mitochondria. *J. Bioenerg. Biomembr.* **2013**, *45*, 177–188. [CrossRef] [PubMed]
43. Zoccarato, F.; Nicholls, D. The role of phosphate in the regulation of the independent calcium-efflux pathway of liver mitochondria. *Eur. J. Biochem.* **1982**, *127*, 333–338. [CrossRef] [PubMed]
44. Wei, A.C.; Liu, T.; O'Rourke, B. Dual Effect of Phosphate Transport on Mitochondrial Ca2+ Dynamics. *J. Biol. Chem.* **2015**, *290*, 16088–16098. [CrossRef] [PubMed]
45. Wei, A.C.; Liu, T.; Winslow, R.L.; O'Rourke, B. Dynamics of matrix-free Ca2+ in cardiac mitochondria: Two components of Ca2+ uptake and role of phosphate buffering. *J. Gen. Physiol.* **2012**, *139*, 465–478. [CrossRef] [PubMed]
46. Glancy, B.; Balaban, R.S. Role of mitochondrial Ca2+ in the regulation of cellular energetics. *Biochemistry* **2012**, *51*, 2959–2973. [CrossRef] [PubMed]
47. Vasington, F.D.; Murphy, J.V. Ca ion uptake by rat kidney mitochondria and its dependence on respiration and phosphorylation. *J. Biol. Chem.* **1962**, *237*, 2670–2677. [PubMed]
48. Chinopoulos, C.; Adam-Vizi, V. Mitochondrial Ca2+ sequestration and precipitation revisited. *FEBS J.* **2010**, *277*, 3637–3651. [CrossRef] [PubMed]
49. Harris, E.J.; Zaba, B. The phosphate requirement for Ca2+-uptake by heart and liver mitochondria. *FEBS Lett.* **1977**, *79*, 284–290. [CrossRef]
50. Nicholls, D.G.; Chalmers, S. The integration of mitochondrial calcium transport and storage. *J. Bioenerg. Biomembr.* **2004**, *36*, 277–281. [CrossRef]
51. Kristian, T.; Pivovarova, N.B.; Fiskum, G.; Andrews, S.B. Calcium-induced precipitate formation in brain mitochondria: Composition, calcium capacity, and retention. *J. Neurochem.* **2007**, *102*, 1346–1356. [CrossRef]
52. Kushnareva, Y.E.; Haley, L.M.; Sokolove, P.M. The role of low (<or = 1 mM) phosphate concentrations in regulation of mitochondrial permeability: Modulation of matrix free Ca2+ concentration. *Arch. Biochem. Biophys.* **1999**, *363*, 155–162. [CrossRef] [PubMed]
53. Malyala, S.; Zhang, Y.; Strubbe, J.O.; Bazil, J.N. Calcium phosphate precipitation inhibits mitochondrial energy metabolism. *PLoS Comput. Biol.* **2019**, *15*, e1006719. [CrossRef] [PubMed]
54. Abramov, A.Y.; Fraley, C.; Diao, C.T.; Winkfein, R.; Colicos, M.A.; Duchen, M.R.; French, R.J.; Pavlov, E. Targeted polyphosphatase expression alters mitochondrial metabolism and inhibits calcium-dependent cell death. *Proc. Natl. Acad. Sci. USA* **2007**, *104*, 18091–18096. [CrossRef]
55. Seidlmayer, L.K.; Gomez-Garcia, M.R.; Blatter, L.A.; Pavlov, E.; Dedkova, E.N. Inorganic polyphosphate is a potent activator of the mitochondrial permeability transition pore in cardiac myocytes. *J. Gen. Physiol.* **2012**, *139*, 321–331. [CrossRef]
56. Chavez, E.; Moreno-Sanchez, R.; Zazueta, C.; Rodriguez, J.S.; Bravo, C.; Reyes-Vivas, H. On the protection by inorganic phosphate of calcium-induced membrane permeability transition. *J. Bioenerg. Biomembr.* **1997**, *29*, 571–577. [CrossRef] [PubMed]
57. Basso, E.; Petronilli, V.; Forte, M.A.; Bernardi, P. Phosphate is essential for inhibition of the mitochondrial permeability transition pore by cyclosporin A and by cyclophilin D ablation. *J. Biol. Chem.* **2008**, *283*, 26307–26311. [CrossRef] [PubMed]

58. McGee, A.M.; Baines, C.P. Phosphate is not an absolute requirement for the inhibitory effects of cyclosporin A or cyclophilin D deletion on mitochondrial permeability transition. *Biochem. J.* **2012**, *443*, 185–191. [CrossRef]
59. Varanyuwatana, P.; Halestrap, A.P. The roles of phosphate and the phosphate carrier in the mitochondrial permeability transition pore. *Mitochondrion* **2012**, *12*, 120–125. [CrossRef]
60. Carafoli, E.; Rossi, C.S.; Lehninger, A.L. Uptake of Adenine Nucleotides by Respiring Mitochondria during Active Accumulation of Ca++ and Phosphate. *J. Biol. Chem.* **1965**, *240*, 2254–2261.
61. Michailova, A.; McCulloch, A. Model study of ATP and ADP buffering, transport of Ca(2+) and Mg(2+), and regulation of ion pumps in ventricular myocyte. *Biophys. J.* **2001**, *81*, 614–629. [CrossRef]
62. Litsky, M.L.; Pfeiffer, D.R. Regulation of the mitochondrial Ca2+ uniporter by external adenine nucleotides: The uniporter behaves like a gated channel which is regulated by nucleotides and divalent cations. *Biochemistry* **1997**, *36*, 7071–7080. [CrossRef] [PubMed]
63. Traba, J.; Del Arco, A.; Duchen, M.R.; Szabadkai, G.; Satrustegui, J. SCaMC-1 promotes cancer cell survival by desensitizing mitochondrial permeability transition via ATP/ADP-mediated matrix Ca(2+) buffering. *Cell Death Differ.* **2012**, *19*, 650–660. [CrossRef] [PubMed]
64. Devenish, R.J.; Prescott, M.; Boyle, G.M.; Nagley, P. The oligomycin axis of mitochondrial ATP synthase: OSCP and the proton channel. *J. Bioenerg. Biomembr.* **2000**, *32*, 507–515. [CrossRef] [PubMed]
65. Genge, B.R.; Wu, L.N.; Wuthier, R.E. In vitro modeling of matrix vesicle nucleation: Synergistic stimulation of mineral formation by annexin A5 and phosphatidylserine. *J. Biol. Chem.* **2007**, *282*, 26035–26045. [CrossRef] [PubMed]
66. Bandorowicz-Pikula, J.; Buchet, R.; Pikula, S. Annexins as nucleotide-binding proteins: Facts and speculations. *Bioessays* **2001**, *23*, 170–178. [CrossRef]
67. McCormack, J.G.; Denton, R.M. Intracellular calcium ions and intramitochondrial Ca2+ in the regulation of energy metabolism in mammalian tissues. *Proc. Nutr. Soc.* **1990**, *49*, 57–75. [CrossRef] [PubMed]
68. Rutter, G.A. Ca2(+)-binding to citrate cycle dehydrogenases. *Int. J. Biochem.* **1990**, *22*, 1081–1088. [CrossRef]
69. Territo, P.R.; Mootha, V.K.; French, S.A.; Balaban, R.S. Ca(2+) activation of heart mitochondrial oxidative phosphorylation: Role of the F(0)/F(1)-ATPase. *Am. J. Physiol. Cell Physiol.* **2000**, *278*, C423–C435. [CrossRef] [PubMed]
70. Chinopoulos, C.; Adam-Vizi, V. The 'ins and outs' of Ca2+ in mitochondria. *FEBS J.* **2010**, *277*, 3621. [CrossRef] [PubMed]
71. Jung, D.W.; Baysal, K.; Brierley, G.P. The sodium-calcium antiport of heart mitochondria is not electroneutral. *J. Biol. Chem.* **1995**, *270*, 672–678. [CrossRef] [PubMed]
72. Kim, B.; Matsuoka, S. Cytoplasmic Na+-dependent modulation of mitochondrial Ca2+ via electrogenic mitochondrial Na+-Ca2+ exchange. *J. Physiol.* **2008**, *586*, 1683–1697. [CrossRef] [PubMed]

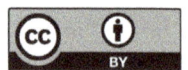

© 2019 by the authors. Licensee MDPI, Basel, Switzerland. This article is an open access article distributed under the terms and conditions of the Creative Commons Attribution (CC BY) license (http://creativecommons.org/licenses/by/4.0/).

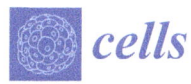

Article

Fatty Acid Oxidation and Mitochondrial Morphology Changes as Key Modulators of the Affinity for ADP in Rat Heart Mitochondria

Adolfas Toleikis [1], Sonata Trumbeckaite [1,2], Julius Liobikas [1,3], Neringa Pauziene [4], Lolita Kursvietiene [3] and Dalia M. Kopustinskiene [5],*

[1] Neuroscience Institute, Lithuanian University of Health Sciences, Eiveniu 4, LT-50161 Kaunas, Lithuania; tadolfas@yahoo.co.uk (A.T.); Sonata.Trumbeckaite@lsmuni.lt (S.T.); Julius.Liobikas@lsmuni.lt (J.L.)
[2] Department of Pharmacognosy, Medical Academy, Lithuanian University of Health Sciences, Sukileliu pr. 13, LT-50166 Kaunas, Lithuania
[3] Department of Biochemistry, Medical Academy, Lithuanian University of Health Sciences, Eiveniu 4, LT-50161 Kaunas, Lithuania; Lolita.Kursvietiene@lsmuni.lt
[4] Institute of Anatomy, Lithuanian University of Health Sciences, Mickeviciaus 9, LT-44307 Kaunas, Lithuania; Neringa.Pauziene@lsmuni.lt
[5] Institute of Pharmaceutical Technologies, Medical Academy, Lithuanian University of Health Sciences, Sukileliu pr. 13, LT-50161 Kaunas, Lithuania
* Correspondence: DaliaMarija.Kopustinskiene@lsmuni.lt

Received: 16 December 2019; Accepted: 27 January 2020; Published: 1 February 2020

Abstract: Fatty acids are the main respiratory substrates important for cardiac function, and their oxidation is altered during various chronic disorders. We investigated the mechanism of fatty acid–oxidation-induced changes and their relations with mitochondrial morphology and ADP/ATP carrier conformation on the kinetics of the regulation of mitochondrial respiration in rat skinned cardiac fibers. Saturated and unsaturated, activated and not activated, long and medium chain, fatty acids similarly decreased the apparent K_m^{ADP}. Addition of 5% dextran T-70 to mimic the oncotic pressure of the cellular cytoplasm markedly increased the low apparent K_m^{ADP} value of mitochondria in cardiac fibers respiring on palmitoyl-L-carnitine or octanoyl-L-carnitine, but did not affect the high apparent K_m^{ADP} of mitochondria respiring on pyruvate and malate. Electron microscopy revealed that palmitoyl-L-carnitine oxidation-induced changes in the mitochondrial ultrastructure (preventable by dextran) are similar to those induced by carboxyatractyloside. Our data suggest that a fatty acid oxidation-induced conformational change of the adenosine diphosphate (ADP)/adenosine triphosphate (ATP) carrier (M-state to C-state, condensed to orthodox mitochondria) may affect the oxidative phosphorylation affinity for ADP.

Keywords: ADP/ATP carrier; K_m^{ADP}; mitochondria; fatty acid oxidation; dextran; morphology

1. Introduction

The major part of energy supply in cells comes from the fatty acid oxidation in mitochondria. Fatty acids as the main respiratory substrates are important, not only for cardiac function [1,2], but also they recently have been shown to provide energy for the proliferation and survival of tumors [3]. An increased fatty acid consumption reduces cardiac efficiency, and among the mechanisms involved, a modulation of the ADP/ATP carrier has been suggested [4–6].

The studies of saponin-permeabilized heart and skeletal muscle fibers demonstrated that, in contrast to isolated mitochondria, the mitochondrial outer membrane in situ possesses a low permeability for exogenous ADP (high apparent K_m^{ADP} of oxidative phosphorylation for external

ADP), and therefore, is crucial in the mechanism of regulation of mitochondrial respiration in vivo [7,8]. K_m^{ADP} is drastically (up to 10-fold) decreased in the case of the oxidation of saturated fatty acids (CoA- or carnitine-esters of palmitate and octanoate; alone or in combination with pyruvate), but not during the transport of fatty acids into mitochondria [9]; however, the mechanism of this phenomenon has not been elucidated yet.

Mitochondria and intracellular ATPases in cardiomyocytes are in close proximity, and are arranged into tightly coupled structural and functional complexes known as intracellular, energetic units [8,10,11]. Strict interpositions of mitochondrion optimizes the energy fluxes and interactions of mitochondria with surrounding organelles; however, at high workload the direct ATP transfer does not fulfil the energy need in heart cells [12,13]. In these conditions, the creatine kinase–phosphocreatine system is useful: creatine (the substrate of mitochondrial creatine kinase) significantly stimulates the production of ADP (when the concentration of ADP is suboptimal, i.e., about 50–10 µM) by mitochondrial creatine kinase functionally coupled with the ADP/ATP carrier. This significantly enhances the respiration of heart mitochondria and ATP production. The stimulating effect of creatine on respiration decreases when the permeability of the mitochondrial outer membrane for ADP increases (the apparent K_m^{ADP} decreases) due to the treatment of cardiac cells with proteolytic enzymes (trypsin or collagenase) [14,15], after the isolation of mitochondria [16,17], or due to some clustering of mitochondria possessing an intact mitochondrial outer membrane and the alteration of their position within the cells of the non-ischemic zone of the low-flow-perfused rat heart [18].

Fatty acids have been demonstrated to change the conformation of uncoupling protein [19]. Furthermore, other studies revealed structural, and to some extent functional, homology between the uncoupling protein and the ADP/ATP carrier [20,21]. There is also an indirect evidence that low apparent K_m^{ADP} in mitochondria from cancerous cells [22,23] and fetal or neonatal mitochondria [24] could be related to mitochondrial ultrastructural changes, namely increased, diffuse the mitochondrial matrix volume corresponding to orthodox mitochondrial conformation [25,26].

Mitochondria are significantly more abundant in hearts compared to skeletal muscle, brain, kidney and liver [27]. Furthermore, cardiac mitochondria primarily use fatty acids as respiratory substrates, whereas most other organs use glucose as the major energy substrate [28], and therefore, we have chosen skinned cardiac fibers as the experimental object in our study. We investigated the mechanism of fatty acid–oxidation-induced changes and their relations with mitochondrial morphology and ADP/ATP carrier conformation on the kinetics of the regulation of mitochondrial respiration (the apparent K_m^{ADP}) in situ; i.e., in the mitochondria of saponin-permeabilized rat heart muscle fibers, where mitochondria and the ATPases in myofibrils and in the sarcoplasmic reticulum remain intact, corresponding to the physiological conditions in the cell [8,10].

2. Materials and Methods

All chemicals used in this work were from Sigma-Aldrich (St. Louis, MO, USA).

The male Wistar rats ~3 months old and weighing 250–300 g were obtained from the Vivarium of the Lithuanian University of Health Sciences, where they were housed at 23 ± 2 °C with a 12-h light/dark cycle and free access to food and water. The experimental procedures used in the present study were performed according to the permission of the Lithuanian Committee of Good Laboratory Animal Use Practice (number 0228/2012). Rats were killed by cervical dislocation. Rat hearts were excised and rinsed in ice-cold 0.9% KCl solution. The bundles of cardiac fibers, approximately 0.3–0.4 mm in diameter, were prepared by using sharp-ended needles from the muscle strips cut out from the left ventricular endocardium in an ice-cold preparation solution containing 20 mM imidazole, 20 mM taurine, 0.5 mM dithiothreitol, 7.1 mM $MgCl_2$, 50 mM 2-(NMorpholino)ethanesulfonic acid (MES), 5 mM adenosine triphosphate (ATP), 15 mM phosphocreatine, 2.62 mM CaK_2EGTA and 7.38 mM K_2EGTA (ionic strength of the solution 160 mM, free Ca^{2+} 0.1 µM, free Mg^{2+} 3 mM; pH 7.0, adjusted with KOH), then permeabilized by saponin (50 µg/mL, 30 min), washed for 10 min in a physiological salt solution containing 20 mM imidazole, 20 mM taurine, 0.5 mM dithiothreitol,

1.61 mM MgCl$_2$, 100 mM MES, 3 mM KH$_2$PO$_4$, 2.95 mM CaK$_2$EGTA and 7.05 mM K$_2$EGTA (ionic strength of the solution 160 mM, free Ca^{2+} 0.1 µM, free Mg^{2+} 1 mM; pH 7.1, adjusted with KOH) [29]. All procedures were carried out under intensive shaking (120 times/min). The washed bundles of fibers were rinsed once in the physiological salt solution, transferred into the tubes with the same solution and then kept on ice.

Respiration rates of skinned cardiac fibers were determined in the closed respiration chamber in physiological salt solution at 37 °C or 25 °C by the means of the Clark-type oxygen electrode. Pyruvate + malate (6 mM + 6 mM), glutamate 6 mM + malate (6 mM + 6 mM), palmitoyl-L-carnitine+malate (9 µM + 0.24 mM), oleoyl-CoA + L-carnitine + malate (6 µM + 2.5 mM + 0.24 mM) or decanoic acid + pyruvate + malate (0.3 mM + 6 mM + 6 mM) were used as respiratory substrates as indicated in the Results section or in the Figure legends. Respiration rates were expressed as nmol O/min/mg fibers' dry weight. Dry weight = wet weight before respiration measurement/factor 'W'. The factor 'W' was calculated to be 4.85 for heart muscle fibers [14]. The solubility of oxygen was taken to be 422 nmol O/mL at 37 °C and 452 nmol O/mL at 25 °C [30]. The adenosine diphosphate (ADP) regenerative system, consisting of 1.2 IU/mL lyophilized yeast hexokinase (Type V; EC 2.7.1.1) and 24 mM glucose, was added to the chamber before the addition of heart muscle fibers. Titration was made by different ADP concentrations in each separate probe. ΔV was expressed as a difference between respiration rates in the presence and in the absence of added ADP. The apparent K_m^{ADP} and V_{max} were estimated from the least-squares fit to the Michaelis–Menten equation (ΔV vs. ADP concentration).

Mitochondria were isolated by a differential centrifugation procedure. Hearts were excised and rinsed in ice-cold isolation medium, containing 160 mM KCl, 10 mM NaCl, 20 mM Tris, 5 mM EGTA (pH 7.7, adjusted with KOH at 2 °C). Mitochondria were isolated in the same medium supplemented with 2 mg/mL bovine serum albumin (BSA). Homogenate was centrifuged for 5 min at 750× g, then the supernatant was centrifuged for 10 min at 6740× g and the pellet was washed once in the medium containing 180 mM KCl, 20 mM Tris, 3 mM EGTA (pH 7.3 adjusted with KOH at 2 °C), suspended in it and kept on ice. The mitochondrial protein concentration was determined by the biuret method (Piotrowski's test) [31]. The final mitochondrial protein concentration was 0.5 mg/mL. Mitochondrial swelling was recorded as the decrease of light scattering at 540 nm with the Heλios α spectrophotometer in physiological salt solution supplemented with 24 mM glucose and 1.2 IU/mL hexokinase, 0.24 mM malate and palmitoyl-L-carnitine (9–80 µM).

An exogenous ADP-trapping system consisting of pyruvate kinase + phosphoenolpyruvate (PK + PEP), which effectively competes with mitochondria for the extramitochondrial ADP, and therefore, decreases the respiration rate in the State 3, was used to investigate the interactions of the functional complexes of mitochondria with Ca, the MgATPases of myofibrils and the sarcoplasmic reticulum under the different conditions (25 °C and 37 °C; mitochondria oxidizing different substrates: glutamate 6 mM + malate 6 mM or palmitoyl-L-carnitine 9 µM + malate 0.24 mM). The sequence of additions to the respiration chamber: 8 mM PEP, ~3 mg of cardiac fibers, 2 mM ATP, 20 + 20 U/mL (or 40 U/mL) PK, 20 mM creatine, 35 µM cytochrome c, 125 µM atractyloside. After each addition, the respiration rate was estimated. The cytochrome c test was used to evaluate the intactness of the mitochondrial outer membrane.

The coupling of mitochondrial creatine kinase (mi-CK) and the ADP/ATP carrier was estimated using two approaches. (1) The apparent K_m^{ADP} and V_{max} values were estimated from ΔV vs. ADP concentration relationships in the presence or in the absence of 20 mM creatine; the results were compared with corresponding kinetic parameters without creatine; (2) 60 µM ADP was added into the respiration chamber followed by the addition of 20 mM of creatine. The stimulation of respiration by creatine, i.e., the creatine effect, was expressed as the ratio of the respiration rates with creatine and with 60 µM of ADP without creatine.

For the electron microscopy studies, the saponin-permeabilized rat cardiac fibers were incubated aerobically in the physiological salt solution containing pyruvate and malate, 6 mM both (without, as control, or with carboxyatractyloside 1.3 µM or bongkrekic acid 17.6 µM), or palmitoyl-L-carnitine 9 µM, or palmitoyl-L-carnitine 9 µM plus 5% dextran T-70, for 5 min at 37 °C under intensive stirring. Subsequently, the fibers were placed into 2.5% glutaraldehyde solution in 0.1 M cacodylate buffer (pH 7.4) and kept in it for 5 min at room temperature under gentle shaking. Afterwards, the fibers were left in the same fixative overnight at 4 °C. Later on, the fibers were washed several times in cacodylate buffer and post-fixed for 1 h at 4 °C with 1% osmium tetraoxide solution in the same buffer. After that, they were dehydrated through a graded ethanol series and embedded in a mixture of resins Epon 812 and Araldite. Ultrathin sections were cut with a with ultra-microtome, stained with uranyl acetate and lead citrate, and examined with a PHILIPS EM300 electron microscope, using AGFA electron image films.

The results are presented as means ± S.E. The data were analyzed with one-way analysis of variance (ANOVA) by Prism v. 5.04 (GraphPad Software Inc., La Jolla, CA, USA). Then $p < 0.05$ was taken as the level of significance.

3. Results

3.1. Role of Oxidation of Fatty Acids in Regulation of Oxidative Phosphorylation and Mitochondrial Swelling

Oxidation of fatty acids, the major myocardial respiratory substrates (palmitoyl-L-carnitine, palmitoyl-CoA + L-carnitine and octanoyl-L-carnitine) caused the drastic decrease of the apparent K_m^{ADP} specific for pyruvate+malate oxidation [9], but the mechanisms of this effect have not been elucidated yet. In this study, we investigated which factors are responsible for the low apparent K_m^{ADP} observed during fatty acid oxidation. Firstly, we evaluated if the fatty acid related decrease of the apparent K_m^{ADP} depend on the different fatty acid chain length and degree of saturation. The principal scheme of fatty acid and pyruvate and malate oxidation in mitochondria is presented in Figure 1.

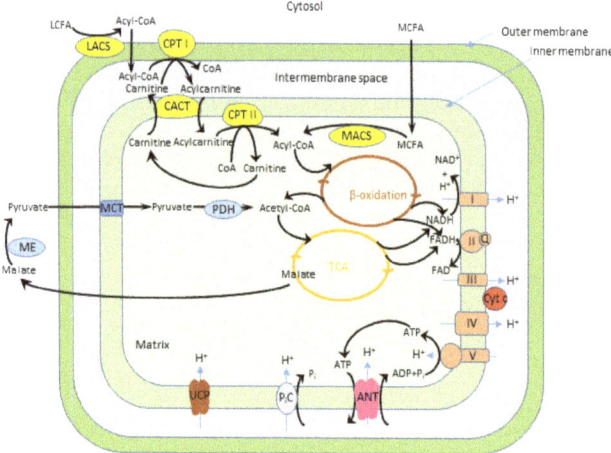

Figure 1. The principal scheme of the fatty acid and pyruvate and malate oxidation in mitochondria. LCFA—long chain fatty acids, MCFA—medium chain fatty acids, LACS—long chain acyl-CoA synthetase, CPT—carnitine palmitoyl-transferase, CACT—carnitine acylcarnitine translocase, MACS—medium chain acyl-CoA synthetase, ME—malic enzyme, MCT—monocarboxylate transporter, PDH—pyruvate dehydrogenase, TCA—tricarboxylic acid cycle, NAD—nicotinamide adenine dinucleotide, FAD—flavin adenine dinucleotide, I-V—mitochondrial electron transport chain complexes, Q—coenzyme Q, Cyt c—cytochrome c, ANT—ADP/ATP carrier, P_iC—inorganic phosphate carrier, UCP—uncoupling protein.

In the case of pyruvate+malate oxidation the apparent K_m^{ADP} of mitochondria in saponin-permeabilized rat cardiac fibers (K_m^{ADP} = 217.8 ± 8 µM) is by 3–10 folds higher if compared with the apparent K_m^{ADP} for oleoyl-CoA + L-carnitine+malate (55.7 ± 5.1 µM ADP), decanoic acid + pyruvate + malate (75.8 ± 7.6 µM ADP) or isolated rat heart mitochondria (K_m^{ADP} = 23 µM, Liobikas et al., 2001) (Figure 2). It is evident that the oxidation of both decanoic acid and oleoyl-CoA in situ induces a marked increase in the affinity of mitochondrial oxidative phosphorylation system for ADP.

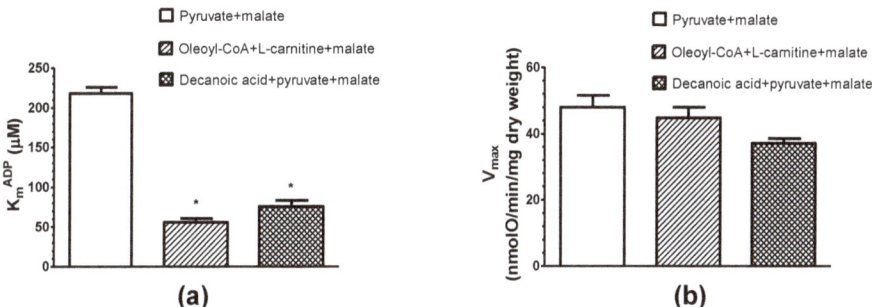

Figure 2. Influence of different respiratory substrates: pyruvate + malate (6 mM + 6 mM), oleoyl-CoA + L-carnitine+malate (6 µM + 2.5mM + 0.24mM) and decanoic acid + pyruvate + malate (0.3 mM + 6 mM + 6 mM) on the apparent K_m^{ADP} (**a**) and V_{max} (**b**) of saponin-permeabilized rat cardiac fibers. n = 5; 37 °C; * p < 0.05 vs. control (pyruvate + malate). The results were analyzed with one-way analysis of variance (ANOVA) followed by the Dunnett post hoc test.

In the next series of experiments on different skinned cardiac fiber samples we tested the concentration dependence of the effect of fatty acids on the apparent K_m^{ADP} (Figure 3). The high apparent K_m^{ADP} with pyruvate + malate decreased to 30% and 33% of control values, when pyruvate + malate was supplemented with 2.2 µM or 9 µM palmitoyl-L-carnitine.

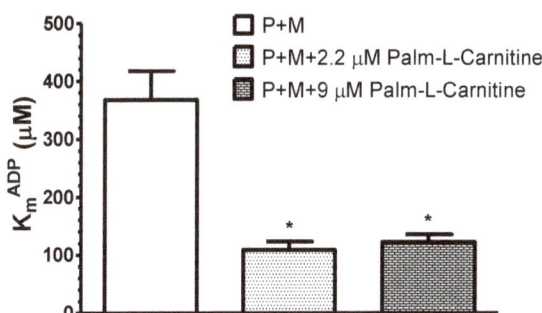

Figure 3. Influence of different respiratory substrates: pyruvate + malate (P + M, 6 mM + 6 mM), pyruvate + malate + palmitoyl-L-carnitine (6 mM + 6 mM + 2.2 µM) and pyruvate + malate + palmitoyl-L-carnitine (6 mM + 6 mM + 9 µM) on the apparent K_m^{ADP} of saponin-permeabilized rat cardiac fibers. Here, n = 5; 37 °C; * p < 0.05 vs. control (pyruvate + malate). The results were analyzed with one-way analysis of variance (ANOVA) followed by the Dunnett post hoc test.

Thus, four times lower concentration of palmitoyl-L-carnitine (2.2 µM) also effectively decreased the apparent K_m^{ADP}. Noteworthy, at 2.2 µM palmitoyl–L-carnitine (alone) the State 3 respiration rate was equal to 30–40% of that estimated at 9 µM. In the separate set of experiments, we revealed also that even 0.5 µM of palmitoyl-L-carnitine (used together with pyruvate+malate) decreased the apparent K_m^{ADP} ($p < 0.05$) to similar level as 9 µM of palmitoyl-L-carnitine (94.6 ± 13 µM and 77.9 ± 11 µM, respectively, compared with pyruvate+malate alone, 253.3 ± 23 µM; data of 4–6 paired experiments; 37 °C). Essentially similar results were obtained in the separate group of experiments when octanoyl-L-carnitine at two different concentrations (0.36 and 0.1 mM) was used as respiratory substrate in the presence of pyruvate + malate (Figure 4).

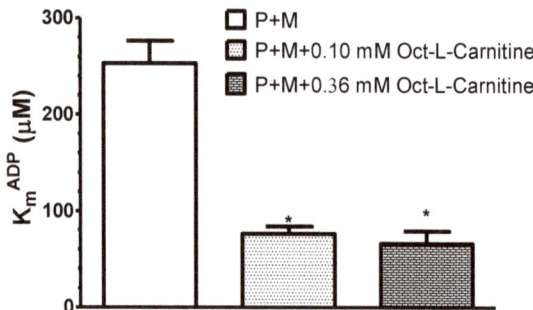

Figure 4. Influence of different respiratory substrates: pyruvate + malate (P + M, 6 mM + 6 mM), pyruvate + malate + octanoyl-L-carnitine (6 mM + 6 mM + 0.36 mM) and pyruvate + malate + octanoyl-L-carnitine (6 mM + 6 mM + 0.1 mM) on the apparent K_m^{ADP} of saponin-permeabilized rat cardiac fibers. In this case, $n = 4$; 37 °C; * $p < 0.05$ vs. control (pyruvate + malate). The results were analyzed with one-way analysis of variance (ANOVA) followed by the Dunnett post hoc test.

In this case, the apparent K_m^{ADP} decreased, respectively, to 34% and 26% of control values estimated with pyruvate+malate ($p < 0.05$, $n = 4$, 37 °C). Thus, our results showed that the decrease in the apparent K_m^{ADP} value did not depend upon the concentration of fatty acids.

Interestingly, during palmitoyl-L-carnitine oxidation, the apparent K_m^{ADP} decreased by about 2.6-fold with elevation of temperature from 25 °C to 37 °C, i.e., from 123 ± 22 µM ADP to 48 ± 5 µM ADP, respectively (Figure 5).

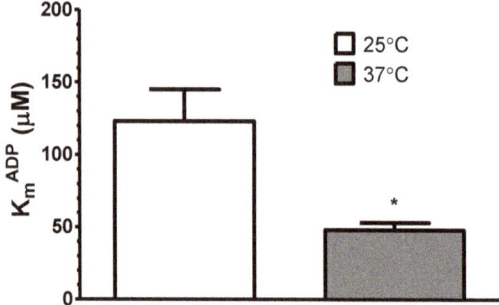

Figure 5. Influence of temperature on the apparent K_m^{ADP} of saponin-permeabilized rat cardiac fibers oxidizing palmitoyl-L-carnitine (9 µM) in the presence of malate (0.24 mM). The results were analyzed with paired t test; $n = 7$; * $p < 0.05$.

When pyruvate+malate were added immediately after the complete oxidation of a limited quantity (1.6 nmol) of palmitoyl-L-carnitine (Figure 6), the apparent K_m^{ADP} of mitochondria in cardiac fibers remained at a high level (211 ± 40 µM ADP), similar as in the case of pyruvate+malate oxidation alone (223 ± 56 µM ADP) (data of five paired experiments, 37 °C). Thus, the effect of fatty acids on the apparent K_m^{ADP} of mitochondria in permeabilized rat cardiac fibers is reversible.

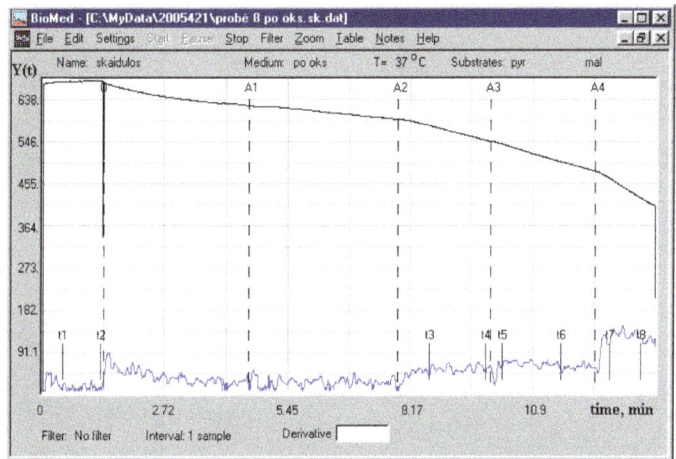

Figure 6. Representative respiration curve after the complete oxidation of a limited quantity of palmitoyl-L-carnitine. The black curve—oxygen consumption, the blue curve—oxygen consumption derivative. Additions: O—skinned rat cardiac fibers (registration of respiration on endogenous substrates), then A1—1.6 nmol of palmitoyl-L-carnitine, A2—pyruvate + malate (6 mM + 6 mM, respiration rate: 24.8 nmol/O/min/mg dry weight), A3—10 µM ADP (respiration rate: 32 nmol/O/min/mg dry weight), A4—1.2 mM ADP (respiration rate: 57.7 nmol/O/min/mg dry weight).

To exclude that the decrease in the apparent K_m^{ADP} during fatty acid oxidation is related to the detergent activity of palmitoyl-L-carnitine (reviewed in Goni FM et al. 1966) and its damage to mitochondrial membranes, we measured the swelling of isolated rat heart mitochondria oxidizing palmitoyl-L-carnitine (9, 27 and 80 µM) and malate (0.24 mM). Our data (Figure 7) showed that palmitoyl-L-carnitine at a concentration of 9 µM did not induce mitochondrial swelling.

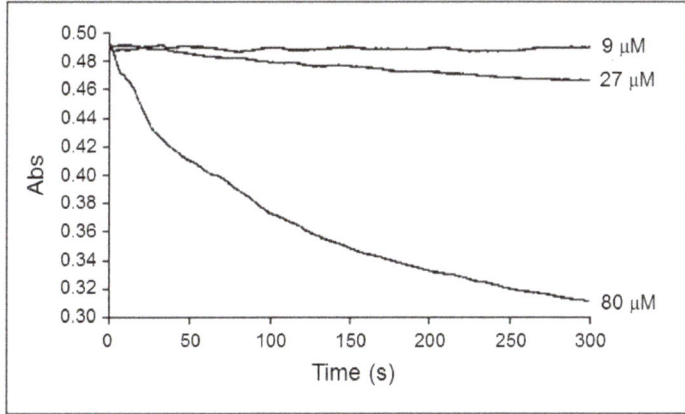

Figure 7. Swelling of isolated rat heart mitochondria respiring on palmitoyl-L-carnitine (9–80 µM) and malate (0.24 mM). $n = 3$, typical absorption traces are shown.

However, the higher concentrations (starting from 27 µM) of a palmitoyl-L-carnitine-induced concentration–dependent increase in mitochondrial swelling. Importantly, palmitoyl-L-carnitine did not change the mitochondrial outer membrane integrity (external cytochrome c did not stimulate the

State 3 respiration; its effect varied between 0.98 and 1.02 at distinct palmitoyl-L-carnitine concentrations; n = 8).

3.2. Regulation of Mitochondrial Respiration by Endogenous versus Exogenous ADP: Influence of Palmitoyl-L-Carnitine

The endogenous ADP is produced from exogenous ATP by ATPases in the myofibrils and in the sarcoplasmic reticulum, and is delivered directly to the mitochondria [8]. In the next series of experiments, the respiration of fibers was supported by palmitoyl-L-carnitine or pyruvate + malate (control), and titrated by ADP and ATP (Figure 8).

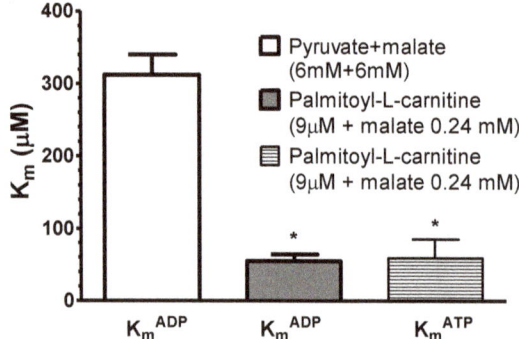

Figure 8. Influence of the adenosine diphosphate (ADP) source (endogenous (from exogenous adenosine triphosphate (ATP)) or exogenous) on the apparent K_m^{ADP} of saponin-permeabilized rat cardiac fibers oxidizing palmitoyl-L-carnitine (9 µM) in the presence of malate (0.24 mM) or pyruvate + malate (control, 6 mM + 6 mM). Experiments were performed at 37 °C. * $p < 0.05$ vs. control. $n = 5$ (paired experiments). The results were analyzed with one-way analysis of variance (ANOVA) followed by Dunnett post hoc test.

The apparent K_m^{ADP} and K_m^{ATP} were very low with palmitoyl-L-carnitine as the substrate (55 ± 9 and 59 ± 26 µM, respectively compared to pyruvate+malate (K_m^{ADP}, 312 ± 28 µM). Thus, in our study the decrease in the apparent K_m^{ADP} during fatty acid oxidation did not depend on the exogenous or endogenous supply of ADP.

3.3. Influence of Palmitoyl-L-Carnitine on the Permeability of Mitochondrial Outer Membrane for ADP

Using an exogenous ADP-trapping system consisting of pyruvate kinase + phosphoenolpyruvate (PK + PEP), which effectively competes with mitochondria for extramitochondrial ADP [8], we investigated the interactions of functional complexes of mitochondria with Ca, Mg ATPases of myofibrils and sarcoplasmic reticulum under different conditions (25 and 37 °C), and mitochondrial outer membrane permeability for ADP. The results of these experiments are presented in Figure 9. By the addition of 2 mM ATP we stimulated the basal respiration of mitochondria (similarly with both substrates, glutamate + malate and palmitoyl-L-carnitine), due to endogenously generated ADP. Consecutive addition of PK (40 U/mL, in the presence of PEP in the medium) suppressed respiration by about 30%; a similar effect (23%) was observed with palmitoyl-L-carnitine at 25 °C. The inhibitory effect of PK + PEP at 37 °C was equal with both respiratory substrates, glutamate + malate (33%) and palmitoyl-L-carnitine+malate (31%).

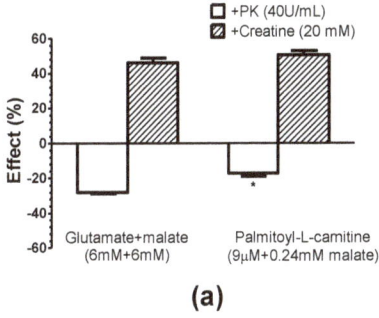
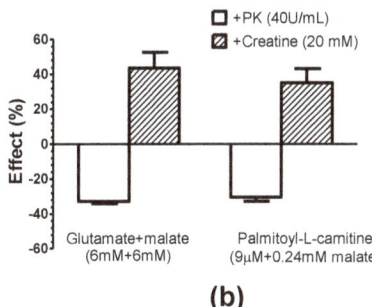

Figure 9. Influence of pyruvate kinase + phosphoenolpyruvate (PK + PEP) ADP-consuming system and creatine on the respiration of rat cardiac fibers using glutamate+malate and palmitoyl-L-carnitine + malate as respiratory substrates at (**a**) 25 °C and (**b**) 37 °C. The effect of pyruvate kinase (PK) (40 U/mL) on V_{ATP} and the effect of creatine on V_{PK} (40 U/mL) are shown. * $p < 0.05$ versus 37 °C with palmitoyl-L-carnitine, $n = 5$ (paired experiments). The results were analyzed with one-way analysis of variance (ANOVA) followed by Tukey's multiple comparison test.

It is important to note that the exogenous cytochrome c test showed the intactness of the mitochondrial outer membrane (no stimulation of respiration in State 3 by cytochrome c was observed; its effect on respiration varied from 0.90 ± 0.02 to 1.04 ± 0.01; $n = 5$, paired experiments) and inaccessibility of PK to ADP localized in the intermembrane space of mitochondria. Thus, neither the increase in temperature (from 25 to 37 °C) nor fatty acid oxidation, which both largely increased the affinity of mitochondrial oxidative phosphorylation for exogenous and endogenous ADP (i.e., decrease in the apparent K_m^{ADP} and K_m^{ATP}), affected the inhibitory effects of exogenous ADP-trapping system, and possibly, the concentration of ADP in the medium. In case palmitoyl-L-carnitine could increase the mitochondrial outer membrane permeability to ADP or ATP, the inhibitory effect of PK + PEP would have been different during palmitoyl-L-carnitine oxidation compared to the oxidation of pyruvate + malate. Our data show that the effect was similar during the oxidation of either substrate. Thus, the data presented above mean that the oxidation of palmitoyl-L-carnitine does not increase the mitochondrial outer membrane permeability to ADP or ATP.

3.4. Influence of Creatine Kinase on Regulation of Mitochondrial Respiration Supported by Fatty Acids

In the next series of experiments, we investigated the effect of fatty acid oxidation on the functional coupling between mitochondrial creatine kinase (mi-CK) and the ADP/ATP carrier.

The addition of 20 mM creatine in the presence of 2 mM ATP and exogenous PK + PEP system give notable and similar (1.35–1.56-fold) increase in the respiration rate in all conditions investigated (with both substrates, glutamate and palmitoyl-L-carnitine, at two different temperatures 25 and 37 °C, Figure 9).

Furthermore, the exogenous creatine, in the medium devoid of PK and PEP, stimulated the respiration of cardiac fibers oxidizing pyruvate + malate or palmitoyl-L-carnitine in presence of low 60 µM ADP concentration, accordingly by 1.37 ± 0.05 times and 1.42 ± 0.04 times (data of six unpaired experiments, 20 °C) with a similar efficacy as in the medium containing PK + PEP (Figure 9). It should be noted that in these experiments, exogenous cytochrome c had no significant stimulating effect on the mitochondrial respiration in State 3 with both substrates, indicating the intactness of the mitochondrial outer membrane.

In other series of experiments, fibers respiration supported by palmitoyl-L-carnitine was stimulated by exogenous ATP. In these conditions, endogenous ADP is produced from exogenous ATP by ATPases in myofibrils and the sarcoplasmic reticulum, and it is delivered directly to the mitochondria [13]. This approach should be regarded as more physiological. In this case the stimulating effect of creatine on mitochondrial respiration appeared to be very close to that observed in the above described experiments with the exogenous ADP; i.e., 1.38 ± 0.06 and 1.47 ± 0.05 times, respectively, with 23 and 37 µM of ATP (data of five unpaired experiments, 20 °C).

The maximal effect of creatine on mitochondrial respiration with octanoyl-DL-carnitine, similarly to palmitoyl-L-carnitine, was observed at 60 µM concentration of exogenous ADP (n = 3–5; Figure 10). Similar results (ADP concentration) were obtained also in the case of pyruvate + malate oxidation. When octanoyl-DL-carnitine was used as a respiratory substrate, the estimated apparent K_m^{ADP} values were significantly different in the presence and absence of creatine, accordingly 98 ± 11 µM ADP and 235 ± 16 µM ADP (Figure 10).

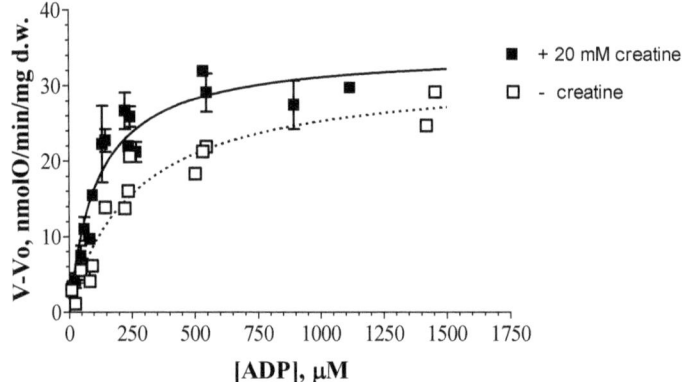

Figure 10. The dependence of the respiration rates of rat cardiac fibers on the external ADP concentration: the effect of creatine. The substrate: octanoyl-DL-carnitine 0.36 mM + malate 0.24 mM. The data of five separate paired experiments are presented. V_{max} values (in nmol O/min/mg dry weight) were found to be similar: 29.9 ± 1.8 (the medium without creatine) and 31.1 ± 1.6 (the medium with 20 mM creatine).

Thus, the creatine-induced decrease in the apparent K_m^{ADP} reflects the maintenance of functional coupling in the intermembrane space between ADP/ATP carrier and mi-CK in the mitochondria respiring on fatty acids.

3.5. Effects of Oncotic Pressure on Mitochondrial Fatty Acid Oxidation

In our further study, 5% of dextran T-70 was added to the respiration medium to mimic the oncotic pressure of the cellular cytoplasm and to test its effect on the respiration of saponin-permeabilized rat cardiac fibers oxidizing pyruvate + malate or palmitoyl-L-carnitine. 5% dextran T-70 similarly (by 25%) decreased the maximal respiration rate (with ADP) of mitochondria in situ, oxidizing both substrates palmitoyl-L-carnitine and pyruvate + malate (Figure 11). Noteworthy, dextran did not affect the high apparent K_m^{ADP} of mitochondria in cardiac fibers oxidizing pyruvate + malate, but significantly (by 50–60%) increased the low apparent K_m^{ADP} of mitochondria oxidizing palmitoyl-L-carnitine. The apparent K_m^{ADP} values during the oxidation of palmitoyl-L-carnitine in the medium containing 5% dextran (110.6 ± 20.7 µM) were much lower than the high apparent K_m^{ADP} values (255.7 ± 42 µM) characteristic for the oxidation of pyruvate + malate.

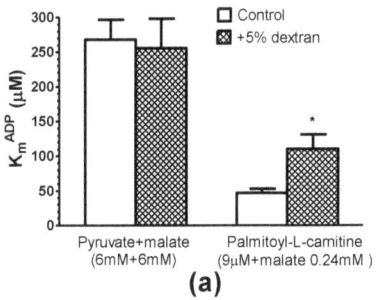 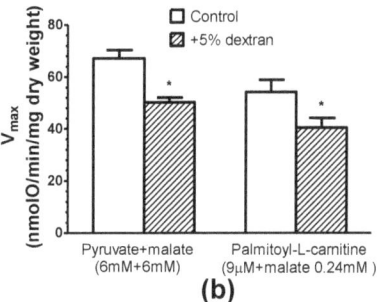

Figure 11. Influence of 5% dextran T70 on the apparent K_m^{ADP} (**a**) and V_{max} (**b**) of saponin-permeabilized rat cardiac fibers using different respiratory substrates. $n = 5$ (paired), 37 °C, * $p < 0.05$ versus control. The results were analyzed with one-way analysis of variance (ANOVA) followed by a Dunnett post hoc test.

3.6. Fatty Acid-Oxidation and Oncotic Pressure-induced Changes of Mitochondrial Morphology

Electron microscopy was used to evaluate morphological changes in mitochondria in situ caused by fatty acids oxidation in presence and absence of 5% dextran T-70 (Figure 12).

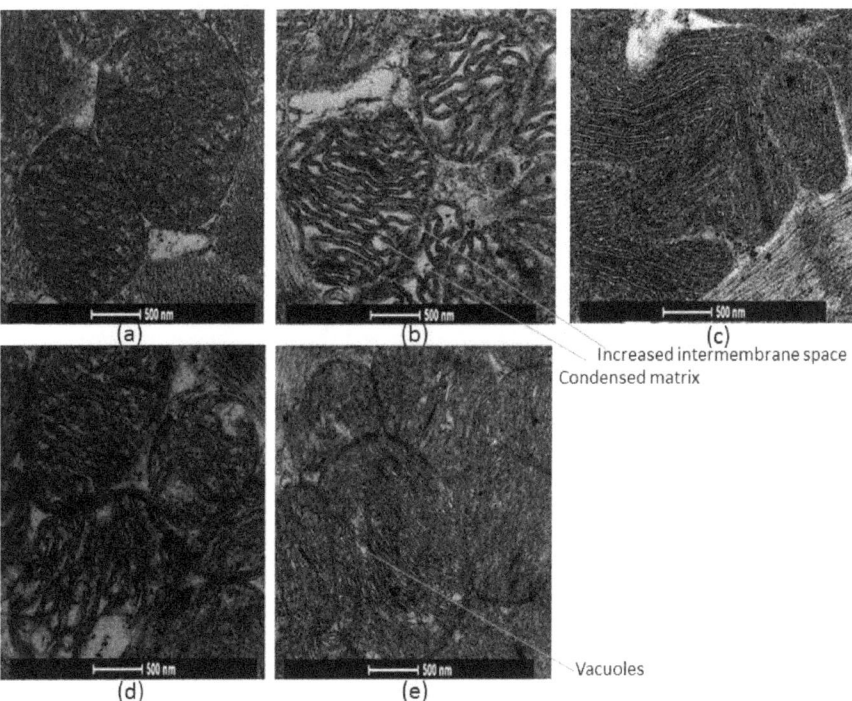

Figure 12. Morphology of mitochondria in skinned rat cardiac fibers. 5 min incubations of saponin-skinned cardiac fibers were performed in physiological salt solution at 37 °C in the presence of: (**a**) pyruvate + malate (6 mM + 6 mM); (**b**) palmitoyl-L-carnitine (9 μM); (**c**) palmitoyl-L-carnitine (9 μM) + 5% dextran T-70; (**d**) pyruvate + malate (6 mM + 6 mM) and ADP/ATP carrier inhibitor carboxyatractyloside (1.3 μM); (**e**) pyruvate + malate (6 mM + 6 mM) and ADP/ATP carrier inhibitor bongkrekic acid (17.6 μM).

The results revealed that mitochondrial morphology in saponin-permeabilized cardiac fibers significantly alters during 5 min oxidation of palmitoyl-L-carnitine in the absence of dextran (Figure 12b); compared with pyruvate and malate oxidation (Figure 12a): increased mitochondrial intermembrane space and condensed mitochondrial matrix were observed.

In fibers treated with dextran (in the presence of palmitoyl-L-carnitine), the whole population of mitochondria was dark (Figure 12c) indicating that they all have intact outer membranes. This finding is in accordance with the functional evaluation of intactness of mitochondrial outer membrane by cytochrome c test. Dextran prevented the palmitoyl-L-carnitine-induced morphological changes of mitochondria, where condensed mitochondria were observed; i.e., the appearance of mitochondria became similar to that in fibers incubated with pyruvate and malate, or similar as with in vivo conditions.

It is noteworthy that the incubation of fibers with carboxyatractyloside (1.3 µM; at this concentration the state 3 respiration with pyruvate and malate was completely inhibited)-induced ultrastructural changes of mitochondria similar to those induced by palmitoyl-L-carnitine, corresponding to the orthodox state of mitochondria; that is, enlarged cristae volume, contracted matrix space (Figure 12d). Bongkrekic acid (17.6 µM) induced completely different changes of mitochondrial ultrastructure; mitochondria were dark, cristae compressed, matrix space enlarged, little vacuoles were noticed, corresponding to the condensed state of mitochondria (Figure 12e). Thus, our results suggest that fatty acid oxidation may cause the morphological changes of mitochondrial ultrastructure, with an orthodox conformation when the ADP/ATP carrier is in the cytosol-oriented state.

4. Discussion

Palmitoyl-L-carnitine and other fatty acids of different chain length and degree of saturation differently affect the various enzymes, carriers and functions of mitochondria [1,2,32]. Therefore, we investigated the role of decanoate, octanoyl-L-carnitine, palmitoyl-L-carnitine and oleoyl-CoA (plus carnitine) in the regulation of mitochondrial respiration. In contrast to oleoyl-CoA, short- and medium-chain fatty acids (up to twelve carbon atoms) can cross mitochondrial membranes bypassing the carnitine dependent transport system [33]. Decanoate is activated to acyl-CoA inside mitochondria before being directed to oxidation. This reaction is catalyzed by the medium-chain acyl-CoA synthetase and requires both CoA and ATP. Meanwhile, oleoyl-CoA does not need activation.

Despite of differences in transport pathways, some reactions preceding β-oxidation and the enzyme systems responsible for β-oxidation, decanoic acid and oleoyl-CoA, similarly decreased the apparent K_m^{ADP} (Figure 2). Based on these findings and the related effects obtained previously with saturated fatty acids [9], it could be concluded that this property is general for all fatty acids. Furthermore, the decrease in the apparent K_m^{ADP} was similar during palmitoyl-L-carnitine oxidation at concentrations resulting in the maximal State 3 respiration rate (9 µM) and the suboptimal one (at 2.2 µM and even at 0.5 µM; Figure 3). In addition, when pyruvate and malate were added immediately after the completion of the oxidation of a limited quantity of palmitoyl-L-carnitine (Figure 6), the apparent K_m^{ADP} of the mitochondria in cardiac fibers remained at a high level, showing that the effect of fatty acids on the apparent K_m^{ADP} of mitochondria in permeabilized rat cardiac fibers was reversible.

Levitsky and Skulachev [34] demonstrated that palmitoyl-L-carnitine, when transported into isolated rat liver mitochondria, induced a swelling of mitochondrial matrix. Neely and Feuvray [35] observed morphological changes of isolated heart mitochondria after incubation with palmitoyl-L-carnitine, and Piper et al. [36], with oleoyl-L-carnitine, and in addition, the surfactant properties of palmitoyl-L-carnitine were revealed (for review, see [37]). We examined in this study the possible influence of palmitoyl-L-carnitine on the swelling of respiring, isolated rat heart mitochondria and the intactness of their outer membrane. Our investigations showed clearly that the decrease of the apparent K_m^{ADP} due to fatty acids oxidation described above cannot be attributed, neither to the increase in the volume of mitochondria (no mitochondrial swelling at 9 µM of palmitoyl-L-carnitine was observed; Figure 7), nor to the injury of mitochondrial outer membrane (no injury of mitochondrial outer membrane was demonstrated neither at 9 µM nor at much higher 80 µM of palmitoyl-L-carnitine, where large swelling was obvious; no injury of the mitochondrial outer membrane was also confirmed electron microscopically using dextran T-70; see Figure 12c and the discussion below).

Under some conditions (starvation, fasting) fatty acids play a major role in the heart energy metabolism. In the other cases, mostly both glucose and fatty acids are used as energy fuel, and as proposed [38], both are required for the optimal function of the failing heart; simultaneous oxidation of these two substrates is the best for heart function [39]. In this regard, our study shows the important effects of fatty acids on the regulation of the kinetics of oxidative phosphorylation (expressed as the apparent K_m^{ADP} value) when they were used alone or in the combination with pyruvate and malate.

We compared the kinetics of the regulation of mitochondrial respiration stimulated both by the exogenous ADP and exogenous ATP. In the latter case, the endogenous ADP is produced by ATPases in the myofibrils and in the sarcoplasmic reticulum, and is delivered directly to the mitochondria [8]. In accordance with the low apparent K_m^{ADP}, also the low apparent K_m^{ATP} values for saponin-permeabilized fibers respiring on palmitoyl-L-carnitine were demonstrated (for the first time with this substrate). In addition, our data are in accordance with the data obtained by Seppet et al. [8], where they demonstrated very similar high (300 µM) apparent K_m values for both exogenous ADP and exogenous ATP for cardiac fibers respiring on non-fatty substrates. Thus, the apparent K_m of oxidative phosphorylation for ADP in saponin-permeabilized rat cardiac fibers did not depend on the external or internal source of ADP.

When endogenous ADP is produced by ATPases in the myofibrils and in the sarcoplasmic reticulum, it is directly channeled to mitochondria without significant release into the medium if the mitochondrial oxidative phosphorylation is active [8]. This evidence was obtained by using an exogenous ADP-trapping system consisting of PK + PEP, which effectively competes with mitochondria for the extramitochondrial ADP, and therefore, decreases the respiration rate in the State 3. In our experiments, the PK effect is exceptionally from the outside of the mitochondria, since the exogenous cytochrome c test (no stimulation of respiration in State 3 by cytochrome c) shows the intactness of the mitochondrial outer membrane and the inaccessibility of PK to ADP localized in the intermembrane space of the mitochondria. Thus, neither the increase in temperature (from 25 to 37 °C), nor fatty acid oxidation, which both largely increase the affinity of mitochondrial oxidative phosphorylation for exogenous and endogenous ADP (decrease in the apparent K_m^{ADP} and apparent K_m^{ATP}), affect the inhibitory effects of the exogenous ADP-trapping system (Figure 9), and thus did not enhance the permeability of the mitochondrial outer membrane for ADP (Figure 9). The inhibitory effects of PK + PEP on the respiration of saponin-permeabilized rat cardiac fibers oxidizing glutamate+malate (25 °C) obtained by us are in good agreement with the data of other investigators [8,10].

The stimulating effects of creatine on fibers respiration with palmitoyl-L-carnitine assessed at low concentration (60 µM) of ADP reflects maintenance of functional coupling in the intermembrane space between the ADP/ATP carrier and mi-CK. Our data (Figure 10) show that the functional coupling between the ADP/ATP carrier and mi-CK is preserved in mitochondria despite the significant decrease in the apparent K_m^{ADP} induced by fatty acid oxidation. Noteworthy, the latter phenomenon is observed not only at 37 °C [9], but also at lower, i.e., 20 °C temperature. The finding that creatine significantly decreases the apparent K_m^{ADP} in the mitochondria oxidizing octanoyl-DL-carnitine (Figure 5) is in a good agreement with the data of other investigators [40,41], when pyruvate+malate, i.e., non-fatty respiratory substrate, was used.

There are two mechanisms suggested to explain the effective interaction between mi-CK and the ADP/ATP carrier: the dynamic compartmentation of ATP and ADP [42], and the direct transfer of ATP and ADP between the proteins [43,44]. According to the first mechanism, the functional coupling between mi-CK and the ADP/ATP carrier can be explained by differences between the concentrations of ATP and ADP in the intermembrane space and those in the surrounding solution due to some limitations of their diffusion across the outer mitochondrial membrane [42]. Beside dynamic compartmentation, facilitated diffusion was also suggested as the potential mechanism of the action of the phosphocreatine shuttle [45]. According to the second mechanism of coupling, ATP and ADP are directly transferred between mi-CK and the ADP/ATP carrier without leaving the complex of proteins [44]. Kuznetsov et al. [41] investigated the apparent Km for ADP in cardiac, slow-twitch and fast-twitch skeletal muscle fibers, and they provide a strong argument against the possibility that the diffusion problems may be related to the increased apparent K_m for ADP in cardiac and slow-twitch skeletal muscle fibers, as in fast-twitch skeletal muscle fibers, it remains low and comparable to the apparent K_m for ADP in isolated mitochondria [41]. Also, they found that in the ghost fibers where the myosin and 10–20% of cellular proteins were removed from the cells by KC1 treatment, the apparent K_m for ADP remained unchanged [41]. Under their conditions the sarcolemma was almost completely removed, and could not act as a diffusion barrier even for the big protein molecules [41]. Their data together with our results that creatine did not increase V_{max} in skinned cardiac fibers oxidizing octanoyl-DL-carnitine (Figure 10), and that the addition of dextran did not affect the apparent K_m for ADP in the skinned cardiac fibers oxidizing pyruvate and malate (Figure 11a), suggest that the changes in the apparent K_m for ADP are unlikely related to the diffusion problems.

In vivo mitochondria are embedded in the cytoplasm in which the protein content may be as high as 20–30% (m/v) [46]. Macromolecules, like bovine serum albumin, dextran, ficol, polyvinylpyrrolidone, added to the medium, can restore the morphological changes in the outer mitochondrial compartment that occur during the isolation of mitochondria [47–49].

It has been also shown that, in isolated rat heart mitochondria, 10% of bovine serum albumin and 5–25% dextran strongly increase the apparent K_m^{ADP} of oxidative phosphorylation [15,50] and of mitochondrial creatine kinase [50]. Dextrans or other macromolecules decrease the conductivity of porin pores in artificial membranes [48,51], the volume of the intermembrane space in isolated mitochondria, and increase the number of contact sites between both mitochondrial membranes [52]. Morphological changes of isolated mitochondria are accompanied by a reduced permeability of the mitochondrial outer membrane for adenine nucleotides [50]. In this study, respirometric investigation of saponin-permeabilized rat cardiac fibers demonstrated that an addition of 5% dextran into the incubation medium (to mimic the oncotic pressure of the cellular cytoplasm) markedly increased the low apparent K_m^{ADP} value of mitochondria respiring on palmitoyl-L-carnitine, but did not affect the high apparent K_m^{ADP} of mitochondria respiring on pyruvate and malate (Figure 11). Interestingly, the apparent K_m^{ADP} values during the oxidation of palmitoyl-L-carnitine in the medium containing 5% dextran (110.6 ± 20.7 µM ADP), despite some increase (compared with medium devoid of dextran), remained far below high values characteristic for the oxidation of pyruvate + malate (apparent K_m^{ADP}: 255.7 ± 42 µM) (Figure 11).

Electron microscopy was used to evaluate the effects of fatty acid oxidation and dextran T-70 on the morphology of rat heart mitochondria in situ (Figure 12). Palmitoyl-L-carnitine oxidation induced marked alterations in the mitochondrial ultrastructure, which is different from that observed with pyruvate and malate, and similar to the changes induced by the incubation of fibers with the ADP/ATP carrier inhibitor carboxyatractyloside. When mitochondria were incubated with compounds, fixing the ADP/ATP carrier in M (i.e., matrix-oriented) conformation, the cristae were compressed, the matrix space enlarged, and the separation of the inner membrane space forming vacuoles was noticed [53]. We obtained similar results after the incubation of mitochondria with bongkrekic acid. In the contrary, when mitochondria were incubated with compounds, fixing the ADP/ATP carrier in C (i.e., cytosol-oriented) conformation, e.g., with carboxyatractyloside, such that the cristae volume was enlarged at the expense of matrix space, the electron densities increased [53]. Furthermore, these two distinct mitochondrial conformations corresponded to condensed and orthodox mitochondrial conformation, accordingly [25,26]. Ultrastructural changes of mitochondria in cardiac fibers respiring on palmitoyl-L-carnitine were completely prevented by dextran addition into the incubation medium. Furthermore, most mitochondria in the fibers incubated with palmitoyl-L-carnitine in the presence of dextran appeared dark, indicating that their outer membranes were intact (Figure 12c), in accordance with the results of the cytochrome c test, presented in the Results section. Partial "normalization", i.e., the increase by dextran of the apparent K_m^{ADP} and complete "normalization" of the ultrastructure of mitochondria in saponin-permeabilized cardiac fibers respiring on palmitoyl-L-carnitine could be due to fatty acid oxidation-induced alterations of the mitochondrial ultrastructure.

The high apparent K_m for exogenous ADP is determined by low mitochondrial outer membrane permeability for ADP and the concerted action of tight complexes (called as intracellular energetic units) of mitochondria and other cellular ADP-producing systems (ATPases) in myofibrils and sarcoplasmic reticulum [8,10]. A highly organized intracellular structure and the arrangement of mitochondria are also crucial for the increase in the affinity of mitochondrial oxidative phosphorylation for ADP and the decrease in the apparent K_m^{ADP} value [16,18,22].

The calculations by Lizana et al. [54] using a simplistic model suggested that mitochondria (and small biological compartments in general) may regulate the dynamics of interior reaction pathways (e.g., the Krebs cycle) by volume changes. It was hypothesized (for review, see [55]) that the cristae shape can be modulated by different pathways/signaling molecules (ROS, the NADH/NAD ratio, the ATP/ADP ratio, etc.). Even low concentration of long-chain fatty acid palmitoyl-L-carnitine oxidation in skeletal muscle and heart mitochondria has been associated with significantly higher ROS production and increased mitochondrial proton leak (2 times lower respiratory control ratio, i.e., coupling), compared with the oxidation of NADH-linked substrates (pyruvate + malate or glutamate + malate) [56–58].

The greater ROS formation, similar at higher and lower mitochondrial membrane potential, was maintained despite of the activation of the uncoupling mechanisms of the ADP/ATP carrier during palmitoyl-L-carnitine (18 µM) oxidation [56]. Furthermore, functional (and possibly structural) interaction of ADP/ATP carrier and VDAC and its modulation/interruption by the ADP/ATP carrier inhibitor atractyloside-induced change of ADP/ATP carrier conformation has been also demonstrated [59]. Structural changes of mitochondria induced by carboxyatractyloside, similar to those induced by palmitoyl-L-carnitine, were observed by us in this study. The functional interaction of ADP/ATP carrier and VDAC facilitated the channeling of nucleotides and other metabolites between cytosol and mitochondrial matrix [59].

The low apparent K_m^{ADP} in mitochondria from cancerous cells [22,23] and fetal or neonatal mitochondria [24] could be related to mitochondrial ultrastructural changes. Adult mitochondria are usually in condensed conformation, with enlarged mitochondrial matrix volume and the decreased intermembrane space, compared to neonatal mitochondria which are mostly in orthodox conformation [25,26]. Our results showed that palmitoyl-L-carnitine oxidation induced ultrastructural changes of mitochondria, with a marked increase in mitochondrial intermembrane space and decrease of mitochondrial matrix (Figure 12b), and similar changes were obtained in the presence of the ADP/ATP carrier inhibitor carboxyatractyloside (Figure 12d).

Recent studies have revealed that fatty acids could be the cofactors [60] of the newly discovered action mode of the ADP/ATP carrier when protons are transported to mitochondrial matrix [61]. Cytosolic fatty acids could interfere with ADP/ATP transport [60] by activating the proton current to mitochondrial matrix [61]. They are able to bind to the ADP/ATP carrier from the cytosolic side in the C- or M-state, but could not induce C–M conformational change or be transported by the ADP/ATP carrier [61]. It was suggested that the ADP/ATP carrier could have two transport modes: C–M conformational change-related electrogenic ADP/ATP exchange and cytosolic fatty acid-activated conformation-independent proton channel [61]. We have also observed that palmitate, palmitoyl-CoA and palmitoyl-L-carnitine could not induce the decrease of apparent K_m^{ADP} when their oxidation was prevented by the absence of necessary cofactors or blocked with rotenone [9]. The lower apparent K_m^{ADP} was related to the oxidation, but not to the transport of fatty acids into mitochondria [9]. In the study of Divakaruni et al. [19], fatty acids have been demonstrated to change the conformation of the uncoupling protein, that is structurally, and to some extent, functionally, similar with the ADP/ATP carrier [20,21]. ADP/ATP exchange is driven by the mitochondrial membrane potential, which has been shown to affect the distribution of the binding sites of the ADP/ATP carrier between inside and outside, as well as the distribution of ADP/ATP carrier molecules between the M- and the

C-state, respectively [62]. Thus, Krämer and Klingenberg argued that the membrane potential could indirectly influence the C- and M-conformational transition of the ADP/ATP carrier [62]. The tumor and fetal/neonatal mitochondria are not only characterized by the low apparent K_m ADP, but also have higher mitochondrial membrane potential, i.e., are hyperpolarized [63,64]. According to the data of our colleagues, the mitochondrial membrane potential of isolated rat heart mitochondria respiring on pyruvate+malate or palmitoyl-L-carnitine as substrates was accordingly 146 ± 2 mV and 124 ± 1 mV (n = 5, assessed with TPP$^+$ electrode; R. Baniene, unpublished data, 2020); i.e., the membrane potential did not increase, rather it slightly decreased during palmitoyl-L-carnitine oxidation. These values are in line with the data from the study of Seifert et al. where lower energization and lower membrane potential of the skeletal muscle mitochondria were reported in the case of palmitoyl-L-carnitine oxidation compared to pyruvate and malate oxidation [56]; however, it could be related to the higher uncoupling protein content in skeletal muscle mitochondria [65]. It is technically complicated to quantify correctly the mitochondrial membrane potential in skinned cardiac fibers due to the distribution of the cationic potential probes within the cellular structures present in this object. However, it could not be excluded that the mitochondrial membrane potential in the skinned fibers might differ from the mitochondrial potential in the isolated mitochondria.

Thus, the hypothesis that the fatty acid oxidation-induced conformational change of the ADP/ATP carrier (M-state to C-state, condensed to orthodox mitochondria) affecting the oxidative phosphorylation affinity for ADP could be driven by the higher membrane potential generated during fatty acid oxidation might be an interesting question to address in the future research.

Overall, our results imply that the fatty acid oxidation could regulate cellular energy metabolism by increasing oxidative phosphorylation affinity for ADP due to fatty acid oxidation-induced ADP/ATP carrier switch from M- to C-state, and corresponding mitochondrial transition from condensed to orthodox conformation. Furthermore, this mechanism could be responsible for the altered mitochondrial metabolism [66] when fatty acid oxidation is increased during the development of chronic [67,68] and age-associated disorders, such as cardiovascular diseases, diabetes, neurodegenerative diseases and cancer [69,70], and the ADP/ATP carrier modulation could be a promising target in the search of novel therapies to restore the normal mitochondrial function.

Author Contributions: Conceptualization, A.T. and D.M.K.; methodology, A.T., S.T., J.L., N.P.; validation, A.T., J.L., S.T., D.M.K.; formal analysis, J.L., S.T., A.T.; investigation, A.T., S.T., N.P., J.L., L.K.; resources, A.T., D.M.K.; data curation, L.K., D.M.K.; writing—original draft preparation, A.T. and D.M.K.; writing—review and editing, J.L., S.T., A.T., D.M.K.; visualization, N.P., L.K. and D.M.K.; supervision, A.T.; project administration, A.T. All authors have read and agreed to the published version of the manuscript.

Funding: This research received no external funding.

Acknowledgments: The authors wish to thank Vilmante Borutaite and Rasa Baniene for valuable comments and suggestions.

Conflicts of Interest: The authors declare no conflict of interest.

References

1. Vignais, P.V. Molecular and physiological aspects of adenine nucleotide transport in mitochondria. *Biochim. Biophys. Acta* **1976**, *456*, 1–38. [CrossRef]
2. Wojtczak, L. Effect of long-chain fatty acids and acyl-CoA on mitochondrial permeability, transport, and energy-coupling processes. *J. Bioenerg. Biomembr.* **1976**, *8*, 293–311. [PubMed]
3. Qu, Q.; Zeng, F.; Liu, X.; Wang, Q.J.; Deng, F. Fatty acid oxidation and carnitine palmitoyltransferase I: Emerging therapeutic targets in cancer. *Cell Death Dis.* **2016**, *7*, e2226. [CrossRef] [PubMed]
4. Roussel, J.; Thireau, J.; Brenner, C.; Saint, N.; Scheuermann, V.; Lacampagne, A.; Le Guennec, J.Y.; Fauconnier, J. Palmitoyl-carnitine increases RyR2 oxidation and sarcoplasmic reticulum Ca2+ leak in cardiomyocytes: Role of adenine nucleotide translocase. *Biochim. Biophys. Acta* **2015**, *1852*, 749–758. [CrossRef] [PubMed]
5. Lopaschuk, G.D.; Ussher, J.R.; Folmes, C.D.; Jaswal, J.S.; Stanley, W.C. Myocardial fatty acid metabolism in health and disease. *Physiol. Rev.* **2010**, *90*, 207–258. [CrossRef] [PubMed]

6. Klingenberg, M. The ADP and ATP transport in mitochondria and its carrier. *Biochim. Biophys. Acta* **2008**, *1778*, 1978–2021. [CrossRef] [PubMed]
7. Saks, V.A.; Khuchua, Z.A.; Vasilyeva, E.V.; Belikova, O.; Kuznetsov, A.V. Metabolic compartmentation and substrate channelling in muscle cells. Role of coupled creatine kinases in in vivo regulation of cellular respiration—A synthesis. *Mol. Cell Biochem.* **1994**, *133–134*, 155–192. [CrossRef]
8. Seppet, E.K.; Kaambre, T.; Sikk, P.; Tiivel, T.; Vija, H.; Tonkonogi, M.; Sahlin, K.; Kay, L.; Appaix, F.; Braun, U.; et al. Functional complexes of mitochondria with Ca,MgATPases of myofibrils and sarcoplasmic reticulum in muscle cells. *Biochim. Biophys. Acta* **2001**, *1504*, 379–395. [CrossRef]
9. Toleikis, A.; Liobikas, J.; Trumbeckaite, S.; Majiene, D. Relevance of fatty acid oxidation in regulation of the outer mitochondrial membrane permeability for ADP. *FEBS Lett.* **2001**, *509*, 245–249. [CrossRef]
10. Saks, V.A.; Kaambre, T.; Sikk, P.; Eimre, M.; Orlova, E.; Paju, K.; Piirsoo, A.; Appaix, F.; Kay, L.; Regitz-Zagrosek, V.; et al. Intracellular energetic units in red muscle cells. *Biochem. J.* **2001**, *356*, 643–657. [CrossRef]
11. Saks, V.; Kuznetsov, A.V.; Gonzalez-Granillo, M.; Tepp, K.; Timohhina, N.; Karu-Varikmaa, M.; Kaambre, T.; Dos Santos, P.; Boucher, F.; Guzun, R. Intracellular Energetic Units regulate metabolism in cardiac cells. *J. Mol. Cell Cardiol.* **2012**, *52*, 419–436. [CrossRef] [PubMed]
12. Dzeja, P.P.; Hoyer, K.; Tian, R.; Zhang, S.; Nemutlu, E.; Spindler, M.; Ingwall, J.S. Rearrangement of energetic and substrate utilization networks compensate for chronic myocardial creatine kinase deficiency. *J. Physiol.* **2011**, *589*, 5193–5211. [CrossRef] [PubMed]
13. Kaasik, A.; Veksler, V.; Boehm, E.; Novotova, M.; Minajeva, A.; Ventura-Clapier, R. Energetic crosstalk between organelles: Architectural integration of energy production and utilization. *Circ. Res.* **2001**, *89*, 153–159. [CrossRef] [PubMed]
14. Toleikis, A.; Majiene, D.; Trumbeckaite, S.; Dagys, A.; Jasaitis, A. The effect of collagenase and temperature on mitochondrial respiratory parameters in saponin-skinned cardiac fibers. *Biosci. Rep.* **1996**, *16*, 513–519. [CrossRef] [PubMed]
15. Liobikas, J.; Kopustinskiene, D.M.; Toleikis, A. What controls the outer mitochondrial membrane permeability for ADP: Facts for and against the role of oncotic pressure. *Biochim. Biophys. Acta* **2001**, *1505*, 220–225. [CrossRef]
16. Appaix, F.; Kuznetsov, A.V.; Usson, Y.; Kay, L.; Andrienko, T.; Olivares, J.; Kaambre, T.; Sikk, P.; Margreiter, R.; Saks, V. Possible role of cytoskeleton in intracellular arrangement and regulation of mitochondria. *Exp. Physiol.* **2003**, *88*, 175–190. [CrossRef]
17. Guzun, R.; Timohhina, N.; Tepp, K.; Monge, C.; Kaambre, T.; Sikk, P.; Kuznetsov, A.V.; Pison, C.; Saks, V. Regulation of respiration controlled by mitochondrial creatine kinase in permeabilized cardiac cells in situ. Importance of system level properties. *Biochim. Biophys. Acta* **2009**, *1787*, 1089–1105. [CrossRef]
18. Boudina, S.; Laclau, M.N.; Tariosse, L.; Daret, D.; Gouverneur, G.; Bonoron-Adele, S.; Saks, V.A.; Dos Santos, P. Alteration of mitochondrial function in a model of chronic ischemia in vivo in rat heart. *Am. J. Physiol. Heart Circ. Physiol.* **2002**, *282*, H821–H831. [CrossRef]
19. Divakaruni, A.S.; Humphrey, D.M.; Brand, M.D. Fatty acids change the conformation of uncoupling protein 1 (UCP1). *J. Biol. Chem.* **2012**, *287*, 36845–36853. [CrossRef]
20. Aquila, H.; Link, T.A.; Klingenberg, M. The uncoupling protein from brown fat mitochondria is related to the mitochondrial ADP/ATP carrier. Analysis of sequence homologies and of folding of the protein in the membrane. *EMBO J.* **1985**, *4*, 2369–2376. [CrossRef]
21. Klingenberg, M. Mechanism and evolution of the uncoupling protein of brown adipose tissue. *Trends Biochem. Sci.* **1990**, *15*, 108–112. [CrossRef]
22. Anmann, T.; Guzun, R.; Beraud, N.; Pelloux, S.; Kuznetsov, A.V.; Kogerman, L.; Kaambre, T.; Sikk, P.; Paju, K.; Peet, N.; et al. Different kinetics of the regulation of respiration in permeabilized cardiomyocytes and in HL-1 cardiac cells. Importance of cell structure/organization for respiration regulation. *Biochim. Biophys. Acta* **2006**, *1757*, 1597–1606. [CrossRef] [PubMed]
23. Eimre, M.; Paju, K.; Pelloux, S.; Beraud, N.; Roosimaa, M.; Kadaja, L.; Gruno, M.; Peet, N.; Orlova, E.; Remmelkoor, R.; et al. Distinct organization of energy metabolism in HL-1 cardiac cell line and cardiomyocytes. *Biochim. Biophys. Acta* **2008**, *1777*, 514–524. [CrossRef] [PubMed]

24. Anmann, T.; Varikmaa, M.; Timohhina, N.; Tepp, K.; Shevchuk, I.; Chekulayev, V.; Saks, V.; Kaambre, T. Formation of highly organized intracellular structure and energy metabolism in cardiac muscle cells during postnatal development of rat heart. *Biochim. Biophys. Acta* **2014**, *1837*, 1350–1361. [CrossRef] [PubMed]
25. Valcarce, C.; Navarrete, R.M.; Encabo, P.; Loeches, E.; Satrustegui, J.; Cuezva, J.M. Postnatal development of rat liver mitochondrial functions. The roles of protein synthesis and of adenine nucleotides. *J. Biol. Chem.* **1988**, *263*, 7767–7775. [PubMed]
26. Valcarce, C.; Cuezva, J.M. Interaction of adenine nucleotides with the adenine nucleotide translocase regulates the developmental changes in proton conductance of the inner mitochondrial membrane. *FEBS Lett.* **1991**, *294*, 225–228. [CrossRef]
27. Benard, G.; Faustin, B.; Passerieux, E.; Galinier, A.; Rocher, C.; Bellance, N.; Delage, J.P.; Casteilla, L.; Letellier, T.; Rossignol, R. Physiological diversity of mitochondrial oxidative phosphorylation. *Am. J. Physiol. Cell Physiol.* **2006**, *291*, C1172–C1182. [CrossRef]
28. Fernandez-Vizarra, E.; Enriquez, J.A.; Perez-Martos, A.; Montoya, J.; Fernandez-Silva, P. Tissue-specific differences in mitochondrial activity and biogenesis. *Mitochondrion* **2011**, *11*, 207–213. [CrossRef]
29. Kuznetsov, A.V.; Veksler, V.; Gellerich, F.N.; Saks, V.; Margreiter, R.; Kunz, W.S. Analysis of mitochondrial function in situ in permeabilized muscle fibers, tissues and cells. *Nat. Protoc.* **2008**, *3*, 965–976. [CrossRef]
30. Holtzman, J.L. Calibration of the oxygen polarograph by the depletion of oxygen with hypoxanthine-xanthine oxidase-catalase. *Anal. Chem.* **1976**, *48*, 229–230. [CrossRef]
31. Gornall, A.G.; Bardawill, C.J.; David, M.M. Determination of serum proteins by means of the biuret reaction. *J. Biol. Chem.* **1949**, *177*, 751–766. [PubMed]
32. Sultan, A.; Sokolove, P.M. Free fatty acid effects on mitochondrial permeability: An overview. *Arch. Biochem. Biophys.* **2001**, *386*, 52–61. [CrossRef] [PubMed]
33. Kerner, J.; Hoppel, C. Fatty acid import into mitochondria. *Biochim. Biophys. Acta* **2000**, *1486*, 1–17. [CrossRef]
34. Levitsky, D.O.; Skulachev, V.P. Carnitine: The carrier transporting fatty acyls into mitochondria by means of an electrochemical gradient of H+. *Biochim. Biophys. Acta* **1972**, *275*, 33–50. [CrossRef]
35. Neely, J.R.; Feuvray, D. Metabolic products and myocardial ischemia. *Am. J. Pathol.* **1981**, *102*, 282–291. [PubMed]
36. Piper, M.H.; Sezer, O.; Schwartz, P.; Hutter, J.F.; Schweickhardt, C.; Spieckermann, P.G. Acyl-carnitine effects on isolated cardiac mitochondria and erythrocytes. *Basic Res. Cardiol.* **1984**, *79*, 186–198. [CrossRef]
37. Goni, F.M.; Requero, M.A.; Alonso, A. Palmitoylcarnitine, a surface-active metabolite. *FEBS Lett.* **1996**, *390*, 1–5. [CrossRef]
38. Tuunanen, H.; Engblom, E.; Naum, A.; Nagren, K.; Hesse, B.; Airaksinen, K.E.; Nuutila, P.; Iozzo, P.; Ukkonen, H.; Opie, L.H.; et al. Free fatty acid depletion acutely decreases cardiac work and efficiency in cardiomyopathic heart failure. *Circulation* **2006**, *114*, 2130–2137. [CrossRef]
39. Taegtmeyer, H. Metabolism—the lost child of cardiology. *J. Am. Coll. Cardiol.* **2000**, *36*, 1386–1388. [CrossRef]
40. Laclau, M.N.; Boudina, S.; Thambo, J.B.; Tariosse, L.; Gouverneur, G.; Bonoron-Adele, S.; Saks, V.A.; Garlid, K.D.; Dos Santos, P. Cardioprotection by ischemic preconditioning preserves mitochondrial function and functional coupling between adenine nucleotide translocase and creatine kinase. *J. Mol. Cell Cardiol.* **2001**, *33*, 947–956. [CrossRef]
41. Kuznetsov, A.V.; Tiivel, T.; Sikk, P.; Kaambre, T.; Kay, L.; Daneshrad, Z.; Rossi, A.; Kadaja, L.; Peet, N.; Seppet, E.; et al. Striking differences between the kinetics of regulation of respiration by ADP in slow-twitch and fast-twitch muscles in vivo. *Eur. J. Biochem.* **1996**, *241*, 909–915. [CrossRef] [PubMed]
42. Gellerich, F.N.; Schlame, M.; Bohnensack, R.; Kunz, W. Dynamic compartmentation of adenine nucleotides in the mitochondrial intermembrane space of rat-heart mitochondria. *Biochim. Biophys. Acta* **1987**, *890*, 117–126. [CrossRef]
43. Saks, V.A.; Chernousova, G.B.; Gukovsky, D.E.; Smirnov, V.N.; Chazov, E.I. Studies of energy transport in heart cells. Mitochondrial isoenzyme of creatine phosphokinase: Kinetic properties and regulatory action of Mg^{2+} ions. *Eur. J. Biochem.* **1975**, *57*, 273–290. [CrossRef] [PubMed]
44. Jacobus, W.E.; Saks, V.A. Creatine kinase of heart mitochondria: Changes in its kinetic properties induced by coupling to oxidative phosphorylation. *Arch. Biochem. Biophys.* **1982**, *219*, 167–178. [CrossRef]
45. Meyer, R.A.; Sweeney, H.L.; Kushmerick, M.J. A simple analysis of the "phosphocreatine shuttle". *Am. J. Physiol.* **1984**, *246*, C365–C377. [CrossRef]
46. Fulton, A.B. How crowded is the cytoplasm? *Cell* **1982**, *30*, 345–347. [CrossRef]

47. Bakeeva, L.E.; Chentsov, Y.S.; Jasaitis, A.A.; Skulachev, V.P. The effect of oncotic pressure on heart muscle mitochondria. *Biochim. Biophys. Acta* **1972**, *275*, 319–332. [CrossRef]
48. Wicker, U.; Bucheler, K.; Gellerich, F.N.; Wagner, M.; Kapischke, M.; Brdiczka, D. Effect of macromolecules on the structure of the mitochondrial inter-membrane space and the regulation of hexokinase. *Biochim. Biophys. Acta* **1993**, *1142*, 228–239. [CrossRef]
49. Wrogemann, K.; Nylen, E.G.; Adamson, I.; Pande, S.V. Functional studies on in situ-like mitochondria isolated in the presence of polyvinyl pyrrolidone. *Biochim. Biophys. Acta* **1985**, *806*, 1–8. [CrossRef]
50. Gellerich, F.N.; Laterveer, F.D.; Korzeniewski, B.; Zierz, S.; Nicolay, K. Dextran strongly increases the Michaelis constants of oxidative phosphorylation and of mitochondrial creatine kinase in heart mitochondria. *Eur. J. Biochem.* **1998**, *254*, 172–180. [CrossRef]
51. Gellerich, F.N.; Wagner, M.; Kapischke, M.; Wicker, U.; Brdiczka, D. Effect of macromolecules on the regulation of the mitochondrial outer membrane pore and the activity of adenylate kinase in the inter-membrane space. *Biochim. Biophys. Acta* **1993**, *1142*, 217–227. [CrossRef]
52. Gellerich, F.N.; Kapischke, M.; Kunz, W.; Neumann, W.; Kuznetsov, A.; Brdiczka, D.; Nicolay, K. The influence of the cytosolic oncotic pressure on the permeability of the mitochondrial outer membrane for ADP: Implications for the kinetic properties of mitochondrial creatine kinase and for ADP channelling into the intermembrane space. *Mol. Cell Biochem.* **1994**, *133–134*, 85–104. [CrossRef] [PubMed]
53. Nohl, H. Age-dependent changes in the structure-function correlation of ADP/ATP-translocating mitochondrial membranes. *Gerontology* **1982**, *28*, 354–359. [CrossRef] [PubMed]
54. Lizana, L.; Bauer, B.; Orwar, O. Controlling the rates of biochemical reactions and signaling networks by shape and volume changes. *Proc. Natl. Acad. Sci. USA* **2008**, *105*, 4099–4104. [CrossRef]
55. Cogliati, S.; Enriquez, J.A.; Scorrano, L. Mitochondrial Cristae: Where Beauty Meets Functionality. *Trends Biochem. Sci.* **2016**, *41*, 261–273. [CrossRef]
56. Seifert, E.L.; Estey, C.; Xuan, J.Y.; Harper, M.E. Electron transport chain-dependent and -independent mechanisms of mitochondrial H2O2 emission during long-chain fatty acid oxidation. *J. Biol. Chem.* **2010**, *285*, 5748–5758. [CrossRef]
57. St-Pierre, J.; Buckingham, J.A.; Roebuck, S.J.; Brand, M.D. Topology of superoxide production from different sites in the mitochondrial electron transport chain. *J. Biol. Chem.* **2002**, *277*, 44784–44790. [CrossRef]
58. Liesa, M.; Shirihai, O.S. Mitochondrial dynamics in the regulation of nutrient utilization and energy expenditure. *Cell Metab.* **2013**, *17*, 491–506. [CrossRef]
59. Allouche, M.; Pertuiset, C.; Robert, J.L.; Martel, C.; Veneziano, R.; Henry, C.; dein, O.S.; Saint, N.; Brenner, C.; Chopineau, J. ANT-VDAC1 interaction is direct and depends on ANT isoform conformation in vitro. *Biochem. Biophys. Res. Commun.* **2012**, *429*, 12–17. [CrossRef]
60. Bernardi, P. Mitochondrial H+ permeability through the ADP/ATP carrier. *Nat. Metab.* **2019**, *1*, 752–753. [CrossRef]
61. Bertholet, A.M.; Chouchani, E.T.; Kazak, L.; Angelin, A.; Fedorenko, A.; Long, J.Z.; Vidoni, S.; Garrity, R.; Cho, J.; Terada, N.; et al. H(+) transport is an integral function of the mitochondrial ADP/ATP carrier. *Nature* **2019**, *571*, 515–520. [CrossRef] [PubMed]
62. Kramer, R.; Klingenberg, M. Electrophoretic control of reconstituted adenine nucleotide translocation. *Biochemistry* **1982**, *21*, 1082–1089. [CrossRef] [PubMed]
63. Heerdt, B.G.; Houston, M.A.; Augenlicht, L.H. Growth properties of colonic tumor cells are a function of the intrinsic mitochondrial membrane potential. *Cancer Res.* **2006**, *66*, 1591–1596. [CrossRef] [PubMed]
64. Chung, S.; Dzeja, P.P.; Faustino, R.S.; Perez-Terzic, C.; Behfar, A.; Terzic, A. Mitochondrial oxidative metabolism is required for the cardiac differentiation of stem cells. *Nat. Clin. Pr. Cardiovasc. Med.* **2007**, *4*, S60–S67. [CrossRef] [PubMed]
65. Ricquier, D. Mitochondrial uncoupling proteins. *Curr. Opin. Drug Discov. Devel.* **1999**, *2*, 497–504. [PubMed]
66. Porporato, P.E.; Filigheddu, N.; Pedro, J.M.B.; Kroemer, G.; Galluzzi, L. Mitochondrial metabolism and cancer. *Cell Res.* **2018**, *28*, 265–280. [CrossRef] [PubMed]
67. Shammas, M.A.; Neri, P.; Koley, H.; Batchu, R.B.; Bertheau, R.C.; Munshi, V.; Prabhala, R.; Fulciniti, M.; Tai, Y.T.; Treon, S.P.; et al. Specific killing of multiple myeloma cells by (-)-epigallocatechin-3-gallate extracted from green tea: Biologic activity and therapeutic implications. *Blood* **2006**, *108*, 2804–2810. [CrossRef]
68. Braicu, C.; Ladomery, M.R.; Chedea, V.S.; Irimie, A.; Berindan-Neagoe, I. The relationship between the structure and biological actions of green tea catechins. *Food Chem.* **2013**, *141*, 3282–3289. [CrossRef]

69. Majumder, K.; Mine, Y.; Wu, J. The potential of food protein-derived anti-inflammatory peptides against various chronic inflammatory diseases. *J. Sci. Food Agric.* **2016**, *96*, 2303–2311. [CrossRef]
70. Zhang, Y.J.; Gan, R.Y.; Li, S.; Zhou, Y.; Li, A.N.; Xu, D.P.; Li, H.B. Antioxidant Phytochemicals for the Prevention and Treatment of Chronic Diseases. *Molecules* **2015**, *20*, 21138–21156. [CrossRef]

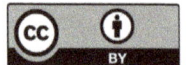

© 2020 by the authors. Licensee MDPI, Basel, Switzerland. This article is an open access article distributed under the terms and conditions of the Creative Commons Attribution (CC BY) license (http://creativecommons.org/licenses/by/4.0/).

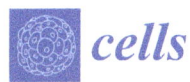

Article

The Role of Adenine Nucleotide Translocase in the Assembly of Respiratory Supercomplexes in Cardiac Cells

Rebecca M. Parodi-Rullán [1,†], Xavier Chapa-Dubocq [1], Roberto Guzmán-Hernández [1], Sehwan Jang [1], Carlos A. Torres-Ramos [1], Sylvette Ayala-Peña [2] and Sabzali Javadov [1,*]

1. Department of Physiology, School of Medicine, University of Puerto Rico, San Juan, PR 00936-5067, USA; rebecca.parodi-rullan@temple.edu (R.M.P.-R.); xavier.chapa@upr.edu (X.C.-D.); roberto.guzman7@upr.edu (R.G.-H.); sehwan.jang@upr.edu (S.J.); carlos.torres27@upr.edu (C.A.T.-R.)
2. Department of Pharmacology and Toxicology, School of Medicine, University of Puerto Rico, San Juan, PR 00936-5067, USA; sylvette.ayala@upr.edu
* Correspondence: sabzali.javadov@upr.edu; Tel.: +1-787-758-2525 (ext. 1-2909)
† Current address: Alzheimer's Center at Temple, Lewis Katz School of Medicine, Temple University, Philadelphia, PA 19140, USA.

Received: 25 June 2019; Accepted: 11 October 2019; Published: 13 October 2019

Abstract: Individual electron transport chain complexes have been shown to assemble into the supramolecular structures known as the respiratory chain supercomplexes (RCS). Several studies reported an associative link between RCS disintegration and human diseases, although the physiological role, structural integrity, and mechanisms of RCS formation remain unknown. Our previous studies suggested that the adenine nucleotide translocase (ANT), the most abundant protein of the inner mitochondrial membrane, can be involved in RCS assembly. In this study, we sought to elucidate whether *ANT* knockdown (KD) affects RCS formation in H9c2 cardiomyoblasts. Results showed that genetic silencing of ANT1, the main ANT isoform in cardiac cells, stimulated proliferation of H9c2 cardiomyoblasts with no effect on cell viability. *ANT1* KD reduced the $\Delta\Psi_m$ but increased total cellular ATP levels and stimulated the production of total, but not mitochondrial, reactive oxygen species. Importantly, downregulation of *ANT1* had no significant effects on the enzymatic activity of individual ETC complexes I–IV; however, RCS disintegration was stimulated in *ANT1* KD cells as evidenced by reduced levels of respirasome, the main RCS. The effects of *ANT1* KD to induce RCS disassembly was not associated with acetylation of the exchanger. In conclusion, our study demonstrates that ANT is involved in RCS assembly.

Keywords: H9c2 cardiomyoblasts; mitochondria; adenine nucleotide translocase; respiratory supercomplexes; ETC complexes

1. Introduction

The adenine nucleotide translocase (ANT), one of the most abundant proteins of the inner mitochondrial membrane, exchanges the matrix ATP for ADP in the intermembrane space and thus, links mitochondrial ATP production with cellular energetics. Several studies have demonstrated a crucial role of ANT in the pathogenesis of cardiac diseases. Downregulation of ANT1, the main ANT isoform in the heart and skeletal muscle [1,2], has been found in patients with hypertrophic cardiomyopathy, and lactic acidosis [3]. Mice lacking *ANT1* developed cardiac hypertrophy and lactic acidosis [2], and a substantial decline in cardiac function compared to wildtype (WT) animals [4]. Heart- and muscle-specific *ANT1* knockout (KO) mice exhibit deficiency in mitochondrial bioenergetics associated with mitochondrial myopathy and hypertrophic cardiomyopathy [5]. Additionally, *ANT1* KO mice display an increase in reactive oxygen species (ROS) production and inhibition of oxidative phosphorylation (OXPHOS) in cardiac mitochondria [6]. Moreover, cardiac ischemia-reperfusion (IR) reduced *ANT1* expression whereas cardiac-specific overexpression of *ANT1* attenuated IR injury and reduced infarct size in rats [7]. In rat neonatal cardiomyocytes, overexpression of ANT1 protected against hypoxia-induced cell death, loss of mitochondrial membrane potential ($\Delta\Psi_m$), and increased ROS production [7]. Therefore, understanding the role of ANT in the regulation of mitochondrial bioenergetics can provide a novel insight into mitochondrial-based cardiac therapies.

ANT has been shown to interact with various subunits of the electron transport chain (ETC) complexes in HEK293 cells [8] and in yeast [9]. Several studies, the earliest one in 2000, demonstrated that ETC individual complexes can be assembled in large supramolecular structures known as respiratory chain supercomplexes (RCS) [10]. The main RCS is the respirasome, which is composed of complexes I, III, and IV in various stoichiometries. It has been proposed that the respirasome facilitates electron transfer, reduces electron leakage and mitochondrial ROS (mtROS) production, maintains structural organization of ETC complexes, and provides an efficient ATP production [11].

The assembly mechanisms and the structural identity of RCS remain to be elucidated. The role of ANT in RCS formation was recently proposed after it was observed that ANT interacts with RCS and that this interaction is conserved from yeast to higher eukaryotes [8], potentially implicating a crucial role of ANT in mitochondrial bioenergetics. However, these studies were mostly done in yeast and HEK293 cells; the RCS and ANT interactome has not been reported in mammalian tissues, particularly, in the heart. We have shown that pharmacological inhibition of ANT by atractyloside provoked RCS disintegration in cardiac mitochondria in vitro [12]. These studies suggest that ANT may have a structural interaction with RCS and/or play a regulatory role in RCS. Furthermore, post-translational modifications on ANT may affect its regulatory and structural capability in RCS assembly. Indeed, acetylation has been demonstrated to regulate the activity of ETC complexes [13,14] and thus, might affect the RCS stability.

Here, we investigated the role of ANT1 in RCS assembly in H9c2 cardiomyoblasts. *ANT1* KD cells demonstrated increased total cellular ATP levels, with a reduction in $\Delta\Psi_m$ and no changes in mitochondrial ATP production. However, *ANT1* KD did not affect the enzymatic activity of individual ETC complexes nor mitochondrial oxygen consumption. Deficiency in *ANT1* expression induced disassembly of RCS, particularly the respirasome, suggesting a potential role of ANT in RCS formation. Also, we found that ANT1 is not hyperacetylated in *SIRT3* KO mice although RCS levels in these animals were lower than in WT counterparts.

2. Materials and Methods

2.1. Animals

Three-month-old male adult WT (129S1/SvImJ) and SIRT3$^{-/-}$ (Sirt3$^{tm1.1Fwa}$) mice (20–25 g) were purchased from Jackson Laboratory (Bar Harbor, ME, USA). All experiments were performed according to protocols approved by the UPR Medical Sciences Campus Animal Care and Use Committee and conformed to the National Research Council Guide for the Care and Use of Laboratory Animals published by the US National Institutes of Health (2011, eighth edition).

2.2. Cell Culture

H9c2 rat embryonic cardiomyoblast cells (American Type Culture Collection, Manassas, VA, USA) were cultured according to the manufacturer's recommendations. The cells were cultured in high-glucose Dulbecco's Modified Eagle's Medium (DMEM, Sigma-Aldrich, St. Louis, MO, USA)-modified solution containing 4 mM L-glutamine, 4.5 g/L glucose, 1 mM sodium pyruvate, and 1.5 g/L sodium bicarbonate (Sigma-Aldrich, St. Louis, MO, USA) supplemented with 10% fetal bovine serum and 1% antibiotic solution (HyClone, GE Healthcare Bio-sciences, Pittsburgh, PA, USA). The cells were maintained in a humidified incubator containing 95% air and 5% CO_2 at 37 °C.

2.3. siRNA Transfection

H9c2 cells were seeded for 40–60% confluency at 24 h. On the day of the experiment, cells were transfected using Lipofectamine RNAiMAX (Invitrogen, Thermo Fisher Scientific, Waltham, MA, USA) and FlexiTube small interfering RNA (siRNA, Qiagen, Germantown, MD, USA) according to the manufacturer's recommendations. Briefly, H9c2 cells were seeded with Opti-MEM™ Reduced Serum Medium, GlutaMAX™ (Thermo Scientific, Thermo Fisher Scientific, Waltham, MA, USA) supplemented with 5% fetal bovine serum and 1% antibiotic solution to reach a 40–60% confluency in 24 h. On the next day, Lipofectamine RNAiMAX (Invitrogen, Thermo Fisher Scientific, Waltham, MA, USA) and FlexiTube siRNA mixtures were added. The following siRNA sequences (sense strand) were used: negative control (NC): UUC UCC GAA CGU GUC ACG, and ANT1: GAC GCA AAG CUU UCU UCA ATT. All experiments were conducted 48 h post-transfection.

Cell viability was determined by the trypan blue exclusion method using the TC20 Automated Cell Counter (Bio-Rad, Hercules, CA, USA).

2.4. Mitochondrial Oxygen Consumption Rate and ATP Production

Oxygen consumption rate and ATP production in H9c2 cells were determined using the Seahorse XFe24 analyzer (Agilent, Santa Clara, CA, USA). An equal number of cells were seeded and transfected at 24 h. Mitochondrial oxygen consumption rate and ATP production were determined 48 h post-transfection following manufacturer's recommendations. Briefly, cell media was changed to Seahorse XF DMEM Medium, pH 7.4, and supplemented with (in mM): 10 glucose, 1 sodium pyruvate, and 2 L-glutamine. Mitochondrial functional parameters were determined after the addition of (in µM): 0.5 oligomycin, 4 carbonyl cyanide-4-(trifluoromethoxy)phenylhydrazone (FCCP), and 0.5 rotenone/antimycin A. Data were extracted using the Seahorse XFe24 report generator and normalized to total protein.

2.5. Isolation of Mitochondria

H9c2 cells were trypsinized and pelleted at 200× g for 7 min. The pellet was resuspended in ice-cold sucrose buffer containing (in mM): 300 sucrose, 10 Tris-HCl, and 2 EGTA; pH 7.4. Cells were centrifuged at 2,500× g for 5 min at 4 °C, the pellet was resuspended in sucrose buffer and incubated on ice for 5 min. To disrupt the plasma membrane and expose mitochondria, cells were plunged using a 27G needle, until all cells were successfully lysed. The cell lysate was then centrifuged at 400× g for 5 min and the supernatant was collected. The mitochondria were concentrated by centrifugation at 10,000× g for 5 min and the final pellet was dissolved in sucrose buffer.

To isolate liver mitochondria, the liver tissue removed from WT and *SIRT3* KO mice was cut and homogenized using a Polytron homogenizer in 2 mL of ice-cold sucrose buffer containing: 300 mM sucrose, 20 mM Tris-HCl, and 2 mM EGTA. Homogenate was then centrifuged at 2,000× g for 3 min, to remove cell debris. The supernatant was then centrifuged at 10,000× g for 15 min to precipitate mitochondria. The final pellet was washed once with sucrose buffer by centrifugation at 10,000× g for 10 min. The mitochondria-enriched pellet was resuspended in 200 µL of sucrose buffer.

2.6. Enzymatic Activity of ETC Complexes in Cultured Cells

Enzymatic activity of ETC complexes was determined as previously described [15], with minor modifications and normalized to mg of mitochondrial protein. All assays were performed at the SpectraMax Microplate Reader (Molecular Devices, San Jose, CA, USA) at 37 °C.

2.7. Total and Mitochondrial ROS Production in Cultured Cells

Total ROS and mtROS production were measured with 2′,7′-dichlorodihydrofluorescein diacetate (H_2DCFDA) and MitoSOX Red, respectively [15]. Briefly, cells were incubated for 30 min with 10 µM H_2DCFDA or 1 µM of MitoSOX and fluorescence intensity was monitored on the SpectraMax

Microplate Reader (Molecular Devices, San Jose, CA, USA) at the excitation/emission of 599 nm/522 nm (for H_2DCFDA) and 510 nm/580 nm (for MitoSOX).

2.8. Mitochondrial Membrane Potential and Total ATP

To measure $\Delta\Psi_m$ in cultured cells, H9c2 cells were incubated with $\Delta\Psi_m$-sensitive dye JC-1 (5,5′,6,6′-tetraethyl-benzimidazolylcarbocyanine iodide; Molecular Probes, Thermo Fisher Scientific, Waltham, MA, USA). Briefly, cells were incubated for 30 min at 37 °C with JC-1 and fluorescence was measured using a SpectraMax Microplate Reader (Molecular Devices, San Jose, CA, USA). J-aggregates (red) and JC-1 dye monomers (green) were monitored at 530 and 590 nm emission (with excitation at 488 nm), respectively. Data are presented as the ratio red/green fluorescence.

ATP levels were measured using the ATP Bioluminescence Assay Kit CLS II (Roche, Indianapolis, IN, USA), according to the manufacturer's recommendations. Luminescence data were normalized to total protein levels.

2.9. SDS-PAGE and Western Blotting

To analyze protein levels, equal amounts of protein were resolved by SDS-PAGE and transferred onto Amersham Hybond ECL nitrocellulose membranes (GE Healthcare Bio-sciences, Pittsburgh, PA, USA). The membranes were immunoblotted with antibodies against ANT1 (Abcam #110322, Cambridge, MA, USA), or ATP5a (Abcam #14748, Cambridge, MA, USA) followed by incubation with IRDye® (LI-COR Biosciences, Lincoln, NE, USA) secondary antibodies. Bands were visualized using an ODYSSEY® CLx (LI-COR Biosciences, Lincoln, NE, USA) infrared scanner. The resulting images were analyzed with Image Studio Lite Software version 5.2.

2.10. Co-Immunoprecipitation

To analyze protein acetylation, immunoprecipitation experiments were performed following the recommended protocol of Dynabeads (Invitrogen-Life Technologies, Thermo Fisher Scientific, Waltham, MA, USA). Proteins containing acetylated lysine (Ac-K) residues were immunoprecipitated from mouse liver mitochondrial extracts using an antibody against acetylated lysine residues (Cell Signaling #9814, Danvers, MA, USA). The immunoprecipitates were separated by SDS-PAGE, blotted onto Amersham Hybond ECL nitrocellulose membranes (GE Healthcare Bio-Sciences, Pittsburgh, PA, USA) and the Western blots developed using antibody against ANT1 (Abcam #110322, Cambridge, MA, USA) and followed by secondary antibodies. Bands were visualized using the ODYSSEY® CLx (LI-COR Biosciences, Lincoln, NE, USA) infrared scanner.

2.11. Analysis of RCS by Blue Native Polyacrylamide Gel Electrophoresis (BN-PAGE)

The RCS in isolated mitochondria were analyzed by BN-PAGE [12,16]. Briefly, NC or ANT1 KD H9c2 mitochondrial protein or rat heart mitochondria treated for 45 min with vehicle (Veh, 0.01% DMSO), 500 nM rotenone (complex I inhibitor), 500 nM antimycin A (complex III inhibitor), or 1 µM FCCP were dissolved in solubilization buffer (50 mM NaCl, 50 mM imidazole-HCl, 2 mM 6-aminohexanoic acid, 1 mM EDTA) supplemented with digitonin, protease and phosphatase inhibitor cocktails (Sigma-Aldrich, St. Louis, MO, USA), and 25U benzonase. Native gels were stained with Coomassie brilliant blue G250 and visualized with the ODYSSEY® CLx (LI-COR Biosciences, Lincoln, NE, USA) infrared scanner. The images were analyzed using Image Studio Lite Software. The respirasome levels were calculated as the pixel density of bands containing complex I, III, and IV and normalized to whole lane densities.

2.12. Statistical Analysis

Data are presented as means ± SEM. Statistical significance was evaluated using Prism Graph Pad (San Diego, CA, USA) using an unpaired two-tailed Student's *t*-test, Mann–Whitney test, or a one-way ANOVA. The BN-PAGE analysis was conducted with a repeated one-way ANOVA analysis. Differences were considered to be statistically significant when $P < 0.05$.

3. Results

3.1. ANT1 KD Increases Cellular Proliferation Without Affecting Cell Viability

Transfection with *ANT1* siRNA significantly reduced ANT1 expression by 37% ($P < 0.001$) 48 h after transfection (Figure 1A). Interestingly, we found that *ANT1* KD increases cell number by 32% ($P < 0.001$, Figure 1B) and the number of alive cells by 22% ($P < 0.05$, Figure 1C) without affecting cell viability (Figure 1D). Altogether, these results suggest that *ANT1* KD does not affect cell viability, but it increases cellular proliferation, possibly as an adaptive response to ANT1 downregulation.

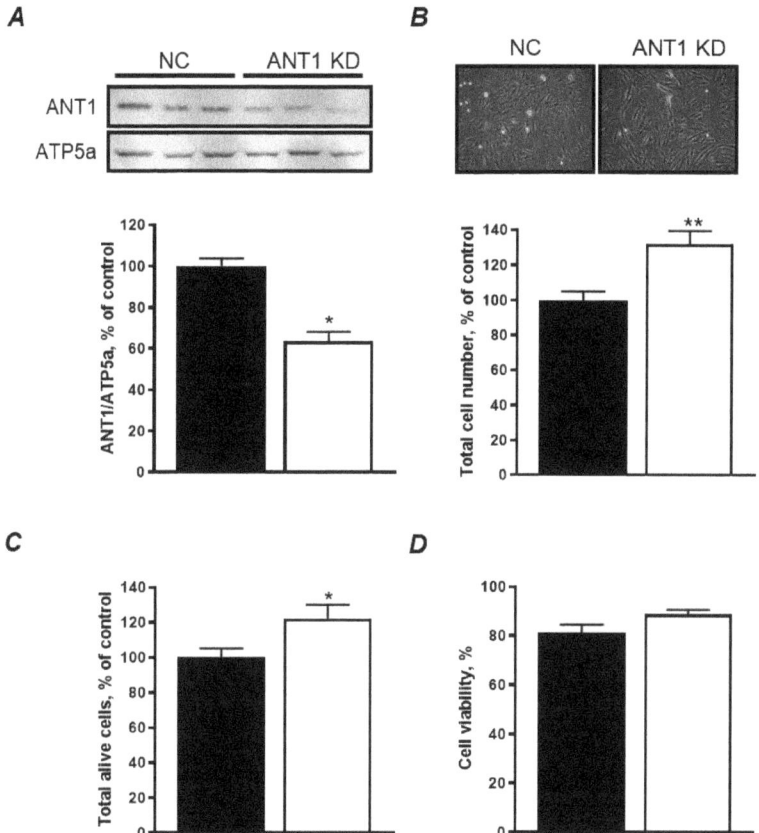

Figure 1. Cell viability is not affected by *ANT* KD in H9c2 cells. (**A**) Protein levels of ANT1 in negative control (NC) and *ANT1* KD cells. *Top panel:* representative immunoblots. *Bottom panel:* quantitative data of ANT1 protein expression normalized to ATP5a (a mitochondrial housekeeping protein); (**B**) Total number of cells 48 h after transfection. *Top panel:* representative images of cells. *Bottom panel:* quantitative data of cells; (**C**) total number of live cells 48 h after transfection; (**D**) cell viability 48 h after transfection calculated as (alive cells/total cells) × 100. * $P < 0.05$ and ** $P < 0.001$ vs. NC. Data represent 4–7 independent experiments.

3.2. ANT1 KD Increased Total ATP and ROS Levels with no Effect on the ETC Activity and mtROS Production

Total ATP levels were elevated by 36% ($P < 0.01$) in *ANT1* KD cells (Figure 2A). Total ATP levels were normalized to μg of total cellular protein to account for the observed increase in cell number (Figure 1B). However, it should be noted that this method does not distinguish glycolytic from mitochondrial ATP. Although these cells appear to have higher levels of total ATP, a decrease in $\Delta\Psi_m$ could hint towards a higher glycolytic ATP production. Results showed that *ANT1* KD cells had significantly lower $\Delta\Psi_m$ compared to NC cells (Figure 2B), suggesting that the elevated ATP levels might result from increased glycolysis but not OXPHOS.

Next, we examined total ROS production using H_2DCFDA fluorescent dye. Results demonstrate that *ANT1* KD cells have a 38% increase ($P < 0.001$) in total ROS generation when compared to NC (Figure 2C). Analysis of mtROS production by MitoSOX shows that *ANT1* KD has no effect on mtROS (Figure 2D). The lack of a difference in mtROS levels can be explained with no significant electron leakage due to low ETC flow in *ANT1* KD cells. In favor of this, analysis of the enzymatic activity of the ETC complexes I, II, III, and IV demonstrated no difference between *ANT1* KD and control cells (Figure 2E–H). Our data are consistent with previous studies where the activity of complexes I, III, and IV were unaffected by ANT expression in HEK293 cells [8]. Altogether, these data demonstrate that ANT1 deficiency has no effect on the enzymatic activity of individual ETC complexes and mtROS production.

3.3. Mitochondrial Oxygen Consumption Rate and OXPHOS is not Affected by ANT1 Downregulation

We measured mitochondrial oxygen consumption rate (OCR) and extracellular acidification rate (ECAR) in H9c2 cells treated with scrambled and *ANT1* siRNA using the Seahorse XFe24 analyzer. Results demonstrate that *ANT1* silencing does not affect the OCR and ECAR in these cells (Figure 3A,B). Likewise, basal and FCCP-induced maximal respiration rates were found unchanged in *ANT1* KD cells (Figure 3C,D). As expected, mitochondrial ATP production was not affected by ANT1 downregulation (Figure 3E). Altogether, these results demonstrate that *ANT1* silencing does not affect OXPHOS in H9c2 cells.

3.4. ANT1 KD in H9c2 Cells Induce RCS Dissociation: the Role of Acetylation

Our recent studies [12] demonstrated that pharmacological inhibition of ANT by atractyloside induces RCS dissociation in isolated cardiac mitochondria. Analysis of RCS in scrambled (NC) or *ANT1* siRNA-treated H9c2 cells demonstrated that ANT1 deficiency induces disassembly of respirasome by 9% ($P < 0.01$) compared to control cells (Figure 4A,B), suggesting that ANT is involved in RCS integrity and stabilization. In order to validate that the decrease in RCS was due to ANT1 downregulation but not $\Delta\Psi_m$ loss (Figure 2B), mitochondria isolated from rat hearts were treated with 1 μM FCCP, an uncoupler, for 45 min [12], prior to RCS analysis. Results demonstrate that loss of $\Delta\Psi_m$ does not affect RCS integrity ($P < 0.1473$, Figure 4C,D). Taken together, these results suggest that the loss of RCS in *ANT1* KD cells is not due to the loss of $\Delta\Psi_m$ and may result from the downregulation of ANT1.

In the following set of experiments, we examined whether ANT1 acetylation is involved in RCS formation. First, we analyzed liver mitochondria isolated from WT and *SIRT3* KO mice to determine the acetylation of total mitochondrial proteins. SIRT3 is the main mitochondrial isoform of sirtuins. Hyperacetylation of mitochondrial proteins due to SIRT3 deficiency has been shown to associate with cardiovascular, neurodegenerative diseases, diabetes, and aging [17–19]. We have previously demonstrated that SIRT3 ablation enhances lysine acetylation (Ac-K) of mitochondrial proteins [20]. However, immunoprecipitation analysis revealed no changes in ANT1 acetylation in the mitochondria of *SIRT3* KO mice (Figure 5A). Interestingly, the mitochondria of *SIRT3* KO mice demonstrated lower RCS levels compared to the WT group (Figure 5B,C). These results suggest that acetylation of mitochondrial proteins, but not ANT1, can stimulate RCS disassembly in mitochondria.

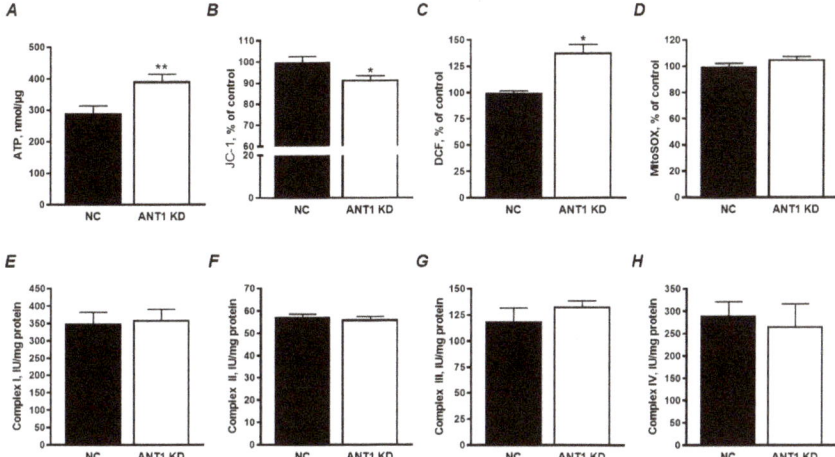

Figure 2. *ANT1* KD disturbs mitochondrial membrane potential (ΔΨm) without affecting enzymatic activity of ETC complexes. (**A**) Total cellular ATP levels normalized to the total amount of protein. (**B**) Mitochondrial membrane potential determined with JC-1 after transfection and calculated as the ratio of J-aggregates to JC-1 monomers. (**C**) Total cellular ROS assessed with H_2DCFDA; (**D**) MtROS assessed using MitoSOX red. Data on the fluorescence activity in the cells (**B–D**) are presented as percent change of negative control (NC). (**E–H**) The enzymatic activity of complexes I, II, III and IV in mitochondria isolated from NC and *ANT1* KD cells. Data were normalized to mitochondrial protein levels. * $P < 0.05$, and ** $P < 0.01$ vs. control (NC). Data represent 3 independent experiments.

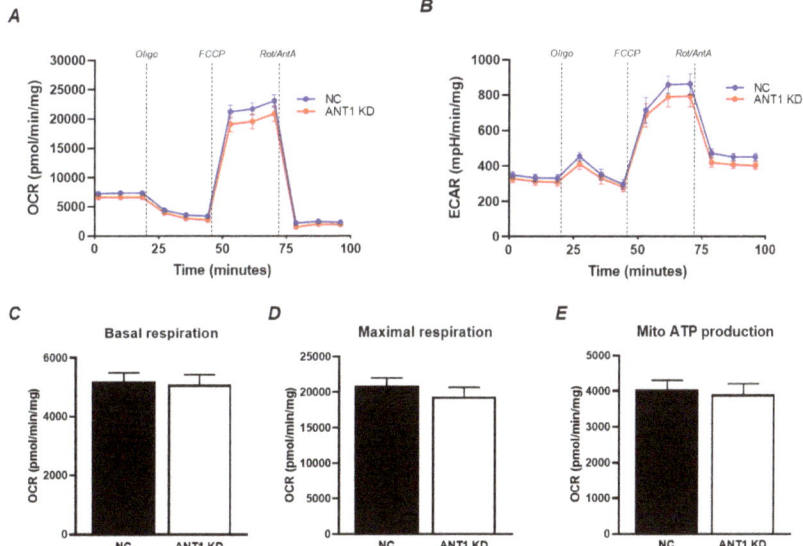

Figure 3. Mitochondrial oxygen consumption and ATP production is not affected by ANT1 downregulation. (**A**) oxygen consumption rate (OCR); (**B**) extracellular acidification rate (ECAR); (**C**) basal respiration; (**D**) maximal respiration; (**E**) mitochondrial ATP production. All parameters were determined using the Seahorse XFe24 analyzer (Agilent) after the addition of (in μM): 0.5 oligomycin (Oligo), 4 FCCP, and 0.5 rotenone/antimycin A (Rot/AntA). The data was extracted using the Seahorse XFe24 report generator and normalized to total protein levels. Data represent 3 independent experiments.

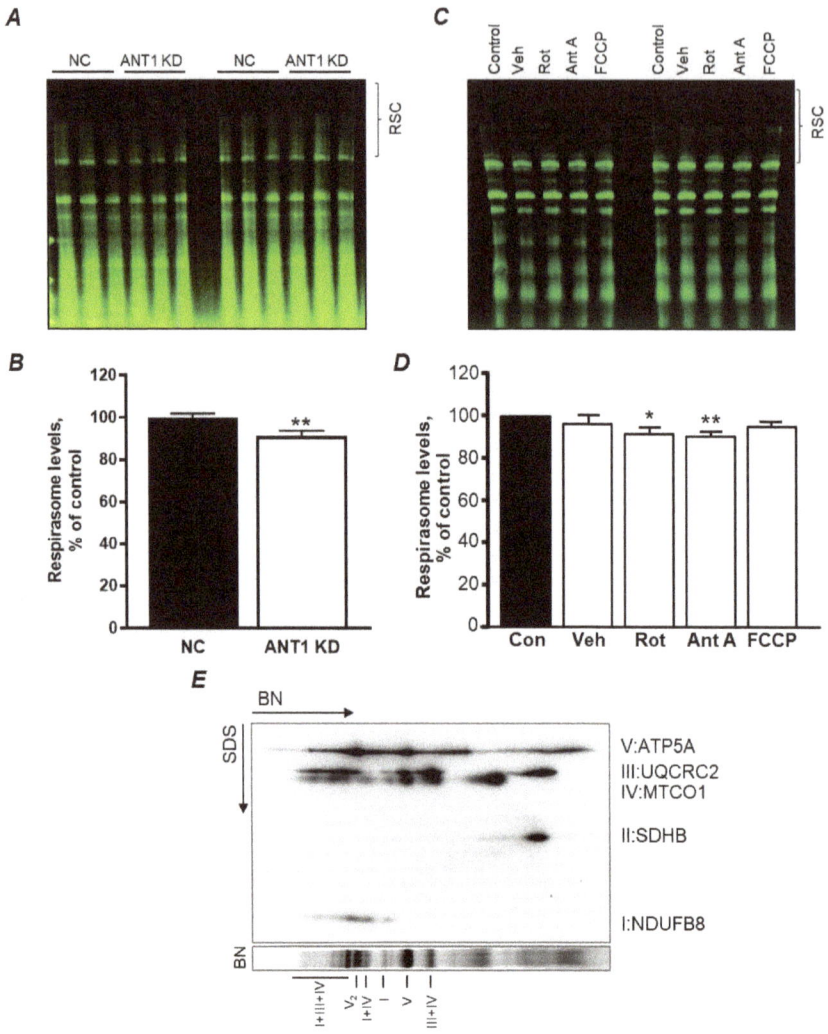

Figure 4. *ANT1* KD stimulates mitochondrial respirasome disintegration in H9c2 cells. (**A**) representative blue native (BN) gel of mitochondria isolated from *ANT1* KD cells and subjected to BN-PAGE; (**B**) quantitative data of respirasome levels; (**C**) representative BN-PAGE gel of mitochondria isolated from rat heart and treated with vehicle (Veh, 0.01% DMSO), 500 nM rotenone (Rot), 500 nM antimycin A (Ant A), or 1 μM FCCP; (**D**) quantitative data of respirasome levels in the groups shown in C; (**E**) representative two-dimensional BN-PAGE of ETC complexes in mitochondria isolated from the rat heart. RCS were analyzed in mitochondria where membrane proteins were solubilized using digitonin and separated by BN-PAGE. ETC complexes were visualized using specific antibodies against the subunits for complexes I (NDUFB8), II (SDHB), III (UQCRC2), IV (MTCO1), and V (ATP5A). Respirasome is shown as I+III+IV. Data in B and D were normalized to mitochondrial protein levels and presented as percent change of negative control (NC) or control (Con). * $P < 0.05$ and ** $P < 0.01$ vs. NC or Con. Data represent 3–4 independent experiments.

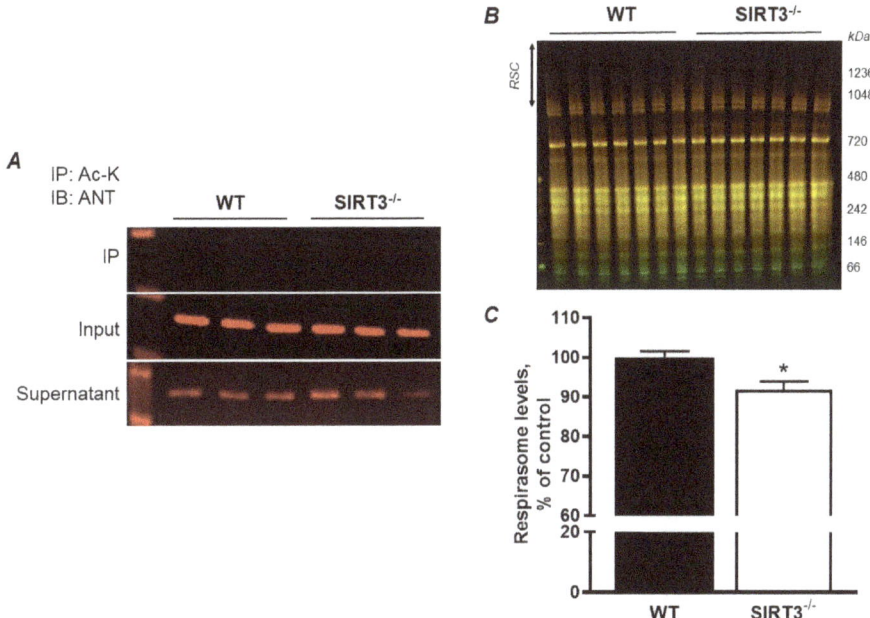

Figure 5. ANT1 is not acetylated but acetylation of mitochondrial proteins stimulates RCS disassembly in *SIRT3* KO mitochondria. (**A**) Immunoprecipitation (IP) of liver mitochondrial proteins with acetylated lysine (Ac-K) antibodies followed by immunoblotting (IB) against ANT1. *Input:* the sample before IP; *Supernatant:* sample that did not bind to Ac-K antibodies; (**B**) BN-PAGE gel of liver mitochondria isolated from WT and *SIRT3* KO⁻ mice. (**C**) Quantitative data of respirasome levels. The data were normalized to total protein levels and presented as percent change from the WT group. * $P < 0.01$ vs. WT; n = 6–7 animals per group.

4. Discussion

The ANT has an important role in maintaining mitochondrial bioenergetics [21] and recently, it has been proposed to play a role in RCS formation [8]. Therefore, in this study, we sought to clarify whether genetic downregulation of ANT1, the main isoform of ANT found in the heart and skeletal muscle cells [1], affects RCS assembly in H9c2 cardioblasts. Our results demonstrate that ANT1 downregulation by 37% does not affect cell viability with no remarkable changes in mitochondria bioenergetics. Furthermore, the activity of all ETC complexes and the mitochondrial OCR was not dependent on ANT1; however, ANT1 appears to be important in the assembly (structural integrity) of the RCS, particularly the respirasome. Additionally, we demonstrate that hyperacetylation of mitochondrial proteins due to SIRT3 ablation stimulates RCS disassembly. The novel role of acetylation on RCS stability may provide additional information as to the mechanism of how acetylation of mitochondrial proteins is involved in the pathogenesis of cardiovascular diseases such as hypertrophy [22–24], IR [20,25,26] and heart failure [27,28]. The current study was performed in H9c2 cardiomyoblasts, but not in primary cardiomyocytes because the latter are quite sensitive to genetic manipulations. It should be noted that H9c2 cardiomyoblasts are more energetically similar (at least, in comparison with atrial HL-1 cells) to primary cardiomyocytes and can be successfully used to simulate an in vitro model of cardiac diseases [29].

Apparently, the role of ANT in the regulation of RCS assembly is not associated with its acetylation as *SIRT3* KO did not increase ANT acetylation in liver mitochondria. Interestingly, we are the first to demonstrate that acetylation per se affects RCS assembly, which could contribute to the mitochondrial dysfunction observed in *SIRT3* KO hearts [20,25]. Disruption of the ANT has been linked to various cardiac diseases. In a mouse model of IR, ANT1 expression was significantly reduced, and cardiac-specific ANT1 overexpression prevented the detrimental effects associated with IR injury [7]. ANT1 KO mice develop cardiac hypertrophy and lactic acidosis [2], similar to that observed in patients. Therefore, ANT1 has an important role in maintaining cardiac function and potentially mediating the detrimental effects associated with heart IR injury [30].

In our studies, *ANT1* KD increased cell number without affecting cell viability (Figure 1B–D). Previous studies have observed an increase in mitochondrial number, size [2,31], and upregulation of mitochondrial genes, including OXPHOS components [31] in *ANT1* KD hearts and skeletal muscle. It is tempting to speculate that *ANT1* KD cells display an increase in cellular proliferation as a reflection of upregulated mitochondrial genes and an increase in mitochondrial number and size as an adaptive response. The lack of any effects of ANT deficiency on cell viability might be explained, at least in part, by (i) insufficient (37%) downregulation of ANT1 to induce mitochondrial dysfunction, or (ii) upregulation of other ANT isoforms, such as ANT2, as a compensatory mechanism, and their functional redundancy. Indeed, ANT2 has been shown to have opposite properties to ANT1 as it has been found capable of importing cytosolic ATP into the mitochondrial matrix [32], possibly maintaining normal mitochondrial function, although these findings are somewhat controversial [33]. In addition, ANT2 is regarded as a proliferative marker and correlated to loss of cell cycle control, which could partially explain why *ANT1* KD cells have an increase in cell number [32].

Interestingly, *ANT1* KD increased the number of total cells by 32% and alive cells by 22% (Figure 1) associated with a 36% increase of ATP levels (Figure 2B). The increase of ATP levels in *ANT1* KD cells might be due to the increase in cell number; however, this suggestion was excluded after normalization of ATP to total cellular protein (Figure 2B). Since aerobic (non-glycolytic) ATP production is coupled to $\Delta\Psi_m$, we sought to examine the possibility of having disturbances in mitochondrial ATP production that could hint towards a glycolytic compensation. Previous studies have reported an increase in anaerobic metabolism and lactic acidosis [2,3] in ANT1 deficiency. Our results demonstrated that *ANT1* KD cells display a decrease in $\Delta\Psi_m$ (Figure 2B), which could be due to an impaired ETC activity and OXPHOS. However, neither we (Figure 2E–H) nor other groups using HEK293 cells [8] reported differences in the activity of individual ETC complexes due to ANT1 downregulation or ablation. In addition, we were unable to detect differences in basal and maximal mitochondrial respiration (Figure 3C,D) and ATP production (Figure 3E). Interestingly, although beyond the scope of our experiments, *ANT1* KD cells displayed a significant increase in cellular ROS levels (Figure 2C) and non-mitochondrial oxygen consumption (*data not shown*). The production of ROS can occur outside the mitochondria, such as in the cytosol (xanthine oxidase, nitric oxide synthase), peroxisomes, and plasma membrane (NADPH oxidases) [34], possibly suggesting a cross-talk between ANT1-deficient mitochondria and other cellular compartments.

The physiological significance of the RCS is still under debate [35]. The mitochondrial RCS have been suggested to increase the effectiveness of electron transport through the ETC complexes, optimize ATP production, and reduce mtROS production by reducing electron leakage [11]. Disassembly of the RCSs, particularly the respirasome, was observed in cardiovascular diseases such as IR [16] and heart failure [36]. However, the mechanisms underlying the assembly of the RCSs, as well as their physiological role in the heart, are not fully understood. Our previous studies demonstrated that high Ca^{2+} and pharmacological/genetic inhibition of complex I (Figure 4C,D) stimulate disruption of the RCS in H9c2 cells and isolated mitochondria [12,37]. These studies suggested crosstalk between RCS assembly and permeability transition pore (PTP) opening as Ca^{2+} is the strong inducer of pore opening and complex I is the PTP regulator. This point is further supported by the current study that demonstrates that genetic downregulation of ANT, a PTP regulator, induces disorganization of the RCS. However, the cause–effect relationship between RCS and PTP seems to be more complex. Despite RCS disassembly, inhibition of complex I by rotenone prevented Ca^{2+}-induced PTP opening in cardiac mitochondria [12], and *ANT1* KD did not increase mtROS, a PTP inducer in H9c2 cells (Figure 2D). Finally, we demonstrate that acetylation of mitochondrial proteins due to SIRT3 deficiency induces

RCS disassembly in an ANT-independent manner because there was no difference in ANT acetylation between WT and SIRT3$^{-/-}$ mitochondria (Figure 5). Disruption of the RCS could be a result of direct mechanisms involving disruption of protein–protein interactions due to changes in lysine residue charges, or indirect mechanisms through inactivation of RCS regulatory proteins (e.g., RCS assembly factors) due to their hyperacetylation.

In conclusion, this study suggests that ANT is involved in RCS assembly, although RCS may not be solely dependent on ANT. ANT may physically interact with ETC complexes I, III, and IV [8] and thus, be involved in the respirasome structure or play a regulatory role in the formation/maintenance of the RCS assembly. Further studies are required to elucidate the role of ANT in the structural integrity and regulation of RCS and other mitochondrial supercomplexes (e.g., ATP synthasome) in cardiac cells.

5. Limitations of the Study

We elucidated the contribution of only *ANT1* downregulation to mitochondrial bioenergetics and RCS assembly. ANT family proteins contain four isoforms (ANT1-4) that play a differential role and perform distinctly opposite functions in cell life and death. We were not able to verify protein expression of other ANT isoforms in *ANT1* KD H9c2 cells due to lack of reliable ANT2, ANT3, and ANT4 antibodies. Functional redundancy of other ANT isoforms could compensate for the effects induced by *ANT1* deficiency.

Author Contributions: Conceptualization: S.J. (Sabzali Javadov); Methodology: R.M.P.-R., S.J. (Sehwan Jang), C.A.T.-R., S.A.-P.; Validation: All authors; Formal analysis: R.M.P.-R., S.J. (Sehwan Jang), X.C.-D.; Investigation: All authors; Writing—original draft: R.M.P.-R.; Writing—review & editing: S.J. (Sabzali Javadov); Supervision: S.J. (Sabzali Javadov); Project administration: S.J. (Sabzali Javadov); Funding acquisition: S.J. (Sabzali Javadov).

Funding: This research was supported by the National Institute of General Medical Sciences (Grants SC1GM128210 and R25GM061838) of the National Institutes of Health.

Conflicts of Interest: The authors declare no conflict of interest.

References

1. Stepien, G.; Torroni, A.; Chung, A.B.; Hodge, J.A.; Wallace, D.C. Differential expression of adenine nucleotide translocator isoforms in mammalian tissues and during muscle cell differentiation. *J. Biol. Chem.* **1992**, *267*, 14592–14597. [PubMed]
2. Graham, B.H.; Waymire, K.G.; Cottrell, B.; Trounce, I.A.; MacGregor, G.R.; Wallace, D.C. A mouse model for mitochondrial myopathy and cardiomyopathy resulting from a deficiency in the heart/muscle isoform of the adenine nucleotide translocator. *Nat. Genet.* **1997**, *16*, 226–234. [CrossRef] [PubMed]
3. Echaniz-Laguna, A.; Chassagne, M.; Ceresuela, J.; Rouvet, I.; Padet, S.; Acquaviva, C.; Nataf, S.; Vinzio, S.; Bozon, D.; Mousson de Camaret, B. Complete loss of expression of the ANT1 gene causing cardiomyopathy and myopathy. *J. Med. Genet.* **2012**, *49*, 146–150. [CrossRef] [PubMed]
4. Narula, N.; Zaragoza, M.V.; Sengupta, P.P.; Li, P.; Haider, N.; Verjans, J.; Waymire, K.; Vannan, M.; Wallace, D.C. Adenine nucleotide translocase 1 deficiency results in dilated cardiomyopathy with defects in myocardial mechanics, histopathological alterations, and activation of apoptosis. *JACC Cardiovasc. Imaging* **2011**, *4*, 1–10. [CrossRef] [PubMed]
5. Palmieri, L.; Alberio, S.; Pisano, I.; Lodi, T.; Meznaric-Petrusa, M.; Zidar, J.; Santoro, A.; Scarcia, P.; Fontanesi, F.; Lamantea, E.; et al. Complete loss-of-function of the heart/muscle-specific adenine nucleotide translocator is associated with mitochondrial myopathy and cardiomyopathy. *Hum. Mol. Genet.* **2005**, *14*, 3079–3088. [CrossRef] [PubMed]
6. Esposito, L.A.; Melov, S.; Panov, A.; Cottrell, B.A.; Wallace, D.C. Mitochondrial disease in mouse results in increased oxidative stress. *Proc. Natl. Acad. Sci. USA* **1999**, *96*, 4820–4825. [CrossRef] [PubMed]
7. Klumpe, I.; Savvatis, K.; Westermann, D.; Tschope, C.; Rauch, U.; Landmesser, U.; Schultheiss, H.P.; Dorner, A. Transgenic overexpression of adenine nucleotide translocase 1 protects ischemic hearts against oxidative stress. *J. Mol. Med. (Berl)* **2016**, *94*, 645–653. [CrossRef] [PubMed]

8. Lu, Y.W.; Acoba, M.G.; Selvaraju, K.; Huang, T.C.; Nirujogi, R.S.; Sathe, G.; Pandey, A.; Claypool, S.M. Human adenine nucleotide translocases physically and functionally interact with respirasomes. *Mol. Biol Cell* **2017**, *28*, 1489–1506. [CrossRef] [PubMed]
9. Claypool, S.M.; Oktay, Y.; Boontheung, P.; Loo, J.A.; Koehler, C.M. Cardiolipin defines the interactome of the major ADP/ATP carrier protein of the mitochondrial inner membrane. *J. Cell Biol.* **2008**, *182*, 937–950. [CrossRef]
10. Schagger, H.; Pfeiffer, K. Supercomplexes in the respiratory chains of yeast and mammalian mitochondria. *EMBO J.* **2000**, *19*, 1777–1783. [CrossRef]
11. Lobo-Jarne, T.; Ugalde, C. Respiratory chain supercomplexes: Structures, function and biogenesis. *Semin. Cell Dev. Biol.* **2017**. [CrossRef] [PubMed]
12. Jang, S.; Javadov, S. Elucidating the contribution of ETC complexes I and II to the respirasome formation in cardiac mitochondria. *Sci. Rep.* **2018**, *8*, 17732. [CrossRef] [PubMed]
13. Cimen, H.; Han, M.J.; Yang, Y.; Tong, Q.; Koc, H.; Koc, E.C. Regulation of succinate dehydrogenase activity by SIRT3 in mammalian mitochondria. *Biochemistry* **2010**, *49*, 304–311. [CrossRef] [PubMed]
14. Wu, Y.T.; Lee, H.C.; Liao, C.C.; Wei, Y.H. Regulation of mitochondrial F(o)F(1)ATPase activity by Sirt3-catalyzed deacetylation and its deficiency in human cells harboring 4977bp deletion of mitochondrial DNA. *Biochim. Biophys. Acta* **2013**, *1832*, 216–227. [CrossRef] [PubMed]
15. Hernandez, J.S.; Barreto-Torres, G.; Kuznetsov, A.V.; Khuchua, Z.; Javadov, S. Crosstalk between AMPK activation and angiotensin II-induced hypertrophy in cardiomyocytes: The role of mitochondria. *J. Cell Mol. Med.* **2014**, *18*, 709–720. [CrossRef] [PubMed]
16. Jang, S.; Lewis, T.S.; Powers, C.; Khuchua, Z.; Baines, C.P.; Wipf, P.; Javadov, S. Elucidating Mitochondrial Electron Transport Chain Supercomplexes in the Heart During Ischemia-Reperfusion. *Antioxid. Redox. Signal.* **2017**, *27*, 57–69. [CrossRef] [PubMed]
17. Parodi-Rullan, R.M.; Chapa-Dubocq, X.R.; Javadov, S. Acetylation of Mitochondrial Proteins in the Heart: The Role of SIRT3. *Front. Physiol.* **2018**, *9*, 1094. [CrossRef]
18. Salvatori, I.; Valle, C.; Ferri, A.; Carri, M.T. SIRT3 and mitochondrial metabolism in neurodegenerative diseases. *Neurochem. Int.* **2017**, *109*, 184–192. [CrossRef]
19. McDonnell, E.; Peterson, B.S.; Bomze, H.M.; Hirschey, M.D. SIRT3 regulates progression and development of diseases of aging. *Trends Endocrinol. Metab.* **2015**, *26*, 486–492. [CrossRef]
20. Parodi-Rullan, R.M.; Chapa-Dubocq, X.; Rullan, P.J.; Jang, S.; Javadov, S. High Sensitivity of SIRT3 Deficient Hearts to Ischemia-Reperfusion Is Associated with Mitochondrial Abnormalities. *Front. Pharmacol.* **2017**, *8*, 275. [CrossRef]
21. Ogunbona, O.B.; Baile, M.G.; Claypool, S.M. Cardiomyopathy-associated mutation in the ADP/ATP carrier reveals translation-dependent regulation of cytochrome c oxidase activity. *Mol. Biol. Cell* **2018**, *29*, 1449–1464. [CrossRef] [PubMed]
22. Sundaresan, N.R.; Gupta, M.; Kim, G.; Rajamohan, S.B.; Isbatan, A.; Gupta, M.P. Sirt3 blocks the cardiac hypertrophic response by augmenting Foxo3a-dependent antioxidant defense mechanisms in mice. *J. Clin. Investig.* **2009**, *119*, 2758–2771. [CrossRef] [PubMed]
23. Pillai, V.B.; Samant, S.; Sundaresan, N.R.; Raghuraman, H.; Kim, G.; Bonner, M.Y.; Arbiser, J.L.; Walker, D.I.; Jones, D.P.; Gius, D.; et al. Honokiol blocks and reverses cardiac hypertrophy in mice by activating mitochondrial Sirt3. *Nat. Commun.* **2015**, *6*, 6656. [CrossRef] [PubMed]
24. Chen, T.; Liu, J.; Li, N.; Wang, S.; Liu, H.; Li, J.; Zhang, Y.; Bu, P. Mouse SIRT3 attenuates hypertrophy-related lipid accumulation in the heart through the deacetylation of LCAD. *PLoS ONE* **2015**, *10*, e0118909. [CrossRef] [PubMed]
25. Porter, G.A.; Urciuoli, W.R.; Brookes, P.S.; Nadtochiy, S.M. SIRT3 deficiency exacerbates ischemia-reperfusion injury: Implication for aged hearts. *Am. J. Physiol. Heart Circ. Physiol.* **2014**, *306*, H1602–H1609. [CrossRef] [PubMed]
26. Koentges, C.; Pfeil, K.; Schnick, T.; Wiese, S.; Dahlbock, R.; Cimolai, M.C.; Meyer-Steenbuck, M.; Cenkerova, K.; Hoffmann, M.M.; Jaeger, C.; et al. SIRT3 deficiency impairs mitochondrial and contractile function in the heart. *Basic Res. Cardiol.* **2015**, *110*, 36. [CrossRef] [PubMed]
27. Parodi-Rullan, R.; Barreto-Torres, G.; Ruiz, L.; Casasnovas, J.; Javadov, S. Direct renin inhibition exerts an anti-hypertrophic effect associated with improved mitochondrial function in post-infarction heart failure in diabetic rats. *Cell Physiol. Biochem.* **2012**, *29*, 841–850. [CrossRef]

28. Horton, J.L.; Martin, O.J.; Lai, L.; Riley, N.M.; Richards, A.L.; Vega, R.B.; Leone, T.C.; Pagliarini, D.J.; Muoio, D.M.; Bedi, K.C., Jr.; et al. Mitochondrial protein hyperacetylation in the failing heart. *JCI Insight* **2016**, *2*. [CrossRef]
29. Kuznetsov, A.V.; Javadov, S.; Sickinger, S.; Frotschnig, S.; Grimm, M. H9c2 and HL-1 cells demonstrate distinct features of energy metabolism, mitochondrial function and sensitivity to hypoxia-reoxygenation. *Biochim. Biophys. Acta* **2015**, *1853*, 276–284. [CrossRef]
30. Borutaite, V.; Mildaziene, V.; Katiliute, Z.; Kholodenko, B.; Toleikis, A. The function of ATP/ADP translocator in the regulation of mitochondrial respiration during development of heart ischemic injury. *Biochim. Biophys. Acta* **1993**, *1142*, 175–180. [CrossRef]
31. Murdock, D.G.; Boone, B.E.; Esposito, L.A.; Wallace, D.C. Up-regulation of nuclear and mitochondrial genes in the skeletal muscle of mice lacking the heart/muscle isoform of the adenine nucleotide translocator. *J. Biol. Chem.* **1999**, *274*, 14429–14433. [CrossRef] [PubMed]
32. Chevrollier, A.; Loiseau, D.; Gautier, F.; Malthiery, Y.; Stepien, G. ANT2 expression under hypoxic conditions produces opposite cell-cycle behavior in 143B and HepG2 cancer cells. *Mol. Carcinog.* **2005**, *42*, 1–8. [CrossRef] [PubMed]
33. Maldonado, E.N.; DeHart, D.N.; Patnaik, J.; Klatt, S.C.; Gooz, M.B.; Lemasters, J.J. ATP/ADP turnover and import of glycolytic ATP into mitochondria in cancer cells is independent of the adenine nucleotide translocator. *J. Biol. Chem.* **2017**, *292*, 16969. [CrossRef] [PubMed]
34. Di Meo, S.; Reed, T.T.; Venditti, P.; Victor, V.M. Role of ROS and RNS Sources in Physiological and Pathological Conditions. *Oxid. Med. Cell Longev.* **2016**, *2016*, 1245049. [CrossRef] [PubMed]
35. Milenkovic, D.; Blaza, J.N.; Larsson, N.G.; Hirst, J. The Enigma of the Respiratory Chain Supercomplex. *Cell Metab.* **2017**, *25*, 765–776. [CrossRef] [PubMed]
36. Rosca, M.G.; Vazquez, E.J.; Kerner, J.; Parland, W.; Chandler, M.P.; Stanley, W.; Sabbah, H.N.; Hoppel, C.L. Cardiac mitochondria in heart failure: Decrease in respirasomes and oxidative phosphorylation. *Cardiovasc. Res.* **2008**, *80*, 30–39. [CrossRef]
37. Jang, S.; Javadov, S. Association between ROS production, swelling and the respirasome integrity in cardiac mitochondria. *Arch. Biochem. Biophys.* **2017**, *630*, 1–8. [CrossRef]

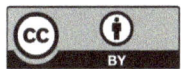

© 2019 by the authors. Licensee MDPI, Basel, Switzerland. This article is an open access article distributed under the terms and conditions of the Creative Commons Attribution (CC BY) license (http://creativecommons.org/licenses/by/4.0/).

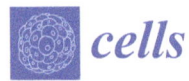

Article

Mutations in *NDUFS1* Cause Metabolic Reprogramming and Disruption of the Electron Transfer

Yang Ni [1,2,3], Muhammad A. Hagras [4,5], Vassiliki Konstantopoulou [6], Johannes A. Mayr [7], Alexei A. Stuchebrukhov [4] and David Meierhofer [1,*]

1. Mass Spectrometry Facility, Max Planck Institute for Molecular Genetics, 14195 Berlin, Germany; yang.ni@kuleuven.vib.be
2. Department of Biology, Chemistry and Pharmacy, Freie Universität Berlin, 14195 Berlin, Germany
3. Present address: Laboratory of Angiogenesis and Vascular Metabolism, VIB-KU Leuven Center for Cancer Biology, 3000 Leuven, Belgium
4. Department of Chemistry, University of California Davis, Davis, CA 95616, USA; mahagras@ucdavis.edu (M.A.H.); aastuchebrukhov@ucdavis.edu (A.A.S.)
5. Present address: Department of Chemical Engineering, Massachusetts Institute of Technology, Cambridge, MA 02142, USA
6. Department of Pediatrics and Adolescent Medicine, Medical University of Vienna, 1090 Vienna, Austria; vassiliki.konstantopoulou@meduniwien.ac.at
7. Department of Pediatrics, Paracelsus Medical University Salzburg, 5020 Salzburg, Austria; H.Mayr@salk.at
* Correspondence: meierhof@molgen.mpg.de; Tel.: +49-30-8413-1567

Received: 24 July 2019; Accepted: 20 September 2019; Published: 25 September 2019

Abstract: Complex I (CI) is the first enzyme of the mitochondrial respiratory chain and couples the electron transfer with proton pumping. Mutations in genes encoding CI subunits can frequently cause inborn metabolic errors. We applied proteome and metabolome profiling of patient-derived cells harboring pathogenic mutations in two distinct CI genes to elucidate underlying pathomechanisms on the molecular level. Our results indicated that the electron transfer within CI was interrupted in both patients by different mechanisms. We showed that the biallelic mutations in *NDUFS1* led to a decreased stability of the entire N-module of CI and disrupted the electron transfer between two iron–sulfur clusters. Strikingly interesting and in contrast to the proteome, metabolome profiling illustrated that the pattern of dysregulated metabolites was almost identical in both patients, such as the inhibitory feedback on the TCA cycle and altered glutathione levels, indicative for reactive oxygen species (ROS) stress. Our findings deciphered pathological mechanisms of CI deficiency to better understand inborn metabolic errors.

Keywords: complex I (CI) deficiency; metabolome and proteome profiling; reactive oxygen species (ROS); respirasome assembly; electron tunneling (ET)

1. Introduction

Complex I (CI, NADH:ubiquinone oxidoreductase) is the first and largest enzyme of the mitochondrial respiratory chain in humans. It catalyzes the transfer of electrons from NADH to coenzyme Q10, which is coupled to the translocation of protons from the mitochondrial matrix into the intermembrane space. Recently, the structures of the entire CI in *Yarrowia lipolytica*, *Ovis aries*, and *Bos taurus* were reported at a resolution of 3.6 to 4.2 Å, describing in detail the central subunits that execute this bioenergetic function [1–3]. Mammalian CI consists of 45 subunits, seven of which are encoded by the genes localized in mitochondrial DNA [4–6]. Therefore, CI deficiency can originate from both mitochondrial or nuclear DNA mutations, which leads to its heterogeneous features [7,8].

Since the discovery of pathogenic mitochondrial DNA (mtDNA) point mutations [9,10] and deletions [11] in the year 1988, more than 309 gene defects have been reported to date, and this number continues to grow [12]. Mitochondrial diseases can be grouped into (i) disorders of oxidative phosphorylation (OXPHOS) subunits and their assembly factors; (ii) defects of mitochondrial DNA, RNA, and protein synthesis; (iii) defects in the substrate-generating upstream reactions of OXPHOS; (iv) defects in relevant cofactors; and (v) defects in mitochondrial homeostasis [13]. Mitochondrial diseases occur at an estimated prevalence of 1 in 5000 live births, and are collectively the most common inborn error of metabolism [14,15]. CI deficiency is the most frequent mitochondrial disorder among inborn errors of metabolism, and is characterized by clinical and genetic heterogeneity [16] including Leber's hereditary optic neuropathy (LHON) [10], mitochondrial encephalomyopathy, lactic acidosis, stroke-like episodes (MELAS) [17], and Leigh syndrome (LS) [18]. In addition, the level of heteroplasmy of mtDNA mutations can vary and is dynamic between cells in the same organism or tissue, and the proportion of mutant mtDNA molecules determines both the penetrance and severity of expression of disease [19]. Recently, Idebenone was designated as the first orphan drug to treat LHON by the European Medicines Agency (EMA product number: EMEA/H/C/3834). Idebenone functions as a mitochondrial electron carrier and bypasses CI to directly transfer electrons to mitochondrial complex III (CIII) [20].

In this study, we applied an integrative proteome and metabolome profiling approach to investigate the molecular and cellular consequences of pathogenic mutations in two core subunits of mitochondrial CI. The first nuclear gene, *NDUFS1*, encodes the NADH-ubiquinone oxidoreductase 75 kDa subunit, the largest subunit of CI that accommodates three iron–sulfur clusters in the N-module, which binds and oxidizes NADH [21,22]. The second gene, *MT-ND5*, is located in the mtDNA and encodes NADH-ubiquinone oxidoreductase chain 5, which represents one of the core subunits in the P-module, wherein the proton translocation takes place. It is located at the distal end of the CI transmembrane arm and facilitates proton translocation [23,24].

The first patient was a girl, who carried a mutation in the mitochondrial gene *MT-ND5* (m.12706T>C). This missense mutation caused a single amino acid substitution of p.Phe124Leu. The second patient was a boy. He carried point mutations in *NDUFS1* (c.683T>C and 755A>G, compound heterozygous), which caused amino acid substitutions of p.Val228Ala and p.Asp252Gly. Identical mutations in both genes have been previously reported to cause a pathogenic phenotype [25–30]; however, the molecular and cellular consequences of these mutations were largely unknown. Here, we explored and compared the proteome and metabolome profiles of patients and control skin fibroblasts to elucidate (i) if the global and OXPHOS-specific protein and metabolite abundances were altered, (ii) if the assembly of CI and the formation of the mitochondrial respirasome was influenced, (iii) if enzymatic activities of OXPHOS were regulated, (iv) if reactive oxygen species (ROS) production was changed in these distinct CI mutations versus unaffected controls, and (v) whether the electron tunneling rate in NDUFS1 was impaired because of the mutation between iron–sulfur clusters N4 and N5.

2. Materials and Methods

2.1. Ethics Statement

The study protocol conformed to the guidelines of the Declaration of Helsinki. Studies with primary human cell lines were approved by the local ethics committee "Ethikkommission Land Salzburg" and written informed consent was provided by the patients' guardians for skin biopsies.

2.2. Mutations in Patients

The first patient carried a missense mutation in the mitochondrial DNA (gene *MT-ND5*, m.12706T>C), which lead to an amino acid substitution (p.Phe124Leu) in the ND5 subunit of complex I. Sanger sequencing revealed a 70% mutation load in cultivated skin fibroblasts. This mutation has been reported in patients with Leigh syndrome [25–27]. The second patient carried two distinct point mutations (c.[683T>C];[755A>G]) in the nuclear gene *NDUFS1* (NM_005006.7), which caused amino acid substitutions (p.[Val228Ala];[Asp252Gly]) in the NDUFS1 subunit of complex I. This patient was compound heterozygous for these two missense mutations.

2.3. Patients

Patient *MT-ND5*: During pregnancy aortic stenosis was diagnosed by sonography. The mother suffered from epilepsy and was treated with Levetiracetam during pregnancy. On the first day of life, the girl presented with right ventricular hypertrophic cardiomyopathy. Sonography of the brain showed partial agenesis of the corpus callosum. At the age of 9 months and during an upper airway infection, the girl was admitted to intensive care because of apnea and insufficient spontaneous breathing. In addition, a brain magnetic resonance imaging showed symmetric signal alterations in the basal ganglia and the brain stem. At the age of $9\frac{1}{2}$ months, the girl died from respiratory failure. Investigation of an unfrozen muscle biopsy revealed a decrease in CI: 20 nmol/min/mg protein (normal 28–76 nmol/min/mg protein, Table 1). Lactate was elevated in blood between 41–50 mg/dL (normal 6–22 mg/dL). Urine organic acid analysis revealed elevated lactate (262 mmol/mol creatinine), 3-hydroxybutyrate, and acetoacetate.

Table 1. Enzyme activities of oxidative phosphorylation (OXPHOS) complexes in muscle biopsies.

Activity Ratio Versus CS	CI	CI + III	CII	CII + III	CIII	CIV	F_1F_0 ATP Synthase
Patient *MT-ND5*	0.04	0.07	0.29	0.39	2.10	1.87	0.96
Patient *NDUFS1*	0.05	0.14	0.29	0.36	2.20	0.97	1.16
Reference range	0.14–0.35	0.24–0.81	0.23–0.41	0.30–0.67	1.45–3.76	0.82–2.04	0.42–1.26

Clinical reference ranges are referred to a previous publication [31]. CS: citrate synthase, C: complex. Enzyme-specific activities were expressed as nanomoles of substrate per minute per milligram of protein (nmol/min/mg protein) and were normalized to the enzyme activity of CS. Indicated are ratios.

Patient *NDUFS1*: At the age of 7 months, this boy presented with muscular hypotonia. He lost skills such as head control and rolling over. Furthermore, he failed to thrive and lost body weight. A muscle biopsy was performed at the age of 9 months and showed decreased activity of respiratory chain CI: 20 nmol/min/mg protein (normal 28–76 nmol/min/mg protein, Table 1).

2.4. Cell Culture

Human-derived primary skin fibroblast cells (patients and controls) were obtained from the Department of Pediatrics, Salzburger Landeskliniken, Salzburg, Austria. Fibroblasts were obtained by a superficial punch skin biopsy, collected from the patient under local anesthesia. Two individuals, from whom the skin fibroblasts were taken as controls, had no genetic defects and were hospitalized for sepsis. In order to meet the requirement of individual experiments, cells were grown in slightly different media. For proteome and metabolome profiling, as well as blue native-polyacrylamide gel electrophoresis (BN-PAGE), cell lines were cultivated in high glucose Dulbecco's modified eagle medium (DMEM, Thermo Scientific, Waltham, MA, USA, # 31966) containing 4.5 g/L glucose, 1 mM pyruvate, and GlutaMAX, and supplemented with 10% fetal bovine serum (FBS, Merck, Darmstadt, Germany, # F7524), 1% penicillin-streptomycin-neomycin (PSN) antibiotic mixture (Thermo, # 15640055) at 37 °C in a normoxia incubator with a humidified atmosphere of 5% CO_2. Cells were grown to 90% confluency in one T75 or one T300 polystyrene flask (TPP, Trasadingen, Switzerland) in biological triplicates for proteome and metabolome experiments, respectively. For the live-cell respiration assay with the Seahorse XFe96 Analyzer (Agilent, Santa Clara, CA, USA), fibroblasts were cultured in basic DMEM (Thermo, # A14430), supplemented with 1 mM sodium pyruvate (Merck, # P2256), 2 mM L-glutamine (Merck, # G3126), 1% PSN antibiotic mixture (Thermo, # 15640055), 10% dialyzed FBS (Silantes, # 281000900), and 25 mM glucose (Merck, # G7021) in three biological replicates in T150 flasks.

2.5. Metabolite Extraction and Profiling by Targeted LC-MS

Metabolite extraction was done as reported previously with a minor modification for cell culture samples [32]. In brief, T300 flasks with fibroblasts between the passages of 11–15 at 90% confluence were harvested in triplicates for each experiment. Twenty-four hours before harvest, the cell culture was replenished with fresh medium. In order to keep the original metabolic state of the cell and minimize metabolite degradation, cells were harvested within 2 minutes. Culture medium was aspirated and the cells were rinsed quickly twice with ice-chilled 1× phosphate-buffered saline, pH 7.4. Then, 1 mL water was added into the flask, which was immediately shock-frozen in liquid nitrogen. The flask was kept on ice, and cell lysates were collected with a cell scraper (TPP) and transferred into a 15 mL tube for three thaw-and-freeze cycles to extract the metabolites. Metabolites were extracted with methyl tert-butyl ether (MTBE), methanol, and water [32]. The remaining protein pellet was used in the bicinchoninic acid (BCA) protein assay for normalization among samples. Extracts were aliquoted equally into three tubes for later reconstitution in water, acetonitrile, and 50% methanol in acetonitrile, respectively. Additionally, an internal standard mixture, containing chloramphenicol and C^{13}-labeled L-glutamine, L-arginine, L-proline, L-valine, and uracil was added to each sample (10 µM final concentration). A SpeedVac was used to dry the aliquots. Dry residuals were dissolved in three different solvents (1) 100 µL 50% acetonitrile in MeOH with 0.1% formic acid, (2) 100 µL MeOH with 0.1% formic acid for analysis by hydrophilic interaction liquid chromatography (HILIC) column, or (3) 100 µL water with 0.1% formic acid for C18 column mode. The supernatants were transferred to micro-volume inserts. Then, 20 µL per run was injected for subsequent LC-MS analysis.

Over 400 metabolites were selected to cover most of the important metabolic pathways in mammals. Metabolites are very diverse in their chemical properties. Therefore, two different LC columns have been used for metabolite separation: a Reprosil-PUR C18-AQ (1.9 µm, 120 Å, 150 × 2 mm ID; Dr. Maisch, Ammerbuch, Germany) column, and a zicHILIC (3.5 µm, 100 Å, 150 × 2.1 mm ID; Merck). The settings of the LC-MS instrument, 1290 series ultra high pressure liquid chromatography (UHPLC) (Agilent) online coupled to a QTRAP 6500 (Sciex, Foster City, CA) were reported previously [33]. The buffer conditions were A1—10 mM ammonium acetate, pH 3.5 (adjusted with acetic acid); B1—99.9% acetonitrile with 0.1% formic acid; A2—10 mM ammonium acetate, pH 7.5 (adjusted with ammonia solution); and B2—99.9% methanol with 0.1% formic acid. All buffers were prepared in LC-MS grade water and organic solvents.

A list of all metabolites, including multiple reaction monitoring (MRM) ion ratios, retention times, and Kyoto Encyclopedia of Genes and Genomes (KEGG) or Human Metabolome Database (HMDB) metabolite identifiers can be found in Table S6. Peak integration was performed using MultiQuant software v.2.1.1 (Sciex, Foster City, CA) without any smoothing and reviewed manually. Peak intensities were normalized, first against the internal standards, and subsequently against protein abundances obtained from the BCA assay. The first transition of each metabolite was used for relative quantification between samples and controls. All original LC-MS-generated QTrap wiff- files, as well as MultiQuant processed peak integration q.session files can be downloaded via http://www.peptideatlas.org/PASS/PASS01195.

2.6. Proteomics Sample Preparation with Label-Free Quantification (LFQ)

Proteomics sample preparation was done according to a published protocol with minor modifications [34]. Three biological replicates of each patient and control fibroblast cell lines between the passages of 8–11 were harvested from T75 flasks and lysed under denaturing conditions in a buffer containing 6 M guanidinium chloride (GdmCl), 5 mM tris(2-carboxyethyl)phosphine, 20 mM chloroacetamide, and 50 mM Tris-HCl pH 8.5. Lysates were denatured at 95 °C for 15 min shaking at 800 rpm in a thermal shaker and sonicated in a water bath for 15 min. A small aliquot of cell lysate was used for the BCA assay to quantify the protein concentration. Lysates (100 µg proteins) were diluted with a dilution buffer containing 10% acetonitrile and 25 mM Tris-HCl, pH 8.5, to reach a 1 M GdmCl concentration. Then, proteins were digested with 2 µg LysC (MS-grade, Roche, enzyme to protein ratio 1:50) shaking at 800 rpm at 25 °C for 2 h. The digestion mixture was diluted again with the same dilution buffer to reach 0.5 M GdmCl. Then, 2 µg trypsin (MS-grade, Roche, enzyme to protein ratio 1:50) was added and the digestion mixture was incubated at 37 °C overnight in a thermal shaker at 800 rpm for 14 h. Solid phase extraction (SPE) disc cartridges (C18-SD, Waters, Milford, MA) were used for peptide desalting according to the manufacturer's instructions. Desalted peptides were reconstituted in 0.1% formic acid in water and further separated into four fractions by strong cation exchange chromatography (SCX, 3M Purification, Meriden, CT). Eluates were first dried in a SpeedVac, then dissolved in 20 µL 5% acetonitrile and 2% formic acid in water, briefly vortexed, and sonicated in a water bath for 30 seconds prior injection to nano-LC-MS.

2.7. LC-MS Instrument Settings for Shotgun Proteome Profiling and Data Analysis

LC-MS/MS was carried out by nanoflow reverse-phase liquid chromatography (Dionex Ultimate 3000, Thermo) coupled online to a Q-Exactive Plus Orbitrap mass spectrometer (Thermo). Briefly, the LC separation was performed using a PicoFrit analytical column (75 µm ID × 55 cm long, 15 µm Tip ID; New Objectives, Woburn, MA) in-house packed with 2.1 µm C18 resin (Reprosil-AQ Pur, Dr. Maisch, Ammerbuch, Germany). Peptides were eluted using a non-linear gradient from 2% to 40% solvent B over 101 min at a flow rate of 266 nL/min (solvent A: 99.9% water, 0.1% formic acid; solvent B: 79.9% acetonitrile, 20% water, 0.1% formic acid). 3.5 kilovolts were applied for nanoelectrospray ionization. A cycle of one full fourier transformation scan mass spectrum (300–1750 m/z, resolution of 60,000 at m/z 200, automatic gain control (AGC) target 1×10^6) was followed by 12 data-dependent MS/MS scans (200–2000 m/z, resolution of 30,000, AGC target 5×10^5, isolation window 2 m/z) with normalized collision energy of 25 eV. Target ions already selected for MS/MS were dynamically excluded for 15 s. In addition, only peptide charge states between two to eight were allowed.

Raw MS data were processed with MaxQuant software (v1.6.0.1) and searched against the human proteome database UniProtKB with 21,074 entries, released in December 2018. Parameters of MaxQuant database searching were a false discovery rate (FDR) of 0.01 for proteins and peptides, a minimum peptide length of seven amino acids, a first search mass tolerance for peptides of 20 ppm and a main search tolerance of 4.5 ppm, and using the function "match between runs". A maximum of two missed cleavages was allowed for the tryptic digest. Cysteine carbamidomethylation was set as fixed modification, while N-terminal acetylation and methionine oxidation were set as variable modifications. Contaminants, as well as proteins identified by site modification and proteins derived from the reversed part of the decoy database, were strictly excluded from further analysis. The MaxQuant processed output files can be found in Table S2, showing peptide and protein identification, accession numbers, percentage of sequence coverage of the protein, q-values, and LFQ intensities. The mass spectrometry data have been deposited to the ProteomeXchange Consortium (http://proteomecentral.proteomexchange.org) via the PRIDE partner repository [35] with the dataset identifier PXD009743.

2.8. Experimental Design, Statistical Rationale, Pathway, and Data Analyses

The correlation analysis of biological replicates and the calculation of significantly different metabolites and proteins were done with Perseus (v1.6.0.2). LFQ intensities, originating from at least two different peptides per protein group, were transformed by $\log_2$. Only protein groups with valid values within compared experiments were used for further data evaluation. Statistical analysis was done by a two-sample *t*-tests with Benjamini–Hochberg (BH, FDR of 0.05) correction for multiple testing. Significantly regulated metabolites and proteins between patients and controls were indicated by a plus sign in Tables S1 and S3.

One-way ANOVA with Tukey's multiple comparison test (significance level, alpha = 0.05) was performed using GraphPad Prism 5 to compare concentration ratios of reduced and oxidized glutathione (GSH/GSSG) in patients and controls, as well as data from live cell respiration assay.

For comprehensive proteome data analyses, we applied gene set enrichment analysis (GSEA, v2.2.3) [36] in order to see if a priori defined sets of proteins showed statistically significant, concordant differences between mutations and controls. All proteins with ratios calculated by Perseus were used for GSEA analysis. The Galaxy online tool (https://usegalaxy.org/) was used to calculate the average of the ratios of the few duplicate gene names. We used GSEA standard settings, except that the minimum size exclusion was set to 5 and Reactome v5.2 and KEGG v5.2 were used as gene set databases. The cutoff for significantly regulated pathways was set to be p-value ≤ 0.05 and FDR ≤ 0.05.

2.9. Simulations of Electron Transfer between the Iron–Sulfur Clusters of NDUFS1 and Prediction of Protein Stability of p.Phe124Leu in ND5

We have applied tunneling calculations of electron transfer between N4 and N5 iron–sulfur clusters of the NDUFS1 subunit and studied the consequences of mutations of the key residues involved in the process using a method described previously [37].

The change of the Gibbs free-energy gap, $\Delta\Delta G$, which measures the gain or loss of protein stability upon mutations, was calculated by the online tool STRUM for the p.Phe124Leu substitution in ND5 [38].

2.10. Measurement of Respiratory Chain Enzyme Activities

Sample preparation of muscle homogenates for the spectrophotometric assay of enzyme activities was done as reported previously [39–41].

2.11. Live Cell Respiration Assay by Seahorse XFe96

The operation and the calibration of sensor cartridges of the Seahorse XFe96 instrument were done according to the manufacturer's instructions. A pilot experiment was performed to optimize the cell number at seeding and the concentration of carbonyl cyanide-4-(trifluoromethoxy)phenylhydrazone (FCCP), an uncoupling agent of the mitochondrial electron transfer chain and the ATP synthase. In the final assay, fibroblasts were seeded at 40,000 cells per well and cultured under normoxic condition (5% CO_2) for 6 h in order to allow them to attach to the bottom of the culture plate. Then, the culture medium was replaced with the Seahorse assay medium and the plate was transferred to a non-CO_2 incubator for 45 min right before the start of the assay. The Mito Stress Test Kit (Agilent, #103015-100) and the Glycolytic Rate Assay Kit (Agilent, #103344-100) were used according to the user manuals. Inhibitor concentrations were used as followed: oligomycin (2 µM), FCCP (1.5 µM), rotenone (0.5 µM), antimycin (0.5 µM), and 2-deoxy-glucose (500 mM).

2.12. Blue Native PAGE, Western Blot, and In-Gel Activity Assay of CI

Fibroblasts were trypsinized, collected by centrifugation, and lysed in mitochondria isolation and storage buffer (83 mM sucrose, 3.3 mM Tris-HCl, pH 7.0, 0.3 mM ethylenediaminetetraacetic acid (EDTA), 1.7 mM 6-aminohexanoic acid, and protease inhibitor cocktails) by passing them through a needle (Ø 0.45 × 25 mm, 26 G × 1") 30 times on ice, on the basis of published protocols with minor modifications [42,43]. In brief, crude mitochondria fractions were solubilized with digitonin in a ratio of 10 µL 20% digitonin per 20 mg cell pellet. Next, 8 µg solubilized mitochondria per lane were loaded onto the precast NativePAGE 3%–12% gradient Bis-Tris protein gels (Thermo, # BN1001BOX) and run at 4 °C with pre-chilled buffers. The blue native PAGE was first run with the dark blue cathode buffer (0.02 % Coomassie Blue G-250) until the running front reached one-third of the gel length. Then, the light blue cathode buffer (0.002% Coomassie Blue G-250) was used to finish the gel running. The gel was further processed for western blot or in-gel activity assay of CI.

Immunodetection of OXPHOS enzymes on blue native gels was performed following an established protocol [43]. The antibodies used in western blot were anti-NDUFS1 (Proteintech, Rosemont, IL, USA, # 12444-1-AP) and all others were purchased from Merck: anti-NDUFS2 (# SAB2702088), anti-NDUFB8 (# HPA003886), anti-UQCRC2 (# HPA007998), and anti-SDHB (# HPA002868).

In-gel activity assays of CI were conducted as described previously [43]. Briefly, blue native gels were incubated in the assay buffer directly after electrophoresis. One half of the gel piece was cut out and incubated in the assay buffer for 1 hour and documented. The other half, as an identical replicate, was stained with Coomassie G-250 following a published protocol [44].

2.13. Protein Sequence Alignment

Protein sequences of NDUFS1 and ND5 were aligned using T-Coffee [45] and visualized in Espript 3.0 [46].

3. Results

3.1. Substituted Amino Acids in ND5 and NDUFS1 are Highly Conserved from Bacteria to Human

A protein sequence alignment across multiple species showed a highly conserved phenylalanine at position 124 in the subunit ND5, which was substituted to leucine in one patient (Figure S1A). The heteroplasmy level of this mutation was 70% in cultivated skin fibroblasts, which is in agreement with other reports, displaying a very severe phenotype [25–27]. Furthermore, Phe124 is localized in the fourth transmembrane helix of subunit ND5, which is close to the proposed proton translocation channel [27] and thus may influence its structure and catalytic function. In the other patient, two highly conserved amino acids, valine at position 228 and aspartate at position 252, were substituted to alanine and glycine in NDUFS1, respectively (Figure S1B). Val228 is located between the two iron–sulfur clusters N4 and N5 in subunit NDUFS1 (protein data bank, PDB: 5XTD, human CI).

3.2. Metabolome Profiling Revealed a Decrease of the GSH/GSSG Ratio in Both Patients

To quantify relative differences in metabolite changes and to elucidate key metabolic alterations caused by mutating the *MT-ND5* and *NDUFS1* genes, we applied a targeted liquid chromatography-mass spectrometry (LC-MS/MS) approach based on multiple reaction monitoring (MRM) [33]. In total, 121 metabolites were quantified relatively (Table S1). The Pearson correlation coefficients were highly similar, ranging from 0.968 to 0.996 in the controls, 0.984 to 0.996 in the *MT-ND5* mutation, and 0.985 to 0.991 in the *NDUFS1* mutations (Figure S2), suggesting a very good quality of the metabolite data sets. Statistical analysis by an unpaired two-sample *t*-test identified significantly regulated metabolites, and six of them were significant after Benjamini–Hochberg (BH, FDR ≤ 0.05) correction for multiple testing (*p*-value ≤ 0.05) in the *MT-ND5* mutation versus controls (Figure 1A). In the case of the *NDUFS1* mutations, 11 significant metabolites were found after the *t*-test and six were identified upon BH correction (*p*-value ≤ 0.05, FDR ≤ 0.05) (Figure 1B). Interestingly, the same metabolites were found to be significantly regulated in both patients.

Glutathione (GSH) was the metabolite with the highest decrease in both patients (12-fold in ND5, 16-fold in NDUFS1, Figure 1A,B). In contrast, oxidized glutathione (GSSG) levels were increased in both patients. The ratio between reduced and oxidized glutathione (GSH/GSSG ratio) can be used as a marker for the redox status of a cell [47–49]. The concentration ratios of GSH/GSSG between patients and controls decreased significantly (more than 35-fold) for both patients' fibroblast cells (Figure 2), thus indicating a higher level of oxidative stress. Furthermore, the polyamine N-acetylputerescine was significantly increased in both patients, also indicative for higher stress levels [50,51].

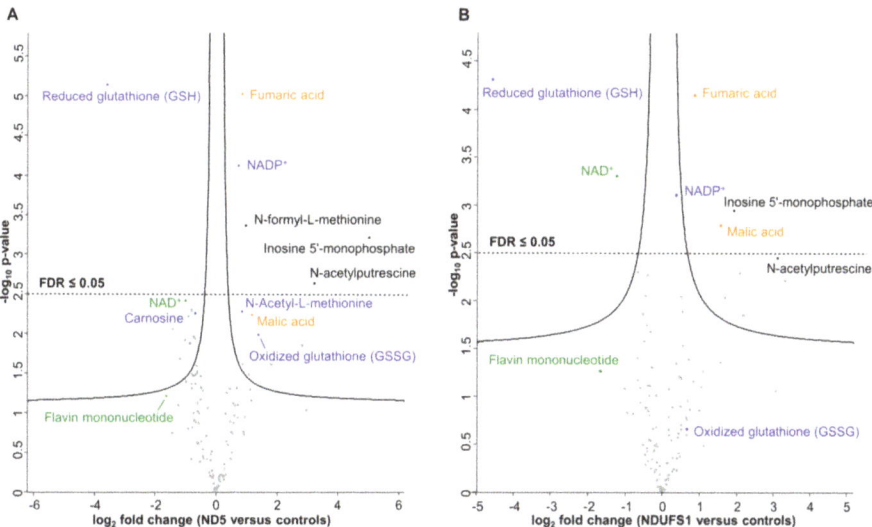

Figure 1. Significantly regulated metabolites between mutated *MT-ND5* and *NDUFS1* versus controls, respectively. (**A**) Abundance ratios of metabolites between mutated *MT-ND5* and controls. (**B**) Abundance ratios of metabolites between mutated *NDUFS1* and controls. Metabolites above the solid lines were considered significant after the *t*-test. Metabolites above the dashed horizontal line were significant after Benjamini–Hochberg correction (false discovery rate (FDR) ≤0.05) for multiple testing. Log$_2$ fold changes were plotted against the -Log10 (*p*-value). Blue: metabolites involved in cellular oxidative stress response; orange: metabolites of the TCA cycle; green: CI-related metabolites.

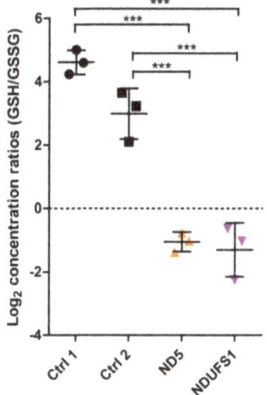

Figure 2. Reduced and oxidized glutathione (GSH/GSSG) ratios of controls, ND5, and NDUFS1 mutant fibroblast cells. The log$_2$ concentration ratios (GSH/GSSG) were compared between patients and controls. One-way ANOVA of log$_2$ ratios was performed (*p*-value < 0.001, labeled as ***). Error bars: mean ± SD.

3.3. The TCA Cycle Metabolites—Fumaric and Malic Acid—Significantly Increased in Both Patients

Malate and fumarate are two TCA cycle intermediates that were significantly upregulated in both patients. Similar findings have been reported in patients' urine samples [52]. Lactic acid, which is converted from pyruvate, was elevated twofold in both patients. This is in concordance with frequently observed lactic acidosis in patient blood [53]. The ability of CI to oxidize NADH in both patients seems to be limited and, as a consequence, the level of NAD$^+$ was found to be significantly reduced (Figure 1A,B).

Furthermore, flavin mononucleotide (FMN) and riboflavin (vitamin B2, a precursor of FMN) were both decreased threefold in patient fibroblasts carrying the *MT-ND5* mutation. FMN is a prosthetic group of mitochondrial CI and accepts electrons from NADH.

The metabolome survey identified that the same metabolites were significantly regulated in both patients. These metabolites, such as GSH, GSSG, NAD$^+$, NADP$^+$, FMN, malate, and fumarate, are all directly or indirectly involved in, or dependent on the functionality of CI.

3.4. Proteome Profiling

Fibroblasts harboring the *MT-ND5* and *NDUFS1* mutations were compared to two individual healthy controls in triplicates by label-free quantification (LFQ) in a total of 60 LC-MS/MS runs. We identified more than 5363 protein groups with at least two peptides per protein group (Table S2). We then compared both mutations individually to controls and filtered for 100% valid values in at least one group and replaced missing values from the normal distribution. This resulted in a total of 4030 protein groups for the *MT-ND5* patient and 3893 for the *NDUFS1* patient versus controls (Table S3).

The reproducibility of the biological replicates was tested by Pearson correlation and visualized in a multi-scatter plot for all experiments. The Pearson correlation coefficients were highly similar, ranging from 0.959 to 0.994 in controls, 0.989 to 0.992 in the *MT-ND5* mutation, and 0.988 to 0.994 in the *NDUFS1* biallelic mutations (Figure S3), indicating very robust replicates.

Statistical analysis by an unpaired two-sample *t*-test identified 1535 significant proteins and 1090 significantly regulated proteins after Benjamini–Hochberg (BH) correction for multiple testing (p-value ≤ 0.05, FDR ≤ 0.05) in the *MT-ND5* mutation versus controls, as visualized in a volcano plot (Figure 3A). In the case of the *NDUFS1* mutations, 324 significantly deregulated proteins were found after the *t*-test, and 145 were identified upon BH correction (p-value ≤ 0.05, FDR ≤ 0.05) (Figure 3B).

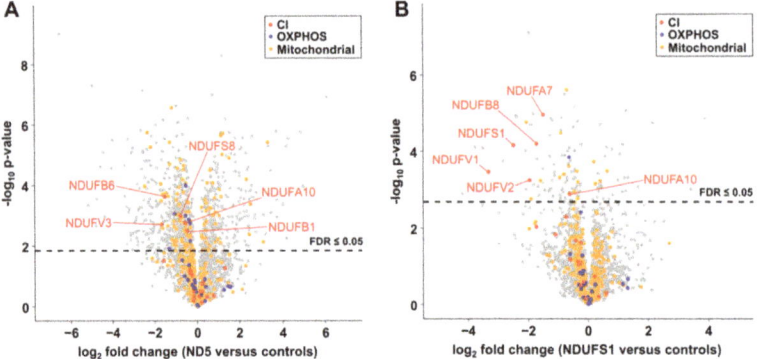

Figure 3. *Cont.*

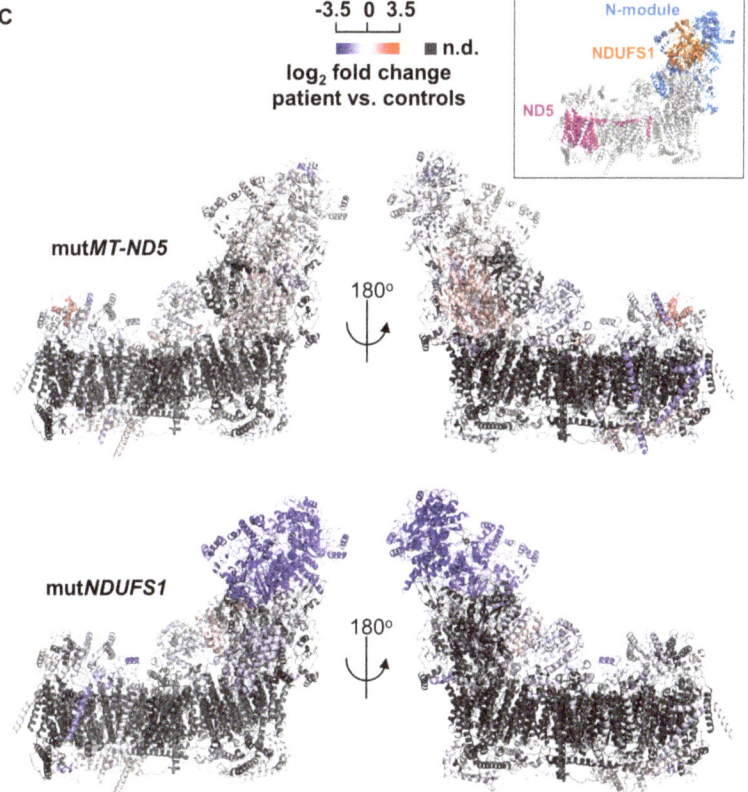

Figure 3. Abundance ratios of CI subunits mapped onto the CryoEM structure of human CI, PDB: 5XTD. (**A**) Protein abundance ratios between mutND5 and controls. Mitochondrial proteins according to Human MitoCarta2.0 are shown in orange, OXPHOS proteins in blue, and CI subunits in red. The dotted line indicated the threshold of significance (FDR ≤0.05) in the two-sample *t*-test after Benjamini–Hochberg correction. Protein names are presented for significantly regulated CI subunits. (**B**) Protein abundance ratios between mutNDUFS1 and controls. Same legend as in (**A**). (**C**) The mutation in *MT-ND5* did not lead to a general change of the abundance of CI subunits, but a specific loss of the N-module was identified in the *NDUFS1* patient. The inset indicates the relative position of the N-module, NDUFS1, and ND5 in CI. n.d., no data.

3.5. Gene Set Enrichment Analyses Reveal Glycolysis is Upregulated in the MT-ND5 Mutation and the Respiratory Chain is Down-Regulated in the NDUFS1 Mutations

We applied the pathway enrichment tool GSEA to assess whether a priori defined sets of proteins showed statistically significant, concordant differences between *MT-ND5* and *NDUFS1* versus controls, respectively. Pathways with significant *p*-values (≤0.05) and FDR q-values (≤0.05) are listed in Tables S4 and S5. In the patient with the *MT-ND5* mutation, pathways comprising proteins of the cytoskeleton, the extracellular matrix, cytosolic tRNA aminoacylation, and glycolysis and gluconeogenesis were significantly upregulated (Table S4).

Many structural and cytoskeleton proteins were enriched in the *MT-ND5* patient, such as myosins MYL9 and MYLK, actin ACTA2, tropomyosins, TPM1, CALD1, MYL6, TPM4, FN1, and collagens, reflected in the respective pathways of muscle contraction, focal adhesion, and collagen formation.

The pathway "cell cycle" was significantly down-regulated in cells harboring the *MT-ND5* mutation, including six of the proteins of the mini-chromosome maintenance complex (MCM) responsible for DNA replication, (threefold, see Table S4).

In the case of the patient with *NDUFS1* mutations, the pathway including cytoskeleton components was only significantly increased at a nominal *p*-value (Table S5).

The respiratory electron chain was the only significantly down-regulated pathway in the patient carrying *NDUFS1* mutations (Table S5). To further shed light on the substructures of CI, we performed a pathway analysis with manually created gene lists for all modules of CI. This analysis identified a significant and specific decrease only in the N-module ($p \leq 0.001$, q-value ≤ 0.05, Table S5), including the subunits NDUFA7 (threefold), NDUFV2 (fourfold), NDUFS1 (sixfold), and NDUFV1 (tenfold) (Figure 3B).

To visualize this dysregulation, all protein abundance ratios of CI subunits between patients and controls were mapped in a three dimensional structure of CI (PDB: 5XTD). The inlet indicated the position of subunit ND5 and NDUFS1 in CI (Figure 3C). Indeed, the N-module in the *NDUFS1* patient was the only region to be severely reduced, whereas the *MT-ND5* patient showed no changes (Figure 3C). This indicated that the stability of the entire N-module was affected, most likely because of fast degradation of misfolded or not integrated subunits of CI.

3.6. The Rate of Electron Tunneling between the Iron–Sulfur Clusters N4 and N5 of NDUFS1 Was Predicted to Decrease Dramatically in a V228A Mutant

We examined the electron transfer between the iron–sulfur clusters N4 and N5 in subunit NDUFS1 using the method of tunneling current theory, as was previously described for a bacterial enzyme [37]. It revealed that the residue Val228 was critical for bridging the electron transfer between the N4 and N5 clusters, as electrons tunnelled primarily through this relatively bulky residue. Our simulations for an ovine enzyme showed that the mutation p.Val205Ala, with a smaller alanine substitution, had a dramatic effect on the rate of electron transfer by reducing it by 35-fold (Figure 4). It is interesting that the effect of mutation of this critical valine residue was predicted to occur earlier in *Thermus thermophilus* [37]. These changes were predicted to occur in the remaining small fraction of fully assembled CI.

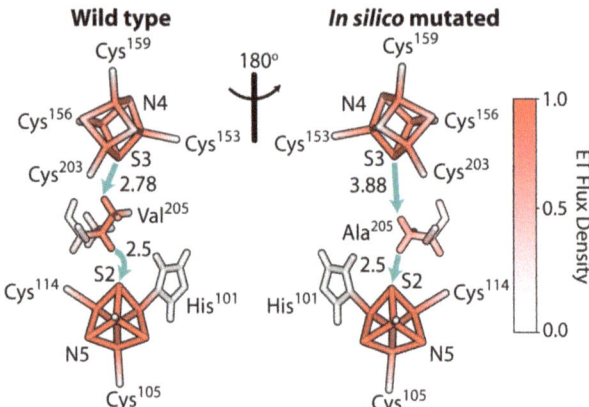

Figure 4. Electron tunneling pathway of the electron transfer reaction between iron–sulfur clusters N4→N5 of the wild-type and *in silico* mutated CI in *Ovis aries*, PDB 5LNK. Solid blue arrows indicate through-space jumps in the primary electron tunneling pathways. Through-space distances in Ångstrom are shown next to the arrows. Relative color density indicates the contribution of the corresponding atom/bond in electron transfer reaction. The mutation resulted in a reduced rate of electron transfer $k_{ET}^{WT}/k_{ET}^{V205A} = 35$ for the ovine enzyme.

3.7. Decreased Stability of CI in Mutated NDUFS1 Prevents the Formation of Supercomplexes

To elucidate the consequences of the specific loss of the N-module in the mutated *NDUFS1* cell line for the formation of supercomplexes, we solubilized OXPHOS proteins under mild conditions using digitonin, and performed blue native PAGE followed by western blot. Only a small fraction of supercomplexes were formed compared to controls (Figure 5A–D). In addition, a major part of CIII was not incorporated into supercomplexes, which was the stoichiometric assembly of CI, III, and IV (Figure 5D). In contrast, no assembly errors were identified in the *MT-ND5* patient. Succinate dehydrogenase (complex II, CII) was used as a loading control and showed no differences between samples (Figure 5E).

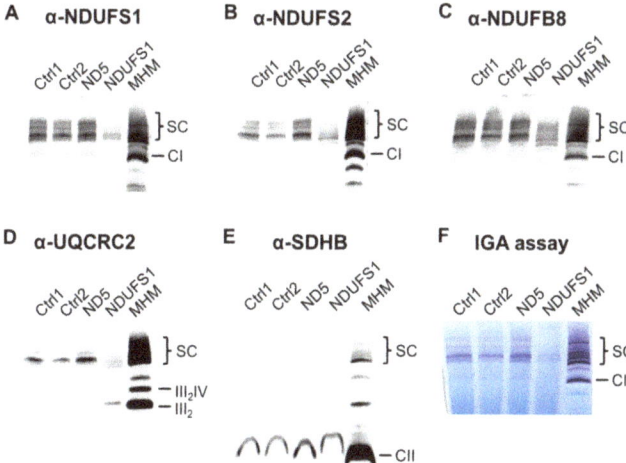

Figure 5. Formation of respiratory chain supercomplexes and in-gel activity assay of CI. Blue native PAGE and western blot detection of respiratory chain enzymes solubilized with digitonin. (**A**) Antibody against NDUFS1, a core subunit of the N-module in CI; (**B**) antibody against NDUFS2, a core subunit of the Q-module in CI; (**C**) antibody against NDUFB8, an accessary subunit of the P-module in CI; (**D**) antibody against UQCRC2, a core subunit of CIII; (**E**) antibody against SDHB, a subunit of complex II (CII), which serves as a loading control. (**F**) In-gel activity assay (IGA) of CI. Ctrl: control; MHM: mouse heart mitochondria, as molecular weight marker and positive control; SC: supercomplexes; III, complex III (CIII); IV, complex IV (CIV).

To test the functionality of the partly assembled respirasome, an in-gel activity assay of CI was performed and revealed that there was almost no enzymatic activity in the patient with *NDUFS1* mutations (Figure 5F).

3.8. Isolated CI Deficiency in Both Patients

Enzymatic measurements of the respiratory chain enzymes and citrate synthase (CS) were performed in the homogenates of muscle biopsies for both patients [40,54]. These were normalized to CS and were compared to reference values (Table 1) [31]. In both cases, the CI enzyme activity was below the reference values, while all other complexes showed values within the range of the references, indicating an isolated CI deficiency.

3.9. Live Cell Respiration Assays Revealed a Low Oxygen Consumption Rate in Both Patients

The respiration rate measurements in live cells (Figure 6A) elucidated that the basal respiration, ATP-linked respiration, maximal respiration, and the spare respiration capacity were less than 50% compared with controls (Figure 6C–F). In contrast, the basal glycolysis rate was significantly higher

(p-value ≤ 0.05) in patients than in the controls (Figure 6G). The glycoPER (Figure 6B), which is the PER (proton efflux rate) contributed by glycolysis, was significantly higher (p-value ≤ 0.05) in the patients (Figure 6H,I). Thus, a clear metabolic shift from aerobic respiration to glycolysis was observed in both mutated cell lines (Figure 6J), which is in concordance with our proteomics data for the patient with the *MT-ND5* mutation, where the glycolytic pathway was upregulated.

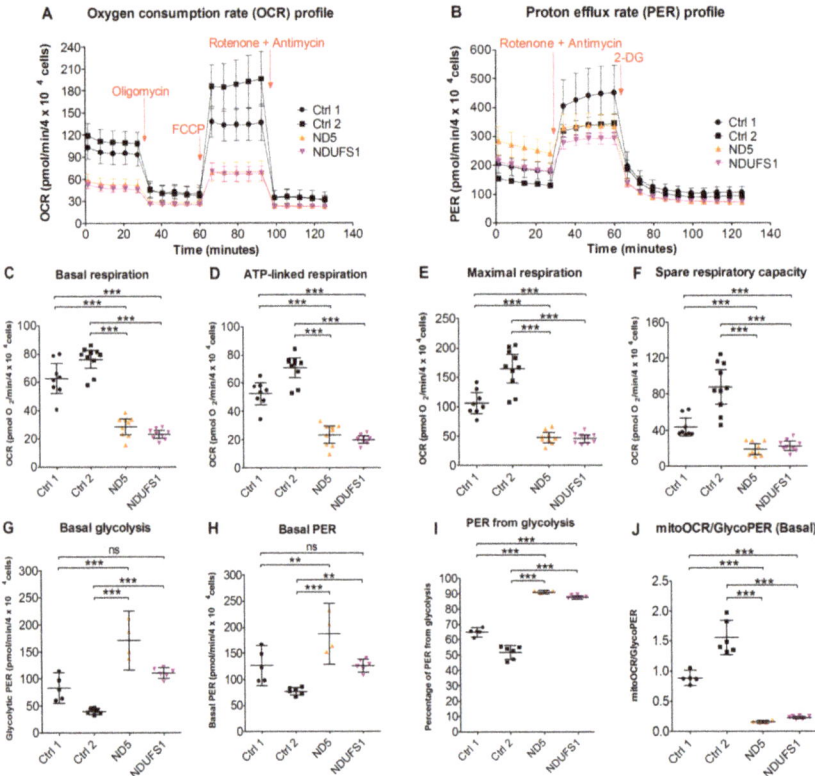

Figure 6. Cellular respiration assays showing mitochondrial dysfunction and increased glycolytic activities in both patients. (**A**) Oxygen consumption rate profile. (**B**) Proton efflux rate (PER) profile. (**C**) Basal respiration rate at the beginning of the assay. (**D**) ATP-linked respiration before the addition of the inhibitors. (**E**) Maximal respiration after carbonyl cyanide-4-(trifluoromethoxy)phenylhydrazone (FCCP) was added. (**F**) Calculated spare respiratory capacity. (**G**) Basal glycolysis rate at the beginning of the assay. (**H**) Total PER before the addition of the inhibitors. (**I**) Percentage of PER from glycolysis. (**J**) The ratio between mitochondrial oxygen consumption rate (OCR) and glycolytic PER as an indicator of the cellular energetic profile. Error bars: (**A**) and (**B**): mean ± SD; (**C–J**): mean ± 95% confidence intervals. One-way ANOVA: p-value < 0.01 (******); p-value < 0.001 (*******); ns, not significant.

4. Discussion

Mitochondrial dysfunction is the most common type of metabolic disorder and can be caused by either mitochondrial or nuclear gene mutations. Here, we applied proteome and metabolome profiling to reveal the molecular consequences of gene mutations in *NDUFS1* and *MT-ND5*, which respectively encode for the two core subunits in the hydrophilic and transmembrane arms of CI.

4.1. Specific Disassembly of the N-Module and the Entire Respirasome in Mutated NDUFS1

Our proteome screening indicated a specific loss of the entire N-module for the *NDUFS1* patient (Figure 3C). For validation, we applied BN-PAGE in combination with western blot to reveal a disrupted assembly for CI. An in-gel activity assay showed a missing band only in this patient, which may either derive from a diminished stability of CI or by the lack of FMN in the protein (Figure 5F). The CI N-module consisted of three core subunits, NDUFS1, NDUFV1, and NDUFV2, which were encoded by nuclear genes and accommodate the FMN prosthetic group, as well as the iron–sulfur clusters N1a, N3, N1b, N4, and N5 [55,56]. The N-module in the patient with mutated *NDUFS1* hence disintegrated easily, resulting in strongly reduced amounts of fully assembled CI, causative for to the observed enzymatic dysfunction. The homozygous mutation p.Asp252Gly in NDUFS1 alone was shown to cause the disassembly of CI in a patient with mild cavitating leukoencephalopathy [30]. Recent studies support a model that functional modules of CI are first assembled independently and then gradually form a mature CI, in which the N-module joins in the final step [57–59]. Over the past two decades, several possible formations of structures for respiratory chain supercomplexes have been identified and resolved at high resolution [60–66]. It has been reported that about 80–90% of the CI population is indeed bound to other OXPHOS complexes in stoichiometry to form supercomplexes (SC), which is named the mitochondrial respirasome and is composed of CI, CIII and CIV [67–69]. The formation of SC was severely reduced in the *NDUFS1* patient compared with the controls (Figure 5A–D). This was further confirmed by the detection of large amounts of individual CIII, which could not be assembled into a mature SC in the *NDUFS1* patient (Figure 5D). Whether the formation of respirasomes indeed enhances the efficiency of electron transfer and minimizes the electron leakage and thus ROS production is still controversially debated [63,64,70,71]. It can be concluded that the N-module disintegrated easily due to the substitutions of two amino acids in the *NDUFS1* patient, which severely affected the maturation and structural stability of CI and, hence, the formation of SC.

4.2. Disruption of The Electron Flow in Mutated NDUFS1

In the patient with *NDUFS1* mutations, the valine at position 228 was changed to alanine. This valine was located between the iron–sulfur cluster N4 and N5 (Figure 4). A previous study modeled the effect of this Val232Gly substitution in bacterial CI and showed that the "Y"-shaped side chain of valine is crucial as a bridge for electron transfer between N4 and N5. The replacement of valine to glycine caused a decrease in the electron transfer efficiency to about one-thousandth in bacterial CI [37]. Our *in silico* modeling of the ovine enzyme with the specific substitution p.Val205Ala again confirmed the dramatically reduced electron transfer, which was expected in the *NDUFS1* patient. The decreased rate of electron transfer between the N4 and N5 clusters should affect the overall rate of electron transfer from NADH via FMN and iron–sulfur clusters to Co-Q10 in CI, with an elevated level of FMN in its reduced state and a consequential increase in the level of ROS production by the enzyme [72–75]. Therefore, both defects, the Val228Ala substitution disrupting electron transfer between the N4 and N5 clusters and the partial disintegration of the N-module due to the Asp252Gly substitution [30], might be the cause of the elevated ROS production, indicated by the decreased GSH/GSSG ratio in the patient (Figure 2). Elevated ROS has been reported in cells with CI assembly defects previously [76]. The reported case, carrying only the p.Asp252Gly substitution, presented a very mild phenotype [30], indicating that the additional interruption of the electron flow between N4 and N5 in our case significantly contributed to the severity of the phenotype.

Regarding tunneling calculations, however, several important points should be mentioned. The change of electron transfer coupling between N4 and N5 was quite significant in all enzymes that we have examined. However, given all the uncertainties in the structure, and difficulties of theoretical modeling of FeS clusters, these results should be regarded only as qualitative trends. It was also recognized that a slower electron transfer rate will only be important if this is the rate-determining step. Furthermore, we cannot exclude that additional water molecules will occupy the mutated site, possibly changing the rates of electron transfer. Generally, it should be recognized that the accurate quantitative predictions on human enzymes is still a significant challenge. However, the calculated dramatic disruption of electronic coupling reported here, and in the emerging picture, appears to be in agreement with overall experimental evidence collected in this work on the NDUFS1 mutant.

4.3. The Stalling of Proton Translocation in Mutated ND5 Is Assumed to Stop Electron Flow Without Any Consequences for Respirasome Formation

In contrast, the other patient with the MT-ND5 mutation, harboring a heteroplasmy level of 70%, had a fully assembled CI (Figure 5). The amino acid substitution in the ND5 subunit, which was located on the distal end of the transmembrane arm, thus had no effect on the assembly of CI. The crystal structure of CI suggests that a unique, out-of-the-membrane quinone-reaction chamber enables redox energy to drive concerted long-range conformational changes, resulting in the translocation of four protons upon oxidation of one NADH molecule [77–79]. A study in *Escherichia coli* showed that amino acid substitutions close to the proton translocation channel indeed reduced the functionality of CI [80]. Thus, we expect that the proton pumping activity in the MT-ND5 patient to be impaired in a similar way. In silico modeling of this effect by the online tool STRUM, a structure-based prediction of protein stability changes upon single-point mutation [38], indeed showed increased stability for the p.Phe124Leu mutation in subunit ND5. Hence, the stabilizing effect of this mutation for the proton channel might hamper its functionality by losing its flexibility. However, the details of the conformational coupling to electron flow remain unknown. It is worth mentioning that the mutation in proton pumping regions hindering electron transfer far away is one of the marvels of CI, and this has been demonstrated by earlier experiments on isolated proteins. One can argue that if the MT-ND5 mutation indeed results in disrupted conformational coupling and affects the electron transfer chain, the immediate consequence of this may be an elevated production of ROS, either by reduced FMN or by a reversed electron transfer mechanism [81–84].

4.4. A Similar Pattern of Regulated Metabolites Was Identified in Both Patients, Mainly for ROS Defense and TCA Cycle Metabolites

Interestingly, an almost identical set of significantly regulated metabolites was identified in both patients (Figure 1). The shortage of NAD^+ may reflect the deficiency of CI, one of the major consumers that oxidizes NADH and generates NAD^+. We further want to mention that an imbalance of the $NADH/NAD^+$ ratio in itself may affect all aspects of impaired metabolism [85,86]. A stable $NADH/NAD^+$ ratio is critical toward maintaining the homeostasis of metabolic process in both the cytoplasm and mitochondria [85,87]. An increased $NADH/NAD^+$ ratio might thus affect the TCA cycle, since previous studies have shown that the inhibition of CI increased succinate oxidation rates [33,88]. The TCA cycle is primarily regulated by product feedback inhibition by NADH and by ADP/ATP and $NAD^+/NADH$ ratios [89]. The lack of NAD^+, required for the conversion of malate to oxaloacetate, resulted in the elevated malate levels. Secondary metabolic alterations caused by CI deficiency were found previously in urine and may play an important role in the pathogenesis of CI deficiency [52]. Fumaric, malic, and also lactic acid, were found to be dramatically increased in some patients' urine, matching our cell culture results [53]. We therefore believe that NADH cannot efficiently transfer electrons to CI, either because of disassembly or because of dramatic disruption of the electron tunneling flow, and thus a jam of unused NADH was created, leading to dysregulation of these TCA cycle metabolites.

The N-module of CI binds and oxidizes NADH and generates two electrons that are transferred through FMN and seven iron–sulfur clusters to ubiquinone in the Q-module [24]. The fundamental role of FMN for the enzymatic functionality of CI has been demonstrated for specific mutations within the FMN docking side carrying subunit NDUFV1. Mutants lacking FMN were fully assembled, but enzymatically inactive [90]. FMN was diminished threefold in both of our cases and previously in rotenone inhibited cells [33], indicating that the electron transfer to quinone was interrupted. It has been reported for both prokaryotes and eukaryotes that the non-covalently bonded prosthetic group

FMN dissociated reversibly from CI when the later one was reduced by NADH and no suitable electron acceptor was available [91,92]. The dissociation of FMN was proposed as a protective mechanism to decrease ROS production [92], as FMN was shown to be a direct site for superoxide radical formation in the CI N-module [73,74,93,94].

Mitochondria are a major source for ROS [81], which can be eliminated by ROS scavengers such as glutathione (GSH) [95]. Apparently, the more than 35-fold decrease in the GSH/GSSG ratio observed in both patients (Figure 2) was a strong indicator of elevated ROS levels because of a stalled electron flow. In addition, N-acetylputrescine, the inactive form of putrescine, was significantly increased in both patients. Putrescine is known to be a main ROS scavenger as well [50,51].

4.5. CI Deficiency Leads to a Glycolytic Phenotype

The cell respiration assay confirmed that both patients were indeed more glycolytic in their bioenergetics profiles, compared with the two controls (Figure 6B). The oxygen consumption rate (OCR) linked with ATP synthesis showed severe decreases in both patients' fibroblasts (Figure 6D), which confirmed the dysfunction of the mitochondrial OXPHOS caused by CI mutations. This was in agreement with the clinical data from patient muscle biopsies, in which the CI activities were found to be below the reference range and matched the elevated lactate levels in the fibroblasts and plasma samples of the patients (Table 1). Furthermore, the maximal and spare respiration capacities were significantly lower in both patients (Figure 6E,F). In order to compensate for the mitochondrial shortage of ATP, the patients' cells exhibited an increased rate of glycolysis, as indicated by the glycolysis-contributed proton efflux rate measurement (glycoPER, Figure 6G).

4.6. Accumulation of Structural Proteins in Patients

An increase of proteins involved in the cytoskeleton and the extracellular matrix (ECM) was found in both patients, in agreement with the diagnosis of ventricular hypertrophic cardiomyopathy in the *MT-ND5* patient. CI deficiency frequently resulted in remodeling of the extracellular matrix, causing cardiomyopathy [96–98]. A relationship between a compromised respiratory chain and alterations in structural proteins has been shown previously [99], and OXPHOS deficiencies have also been linked to the development of hypertrophic cardiomyopathy [100]. Thus, our proteome survey indicated that an insufficient cellular bioenergetic status led to an increase in the ECM and cytoskeletal mass, but further studies are necessary to provide mechanistic links.

5. Conclusions

We have characterized the molecular consequences of two distinct CI mutations that result in the stalling of electron flow within CI by two different mechanisms. In the *NDUFS1* patient, destabilization of the N-module and, in addition, an interruption of electron tunneling between the iron–sulfur clusters N4–N5 of the remaining assembled CI was observed. In the *MT-ND5* patient, a dysfunctional proton channel might be less efficient to translocate protons utilizing the energy provided by the electron transfer. The interruption of the electron flow led to electron leakage and, in turn, to increased ROS generation, as seen by the reduced GSH/GSSG ratios in both cases. Furthermore, the isolated CI deficiency induced a metabolic switch towards a glycolytic phenotype, and the imbalance of the $NADH/NAD^+$ ratio caused an identical feedback on the regulation of TCA cycle metabolites in both mutations.

Supplementary Materials: The following are available online at http://www.mdpi.com/2073-4409/8/10/1149/s1, Figure S1: Protein sequence alignment of ND5 and NDUFS1. Mutated amino acids in patients were indicated with red triangles. Secondary structure elements are shown above the alignments. (**A**) Sequence alignments for ND5. (**B**) Sequence alignments for NDUFS1. Figure S2: Pearson correlation of MRM-targeted metabolome data among patients and controls. Correlation coefficients are shown in the squares. Ctrl, control; rep, replicate. Figure S3: Pearson correlation of label-free quantification (LFQ) proteome data among patients and controls. Correlation coefficients are shown in the squares. Ctrl, control; rep, replicate. Table S1: Identified metabolite ratios between patients and controls. Fold changes for each metabolite and Benjamini–Hochberg (BH) corrected two-sample *t*-test values are indicated. Table S2: MaxQuant output file featuring the proteome profiles of fibroblasts harboring the *MT-ND5* and *NDUFS1* mutations, as well as healthy controls with LFQ intensities. Table S3: Proteome analysis by Perseus with fold changes between mutations versus controls and two-sample *t*-test significances. Table S4: Gene set enrichment analysis (GSEA) report of all upregulated (sheet 1) and downregulated (sheet 2) pathways in the patient carrying the *MT-ND5* mutation. The significant threshold was set to *p*-value ≤ 0.05, FDR ≤0.05, and is highlighted in green. Table S5: GSEA report of all upregulated (sheet 1) and downregulated (sheet 2) pathways in the patient carrying the *NDUFS1* mutations. The significant threshold was set to *p*-value ≤ 0.05, FDR ≤0.05, and is highlighted in green. Table S6: Mass spectrometry transition settings for metabolites and MRM ion ratios. RT of 0 min indicates that the metabolite was measured continuously because of the long elution time of the compound.

Author Contributions: Y.N. performed the experiments, analyzed the data, and prepared the figures. D.M. conceived the study. Y.N. and D.M. wrote the paper. M.A.H. and A.A.S. modeled the electron tunneling. J.A.M. provided enzymatic analyses of muscle biopsies. V.K. performed organic acid analysis and took care of a patient.

Funding: This research was supported by the NIH grant GM054052 to A.A.S.

Acknowledgments: We appreciate David Stroud (University of Melbourne, Australia) for providing the Python script to prepare Figure 3. We thank Rainer Glauben (Charité - Universitätsmedizin Berlin) for kindly sharing the Seahorse XFe96 Analyzer. We also wish to thank the referees for a number of insightful suggestions. Our work is supported by the Max Planck Society. The work in UC Davis (A.A.S. and M.A.H.) was supported by the NIH grant GM054052.

Conflicts of Interest: The authors declare no conflict of interest.

References

1. Zickermann, V.; Wirth, C.; Nasiri, H.; Siegmund, K.; Schwalbe, H.; Hunte, C.; Brandt, U. Mechanistic insight from the crystal structure of mitochondrial complex I. *Science* **2015**, *347*, 44–49. [CrossRef] [PubMed]
2. Zhu, J.; Vinothkumar, K.R.; Hirst, J. Structure of mammalian respiratory complex I. *Nature* **2016**, *536*, 354–358. [CrossRef] [PubMed]
3. Fiedorczuk, K.; Letts, J.A.; Degliesposti, G.; Kaszuba, K.; Skehel, M.; Sazanov, L.A. Atomic structure of the entire mammalian mitochondrial complex I. *Nature* **2016**, *538*, 406–410. [CrossRef] [PubMed]
4. Carroll, J.; Fearnley, I.M.; Skehel, J.M.; Shannon, R.J.; Hirst, J.; Walker, J.E. Bovine complex I is a complex of 45 different subunits. *J. Biol. Chem.* **2006**, *281*, 32724–32727. [CrossRef] [PubMed]
5. Carroll, J.; Fearnley, I.M.; Shannon, R.J.; Hirst, J.; Walker, J.E. Analysis of the subunit composition of complex I from bovine heart mitochondria. *Mol. Cell. Proteomics MCP* **2003**, *2*, 117–126. [CrossRef] [PubMed]
6. Letts, J.A.; Degliesposti, G.; Fiedorczuk, K.; Skehel, M.; Sazanov, L.A. Purification of ovine respiratory complex I results in a highly active and stable preparation. *J. Biol. Chem.* **2016**, *291*, 24657–24675. [CrossRef]
7. Alston, C.L.; Rocha, M.C.; Lax, N.Z.; Turnbull, D.M.; Taylor, R.W. The genetics and pathology of mitochondrial disease. *J. Pathol.* **2017**, *241*, 236–250. [CrossRef] [PubMed]
8. Tuppen, H.A.; Blakely, E.L.; Turnbull, D.M.; Taylor, R.W. Mitochondrial DNA mutations and human disease. *Biochim. Biophys. Acta* **2010**, *1797*, 113–128. [CrossRef]
9. Wallace, D.C.; Zheng, X.X.; Lott, M.T.; Shoffner, J.M.; Hodge, J.A.; Kelley, R.I.; Epstein, C.M.; Hopkins, L.C. Familial mitochondrial encephalomyopathy (MERRF): Genetic, pathophysiological, and biochemical characterization of a mitochondrial DNA disease. *Cell* **1988**, *55*, 601–610. [CrossRef]
10. Wallace, D.C.; Singh, G.; Lott, M.T.; Hodge, J.A.; Schurr, T.G.; Lezza, A.M.; Elsas, L.J., 2nd; Nikoskelainen, E.K. Mitochondrial DNA mutation associated with Leber's hereditary optic neuropathy. *Science* **1988**, *242*, 1427–1430. [CrossRef]
11. Holt, I.J.; Harding, A.E.; Morgan-Hughes, J.A. Deletions of muscle mitochondrial DNA in patients with mitochondrial myopathies. *Nature* **1988**, *331*, 717–719. [CrossRef] [PubMed]
12. Stenton, S.L.; Prokisch, H. Advancing genomic approaches to the molecular diagnosis of mitochondrial disease. *Essays Biochem.* **2018**, *62*, 399–408. [CrossRef] [PubMed]
13. Mayr, J.A.; Haack, T.B.; Freisinger, P.; Karall, D.; Makowski, C.; Koch, J.; Feichtinger, R.G.; Zimmermann, F.A.; Rolinski, B.; Ahting, U.; et al. Spectrum of combined respiratory chain defects. *J. Inherit. Metab. Dis.* **2015**, *38*, 629–640. [CrossRef] [PubMed]
14. Schaefer, A.M.; Taylor, R.W.; Turnbull, D.M.; Chinnery, P.F. The epidemiology of mitochondrial disorders—Past, present and future. *Biochim. Biophys. Acta* **2004**, *1659*, 115–120. [CrossRef] [PubMed]
15. Skladal, D.; Halliday, J.; Thorburn, D.R. Minimum birth prevalence of mitochondrial respiratory chain disorders in children. *Brain J. Neurol.* **2003**, *126*, 1905–1912. [CrossRef] [PubMed]

16. Fassone, E.; Rahman, S. Complex I deficiency: Clinical features, biochemistry and molecular genetics. *J. Med. Genet.* **2012**, *49*, 578–590. [CrossRef] [PubMed]
17. Pavlakis, S.G.; Phillips, P.C.; DiMauro, S.; De Vivo, D.C.; Rowland, L.P. Mitochondrial myopathy, encephalopathy, lactic acidosis, and strokelike episodes: A distinctive clinical syndrome. *Ann. Neurol.* **1984**, *16*, 481–488. [CrossRef] [PubMed]
18. Van Erven, P.M.; Gabreels, F.J.; Ruitenbeek, W.; Den Hartog, M.R.; Fischer, J.C.; Renier, W.O.; Trijbels, J.M.; Slooff, J.L.; Janssen, A.J. Subacute necrotizing encephalomyelopathy (Leigh syndrome) associated with disturbed oxidation of pyruvate, malate and 2-oxoglutarate in muscle and liver. *Acta Neurol. Scand.* **1985**, *72*, 36–42. [CrossRef]
19. Stewart, J.B.; Chinnery, P.F. The dynamics of mitochondrial DNA heteroplasmy: Implications for human health and disease. *Nat. Rev. Genet.* **2015**, *16*, 530–542. [CrossRef]
20. Lyseng-Williamson, K.A. Idebenone: A review in Leber's hereditary optic neuropathy. *Drugs* **2016**, *76*, 805–813. [CrossRef]
21. Brink, J.; Hovmoller, S.; Ragan, C.I.; Cleeter, M.W.; Boekema, E.J.; van Bruggen, E.F. The structure of NADH:ubiquinone oxidoreductase from beef-heart mitochondria: Crystals containing an octameric arrangement of iron-sulphur protein fragments. *Eur. J. Biochem.* **1987**, *166*, 287–294. [CrossRef]
22. Hirst, J.; Carroll, J.; Fearnley, I.M.; Shannon, R.J.; Walker, J.E. The nuclear encoded subunits of complex I from bovine heart mitochondria. *Biochim. Biophys. Acta* **2003**, *1604*, 135–150. [CrossRef]
23. Baranova, E.A.; Morgan, D.J.; Sazanov, L.A. Single particle analysis confirms distal location of subunits NuoL and NuoM in Escherichia coli complex I. *J. Struct. Biol.* **2007**, *159*, 238–242. [CrossRef] [PubMed]
24. Zickermann, V.; Kerscher, S.; Zwicker, K.; Tocilescu, M.A.; Radermacher, M.; Brandt, U. Architecture of complex I and its implications for electron transfer and proton pumping. *Biochim. Biophys. Acta* **2009**, *1787*, 574–583. [CrossRef] [PubMed]
25. Taylor, R.W.; Morris, A.A.; Hutchinson, M.; Turnbull, D.M. Leigh disease associated with a novel mitochondrial DNA ND5 mutation. *Eur. J. Hum. Genet.* **2002**, *10*, 141–144. [CrossRef]
26. Lebon, S.; Chol, M.; Benit, P.; Mugnier, C.; Chretien, D.; Giurgea, I.; Kern, I.; Girardin, E.; Hertz-Pannier, L.; de Lonlay, P.; et al. Recurrent de novo mitochondrial DNA mutations in respiratory chain deficiency. *J. Med. Genet.* **2003**, *40*, 896–899. [CrossRef]
27. Zhadanov, S.I.; Grechanina, E.Y.; Grechanina, Y.B.; Gusar, V.A.; Fedoseeva, N.P.; Lebon, S.; Munnich, A.; Schurr, T.G. Fatal manifestation of a de novo ND5 mutation: Insights into the pathogenetic mechanisms of mtDNA ND5 gene defects. *Mitochondrion* **2007**, *7*, 260–266. [CrossRef]
28. Benit, P.; Chretien, D.; Kadhom, N.; de Lonlay-Debeney, P.; Cormier-Daire, V.; Cabral, A.; Peudenier, S.; Rustin, P.; Munnich, A.; Rotig, A. Large-scale deletion and point mutations of the nuclear NDUFV1 and NDUFS1 genes in mitochondrial complex I deficiency. *Am. J. Hum. Genet.* **2001**, *68*, 1344–1352. [CrossRef]
29. Pagniez-Mammeri, H.; Lombes, A.; Brivet, M.; Ogier-de Baulny, H.; Landrieu, P.; Legrand, A.; Slama, A. Rapid screening for nuclear genes mutations in isolated respiratory chain complex I defects. *Mol. Genet. Metab.* **2009**, *96*, 196–200. [CrossRef]
30. Kashani, A.; Thiffault, I.; Dilenge, M.E.; Saint-Martin, C.; Guerrero, K.; Tran, L.T.; Shoubridge, E.; van der Knaap, M.S.; Braverman, N.; Bernard, G. A homozygous mutation in the NDUFS1 gene presents with a mild cavitating leukoencephalopathy. *Neurogenetics* **2014**, *15*, 161–164. [CrossRef]
31. Mayr, J.A.; Haack, T.B.; Graf, E.; Zimmermann, F.A.; Wieland, T.; Haberberger, B.; Superti-Furga, A.; Kirschner, J.; Steinmann, B.; Baumgartner, M.R.; et al. Lack of the mitochondrial protein acylglycerol kinase causes Sengers syndrome. *Am. J. Hum. Genet.* **2012**, *90*, 314–320. [CrossRef] [PubMed]
32. Matyash, V.; Liebisch, G.; Kurzchalia, T.V.; Shevchenko, A.; Schwudke, D. Lipid extraction by methyl-tert-butyl ether for high-throughput lipidomics. *J. Lipid Res.* **2008**, *49*, 1137–1146. [CrossRef] [PubMed]
33. Gielisch, I.; Meierhofer, D. Metabolome and proteome profiling of complex I deficiency induced by rotenone. *J. Proteome Res.* **2015**, *14*, 224–235. [CrossRef]
34. Kulak, N.A.; Pichler, G.; Paron, I.; Nagaraj, N.; Mann, M. Minimal, encapsulated proteomic-sample processing applied to copy-number estimation in eukaryotic cells. *Nat. Methods* **2014**, *11*, 319–324. [CrossRef] [PubMed]
35. Martens, L.; Hermjakob, H.; Jones, P.; Adamski, M.; Taylor, C.; States, D.; Gevaert, K.; Vandekerckhove, J.; Apweiler, R. PRIDE: The proteomics identifications database. *Proteomics* **2005**, *5*, 3537–3545. [CrossRef] [PubMed]

36. Subramanian, A.; Tamayo, P.; Mootha, V.K.; Mukherjee, S.; Ebert, B.L.; Gillette, M.A.; Paulovich, A.; Pomeroy, S.L.; Golub, T.R.; Lander, E.S.; et al. Gene set enrichment analysis: A knowledge-based approach for interpreting genome-wide expression profiles. *Proc. Natl. Acad. Sci. USA* **2005**, *102*, 15545–15550. [CrossRef] [PubMed]
37. Hayashi, T.; Stuchebrukhov, A.A. Electron tunneling in respiratory complex I. *Proc. Natl. Acad. Sci. USA* **2010**, *107*, 19157–19162. [CrossRef] [PubMed]
38. Quan, L.; Lv, Q.; Zhang, Y. STRUM: Structure-based prediction of protein stability changes upon single-point mutation. *Bioinformatics* **2016**, *32*, 2936–2946. [CrossRef]
39. Feichtinger, R.G.; Zimmermann, F.; Mayr, J.A.; Neureiter, D.; Hauser-Kronberger, C.; Schilling, F.H.; Jones, N.; Sperl, W.; Kofler, B. Low aerobic mitochondrial energy metabolism in poorly- or undifferentiated neuroblastoma. *BMC Cancer* **2010**, *10*, 149. [CrossRef]
40. Meierhofer, D.; Mayr, J.A.; Foetschl, U.; Berger, A.; Fink, K.; Schmeller, N.; Hacker, G.W.; Hauser-Kronberger, C.; Kofler, B.; Sperl, W. Decrease of mitochondrial DNA content and energy metabolism in renal cell carcinoma. *Carcinogenesis* **2004**, *25*, 1005–1010. [CrossRef]
41. Berger, A.; Mayr, J.A.; Meierhofer, D.; Fotschl, U.; Bittner, R.; Budka, H.; Grethen, C.; Huemer, M.; Kofler, B.; Sperl, W. Severe depletion of mitochondrial DNA in spinal muscular atrophy. *Acta Neuropathol.* **2003**, *105*, 245–251. [PubMed]
42. Aretz, I.; Hardt, C.; Wittig, I.; Meierhofer, D. An Impaired Respiratory Electron Chain Triggers Down-regulation of the Energy Metabolism and De-ubiquitination of Solute Carrier Amino Acid Transporters. *Mol. Cell. Proteomics MCP* **2016**, *15*, 1526–1538. [CrossRef] [PubMed]
43. Heidler, J.; Strecker, V.; Csintalan, F.; Bleier, L.; Wittig, I. Quantification of protein complexes by blue native electrophoresis. *Methods Mol. Biol.* **2013**, *1033*, 363–379. [PubMed]
44. Wittig, I.; Carrozzo, R.; Santorelli, F.M.; Schagger, H. Functional assays in high-resolution clear native gels to quantify mitochondrial complexes in human biopsies and cell lines. *Electrophoresis* **2007**, *28*, 3811–3820. [CrossRef] [PubMed]
45. Di Tommaso, P.; Moretti, S.; Xenarios, I.; Orobitg, M.; Montanyola, A.; Chang, J.M.; Taly, J.F.; Notredame, C. T-Coffee: A web server for the multiple sequence alignment of protein and RNA sequences using structural information and homology extension. *Nucleic Acids Res.* **2011**, *39*, W13–W17. [CrossRef] [PubMed]
46. Robert, X.; Gouet, P. Deciphering key features in protein structures with the new ENDscript server. *Nucleic Acids Res.* **2014**, *42*, W320–W324. [CrossRef] [PubMed]
47. Enns, G.M.; Moore, T.; Le, A.; Atkuri, K.; Shah, M.K.; Cusmano-Ozog, K.; Niemi, A.K.; Cowan, T.M. Degree of glutathione deficiency and redox imbalance depend on subtype of mitochondrial disease and clinical status. *PLoS ONE* **2014**, *9*, e100001. [CrossRef] [PubMed]
48. Zitka, O.; Skalickova, S.; Gumulec, J.; Masarik, M.; Adam, V.; Hubalek, J.; Trnkova, L.; Kruseova, J.; Eckschlager, T.; Kizek, R. Redox status expressed as GSH:GSSG ratio as a marker for oxidative stress in paediatric tumour patients. *Oncol. Lett.* **2012**, *4*, 1247–1253. [CrossRef] [PubMed]
49. Santa, T. Recent advances in analysis of glutathione in biological samples by high-performance liquid chromatography: A brief overview. *Drug Discov. Ther.* **2013**, *7*, 172–177. [CrossRef]
50. Das, K.C.; Misra, H.P. Hydroxyl radical scavenging and singlet oxygen quenching properties of polyamines. *Mol. Cell. Biochem.* **2004**, *262*, 127–133. [CrossRef]
51. Fujisawa, S.; Kadoma, Y. Kinetic evaluation of polyamines as radical scavengers. *Anticancer Res.* **2005**, *25*, 965–969. [PubMed]
52. Esteitie, N.; Hinttala, R.; Wibom, R.; Nilsson, H.; Hance, N.; Naess, K.; Tear-Fahnehjelm, K.; von Dobeln, U.; Majamaa, K.; Larsson, N.G. Secondary metabolic effects in complex I deficiency. *Ann. Neurol.* **2005**, *58*, 544–552. [CrossRef] [PubMed]
53. Robinson, B.H. Lactic acidemia and mitochondrial disease. *Mol. Genet. Metab.* **2006**, *89*, 3–13. [CrossRef] [PubMed]
54. Feichtinger, R.G.; Weis, S.; Mayr, J.A.; Zimmermann, F.; Geilberger, R.; Sperl, W.; Kofler, B. Alterations of oxidative phosphorylation complexes in astrocytomas. *Glia* **2014**, *62*, 514–525. [CrossRef] [PubMed]
55. Hinchliffe, P.; Sazanov, L.A. Organization of iron-sulfur clusters in respiratory complex I. *Science* **2005**, *309*, 771–774. [CrossRef]

56. Nakamaru-Ogiso, E. Iron–Sulfur Clusters in Complex I. In *A Structural Perspective on Respiratory Complex I: Structure and Function of NADH:ubiquinone Oxidoreductase*; Sazanov, L., Ed.; Springer: Dordrecht, The Netherland, 2012; pp. 61–79.
57. Lazarou, M.; McKenzie, M.; Ohtake, A.; Thorburn, D.R.; Ryan, M.T. Analysis of the assembly profiles for mitochondrial- and nuclear-DNA-encoded subunits into complex I. *Mol. Cell. Biol.* **2007**, *27*, 4228–4237. [CrossRef]
58. Garcia, C.J.; Khajeh, J.; Coulanges, E.; Chen, E.I.; Owusu-Ansah, E. Regulation of Mitochondrial Complex I Biogenesis in Drosophila Flight Muscles. *Cell Rep.* **2017**, *20*, 264–278. [CrossRef] [PubMed]
59. Guerrero-Castillo, S.; Baertling, F.; Kownatzki, D.; Wessels, H.J.; Arnold, S.; Brandt, U.; Nijtmans, L. The Assembly Pathway of Mitochondrial Respiratory Chain Complex I. *Cell Metab.* **2017**, *25*, 128–139. [CrossRef] [PubMed]
60. Schägger, H.; Pfeiffer, K. Supercomplexes in the respiratory chains of yeast and mammalian mitochondria. *EMBO J.* **2000**, *19*, 1777–1783. [CrossRef]
61. Eubel, H.; Heinemeyer, J.; Braun, H.P. Identification and characterization of respirasomes in potato mitochondria. *Plant Physiol.* **2004**, *134*, 1450–1459. [CrossRef] [PubMed]
62. Acin-Perez, R.; Fernandez-Silva, P.; Peleato, M.L.; Perez-Martos, A.; Enriquez, J.A. Respiratory active mitochondrial supercomplexes. *Mol. Cell* **2008**, *32*, 529–539. [CrossRef] [PubMed]
63. Letts, J.A.; Fiedorczuk, K.; Sazanov, L.A. The architecture of respiratory supercomplexes. *Nature* **2016**, *537*, 644–648. [CrossRef] [PubMed]
64. Gu, J.; Wu, M.; Guo, R.; Yan, K.; Lei, J.; Gao, N.; Yang, M. The architecture of the mammalian respirasome. *Nature* **2016**, *537*, 639–643. [CrossRef] [PubMed]
65. Wu, M.; Gu, J.; Guo, R.; Huang, Y.; Yang, M. Structure of Mammalian Respiratory Supercomplex I1III2IV1. *Cell* **2016**, *167*, 1598–1609. [CrossRef] [PubMed]
66. Guo, R.; Zong, S.; Wu, M.; Gu, J.; Yang, M. Architecture of Human Mitochondrial Respiratory Megacomplex I2III2IV2. *Cell* **2017**, *170*, 1247–1257. [CrossRef]
67. Schägger, H.; Pfeiffer, K. The Ratio of Oxidative Phosphorylation Complexes I–V in Bovine Heart Mitochondria and the Composition of Respiratory Chain Supercomplexes. *J. Biol. Chem.* **2001**, *276*, 37861–37867.
68. Vartak, R.; Porras, C.A.; Bai, Y. Respiratory supercomplexes: Structure, function and assembly. *Protein Cell* **2013**, *4*, 582–590. [CrossRef] [PubMed]
69. Schägger, H.; de Coo, R.; Bauer, M.F.; Hofmann, S.; Godinot, C.; Brandt, U. Significance of respirasomes for the assembly/stability of human respiratory chain complex I. *J. Biol. Chem.* **2004**, *279*, 36349–36353. [CrossRef]
70. Milenkovic, D.; Blaza, J.N.; Larsson, N.G.; Hirst, J. The Enigma of the Respiratory Chain Supercomplex. *Cell Metab.* **2017**, *25*, 765–776. [CrossRef]
71. Fedor, J.G.; Hirst, J. Mitochondrial Supercomplexes Do Not Enhance Catalysis by Quinone Channeling. *Cell Metab.* **2018**, *28*, 525–531. [CrossRef]
72. Hirst, J.; Roessler, M.M. Energy conversion, redox catalysis and generation of reactive oxygen species by respiratory complex I. *Biochim. Biophys. Acta* **2016**, *1857*, 872–883. [CrossRef] [PubMed]
73. Esterhazy, D.; King, M.S.; Yakovlev, G.; Hirst, J. Production of reactive oxygen species by complex I (NADH:Ubiquinone oxidoreductase) from Escherichia coli and comparison to the enzyme from mitochondria. *Biochemistry* **2008**, *47*, 3964–3971. [CrossRef] [PubMed]
74. Kussmaul, L.; Hirst, J. The mechanism of superoxide production by NADH:ubiquinone oxidoreductase (complex I) from bovine heart mitochondria. *Proc. Natl. Acad. Sci. USA* **2006**, *103*, 7607–7612. [CrossRef] [PubMed]
75. King, M.S.; Sharpley, M.S.; Hirst, J. Reduction of hydrophilic ubiquinones by the flavin in mitochondrial NADH:Ubiquinone oxidoreductase (Complex I) and production of reactive oxygen species. *Biochemistry* **2009**, *48*, 2053–2062. [CrossRef] [PubMed]
76. Leman, G.; Gueguen, N.; Desquiret-Dumas, V.; Kane, M.S.; Wettervald, C.; Chupin, S.; Chevrollier, A.; Lebre, A.S.; Bonnefont, J.P.; Barth, M.; et al. Assembly defects induce oxidative stress in inherited mitochondrial complex I deficiency. *Int. J. Biochem. Cell Biol.* **2015**, *65*, 91–103. [CrossRef] [PubMed]
77. Baradaran, R.; Berrisford, J.M.; Minhas, G.S.; Sazanov, L.A. Crystal structure of the entire respiratory complex I. *Nature* **2013**, *494*, 443–448. [CrossRef] [PubMed]
78. Brandt, U. A two-state stabilization-change mechanism for proton-pumping complex I. *Biochim. Biophys. Acta* **2011**, *1807*, 1364–1369. [CrossRef] [PubMed]

79. Jones, A.J.; Blaza, J.N.; Varghese, F.; Hirst, J. Respiratory Complex I in Bos taurus and Paracoccus denitrificans Pumps Four Protons across the Membrane for Every NADH Oxidized. *J. Biol. Chem.* **2017**, *292*, 4987–4995. [CrossRef] [PubMed]
80. Narayanan, M.; Sakyiama, J.A.; Elguindy, M.M.; Nakamaru-Ogiso, E. Roles of subunit NuoL in the proton pumping coupling mechanism of NADH:ubiquinone oxidoreductase (complex I) from *Escherichia coli*. *J. Biochem.* **2016**, *160*, 205–215. [CrossRef] [PubMed]
81. Murphy, M.P. How mitochondria produce reactive oxygen species. *Biochem. J.* **2009**, *417*, 1–13. [CrossRef] [PubMed]
82. Willems, P.H.; Rossignol, R.; Dieteren, C.E.; Murphy, M.P.; Koopman, W.J. Redox Homeostasis and Mitochondrial Dynamics. *Cell Metab.* **2015**, *22*, 207–218. [CrossRef] [PubMed]
83. Robb, E.L.; Hall, A.R.; Prime, T.A.; Eaton, S.; Szibor, M.; Viscomi, C.; James, A.M.; Murphy, M.P. Control of mitochondrial superoxide production by reverse electron transport at complex I. *J. Biol. Chem.* **2018**, *293*, 9869–9879. [CrossRef] [PubMed]
84. Sazanov, L.A. Structure of Respiratory Complex I: "Minimal" Bacterial and "De luxe" Mammalian Versions. In *Mechanisms of Primary Energy Transduction in Biology*; The Royal Society of Chemistry: Cambridge, UK, 2018; pp. 25–59.
85. Canto, C.; Menzies, K.J.; Auwerx, J. NAD(+) Metabolism and the Control of Energy Homeostasis: A Balancing Act between Mitochondria and the Nucleus. *Cell Metab.* **2015**, *22*, 31–53. [CrossRef] [PubMed]
86. Verdin, E. NAD(+) in aging, metabolism, and neurodegeneration. *Science* **2015**, *350*, 1208–1213. [CrossRef] [PubMed]
87. Houtkooper, R.H.; Canto, C.; Wanders, R.J.; Auwerx, J. The secret life of NAD+: An old metabolite controlling new metabolic signaling pathways. *Endocr. Rev.* **2010**, *31*, 194–223. [CrossRef] [PubMed]
88. Esterhuizen, K.; van der Westhuizen, F.H.; Louw, R. Metabolomics of mitochondrial disease. *Mitochondrion* **2017**, *35*, 97–110. [CrossRef]
89. Williamson, J.R.; Cooper, R.H. Regulation of the citric acid cycle in mammalian systems. *FEBS Lett.* **1980**, *117*, K73–K85. [CrossRef]
90. Varghese, F.; Atcheson, E.; Bridges, H.R.; Hirst, J. Characterization of clinically identified mutations in NDUFV1, the flavin-binding subunit of respiratory complex I, using a yeast model system. *Hum. Mol. Genet.* **2015**, *24*, 6350–6360. [CrossRef]
91. Gostimskaya, I.S.; Grivennikova, V.G.; Cecchini, G.; Vinogradov, A.D. Reversible dissociation of flavin mononucleotide from the mammalian membrane-bound NADH:ubiquinone oxidoreductase (complex I). *FEBS Lett.* **2007**, *581*, 5803–5806. [CrossRef]
92. Holt, P.J.; Efremov, R.G.; Nakamaru-Ogiso, E.; Sazanov, L.A. Reversible FMN dissociation from Escherichia coli respiratory complex I. *Biochim. Biophys. Acta* **2016**, *1857*, 1777–1785. [CrossRef]
93. Kudin, A.P.; Bimpong-Buta, N.Y.; Vielhaber, S.; Elger, C.E.; Kunz, W.S. Characterization of superoxide-producing sites in isolated brain mitochondria. *J. Biol. Chem.* **2004**, *279*, 4127–4135. [CrossRef] [PubMed]
94. Galkin, A.; Brandt, U. Superoxide Radical Formation by Pure Complex I (NADH:Ubiquinone Oxidoreductase) from *Yarrowia lipolytica*. *J. Biol. Chem.* **2005**, *280*, 30129–30135. [CrossRef] [PubMed]
95. Ribas, V.; Garcia-Ruiz, C.; Fernandez-Checa, J.C. Glutathione and mitochondria. *Front. Pharmacol.* **2014**, *5*, 151. [CrossRef] [PubMed]
96. Benit, P.; Beugnot, R.; Chretien, D.; Giurgea, I.; De Lonlay-Debeney, P.; Issartel, J.P.; Corral-Debrinski, M.; Kerscher, S.; Rustin, P.; Rotig, A.; et al. Mutant NDUFV2 subunit of mitochondrial complex I causes early onset hypertrophic cardiomyopathy and encephalopathy. *Hum. Mutat.* **2003**, *21*, 582–586. [CrossRef] [PubMed]
97. Brecht, M.; Richardson, M.; Taranath, A.; Grist, S.; Thorburn, D.; Bratkovic, D. Leigh Syndrome Caused by the MT-ND5 m.13513G>A Mutation: A Case Presenting with WPW-Like Conduction Defect, Cardiomyopathy, Hypertension and Hyponatraemia. *JIMD Rep.* **2015**, *19*, 95–100. [PubMed]
98. Ayalon, N.; Flore, L.A.; Christensen, T.G.; Sam, F. Mitochondrial encoded NADH dehydrogenase 5 (MT-ND5) gene point mutation presents as late onset cardiomyopathy. *Int. J. Cardiol.* **2013**, *167*, e143–e145. [CrossRef]

99. Annunen-Rasila, J.; Ohlmeier, S.; Tuokko, H.; Veijola, J.; Majamaa, K. Proteome and cytoskeleton responses in osteosarcoma cells with reduced OXPHOS activity. *Proteomics* **2007**, *7*, 2189–2200. [CrossRef] [PubMed]
100. Meyers, D.E.; Basha, H.I.; Koenig, M.K. Mitochondrial cardiomyopathy: Pathophysiology, diagnosis, and management. *Tex. Heart Inst. J.* **2013**, *40*, 385–394.

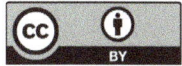

© 2019 by the authors. Licensee MDPI, Basel, Switzerland. This article is an open access article distributed under the terms and conditions of the Creative Commons Attribution (CC BY) license (http://creativecommons.org/licenses/by/4.0/).

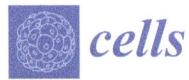

Article

Absence of Uncoupling Protein-3 at Thermoneutrality Impacts Lipid Handling and Energy Homeostasis in Mice

Assunta Lombardi [1,*,†], Rosa Anna Busiello [1,†], Rita De Matteis [2], Lillà Lionetti [3], Sabrina Savarese [1], Maria Moreno [4], Alessandra Gentile [1], Elena Silvestri [4], Rosalba Senese [5], Pieter de Lange [5], Federica Cioffi [4], Antonia Lanni [5] and Fernando Goglia [4,*]

1. Department of Biology, University of Naples "Federico II", 80138 Naples, Italy
2. Department of Biomolecular Sciences, University of Urbino "Carlo Bo", 61029 Urbino, Italy
3. Department of Chemistry and Biology, "Adolfo Zambelli" University of Salerno, 84084 Salerno, Italy
4. Department of Science and Technology, University of Sannio, 82100 Benevento, Italy
5. Department of Environmental, Biological and Pharmaceutical Sciences and Technologies, University of Campania "Luigi Vanvitelli", 81100 Caserta, Italy
* Correspondence: assunta.lombardi@unina.it (A.L.); goglia@unisannio.it (F.G.); Tel.: +39-08-1253-2098 (A.L.)
† These authors equally contributed to the manuscript.

Received: 27 June 2019; Accepted: 15 August 2019; Published: 17 August 2019

Abstract: The role of uncoupling protein-3 (UCP3) in energy and lipid metabolism was investigated. Male wild-type (WT) and UCP3-null (KO) mice that were housed at thermoneutrality (30 °C) were used as the animal model. In KO mice, the ability of skeletal muscle mitochondria to oxidize fatty acids (but not pyruvate or succinate) was reduced. At whole animal level, adult KO mice presented blunted resting metabolic rates, energy expenditure, food intake, and the use of lipids as metabolic substrates. When WT and KO mice were fed with a standard/low-fat diet for 80 days, since weaning, they showed similar weight gain and body composition. Interestingly, KO mice showed lower fat accumulation in visceral adipose tissue and higher ectopic fat accumulation in liver and skeletal muscle. When fed with a high-fat diet for 80 days, since weaning, KO mice showed enhanced energy efficiency and an increased lipid gain (thus leading to a change in body composition between the two genotypes). We conclude that UCP3 plays a role in energy and lipid homeostasis and in preserving lean tissues by lipotoxicity, in mice that were housed at thermoneutrality.

Keywords: uncoupling protein; mitochondria: energy metabolism; lipid handling; fatty acid oxidation

1. Introduction

Uncoupling protein-3 (UCP3) is a mitochondrial protein, first discovered in 1997 [1], and prevalently expressed in skeletal muscle (SkM), the heart and brown and white adipose tissues [2]. The extent of homology between the UCP1 and UCP3 genes led to the proposal that UCP3 might be involved in thermogenic mechanisms, and although it does not appear to contribute to cold-induced thermogenesis [3], it has recently proved to be essential in thermogenic responses that are induced by the endotoxin lipopolysaccharide and by the sympathomimetic methamphetamine [4]. Indeed, the evidence that up-regulation of UCP3 is not always associated with mitochondrial uncoupling/thermogenesis [5], which suggested that uncoupling oxidative phosphorylation is not the primary role of UCP3, but rather a consequence of its true function. Other than thermogenesis, other roles that have been attributed to UCP3 include prevention of damage induced by reactive oxygen species (ROS) and lipid hydroperoxides (LOOH), as well as modulation of lipid handling [6–9]. Indeed, high amounts of UCP3 are present in tissues that are known to metabolize fatty acids (FA) to a high extent, and enhanced levels of UCP3 expression are observed under physiological and pathological conditions, in which the fatty acid oxidation rate is elevated [8–10]. In addition, the expression of UCP3 during heart development is correlated to that of mitochondrial fatty acid oxidation rate markers [11]. Furthermore, the absence of UCP3 negatively influences the ability of SkM mitochondria to oxidize FA [12,13]. In this context, Bouillaud et al. [14] suggested that UCP3 could switch cells from carbohydrate to fatty acid metabolic pathways by promoting mitochondrial pyruvate extrusion, which prevents the use of pyruvate as a substrate. However, mechanistic information on this possible activity is currently lacking.

Although the roles that were proposed for UCP3 suggest that it could play a role in energy homeostasis (EH), the obtained contrasting results have not produced a common and unambiguous conclusion so far. Several lines of experimental evidence supporting the role of UCP3 in EH came from human studies [see 6 and references within] and from mice over-expressing UCP3, being: (i) obesity-resistant mice present higher UCP3 levels than obesity-prone mice [15]; (ii) transgenic mice that over-express UCP3 are metabolically less efficient than their wild-type litter mates, and are protected against high fat diet (HFD)-induced obesity [16,17]; and, (iii) modest UCP3 over-expression in SkM increased mice energy expenditure [18]. Conversely, some studies that were performed on mice lacking UCP3 (KO mice) are discordant, since they did not show alterations in several metabolic parameters, such as the resting metabolic rate, the regulation of body temperature during cold exposure, food intake, body weight regulation, and the total body triglyceride content [3,19]. Nevertheless, KO mice have been shown not to be obese [3] (only showing higher lipid accumulation relative to WT litter mates when fed a HFD for a prolonged period (eight months)). Furthermore, the KO mice showed no alteration in metabolic efficiency [20]. The absence of metabolic alterations in KO mice could be due to the constant thermal stress that is caused by the animal housing conditions. In fact, in most studies, mice (which have a thermoneutrality temperature of 30 °C) are housed at the standard temperature (20–24 °C), which represents cold stress. Thus, mice lacking UCP3 that are exposed to thermal stress may implement compensatory mechanisms to maintain their body temperature, and these mechanisms are likely to affect the overall metabolic rate and other investigated parameters. Such a possibility was previously tested for UCP1 [21]. UCP1 ablation only induced obesity when the mice were housed under thermoneutral conditions. This outcome highlights the importance of avoiding thermal stress in metabolic studies on mice, since housing temperatures significantly influence the outcome of experiments, as well as their translatability to humans that, indeed, create a thermoneutral environment without cold stress for themselves [22]. Here, we investigated the role of UCP3 in metabolic control in situations in which thermal stress was eliminated. We report that, in adult mice acclimated at thermoneutrality for two weeks, UCP3 ablation altered energy and lipid metabolism. Moreover, in standard diet fed mice, which were kept at thermoneutrality since weaning, UCP3 ablation enhanced ectopic fat accumulation in liver and skeletal muscle, and vastly augmented HFD-induced fat accumulation. We conclude that the exposure temperature is determinative for the outcome of metabolic effects elicited by UCP3 and that the protein can be involved in the metabolic control of lipid metabolism in mice and possibly in humans.

2. Materials and Methods

2.1. Materials

All of the chemicals were purchased from Sigma-Aldrich (St. Louis, MO, USA), unless otherwise specified.

2.2. Animals

UCP3-ablated mice were derived from those that were described by Gong et al. [3] and they were backcrossed to the C57BL/6 strain for ten generations.

Male wild type (WT) and UCP3 knockout mice (KO) were used in the present study. Mice were housed in thermoneutrality (30 ± 1 °C) with a 12/12 h light-dark cycle and free access to food and water. This study was carried out in accordance with recommendations in the EU Directive 2010/63/ for the Care and Use of Laboratory Animals. The Committee on the Ethics of Animal Experiments of the University of Napoli Federico II (Italy) and the Italian Minister of Health approved all of the animal protocols. Every effort was made to minimize animal pain and suffering. At the end of the treatments described below, the mice were anesthetized with Zoletil (40 mg/100 g bw) and sacrificed by decapitation.

To detect metabolic parameters and mitochondrial functionality, four–five month-old mice of each genotype acclimated to 30 °C ± 1 for 2–3 weeks and fed a standard diet were used to detect resting metabolic rate (RMR), respiratory quotient (RQ), energy expenditure (EE), and mitochondrial functional parameters. Other groups of WT and KO mice were kept one per cage and were housed at 30 °C ± 1 for 80 days since weaning and fed with a standard diet or a high fat diet (HFD) for 80 days in order to detect body composition and energy gains as well as to perform histological analysis of mice under different "lipid loads". Standard/low fat diet (STD) consisted of 10% lipids, 20% proteins, 70% carbohydrates with a gross energy density of 15.5 kJ/g wet food. HFD consisted of 45% lipid, 20% proteins, and 35% carbohydrates with a gross energy density of 19.2 kJ/g wet food. Both of the diets were from Mucedola (Milano Italy).

2.3. Metabolic Parameters

Oxygen consumption (VO_2) and carbon dioxide production (CO_2) measurements were made using a four-chamber, indirect open-circuit calorimeter (Columbus Instrument), with one mouse per chamber at a room temperature of 30 °C to evaluate basal metabolic parameters. Measurements were performed between 1100 and 1600 h. After a 1-h period of adaptation to the metabolic chamber, VO_2 and VCO_2 were measured when the mice were not moving for at least 10 min. The system settings included a flow rate of 0.5 L/min., a sample line-purge time of 2 min., and a measurement period of 30 s every 12 min. Mice were placed in separate 2.5-L calorimetry chamber with ad libitum access to water. Values of VO_2 and VCO_2 were obtained by means of three different consecutive measurements during which the mice were not moving. These data were used to calculate the respiratory quotient (RQ; VCO_2/VO_2) and the resting energy expenditure (REE) ([3.815 + 1.232 RQ] VO_2). The contribution of fatty acid oxidation to REE was calculated, as described using the following equation: percentage of fat contribution = [468.6 (1 − RQ)]/[5.047 (RQ − 0.707) + 4.686 (1 − RQ)] [23].

2.4. SkM Mitochondrial Respiration

As soon as euthanasia was performed, SkM were excised and all visible contaminating tissues were removed. The tissues were either immediately processed for mitochondria isolation or frozen in liquid nitrogen and then stored at −80 °C for later analysis. Mitochondria from SkM were isolated by differential centrifugation, as reported by Lombardi et al. [24]. The mitochondrial respiration and fatty acid oxidation rate were assessed by the polarographic method while using a Clark-type electrode at 37 °C by using different respiratory substrates. SkM mitochondrial respiration was detected in a final volume of a 0.5 mL respiration medium consisting of 80 mM KCl, 50 mM HEPES (pH 7.0), 1 mM EGTA, 5 mM K2HPO4, and 0.5% fatty acid-free BSA (w/v). The mitochondria were incubated for three min in the respiratory medium, and the respiration was initiated by the addition of succinate (5 mM) in the presence of rotenone (4 µM) or pyruvate (10 mM) in the presence of malate (2 mM), or palmitoyl-carnitine (40 µM) in the presence of malate (2 mM). Once State 2 of respiration was reached, ADP (300 µM) was added to the incubation medium to induce State 3 respiration; when ADP was exhausted, State 4 was reached.

2.5. Separation of Respiratory Complexes by Blue-Native Page (BN-PAGE) and Histochemical Staining for in-Gel Activity

Solubilisation of mitochondrial membranes by detergents, BN-PAGE, staining, and densitometric quantification of oxidative phosphorylation complexes were performed, as described in Scagger et al. [25] and Lombardi et al. [26], with some minor variations. Mitochondria enriched fraction was suspended in a low-salt buffer (50 mM NaCl, 50 mM imidazole, pH 7.0) and solubilised with 10% (w/v) dodecyl-maltoside to solubilise the individual respiratory chain complexes. The electrophoretic run was carried out on 4–13% gradient polyacrylamide gels and enzymatic colorimetric reactions were performed essentially as reported by Zerbetto et al. [27]. The activity of complex I activity was evaluated by incubating the gel slices with 2 mM Tris–HCl, pH 7.4, 0.1 mg/mL NADH, and 2.5 mg/mL nitro blue tetrazolium (NTB) at room temperature. To detect complex II activity, gel slices were incubated at room temperature in a 100 mM Tris/glycine buffer at pH 7.4 containing 1 mg/mL NTB and 1 mM sodium succinate. Complex IV activity was assessed by incubating BN-PAGE gels with 5 mg 3,3'-diaminobenzidine tetrahydrochloride (DAB) that was dissolved in a 9 mL phosphate buffer (0.05 M, pH 7.4), 1 mL catalase (20 µg/mL), 10 mg cytochrome c, and 750 mg sucrose. The original colour of the complex I, II, or IV-reacting bands was preserved by fixing the gels in 50% methanol and 10% acetic acid. In parallel, another electrophoretic run was performed to stain the gels with Coomassie Blue G to obtain the total band pattern of the respiratory complexes. After gel scanning, the areas of the bands were expressed as absolute values (arbitrary units).

2.6. Determination of Glycerol Release from White Adipose Tissue

100 mg of epididymal white adipose tissue samples were removed. Samples were cut into 20 mg sections to evaluate the glycerol diffusion from tissue to the medium better; 100 mg of tissue were incubated at 37 °C in 500 µL of Krebs Ringer buffer (KRB; 12 mM HEPES, 121 mM NaCl, 4.9 mM KCl, 1.2 mM $MgSO_4$, 0.33 mM $CaCl_2$) containing 2% FA-free bovine serum albumin (BSA) and 0.1% glucose in the presence or absence of 10 µM isoproterenol (Sigma). Tissue was incubated for 1 h at 37 °C in a shaking bath and then gassed with 95% O_2-5% CO_2. At the end of the incubation period, an aliquot of the medium was used for the analysis of glycerol. A commercially available absorbance-based enzyme assay for glycerol (Free Glycerol Reagent; Sigma) was converted to fluorescence-based detection by the inclusion of the hydrogen peroxide-sensitive dye Amplex UltraRed, as reported by Clark et al. [28].

2.7. Hystological Analysis

Samples of visceral WAT (mesenteral), liver, and gastrocnemius skeletal muscle were fixed by immersion in 4% formaldehyde in 0.1 M phosphate buffer (overnight at 4 °C). The samples were dehydrated in ethanol, cleared, and then embedded in paraffin blocks. The tissues were cut into serial 6-πm-thick sections and then stained with hematoxylin-eosin for morphological examination. For adipocyte size quantification, evaluations were performed on three different hematoxylin-eosin slides (sections every 400 µm) for each animal and at least 400 adipocytes per animal were analyzed. The sections were viewed with a Nikon Eclipse 80i light microscope (Nikon Instruments, Milan, Italy) at 20× magnification. Images were obtained with a Sony DS-5M camera connected to an ACT-2U image analyzer. The mean surface area and the frequency distribution were calculated from at least four mice for each group, adipocyte size distribution is presented as the percentage of the total amount of cells.

2.8. Body Composition and Energy Gains

Body composition and carcass energy content were evaluated, as reported by Iossa et al. [29]. In brief, after removing the gut contents, the carcasses were autoclaved and homogenized in water. The water content of the carcass was detected by drying the homogenate at 70 °C in a vacuum oven. Small pellets of dried homogenate were then used to evaluate the carcass energy content by bomb calorimetry. Other homogenate aliquots were used to detect the lipid content by the Folch et al. method [30]. Body protein content was determined from a general formula relating to the total energy value of the carcass, the energy derived from fat, and the energy derived from protein [31,32]. The caloric values for body fat and protein were taken as 38.6 and 22.7 kJ/g, respectively. To detect lipid and protein gains, as well as energy efficiency in WT and UCP3 KO mice, six mice from each genotype were euthanatized at weaning (i.e., when they were 24 days old) that corresponded to the beginning of dietary treatments (groups were named WT-time 0 and KO-time 0). Two additional groups of mice for each genotype were individually caged for 80 days since weaning, and feed ad libitum with either a STD diet or a HFD, as described above (groups were named WT-STD, KO-STD, WT-HFD, KO-HFD). The duration of the treatment with the high fat diet was chosen, since it was long enough to induce a HFD induced obesity in mice that were acclimated at thermoneutrality [33]. During the treatment, the body weight and food intake of the mice were monitored twice weekly. Feed spillage was taken into account when calculating the energy intake during the treatment. Body composition and energy content were evaluated, as described above. Carcass total energy gain, as well as the amount of energy that is gained and stored as lipids or as proteins after 80 days of either STD or HFD were determined by subtracting the total carcass energy, the carcass lipid-derived energy, and the carcass protein-derived energy detected in the WT-time 0 and KO-time 0 groups from the respective values detected in the WT-STD, WT-STD, KO-STD, and KO-HFD groups. The efficiencies of energy, lipid, and protein deposition were calculated as: (energy gain/energy consumed by diet) × 100, (lipid gain/lipid-derived energy consumed by diet) × 100, (protein gain/protein-derived energy consumed by diet) × 100, respectively.

2.9. Statistical Analysis

Data are reported as mean ± SEM and have been analyzed by Student's *t*-test or by two-way ANOVA, followed by Tukey's post-hoc test. Analyses have been performed with Graphpad Prism 5 software. Differences have been considered to be statistically significant when $p < 0.05$.

3. Results

3.1. UCP3 Ablation Affects Resting Metabolic Rate, Energy Expenditure, and Fatty Acid Utilization in Adult Mice Acclimated at Thermoneutrality

The resting metabolic rate (RMR), the resting energy expenditure (REE), and the respiratory quotient (RQ) were detected in 4–5 month old animals, which were acclimated at thermoneutrality for at least two weeks. RMR was significantly reduced in KO mice as compared to WT mice (−30%) (Figure 1), both when it was expressed in Litres oxygen/(hour Kg$^{0.75}$) and when expressed in Litres oxygen/(hour g of lean mass). The RQ was increased in KO mice, which indicates a lower use of lipids as metabolic substrates in these animals. Indeed, in KO mice, the contribution of fatty acid oxidation to REE was reduced by about 27% relative to that in WT mice (Figure 1). In addition, in adult KO animals, food intake resulted in a reduction of about 15%, being the values 3.1 ± 0.11 and 2.63 ± 0.014 g food/day, for WT and KO mice, respectively ($n = 6$, $p < 0.05$ by Student's *t*-test).

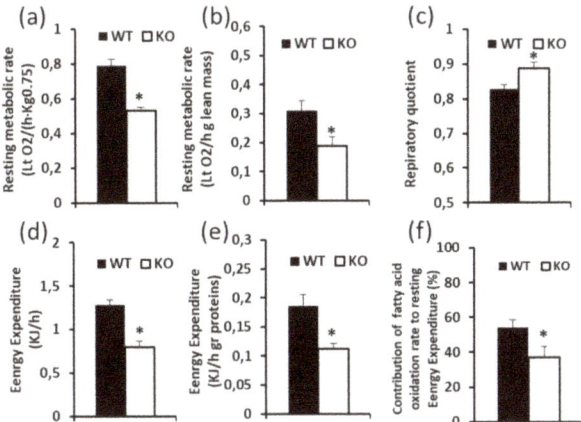

Figure 1. Effect of UCP3 ablation on metabolic parameters detected in WT and KO mice housed at thermoneutrality for 2–3 weeks and fed a standard diet (**a**), (**b**) Resting Metabolic Rate, (**c**) Respiratory Quotient, (**d**), (**e**) Energy Expenditure, (**f**) contribution of fatty acid oxidation to energy expenditure (EE). Values represent mean ± SE of 6–7 animals for WT and KO mice, respectively. Statistical analyses were performed by two-tailed Student's T-test, * $p < 0.05$ vs. WT.

SkM mitochondria that were isolated from WT and KO mice did not show significant differences in respiratory parameters (State 4 and State 3) when using pyruvate + malate or succinate + rotenone as substrate (Figure 2a,b). On the other hand, a significant State 3 inhibition was observed in mitochondria from KO mice when palmitoyl carnitine + malate was used as the substrate, which thus indicated the lower ability of mitochondria to oxidize fatty acids (Figure 2c).

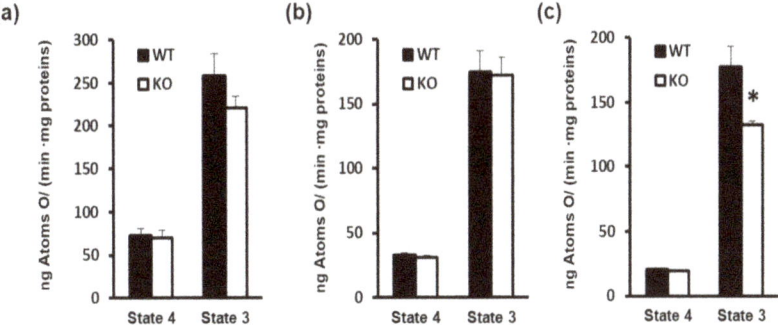

Figure 2. Impact of UCP3 ablation on mitochondrial respiration rate, detected in the presence of different substrates: (**a**) Succinate (+rotenone), (**b**) Pyruvate (+malate), and (**c**) Palmitoyl-carnitine (+malate). Skeletal muscle mitochondria were isolated from WT and KO mice housed at thermoneutrality for 2–3 weeks and fed a standard diet. Values represent mean ± SE of six different animals. Statistical analyses were performed by two-tailed Student's t-test, * $p < 0.05$ vs. WT.

Subsequently, we evaluated whether UCP3 ablation could influence respiratory chain complexes activity. In-gel activity of each individual respiratory complex (I, II, and IV) did not differ between WT and KO mitochondria (Figure 3). In view of the above results, we wondered whether UCP3 ablation would affect body fat accumulation in mice that were housed at thermoneutrality since weaning by determining their metabolic phenotype after feeding for 80 days, either with a standard/low fat diet (STD) or a high fat diet (HFD).

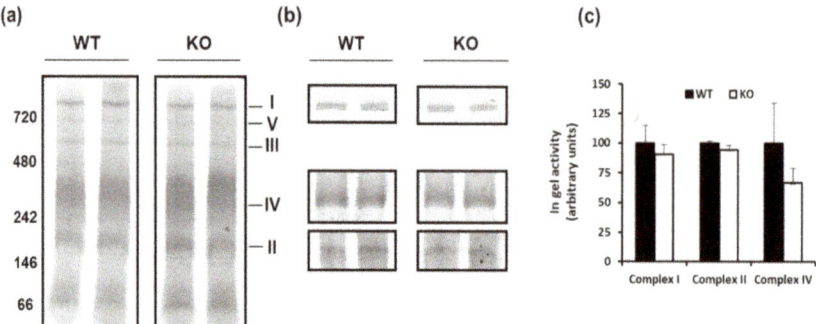

Figure 3. BN-PAGE-based analysis of individual respiratory complexes from dodecylmaltoside-solubilized crude mitochondria from SkM of WT and KO mice housed at thermoneutrality for 2–3 week and fed a standard diet. (**a**) Panels show representative images of Coomassie blue stained BN-PAGE gels. (**b**) Panels show representative images of histochemical staining of complex I (**I**), complex IV (**IV**), and complex II (**II**) in-gel activity. (**c**) Densitomentric quantification of band corresponding to in gel-activity of complex I, complex IV, and complex II. Protein extracts were prepared for each animal, and each individual was separately assessed. Data were normalized to the value obtained for WT animals, set as 100, and separately presented for each genotype (means ± SE; $n = 3$).

3.2. Effect of UCP3 Ablation on Body Weight, Energy Efficiency, and Body Composition in Mice Fed Either with a Standard Low Fat Diet or a High Fat Diet

At weaning, representing the experimental starting condition, KO-time 0 mice tended to have a lower body weight when compared to WT-time 0. However, the two groups showed similar body composition in terms of water, lipid, and protein percentage, as well as in energy content, referring to each gram of animal (Table 1).

Table 1. Body weight, body composition and energy content of each gram of animal weight detected in wild type (WT) and knockout mice (KO) mice at weaning (representing the beginning of the dietary treatment, i.e., time 0 of the experimental procedure).

	WT Time 0	KO Time 0
Body weight (g)	13.6 ± 0.9	11.5 ± 0.8
Body composition Water (%)	65 ± 1.7	67 ± 1.5
Lipids (%)	13.8 ± 0.3	12.7 ± 0.9
Proteins (%)	16.5 ± 2.4	12.8 ± 2.6
Energy content/g of animal	8.9 ± 0.5	7.64 ± 0.5

Values represent mean ± SE of 5 different animals.

WT and KO mice housed at thermoneutrality and fed a standard/low fat diet (STD) for 80 days since weaning (named WT-STD and KO-STD, respectively) gained the same body weight, while consuming the same amount of energy by food (Table 2), thus no differences were observed in the rough energy efficiency between WT-STD and KO-STD (Table 2).

Table 2. Body weight, body weight gain, food intake, body rough energy efficiency and visceral WAT weight detected in WT and KO mice, housed at thermoneutrality, and fed either a standard low fat diet (STD) or a high fat diet (HFD) for 80 days, since weaning.

	WT-WT	KO-STD	WT-HFD	KO-HFD
Initial weight (g)	11.88 ± 1.1 [a]	10.3 ± 1.01 [a]	14.50 ± 1.2 [a]	11.14 ± 1.2 [a]
Final weight (g)	32.4 ± 1.1 [a]	29.3 ± 1.1 [b]	38.44 ± 0.6 [c]	38.98 ± 1.2 [c]
Body weight gain (g)	19.0 ± 1.4 [a]	19.0 ± 1.1 [a]	23.94 ± 1.0 [b]	27.79 ± 0.94 [b]
Food intake (kJ)	3294 ± 85 [a]	3264 ± 107 [a]	4107 ± 72 [b]	3938 ± 96 [b]
Body rough energy efficiency [Body weight gain (g)/food intake (MJ)]	6.33 ± 0.35 [a,b]	5.86 ± 0.24 [a]	5.85 ± 0.29 [a]	7.08 ± 0.29 [b]
Visceral WAT (g)	2.01 ± 0.14 [a]	1.36 ± 0.08 [b]	3.67 ± 0.16 [c]	3.40 ± 0.24 [c]
WAT weight/body weight * 100	6.09 ± 0.28 [a]	4.62 ± 0.17 [b]	9.51 ± 0.31 [c]	9.09 ± 0.67 [c]

Values represent mean ± SE of 7–8 different animals. Differences were evaluated for statistical significance by two-way ANOVA followed by a Tukey's post hoc multiple comparison test. Different letters indicate that differences between mean values are statistically significant, with $p < 0.05$. Two-ways ANOVA test results: Body weight gain: diet effect $p < 0.0001$, genotype effect ns interaction ns; body rough energy efficiency: diet effect ns, genotype effect ns. interaction $p < 0.0089$; Visceral WAT: diet effect $p < 0.0001$, genotype effect $p = 0.0094$, interaction ns; WAT weight/body weight * 100: diet effect $p < 0.0001$, genotype effect $p = 0.0223$, interaction ns.

As expected, mice that were fed a HFD for 80 days since weaning (named WT-HFD and KO-HFD) gained more body weight when compared to mice under STD feeding, independent of the genotype. Body weight gain tended to be higher in KO-HFD mice than WT-HFD mice, although the food that was consumed was similar between the two groups, thus indicating that WT-HFD-mice have lower body rough energy efficiency than KO-HFD ones (Table 2). Indeed, concerning the last parameter, a two-way ANOVA test indicated the effect of the genotype and that of the diet was not statistically significant, while a significant interaction between genotype and diet was observed (see Table 2 legend). Remarkably, in both groups of mice, body rough energy efficiency changed during the treatment with either STD or HFD. Indeed, it was maximal during the first 25 days and then progressively declined (Figure 4). A difference in rough body energy efficiency between WT-HFD and KO-HFD mice was principally observed at the end of treatment, and, also in this case, a two-way ANOVA test indicated a significant interaction effect between genotype and diet (Figure 4 legend).

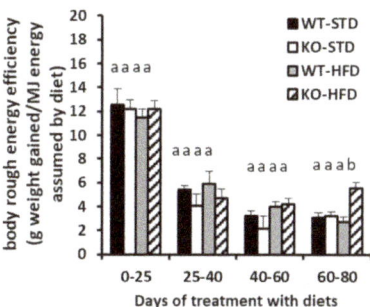

Figure 4. Variation in body rough metabolic energy efficiency during the 80 days of treatment of WT and KO mice with either STD or HFD. Values represent the mean ± SE of 7–8 different animals. The differences were evaluated for statistical significance by two-way ANOVA test, followed by a Tukey's post hoc multiple comparison test. Different letters indicate that differences between mean values are statistically significant, with $p < 0.05$. Two way ANOVA test results: diet effect $p = 0.0162$, genotype effect $p = 0.0037$, interaction $p = 0.0081$.

We then detected body energy, lipid, and protein gains, as well as the efficiency of energy, lipid, and protein deposition. Concerning energy intake (Figure 5a) and whole body energy gain (Figure 5b), no significant differences were observed between WT-STD and KO-STD. HFD feeding induced a significant increase in mouse energy gain, and, despite KO-HFD tending to have higher body energy gains when compared to WT-HFD, statistical analysis revealed a significant effect of the diet, while the genotype effect and genotype/diet interaction were not significant. When looking at the lipid gain (Figure 5b), similar values were detected in WT-STD and KO-STD. As expected, the HFD regimen induced a significant increase in mice lipid gain, which was significantly higher in KO-HFD when compared to WT-HFD. Indeed, the two-way ANOVA test revealed the significant effects of diet, genotype, as well as the interaction between genotype and diet (Figure 5 legend). No differences between WT-STD and KO-STD were observed regarding protein gain (Figure 5b). The HFD regimen significantly enhanced protein gain, and similar values were detected in WT-HFD and KO-HFD mice (Figure 5b). In fact, the two-way ANOVA test revealed the significant effect of the diet but not of genotype or genotype/diet interactions (Figure 5 legend).

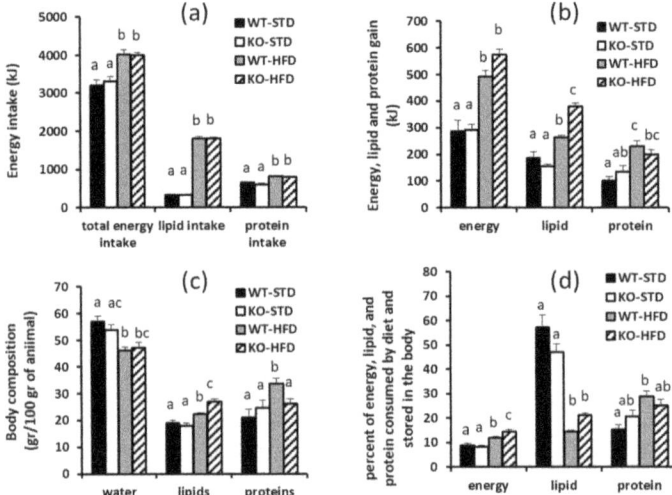

Figure 5. (a) Total energy, lipid and protein consumed by diet (b) Body energy, lipid and protein gains (c) Body composition (d) Efficiency of energy, lipid, and protein deposition of WT and KO mice, housed at thermoneutrality, and fed with either a standard/low fat diet (STD) or a high fat diet (HFD) for 80 days since weaning. Body composition was detected in terms of water, lipids, and proteins percentage. Values represent mean ± SE of 5–6 different animals. Differences were evaluated for statistical significance by two-way ANOVA test followed by a Tukey's post hoc multiple comparison test. Different letters indicate that differences between mean values are statistically significant, with $p < 0.05$. Two way ANOVA test results: - Panel a, for each parameter considered: diet effect $p < 0.0001$, genotype effect ns, interaction ns. - Panel b, energy gain: diet effect $p < 0.0001$, genotype effect ns interaction ns -lipid gain: diet effect $p < 0.0001$, genotype effect $p = 0.0074$, interaction $p < 0.0001$ -protein gain: diet effect $p < 0.0001$, genotype effect ns, interaction ns, Panel c—water: diet effect $p < 0.0001$, genotype effect ns interaction ns -lipids: diet effect $p < 0.0001$, genotype effect $p = 0.0040$, interaction $p < 0.0032$ - protein gain: diet effect $p = 0.0154$, genotype effect ns, interaction ns ($p = 0.0516$), Panel d – Efficiency of energy deposition: diet effect $p < 0.0001$, genotype effect ns ($p = 0.0913$), interaction $p = 0.013$ - Efficiency of lipid deposition: diet effect $p < 0.0001$, genotype effect ns, interaction $p = 0.0118$ - Efficiency of protein deposition: diet effect $p = 0.0016$ genotype effect ns, interaction ns.

In mice that were fed a STD, the efficiency of the energy deposition (evaluated as percent of energy consumed by diet and stored in the body) was similar in WT and KO mice (Figure 5d). The HFD regimen induced a significant increase in the efficiency of the energy deposition, which was significantly higher in KO-HFD as compared to WT-HFD. Indeed, the two-way ANOVA test revealed the significant effects of diet and the interaction between genotype and diet (Figure 5 legend).

The percentage of energy that was consumed by diet as lipids that was stored in the body did not differ between WT-STD and KO-STD (Figure 5d). HFD feeding significantly reduced such a parameter and, despite KO-HFD mice tending to have higher lipid deposition efficiency than WT-HFD (+40%), differences between these two groups did not reach statistical significance. Concerning the efficiency of protein deposition, no difference was observed between WT-STD and KO-STD. The HFD regimen enhances the efficiency of protein deposition and similar values were detected in WT-HFD and KO-HFD (Figure 5d). When considering either lipids or protein deposition (Figure 5d), two-way ANOVA tests revealed a significant effect of the diet, while neither the effect of genotype or the interaction between genotype and diet were significant (Figure 5 legend).

Consistent with what is described above, after 80 days of STD no differences in mouse body composition (evaluated in terms of content of water, lipids and protein in the carcass and expressed in percentage terms) were detected between WT-STD and KO-STD (Figure 5c). As expected, HFD treatment significantly affected mouse body composition, and a reduction in water content was observed independent of the genotype. Regarding the body lipid percentage, HFD treatment significantly enhanced it, with KO-HFD showing values that were higher than WT-HFD. In this case, the two-way ANOVA test reported the significant effects of diet and genotype, as well as a significant interaction effect between diet and genotype (Figure 5 legend). Concerning the body protein percentage (Figure 5c), HFD treatment enhanced it in WT mice, but failed to affect it in KO mice. Indeed, in the WT-HFD mice the protein percentage was higher than in the WT-STD ones, while no differences between KO-HFD and KO-STD were detected. Two-way ANOVA tests revealed a significant diet effect, being that the genotype effect was not significant and the interaction between the diet and genotype effects were at the limit of significance ($p = 0.0516$).

3.3. Effect of UCP3 Ablation on Visceral Adipose Tissue and Lipid Accumulation in Lean Tissue in Mice Fed Either with a Standard/Low Fat Diet or a High Fat Diet

The contribution of metabolically active tissues (liver, heart, gastrocnemius skeletal muscle, brown adipose tissue) to the weight of mice was similar when comparing the WT-STD, KO-STD, WT-HFD, and KO-HFD mice (data not shown). Interestingly, the contribution of total visceral WAT (vWAT) to body weight was lower in KO-STD than in WT-STD mice (about −25%) (Table 2). As expected, in mice under HFD, the contribution of vWAT weight to whole body animal was significantly higher than in mice under STD. Indeed, in WT-HFD the contribution was 56% higher than that of WT-STD, while in KO-HFD it was 97% higher than that observed in KO-STD (Table 2). In this case, a two-way ANOVA test indicated the genotype effect and the diet one as significant, but the interaction effect between genotype and diet as not significant (Table 2 legend).

Variations in vWAT mass, which were detected between WT-STD and KO-STD, were not associated with change in adipocytes size (Figure 6a–c), while WAT basal lipolysis was almost doubled in KO mice as compared to WT (Figure 7). Histological analysis of lean tissues (liver and skeletal muscle) revealed the presence of some lipid droplets in liver from WT-STD exposed at thermoneutrality, in accordance with data present in literature. Interestingly, the same analysis indicated an ectopic accumulation of fat that is associated with the absence of UCP3 in liver and skeletal muscle (Figure 6a). Indeed, H&E staining of skeletal muscle and liver sections from KO-STD at 100× magnification showed many large intracellular lipid droplets (LD) as uncoloured circles. Numerous large (~2 μm) intramyocellular lipid droplets (IMLDs) were only present in the skeletal muscle of KO-STD mice as well as a massive lipid accumulation being shown in the cytoplasm of all the hepatocytes. Mice under HFD presented an accumulation of lipids in liver whatever the genotype, and lipid accumulation in skeletal muscle was more evident in the KO-HFD mice then in the WT-HFD ones.

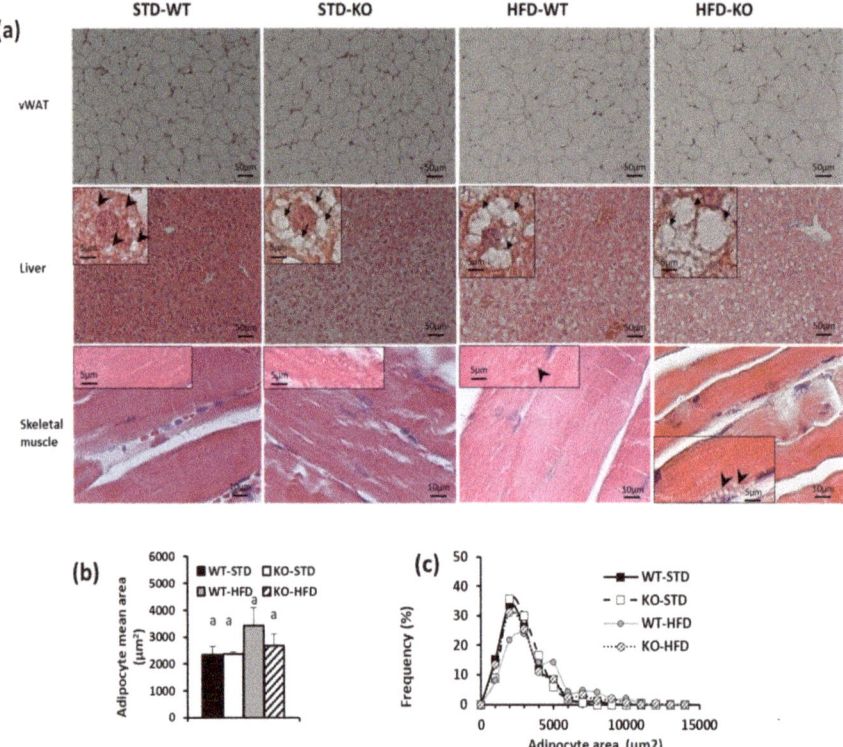

Figure 6. Effect of UCP3 ablation on lipid accumulation in WT and KO mice housed at thermoneutrality and fed with either a standard/low fat diet (STD) or high fat diet (HFD) for 80 days, since weaning. (**a**) Representative histological analysis of visceral WAT, liver and gastrocnemius skeletal muscle isolated from WT and KO mice, housed at thermoneutrality since weaning and fed with a standard/low fat diet for 80 days. Insets: high magnification images (100x) to visualize intracellular LD as uncoloured circles. In liver, arrowheads indicated small LD whereas arrows showed very large LD. (**b**) Mean Surface Area of adipocytes (μm^2), (**c**) frequency distribution for surface area of adipocyte Values represent mean ± SE of 3 different animals. Differences were evaluated for statistical significance by two-way ANOVA test followed by a Tukey's post hoc multiple comparison test. Different letters indicate that differences between mean values are statistically significant, with $p < 0.05$. Two-way ANOVA test results for adipocyte mean area: diet effect, genotype effect and interaction ns.

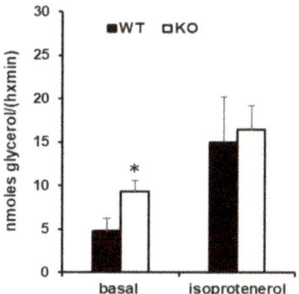

Figure 7. Effect of UCP3 ablation on visceral WAT lipolysis detected in WT and KO mice housed at thermoneutrality and fed with a standard/low fat diet (STD) for 80 days, since weaning. A glycerol release was detected on small pieces of epididymal WAT from WT-STD and KO-STD mice in the absence and in the presence of isoprotenerol. Values represent mean ± SE of 6 different animals. Statistical analyses were performed by two-tailed Student's t-test, * $p < 0.05$ vs. WT.

4. Discussion

In this study, we minimized thermal stress to better define the role of UCP3 in whole energy homeostasis and lipid utilization and we showed that in 4–5 month old mice acclimated for 2–3 weeks at thermoneutrality, the absence of UCP3 significantly depresses the whole animal RMR and REE, the energy intake, and the use of lipids as metabolic substrates. The last effect seems to be the result of the impaired ability of SkM mitochondria to oxidize fatty acid, which confirmed the results of previous studies employing mice that were housed at a standard temperature [11,12,34].

Interestingly, the absence of UCP3 selectively reduces the oxidation of lipid derived substrates, such as palmitoyl carnitine (State 3), while not affecting respiratory parameters (both State 4 and State 3) when pyruvate or succinate was used as substrate, i.e., a complex I- linked substrate and complex II-linked substrate, respectively. It should be considered that the control of State 4 respiration is shared between proton leak and reactions that are involved in the oxidation of substrates (among these respiratory chain). The control of State 3 respiration is shared between the reaction involved in the synthesis and export of ATP and the reaction involved in the oxidation of a substrate [35]. Thus, the absence of variations in State 4 respiration suggest that UCP3 does not impact the respiration that is needed to balance the proton leak in basal condition. These data are in line with some studies showing no differences in basal proton-leak kinetics between WT and KO in skeletal muscle mitochondria from mice that were housed at a standard temperature [36,37] and from mice housed at thermoneutrality (our unpublished observation). They also support the concept that UCP3 could only mediate the proton leak in the presence of activators, plausibly ROS and FA [6,37]. At the same time, we did not observe any variations in State 3, in the presence of either pyruvate or succinate, between WT and KO SkM mitochondria. This finding suggests that the absence of UCP3 does not influence the activities of the reactions that are involved in the synthesis and export of ATP, and that are involved in the oxidation of the above substrates, among these the respiratory chain. The functional data, obtained in isolated mitochondria that are oxidizing pyruvate or succinate, agree with the in gel respiratory complexes activity. The reduced state 3, detected in KO mice mitochondria in the presence of palmitoyl-carnitine, suggests that it is plausibly due to the impaired activity of the reactions that are involved in the oxidation of such a substrate.

Data that were obtained in adult animals acclimated to thermoneutrality for two to three weeks suggest that the absence of UCP3 could influence body lipid accumulation. We tested this hypothesis by chronically exposing mice to different lipid loads when housed at thermoneutrality since weaning.

The absence of UCP3 leads mice to be more susceptible to whole animal lipid accumulation only when they are subject to a HFD lipid overload. In fact, HFD-KO mice showed enhanced body energy efficiency and increased body lipid gain, which, by the end of the treatment, produced a different body composition with KO-HFD mice presenting a higher body lipid percentage and lower protein percentage when compared to HDF-WT mice. Interestingly, the evidence that KO-HFD and HFD-WT mice showed the same energy/lipid intake, but at the same time HFD-KO mice accumulated more lipid, further sustains that the absence of UCP3 reduced fat utilization and increased whole body fat storage. As a whole our data also indicates that lipids overload, as obtained by HFD administration, is important to shed light on the involvement of UCP3 in influencing body composition, since, when mice were fed with a standard/low fat diet, the absence of UCP3 does not influence the whole body lipid accumulation as well as body composition.

The ability of KO mice fed a HFD to accumulate more fat than WT mice was previously demonstrated by Costford et al. [15]. However, this accumulation was observed in mice that were housed at 23 °C that had received HFD for eight months, whereas the treatment was ineffective after only four months of HFD [19]. Notably, our data indicates that, when housing mice under thermoneutral conditions, 80 days (~2.5 month) of HFD was enough to produce a higher lipid gain in KO mice when compared to wild type mice. This finding further supports the critical role of housing temperature for metabolic studies. Interestingly, despite the fact that, in young mice fed with standard/low fat diet, the absence of UCP3 does not change whole body lipid accumulation, redistribution of fat in the body does get affected, since it represses lipid storage in visceral WAT, while promoting accumulation in the liver and skeletal muscle.

Previous studies that were performed on KO mice housed at standard temperature and fed with low fat/standard diet failed to show an increase in intramuscular lipid accumulation. This was only observed when KO mice were fed with a HFD for eight months [15], thus further confirming the importance of the housing temperature for the outcome of this phenomenon in the absence of chronic lipids overload.

It should be considered that, in mice, the inability to adequately promote fatty acid utilization is associated with lipid accumulation in peripheral tissues and it contributes to the development of insulin resistance [38], a condition that is more evident when associated with enhanced WAT lipolysis. This "metabolic picture" is observed in KO mice that were acclimated to thermoneutrality, in which fatty acid oxidation is blunted, release of fatty acids by visceral adipose tissue' depots is enhanced, and the accumulation of lipid in lean tissues (liver and skeletal muscle) takes place. These data suggest that: (i) an alteration in UCP3 activity can also affect the metabolism of tissues that do not express it, such as liver, presumably through changes in systemic metabolite trafficking, and (ii) UCP3 exerts a protective role against lean tissue "lipotoxicity" and insulin resistance, by avoiding ectopic fat accumulation.

The above data are in agreement with our previous studies indicating that a progressive decline in insulin sensitivity in UCP3+/− heterozygous mice and UCP3−/− mice [11] and with clinical observations reporting that (i) a 50% reduction of UCP3 protein in human SkM is correlated with the incidence of T2DM [39], (ii) in humans, the UCP3 protein levels are reduced in the pre-diabetic state of impaired glucose tolerance [40,41], (iii) heterozygous mutations in the UCP3 gene (V56M, A111V, V192I, and Q252X) in children was associated with dyslipidemia and lower insulin sensitivity [42]. Nevertheless, some limitations exist in our study that are to be addressed in the future. These are:

(i)   Mice habitual activity levels have not been evaluated. This is known to influence parameters, such as energy efficiency, body weight gain, and lipid accumulation. Thus, at the moment, it is unclear whether mouse activity levels were altered between gene and or diets, or whether activity levels contributed to study outcomes;
(ii) Whole animal metabolic rate, respiratory quotient, mitochondrial functionality, and WAT lipolysis have only been evaluated in mice that were fed a standard diet. Thus, the estimation of the impact of high fat diet feeding on the above parameters would allow for better clarification of how they are influenced by different diet regimen and the eventual existence of an interaction diet-genotype;
(iii) The evaluation of lipid serum levels, not detected in the present paper, would have provided additional knowledge regarding the role played by UCP3 in influencing lipid metabolism.

5. Conclusions

By carrying out our studies under conditions where thermal stress was eliminated, we have highlighted the protective role of UCP3 against ectopic lipid accumulation in lean tissues. Of relevance, by varying the energy and fat intake through the administration of HFD, the role that is played by UCP3 in contrasting HFD-induced fat accumulation clearly emerged. In addition, results that were obtained from studies performed in animals housed at thermoneutrality could be better translated to humans, which choose to live in a thermoneutral environment.

Author Contributions: A.L. (Assunta Lombardi), F.G., M.M. and A.L. (Antonia Lanni); Conceptualization. A.L. (Assunta Lombardi), R.A.B., R.d.M., L.L., S.S., A.G., E.S., F.C., P.d.L. and R.S.; investigation and data curation, A.L. (Assunta Lombardi), F.G.; original draft preparation; A.L. (Assunta Lombardi), F.G., M.M., L.L., A.L. (Antonia Lanni), P.d.L., E.S., R.D.M. and L.L.; review and editing manuscript.

Funding: This work was supported by University of Sannio (Fondi FRA 2016) and by Department of Biology University of Naples Federico II (Ricerca di Base).

Conflicts of Interest: The authors declare no conflict of interest.

References

1. Boss, O.; Samec, S.; Paoloni-Giacobino, A.; Rossier, C.; Dullo, A.; Seydoux, J.; Muzzin, P.; Giacobino, J.P. Uncoupling protein-3: A new member of the mitochondrial carrier family with tissue-specific expression. *FEBS Lett.* **1997**, *408*, 39–42. [CrossRef]
2. Hilse, K.E.; Kalinovich, A.V.; Rupprecht, A.; Smorodchenko, A.; Zeitz, U.; Staniek, K.; Erben, R.G.; Pohl, E.E. The expression of UCP3 directly correlates to UCP1 abundance in brown adipose tissue. *Biochim. Biophys. Acta (BBA)-Bioenerg.* **2016**, *1857*, 72–78. [CrossRef] [PubMed]
3. Gong, D.W.; Monemdjou, S.; Gavrilova, O.; Leon, L.R.; Marcus-Samuels, B.; Chou, C.J.; Everett, C.; Kozak, L.P.; Li, C.; Deng, C.; et al. Lack of obesity and normal response to fasting and thyroid hormone in mice lacking uncoupling protein-3. *J. Biol. Chem.* **2000**, *275*, 16251–16257. [CrossRef] [PubMed]
4. Riley, C.L.; Dao, C.; Kenaston, M.A.; Muto, L.; Kohno, S.; Nowinski, S.M.; Solmonson, A.D.; Pfeiffer, M.; Sack, M.N.; Lu, Z.; et al. The complementary and divergent roles of uncoupling proteins 1 and 3 in thermoregulation. *J. Physiol.* **2016**, *594*, 7455–7464. [CrossRef] [PubMed]
5. Cadenas, S.; Seydoux, J.J.; Din, N.; Dulloo, A.G.; Brand, M.D. UCP2 and UCP3 rise in starved rat skeletal muscle but mitochondrial proton conductance is unchanged. *FEBS Lett.* **1999**, *462*, 257–260. [CrossRef]
6. Brand, M.D.; Esteves, T.C. Physiological functions of the mitochondrial uncoupling proteins UCP2 and UCP3. *Cell Metab.* **2005**, *2*, 85–93. [CrossRef]
7. Echtay, K.S.; Pakay, J.L.; Esteves, T.C.; Brand, M.D. Hydroxynonenal and uncoupling proteins: A model for protection against oxidative damage. *Biofactors* **2005**, *24*, 119–130. [CrossRef]
8. Cioffi, F.; Senese, R.; de Lange, P.; Goglia, F.; Lanni, A.; Lombardi, A. Uncoupling proteins: A complex journey to function discovery. *Biofactors* **2009**, *35*, 417–428. [CrossRef]
9. Cadenas, S. Mitochondrial uncoupling, ROS generation and cardioprotection. *Biochim. Biophys. Acta (BBA)-Bioenerg.* **2018**, *1859*, 940–950. [CrossRef]
10. Bézaire, V.; Seifert, E.L.; Harper, M.E. Uncoupling protein-3: Clues in an ongoing mitochondrial mystery. *FASEB J.* **2007**, *21*, 312–324. [CrossRef]
11. Hilse, K.E.; Rupprecht, A.; Egerbacher, M.; Bardakji, S.; Zimmermann, L.; Wulczyn, A.E.M.S.; Pohl, E.E. The Expression of Uncoupling Protein 3 Coincides with the Fatty Acid Oxidation Type of Metabolism in Adult Murine Heart. *Front. Physiol.* **2018**, *9*, 747. [CrossRef]
12. Senese, R.; Valli, V.; Moreno, M.; Lombardi, A.; Busiello, R.A.; Cioffi, F.; Silvestri, E.; Goglia, F.; Lanni, A.; de Lange, P.; et al. Uncoupling protein-3 expression levels influence insulin sensitivity, fatty acid oxidation, and related signaling pathways. *Pflug. Arch. Eur. J. Physiol.* **2011**, *461*, 153–164. [CrossRef]
13. McBride, S.; Wei-LaPierre, L.; McMurray, F.; MacFarlane, M.; Qiu, X.; Patten, D.A.; Dirksen, R.T.; Harper, M.E. Skeletal muscle mitoflashes, pH, and the role of uncoupling protein-3. *Arch. Biochem. Biophys.* **2019**, *663*, 239–248. [CrossRef]
14. Bouillaud, F. UCP2, not a physiologically relevant uncoupler but a glucose sparing switch impacting ROS production and glucose sensing. *Biochim. Biophys. Acta (BBA)-Bioenerg.* **2009**, *1787*, 377–383. [CrossRef]

15. Fink, B.D.; Herlein, J.A.; Almind, K.; Cinti, S.; Kahn, C.R.; Sivitz, W.I. Mitochondrial proton-leak in obesity resistant and obesity-prone mice. *Am. J. Physiol. Regul. Integr. Comp. Physiol.* **2007**, *293*, R1773–R1780. [CrossRef]
16. Costford, S.R.; Chaudhry, N.; Salkhordeh, M.; Harper, M.E. Effects of the presence, absence, and overexpression of uncoupling protein-3 on adiposity and fuel metabolism in congenic mice. *Am. J. Physiol. Endocrinol. Metab.* **2006**, *290*, E1304–E1312. [CrossRef]
17. Son, C.; Hosoda, K.; Ishihara, K.; Bevilacqua, L.; Masuzaki, H.; Fushiki, T.; Harper, M.E.; Nakao, K. Reduction of diet-induced obesity in transgenic mice overexpressing uncoupling protein 3 in skeletal muscle. *Diabetologia* **2004**, *47*, 47–54. [CrossRef]
18. Aguer, C.; Fiehn, O.; Seifert, E.L.; Bézaire, V.; Meissen, J.K.; Daniels, A.; Scott, K.; Renaud, J.M.; Padilla, M.; Bickel, D.R.; et al. Muscle uncoupling protein 3 overexpression mimics endurance training and reduces circulating biomarkers of incomplete β-oxidation. *FASEB J.* **2013**, *27*, 4213–4225. [CrossRef]
19. Vidal-Puig, A.J.; Grujic, D.; Zhang, C.Y.; Hagen, T.; Boss, O.; Ido, Y.; Szczepanik, A.; Wade, J.; Mootha, V.; Cortright, R.; et al. Energy metabolism in uncoupling protein 3 gene knockout mice. *J. Biol. Chem.* **2000**, *275*, 16258–16266. [CrossRef]
20. Costford, S.R.; Chaudhry, S.N.; Crawford, S.A.; Salkhordeh, M.; Harper, M.E. Long-term high-fat feeding induces greater fat storage in mice lacking UCP3. *Am. J. Physiol. Endocrinol. Metab.* **2008**, *295*, E1018–E1024. [CrossRef]
21. Feldmann, H.M.; Golozoubova, V.; Cannon, B.; Nedergaard, J. UCP1 ablation induces obesity and abolishes diet-induced thermogenesis in mice exempt from thermal stress by living at thermoneutrality. *Cell Metab.* **2009**, *9*, 203–209. [CrossRef]
22. Fischer, A.W.; Cannon, B.; Nedergaard, J. Optimal housing temperatures for mice to mimic the thermal environment of humans: An experimental study. *Mol. Metab.* **2008**, *7*, 161–170. [CrossRef]
23. Lusk, G. Animal calorimetry: Analysis of the oxidation of mixtures of carbohydrates and fat. *J. Biol. Chem.* **1926**, *59*, 41–42.
24. Lombardi, A.; Lanni, A.; de Lange, P.; Silvestri, E.; Grasso, P.; Senese, R.; Goglia, F.; Moreno, M. Acute administration of 3,5-diiodo-L-thyronine to hypothyroid rats affects bioenergetic parameters in rat skeletal muscle mitochondria. *FEBS Lett.* **2007**, *581*, 5911–5916. [CrossRef]
25. Schagger, H. Native electrophoresis for isolation of mitochondrial oxidative phosphorylation protein complexes. *Methods Enzymol.* **1995**, *260*, 190–202.
26. Lombardi, A.; Silvestri, E.; Cioffi, F.; Senese, R.; Lanni, A.; Goglia, F.; de Lange, P.; Moreno, M. Defining the transcriptomic and proteomic profiles of rat ageing skeletal muscle by the use of a cDNA array, 2D- and Blue native-PAGE approach. *J. Proteomics* **2009**, *72*, 708–721. [CrossRef]
27. Zerbetto, E.; Vergani, L.; Dabbeni-Sala, F. Quantification of muscle mitochondrial oxidative phosphorylation enzymes via histochemical staining of blue native polyacrylamide gels. *Electrophoresis* **1997**, *18*, 2059–2064. [CrossRef]
28. Clark, A.M.; Sousa, K.M.; Jennings, C.; MacDougald, O.A.; Kennedy, R.T. Continuous-flow enzyme assay on a microfluidic chip for monitoring glycerol secretion from cultured adipocytes. *Anal. Chem.* **2009**, *81*, 2350–2356. [CrossRef]
29. Iossa, S.; Lionetti, L.; Mollica, M.P.; Barletta, A.; Liverini, G. Energy intake and utilization vary during development in rats. *J. Nutr.* **1999**, *129*, 1593–1596. [CrossRef]
30. Folch, N.; Leess, M.; Stanley, G.H.S. A simple method for the isolation and purification of total lipids from animal tissues. *J. Biol. Chem.* **1957**, *226*, 497–51011.
31. Dulloo, A.G.; Girardier, L. Adaptive changes in energy expenditure during refeeding following low calorie intake: Evidence for a specific metabolic component favoring fat storage. *Am. J. Clin. Nutr.* **1990**, *52*, 415–420. [CrossRef]
32. Dulloo, A.G.; Seydoux, G.; Girardier, L. Role of corticosterone in adaptive changes in energy expenditure during refeeding after low calorie intake. *Am. J. Physiol. Endocrinol. Metab.* **1990**, *259*, E658–E664. [CrossRef]
33. Giles, D.A.; Moreno-Fernandez, M.E.; Stankiewicz, T.E.; Graspeuntner, S.; Cappelletti, M.; Wu, D.; Mukherjee, R.; Chan, C.C.; Lawson, M.J.; Klarquist, J.; et al. Thermoneutral housing exacerbates nonalcoholic fatty liver disease in mice and allows for sex-independent disease modeling. *Nat. Med.* **2017**, *23*, 829–838. [CrossRef]

34. Nabben, M.; Hoeks, J.; Moonen-Kornips, E.; van Beurden, D.; Briedé, J.J.; Hesselink, M.K.; Glatz, J.F.; Schrauwen, P. Significance of uncoupling protein-3 in mitochondrial function upon mid and long term dietary high-fat exposure. *FEBS Lett.* **2011**, *585*, 4010–4017. [CrossRef]
35. Rolfe, D.F.; Hulbert, A.J.; Brand, M.D. Characteristics of mitochondrial proton leak and control of oxidative phosphorylation in the major oxygen-consuming tissues of the rat. *Biochim. Biophys. Acta (BBA)-Bioenerg.* **1994**, *1188*, 405–416. [CrossRef]
36. Cadenas, S.; Echtay, K.S.; Harper, J.A.; Jekabsons, M.B.; Buckingham, J.A.; Grau, E.; Abuin, A.; Chapman, H.; Clapham, J.C.; Brand, M.D.; et al. The basal proton conductance of skeletal muscle mitochondria from transgenic mice overexpressing or lacking uncoupling protein-3. *J. Biol. Chem.* **2002**, *277*, 2773–2778. [CrossRef]
37. Lombardi, A.; Busiello, R.A.; Napolitano, L.; Cioffi, F.; Moreno, M.; de Lange, P.; Silvestri, E.; Lanni, A.; Goglia, F. UCP3 translocates lipid hydroperoxide and mediates lipid hydroperoxide-dependent mitochondrial uncoupling. *J. Biol. Chem.* **2010**, *285*, 16599–16605. [CrossRef]
38. Schönke, M.; Massart, J.; Zierath, J.R. Effects of high-fat diet and AMP-activated protein kinase modulation on the regulation of whole-body lipid metabolism. *J. Lipid Res.* **2018**, *59*, 1276–1282. [CrossRef]
39. Schrauwen, P.; Hesselink, M.K.; Blaak, E.E.; Borghouts, L.B.; Schaart, G.; Saris, W.H.; Keizer, H.A. Uncoupling protein 3 content is decreased in skeletal muscle of patients with type 2 diabetes. *Diabetes* **2001**, *50*, 2870–2873. [CrossRef]
40. Schrauwen, P.; Messelink, M.K.C. Oxidative capacity, lipotoxicity, and mitochondrial damage in type 2 diabetes. *Diabetes* **2005**, *53*, 412–1417. [CrossRef]
41. Mensink, M.; Hesselink, M.K.; Borghouts, L.B.; Keizer, H.; Moonen-Kornips, E.; Schaart, G.; Blaak, E.E.; Schrauwen, P. Skeletal muscle uncoupling protein-3 restores upon intervention in the prediabetic and diabetic state: Implications for diabetes pathogenesis? *Diabetes Obes. Metab.* **2007**, *9*, 594–596. [CrossRef]
42. Musa, C.V.; Mancini, A.; Alfieri, A.; Labruna, G.; Valerio, G.; Franzese, A.; Pasanisi, F.; Licenziati, M.R.; Sacchetti, L.; Buono, P.; et al. Four novel UCP3 gene variants associated with childhood obesity: Effect on fatty acid oxidation and on prevention of triglyceride storage. *Int. J. Obes.* **2012**, *36*, 207–217. [CrossRef]

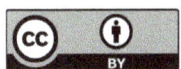 © 2019 by the authors. Licensee MDPI, Basel, Switzerland. This article is an open access article distributed under the terms and conditions of the Creative Commons Attribution (CC BY) license (http://creativecommons.org/licenses/by/4.0/).

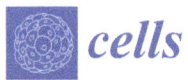

Communication

Critical Impact of Human Amniotic Membrane Tension on Mitochondrial Function and Cell Viability In Vitro

Laura Poženel [1,2], Andrea Lindenmair [2,3], Katy Schmidt [4], Andrey V. Kozlov [1,2], Johannes Grillari [1,2,5], Susanne Wolbank [1,2], Asmita Banerjee [1,2,*,†] and Adelheid Weidinger [1,2,†]

1. Ludwig Boltzmann Institute for Experimental and Clinical Traumatology, AUVA Research Center, Donaueschingenstraße 13, 1200 Vienna, Austria; laura.pozenel@trauma.lbg.ac.at (L.P.); andrey.kozlov@trauma.lbg.ac.at (A.V.K.); johannes.grillari@trauma.lbg.ac.at (J.G.); susanne.wolbank@trauma.lbg.ac.at (S.W.); adelheid.weidinger@trauma.lbg.ac.at (A.W.)
2. Austrian Cluster for Tissue Regeneration, 1200 Vienna, Austria; Andrea.Lindenmair@o.roteskreuz.at
3. Ludwig Boltzmann Institute for Experimental and Clinical Traumatology, AUVA Research Center, Garnisonstraße 21, 4020 Linz, Austria
4. Medical University of Vienna, Center for Anatomy and Cell Biology, Division of Cell and Developmental Biology, Schwarzspanierstraße 17, 1090 Vienna, Austria; katy.schmidt@meduniwien.ac.at
5. University of Natural Resources and Life Sciences Vienna, Department of Biotechnology, Muthgasse 18, 1190 Vienna, Austria
* Correspondence: asmita.banerjee@trauma.lbg.ac.at; Tel.: +43-59-3934-1984
† These authors contributed equally to this work.

Received: 11 November 2019; Accepted: 13 December 2019; Published: 15 December 2019

Abstract: Amniotic cells show exciting stem cell features, which has led to the idea of using living cells of human amniotic membranes (hAMs) in toto for clinical applications. However, under common cell culture conditions, viability of amniotic cells decreases rapidly, whereby reasons for this decrease are unknown so far. Recently, it has been suggested that loss of tissue tension in vivo leads to apoptosis. Therefore, the aim of this study was to investigate the effect of tissue distention on the viability of amniotic cells in vitro. Thereby, particular focus was put on vital mitochondria-linked parameters, such as respiration and ATP synthesis. Biopsies of hAMs were incubated for 7–21 days either non-distended or distended. We observed increased B-cell lymphoma 2-associated X protein (BAX)/B-cell lymphoma (BCL)-2 ratios in non-distended hAMs at day seven, followed by increased caspase 3 expression at day 14, and, consequently, loss of viability at day 21. In contrast, under distention, caspase 3 expression increased only slightly, and mitochondrial function and cellular viability were largely maintained. Our data suggest that a mechano-sensing pathway may control viability of hAM cells by triggering mitochondria-mediated apoptosis upon loss of tension in vitro. Further studies are required to elucidate the underlying molecular mechanisms between tissue distention and viability of hAM cells.

Keywords: apoptosis; human amniotic membrane; mitochondrial cell death; BAX; BCL-2; tensile strength

---

1. Introduction

Despite the over a century old tradition of using the human amniotic membrane (hAM) successfully for tissue regeneration in clinics [1–5], properties of the hAM are still subject of research.

The hAM starts to develop around day 7.5 of human gestation, far earlier than the formation of the three germ layers [6]. Forming the amniotic cavity, the hAM expands during the course of pregnancy and is supposed to rupture at term. It is usually discarded after childbirth, and, although of embryonic origin, the use and application of hAMs does not raise ethical issues. The hAM can be classified into different sub-regions. While both amniotic membranes are attached to the chorion, placental amnion (and chorion) covers the placenta, and reflected amnion (and chorion) is located opposite it. After preparation, the hAM is a thin, flexible and almost translucent membrane, harboring two vital cell populations. Human amniotic epithelial cells (hAECs) form a layer that, in vivo, faces the fetus, and is in direct contact with the amniotic fluid. Underneath, human amniotic mesenchymal stromal cells (hAMSCs) are embedded in a layer of extracellular matrix. Both cell populations have been proven to have stem cell characteristics, such as the ability to differentiate into lineages of all three germ layers in vivo and in vitro [7–10]. Furthermore, the cells express markers of pluripotency, an otherwise solely embryonic feature [11]. Properties of the hAM have been extensively described, as it is known to be anti-inflammatory [12–15] and immune-modulatory [14,15]. Moreover, remarkably, no substantial immune reactions upon application have been reported. We and others, furthermore, showed significantly different properties of cells of placental and reflected amnion in previous studies [16–19].

Up until the turn of the century, the hAM has normally been used in a denuded or decellularized form, making use of the composition of its extracellular matrix (reviewed in [5]). With increasing evidence of the stem cell properties of hAECs and hAMSCs, using hAMs with their original vital cell populations for tissue regeneration has come more and more into focus (reviewed in [5]). In other tissues and cell types, in recent years, researchers have concentrated on mitochondria in particular, as it has been shown that functional mitochondria are required to support tissue regeneration processes [20–22]. While beneficial properties of amniotic cells have been known for more than two decades, sustaining cellular viability of the hAM remains a challenge. For example, cryopreservation of hAMs under conditions reported does not result in any viable cells [23]. However, storage under common cell culture conditions is also not applicable, since several studies have shown decreasing cellular viability of the hAM [9,10,24]. To our knowledge, reasons for this rapid decrease of viability in vitro are not known so far.

However, in vivo, net loss of extracellular matrix [25] and apoptosis of hAECs are involved in the mechanisms leading to rupture of the membranes at term (reviewed in [26]). Parry therefore suggested that apoptosis of amniotic cells in vivo is probably a consequence of loss of tissue tension [26]. Of note, in vivo, the hAM is distended by a factor of 1.75 [27], a tensile strength that, ex vivo, is no longer existent. We therefore hypothesized that for in vitro culture of hAM, tensile strength plays an important role in the maintenance of cellular viability and that mitochondria play a critical role in this process.

The aim of this study was to clarify whether tissue distention controls apoptosis in a mitochondria-dependent manner and whether it can impact the viability of hAMs. To achieve this aim, we examined cellular viability, mitochondrial activity and activation of apoptotic pathways in distended compared to non-distended (floating) hAM samples in culture.

2. Materials and Methods

2.1. Preparation of the Human Amniotic Membrane (hAM)

Human placentae from caesarean sections were collected with informed consent of the patients and approval of the local ethical commission (Ethikkommission des Landes Oberösterreich, 21 May 2014), in accordance to the Declaration of Helsinki. Placentae were transported within 4 h in 500 mL Ringer solution. Placentae from caesarean sections of premature deliveries, emergency caesarean sections and placentae with detached amniotic membranes were excluded from the study. Placental (P) and reflected (RA) regions were separated, the hAM was peeled off the chorion and washed with cold phosphate-buffered saline (PBS).

2.2. Cultivation of hAM Samples

For tissue distention, fresh hAM was mounted on CellCrown™ inserts (Scaffdex, Tampere, Finland) (Figure 1B) and incubated in Dulbecco's Modified Eagle's Medium (DMEM) supplemented with 10% fetal calf serum (FCS), 1% L-glutamine and 1% penicillin/streptomycin ("culture medium") at 37 °C, a humidified atmosphere and 5% CO_2. On the day of measurement or sample freezing, biopsies of 8 mm diameter of distended samples were punched. Non-distended (floating) samples (Figure 1C) were kept under the same conditions. All samples were measured at day 0 and incubated for 7 days (B-cell lymphoma 2-associated X protein (BAX), B-cell lymphoma (BCL)-2), 14 days (mitochondrial morphology, caspase 3), or 21 days (mitochondrial membrane potential, mitochondrial respiration, ATP concentration). The culture medium was changed twice weekly.

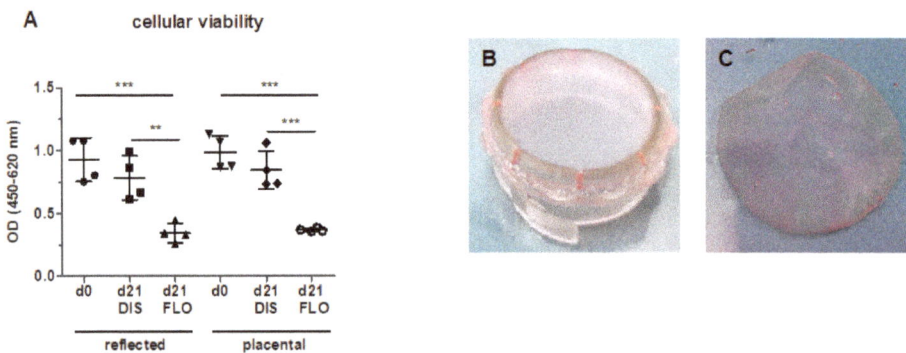

Figure 1. Cellular viability of reflected and placental amnion in fresh biopsies (day 0), biopsies mounted on CellCrown™ inserts (DIS), and biopsies kept floating (FLO) under common cell culture conditions for 21 days (**A**). Viability was measured with the EZ4U assay. Mean ± standard deviation (SD), n = 4 (donors). Samples of human amniotic membrane distended on CellCrown™ inserts (in 6 well plates) (**B**), and non-distended ("floating") (**C**) at day 0. DIS: distended biopsies; FLO: floating biopsies; OD: optical density. **$p < 0.01$, ***$p < 0.001$.

2.3. Cell Viability Assay

Cell viability of hAM biopsies (8 mm diameter) was quantified with the EZ4U—Cell Proliferation and Cytotoxicity Assay (Biomedica, Vienna, Austria). The assay was performed according to the manufacturer's protocol. Briefly, the substrate solution was diluted 1:10 in DMEM without phenol red supplemented with 1% L-glutamine (Sigma-Aldrich, St. Louis, MO, USA). Biopsies were added to the solution and incubated for 3 h 45 min at 37 °C and 5% CO_2. Plates were shaken for 15 min and the optical density (OD) was measured with a microplate reader (BMG Labtech, Polarstar Omega, Ortenberg, Germany) at 450 nm with 620 nm as reference. n = 4 (biological replicates).

2.4. Laser Scanning Confocal Microscopy

hAM samples were placed in 2-well chambered cover glass (Nunc™ Lab-Tek™, St. Louis, MO, USA) and stained with mitochondrial membrane potential sensitive fluorescent dye (500 nM tetramethylrhodamin-methylester (TMRM; VWR, Radnor, PA, USA (excitation/emission: 543 nm/585 nm)) for 45 min at 37 °C and 5% CO_2. Imaging was performed with an inverted confocal microscope (LSM510, Carl Zeiss, Oberkochen, Germany). Image analysis (mean fluorescence) was performed with ZEN2009 Software (release version 6.0 SP2; Carl Zeiss). n = 2–3 (biological replicates).

2.5. High Resolution Respirometry

Mitochondrial respiratory parameters were monitored using high resolution respirometry (Oxygraph-2k, Oroboros Instruments, Innsbruck, Austria). Mitochondrial ROUTINE respiration, reflecting total mitochondrial oxygen consumption, was measured by incubating 14 hAM biopsies (8 mm diameter) in DMEM at pH 7.2 and 37 °C. For details, see Supplementary Material. Mitochondrial states were calculated as the negative time derivative of oxygen concentration (rate of oxygen uptake), and corrected for non-mitochondrial respiration (myxothiazol, 1 µM). Data were calculated in µM O/min/14 biopsies and are displayed in percent of placental amnion at day 0. n = 4 (biological replicates).

2.6. ATP Measurement

Liquid nitrogen frozen hAM biopsies (8 mm diameter) were homogenized in Precellys tubes with ceramic beads (Keramik-Kit 1.4 mm Peqlab VWR, USA) in a ball mill (CryoMill MM301, Retsch, Haan, Germany) with 500 µL of Tris-HCl buffer (20 mM Tris, 135 mM KCl, pH 7.4). Boiling buffer (400 µL of 100 mM Tris/4 mM EDTA, pH 7.75) was added to 100 µL hAM homogenate, incubated for 2 min at 100 °C and centrifuged at 1000× g for 2 min. ATP measurements were performed with the ATP Bioluminescence Assay Kit CLS II (Roche, Basel, Switzerland) in accordance with the manufacturer's protocol using luciferase reagent with Lumat LB 9507 (Berthold, Bad Wildbad, Germany). For details, see Supplementary Material. n = 4 (biological replicates).

2.7. Histology

Amnion biopsies were fixed for 24 h in 4% formalin and samples were embedded in paraffin. Immunohistochemistry against caspase 3 was performed with an anti-cleaved caspase 3 antibody 1:100 (Cell Signaling Technology, Danvers, MA, USA). Immunohistochemical negative controls were performed by replacing the primary antibody with buffer. Immunohistochemical sections were quantified with ImageJ software (National Institutes of Health, version 1.51j8, Bethesda, MD, USA). n = 3 (biological replicates).

2.8. Transmission Electron Microscopy

Biopsies were fixed with 2.5% glutaraldehyde and 2% paraformaldehyde for 2–3 h at room temperature and post-fixed with 1% OsO_4 in 0.1 M cacodylate buffer. Dehydration and embedding in Epon resin were carried out according to standard protocols. Sections (70 nm) were contrasted with 2% uranyl acetate. Images were acquired with an electron microscope (Tecnai20, FEI Europe, Eindhoven, Netherlands) equipped with a 4K EagleCCD camera and processed with Adobe Photoshop. n = 2 (biological replicates).

2.9. Reverse-Transcription Quantitative PCR Analysis

Samples of hAM biopsies (8 mm diameter) were snap-frozen in liquid nitrogen and kept at −80 °C until further analysis. Total RNA extraction, mRNA reverse transcription and qPCR were performed by TAmiRNA GmbH (Vienna, city, Austria). n = 3 (biological replicates).

Total RNA extraction: total RNA was extracted from 10 amnion biopsies (8 mm diameter) using the miRNeasy Mini Kit (Qiagen, Hilden, Germany). Tissue was homogenized with 700 µL Qiazol; following incubation at room temperature for 5 min, 140 µL chloroform was added to the lysates, which were incubated for 3 min at room temperature and centrifuged at 12,000× g for 15 min at 4 °C. Precisely 350 µL of the upper aqueous phase was transferred to a miRNeasy mini column, and RNA was precipitated with 525 µL ethanol followed by automated washing with RPE and RWT buffer in a Qiacube liquid handling robot. Finally, total RNA was eluted in 30 µL nuclease free water and stored at −80 °C until further analysis.

mRNA reverse transcription and qPCR (RT-qPCR): messenger RNA quantification was performed using the TATAA Grandscript cDNA synthesis and SYBR Grandmaster mix kit (TATAA Biocenter, Göteborg, Sweden). Total RNA (500 ng) was used for reverse transcription and all steps were carried out according to recommendations by the manufacturer. PCR amplification was performed in a 96 well format in a Roche LC480 II instrument (Roche, Mannheim, Germany) with the following settings: 95 °C for 30 s followed by 45 cycles of 95 °C for 5 s, 63 °C for 15 s and 72 °C for 10 s and subsequent melting curve analysis. To calculate the cycle of quantification values (Cq-values), the second derivative method was used. Cq-values were subsequently normalized to the geometric mean of glyceraldehyde 3-phosphate dehydrogenase (GAPDH), beta-actin (ACTB), hypoxanthine phosphoribosyltransferase (HPRT1) and ubiquitin C (UBC) mRNA levels, by subtracting the gene of interest Cq-value from the respective geometric mean of the four references. Primer sequences of BAX and BCL-2 used for mRNA reverse-transcription quantitative PCR analysis are shown in Table S1.

2.10. Statistical Analysis

Data were analyzed using GraphPad Prism software (GraphPad Software 5.01, San Diego, CA, USA) by one-way ANOVA followed by Bonferroni post hoc test. In all tests, n (sample size) represents biological replicates (donors). Results are presented as mean ± SD. Level of significance was set at 0.05 and is indicated as *$p < 0.05$, **$p < 0.01$, or ***$p < 0.001$.

3. Results and Discussion

All tests were performed with reflected and placental amnion samples, as we and others already have shown significant differences between reflected and placental amnion [16–19].

3.1. Cellular Viability Strongly Decreased in Floating hAM Samples

In order to test hAM viability in vitro, biopsies kept under floating conditions for 21 days were tested for cell viability with the EZ4U assay. Indeed, cell viability significantly decreased in reflected and placental amnion compared to fresh biopsies at day 0 (Figure 1A), confirming that standard cell culture conditions do not sufficiently maintain cell viability. This is in line with previous studies, where loss of viability was already observed [9,10,24]. Interestingly, in these studies, cells in non-distended hAMs remained viable under osteogenic [9], chondrogenic [24] or Schwann cell-like cell differentiation conditions [10]. This could mean that under differentiation conditions, cells may receive signals that sustain cell viability.

To test our hypothesis (whether mechanical tissue distention could prolong cellular viability and preserve mitochondrial function in in vitro culture), we incubated hAM biopsies for 21 days under two different conditions. For distended samples, the hAM was mounted on CellCrown™ inserts in order to expose the hAM to tensile strength (Figure 1B). For non-distended biopsies, we kept the biopsies "floating" in culture medium (Figure 1C). In contrast to floating biopsies, biopsies mounted on CellCrown™ inserts for 21 days showed no loss of cellular viability (Figure 1A). It has to be taken into account that in floating samples, cells still have close cell–cell contact, however, no mechanical tension on the tissue is present.

3.2. Mitochondrial Membrane Potential Drastically Decreased in Floating hAM Samples

In order to see if mitochondria play a role in this strong decrease of cell viability, mitochondrial membrane potential was visualized after 21 days. Membrane potential was slightly decreased in distended reflected amnion (Figure 2B,G) compared to fresh hAM at day 0 (Figure 2A,G). Distended placental amnion (Figure 2E,G) at day 21 did not show any significant decrease compared to fresh biopsies at day 0 (Figure 2D,G). In contrast, mitochondrial membrane potential was drastically reduced in both reflected amnion (Figure 2C,G) and placental amnion (Figure 2F,G) under floating conditions after 21 days, compared to day 0 (Figure 2A,D,G) or distended biopsies (Figure 2B,E,G). Such changes in mitochondrial membrane potential can be connected to loss of cell viability [28].

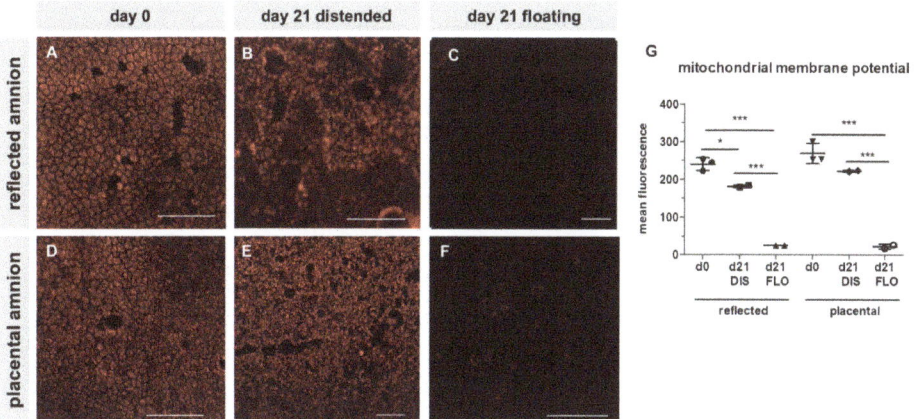

Figure 2. Mitochondrial membrane potential of reflected (**A,B,C**) and placental (**D,E,F**) amnion. Mitochondrial membrane potential (red) was stained with tetramethylrhodamin-methylester (TMRM; 500 nM) at day 0 (**A,D**) and at day 21 in biopsies cultivated while mechanically stretched (DIS; **B,E**) or kept floating (FLO; **C,F**). Imaging was performed with an inverted confocal microscope (LSM510, Zeiss, excitation/emission 543 nm/585 nm). Image analysis was performed with Zeiss ZEN2009 software (**G**). Mean ± standard deviation (SD), n = 3 (donors); representative images of one donor. Scale bar: 100 µm. DIS: distended biopsies; FLO: floating biopsies. Level of significance is indicated as * $p < 0.05$, *** $p < 0.001$

3.3. Mitochondrial Respiration and ATP Concentration Strongly Decreased in Floating hAM Samples

Since mitochondrial membrane potential does not necessarily reflect mitochondrial activity, we determined mitochondrial ROUTINE respiration, a measure for total mitochondrial oxygen consumption. In fresh biopsies (day 0), significantly higher ROUTINE respiration was detected in placental compared to reflected amnion (Figure 3A). This is in line with a previous publication of our group [18]. No difference was observed between day 0 and distended reflected amnion at day 21. Placental amnion biopsies showed an approximately 30% lower ROUTINE respiration at day 21 compared to day 0. This is insofar interesting, as it has been shown that regarding mitochondrial activity, placental amnion is also much more responsive to changes in the microenvironment compared to reflected amnion [29]. In that study, responsiveness of placental amnion to inhibition of ATP synthase was much more pronounced. Furthermore, human amniotic mesenchymal stromal cells of placental amnion were found to be more susceptible to changes in oxygen tension [30]. As expected, ROUTINE respiration of both regions (reflected and placental) dramatically decreased in floating biopsies after 21 days compared to day 0. ROUTINE respiration was also significantly lower in floating compared to distended biopsies in reflected amnion. This effect was again even more pronounced in placental amnion (Figure 3A). The reasons for the repeatedly observed differences between reflected and placental amnion are still not known. We believe that the different anatomical locations of the hAM (one covering the placenta, the other opposite it) influence its properties. It is likely that during pregnancy, the two different amniotic sub-regions have different biological functions. Of note, regarding mechanical forces, the rupture of membranes at term takes place in the zone of altered morphology, an area within the reflected amnion [31].

The drastic decrease of mitochondrial oxygen consumption in floating samples of both amniotic regions, together with the massive loss of mitochondrial membrane potential, indicate severe mitochondrial dysfunction. We assume that this dysfunction is the prerequisite for the loss of cellular viability displayed in Figure 1.

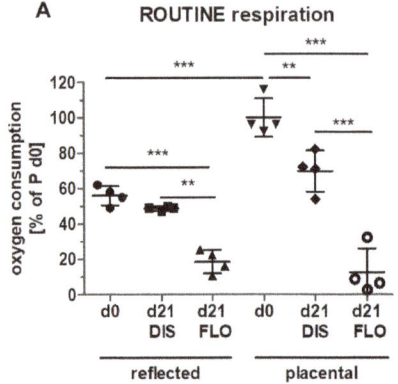 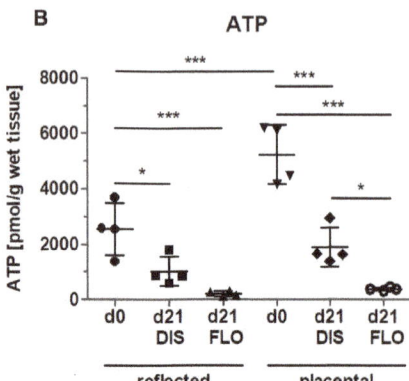

Figure 3. Measurement of mitochondrial activity. (**A**) Mitochondrial ROUTINE respiration (total mitochondrial oxygen consumption) was measured with high resolution respirometry (Oxygraph 2k, Oroboros Instruments) in reflected and placental amnion. Oxygen consumption was determined in fresh biopsies (day 0) and at day 21 in biopsies cultivated while mechanically stretched (DIS) or kept floating (FLO). Measurement of ATP levels. (**B**) ATP levels were determined using the ATP Bioluminescence Assay Kit CLS II (Roche) in fresh biopsies (day 0) and at day 21 in biopsies cultivated while mechanically stretched (DIS) or kept floating (FLO) in reflected and placental amnion. Mean ± SD, n = 4 (donors). P: placental amnion; DIS: distended biopsies; FLO: floating biopsies. Level of significance is indicated as *$p < 0.05$, **$p < 0.01$, ***$p < 0.001$.

Next, we wanted to see whether the changes in mitochondrial respiration also have an effect on ATP levels (Figure 3B). The results showed a similar pattern to the results of ROUTINE respiration. ATP concentrations at day 0 were also higher in placental amnion compared to reflected amnion, which is in line with a previous publication [29]. Distended biopsies after 21 days showed lower ATP concentrations compared to day 0 in both regions. Biopsies kept floating for 21 days showed a strong decrease in ATP concentrations in both regions (reflected and placental) compared to day 0. Floating biopsies of placental amnion showed lower ATP concentrations compared to distended biopsies. These data again indicate mitochondrial dysfunction.

Taken together, floating biopsies seem to have lost most of their viability, whereas in distended biopsies, viability could be sustained to a large extent. The question arose whether the loss of cellular viability was due to apoptosis or necrosis. The very low levels of ATP contradict apoptosis, since induction of apoptosis requires ATP [32,33]. We, however, measured ATP concentrations at a time point at which most of the cells had already lost their viability, meaning that the process of cell death had already been executed. In order to investigate whether apoptosis was involved in the initiation of cell death at an earlier time point, we shortened the incubation period and incubated non-distended and distended amnion biopsies for only 14 days.

3.4. Caspase 3 is Strongly Upregulated in Floating hAM Samples

We first subjected paraffin-embedded hAM biopsies to immunohistochemistry staining with anti-cleaved caspase 3 antibodies. As expected, in fresh biopsies (day 0), no caspase 3 positive cells were detected in either amniotic region (Figure 4A,D,G). After 14 days, in distended biopsies, scattered expression of caspase 3 was found in reflected (Figure 4B,G) and placental samples (Figure 4E,G). In contrast, in floating biopsies, expression of caspase 3 drastically increased in both regions (Figure 4C,F,G), compared to fresh biopsies (Figure 4A,D,G), and distended biopsies (Figure 4B,E,G), indicating the occurrence of apoptotic cell death [34].

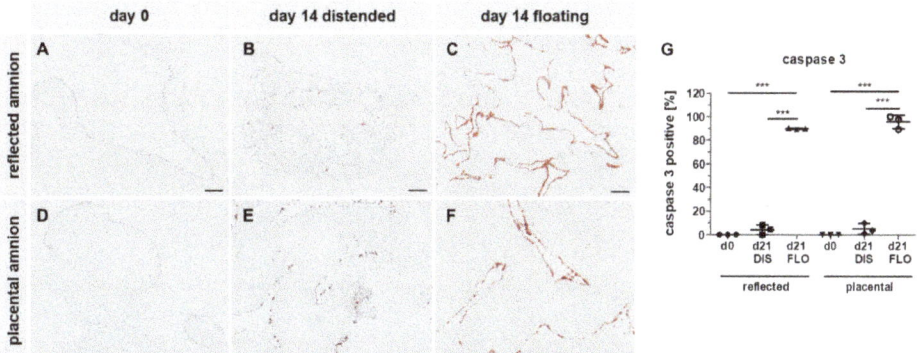

Figure 4. Caspase 3 immunohistochemical staining. Histological sections of reflected (**A,B,C**) and placental (**D,E,F**) amnion at day 0 (**A,D**) and at day 14 in biopsies cultivated while mechanically stretched (**B,E**) or kept floating (**C,F**) were stained for the expression of apoptosis marker caspase 3 (brown). Image analysis was performed with ImageJ software (**G**). Mean ± SD, n = 3 (donors); representative images of one donor. Scale bar: 100 µm. DIS: distended biopsies; FLO: floating biopsies. Level of significance is indicated as ***$p < 0.001$.

3.5. Severe Loss of Mitochondrial Internal Structure under Floating Conditions

In order to see if mitochondria are involved in the process of cell death, we investigated mitochondrial morphology using transmission electron microscopy. In fresh biopsies (day 0) of the hAM, mitochondria displayed well developed cristae within a strongly contrasted matrix in reflected (RA, Figure 5A) and placental (P, Figure 5D) hAM. At day 14, in distended samples, mitochondria of the placental region retained their cristae, however, the mitochondrial matrix appeared less dense (Figure 5E). Most of the mitochondrial cristae in distended reflected amnion were lost (Figure 5B). Floating samples showed mitochondria with severe loss of cristae and overall integrity in both regions (Figure 5C,F). These internal structural changes can be an indication for the onset of apoptosis [35,36].

3.6. Mitochondria-Linked Apoptotic Gene Expression was Upregulated within Seven Days

In order to confirm that apoptosis was mitochondria-linked, we compared BAX and BCL-2 levels. Since we already observed strong upregulation in caspase 3 expression and changes in mitochondrial ultrastructure on day 14, we shortened the incubation time to seven days. Indeed, amnion samples showed higher gene expression of BAX and BCL-2 at day 7 in distended and floating biopsies in both regions compared to day 0 (Figure 6A,B). Moreover, floating placental amnion on day 7 showed significantly higher BAX expression compared to distended biopsies (Figure 6A). Calculating the BAX/BCL-2 ratio revealed that BAX levels in distended samples were higher compared to day 0, but this was only significant in reflected amnion (Figure 6C). As expected, the most pronounced effects were observed between day 0 and floating biopsies of day 7 for both regions (Figure 6C). Additionally, floating placental amnion had a higher BAX/BCL-2 ratio compared to distended biopsies. Although the increase in the BAX/BCL-2 ratio in distended samples also points to the onset of apoptosis, the low number of caspase 3 positive cells (Figure 4) showed that apoptosis was only partly initiated in distended samples. In floating samples, results of BAX/BCL-2 gene expression and caspase 3 immunohistochemistry indicate that the lack of tissue distention initiated mitochondria-mediated apoptosis. The results are in line with studies showing that the mitochondria-linked pathway via BAX is involved in the initiation of apoptosis in hAM in vivo [37,38], a crucial step that leads to the rupture of the membranes at term. Interestingly, it was also shown that chronic stretching of isolated human amniotic epithelial cells (hAECs) cultivated on flexible bottom cell culture plates increased the expression of pre-B cell colony-enhancing factor. This protected isolated hAECs from apoptosis [39], suggesting that distention can prolong cellular life span in vitro.

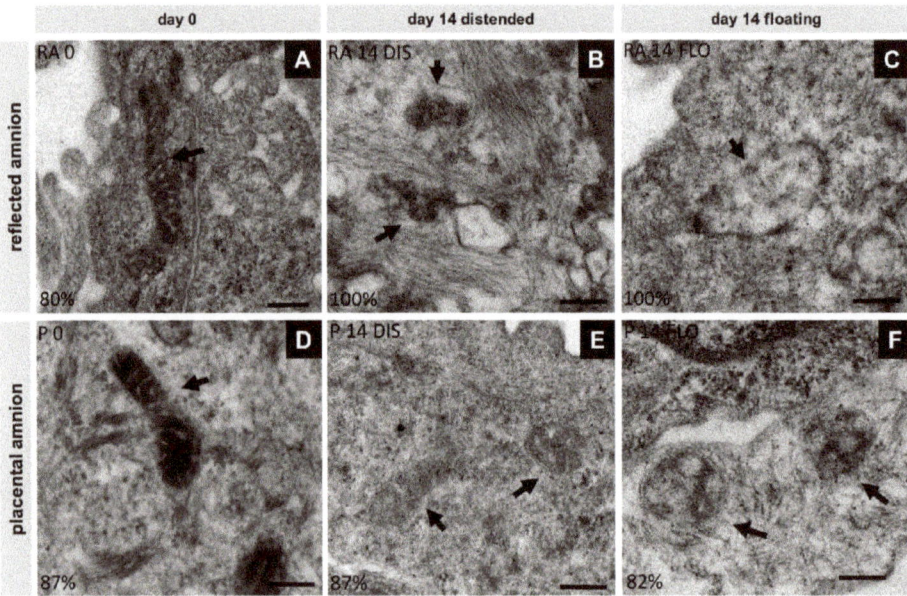

Figure 5. Changes in mitochondrial morphology were analyzed with transmission electron microscopy (Tecnai 20, FEI Europe, Eindhoven, Netherlands) in reflected (RA) (**A,B,C**) and placental (P) (**D,E,F**) amnion at day 0 (**A,D**) and at day 14 in biopsies cultivated while mechanically stretched (**B,E**) or kept floating (**C,F**), n = 2 (donors). Scale bar: 200 nm. Arrows indicate mitochondria. DIS: distended biopsies; FLO: floating biopsies.

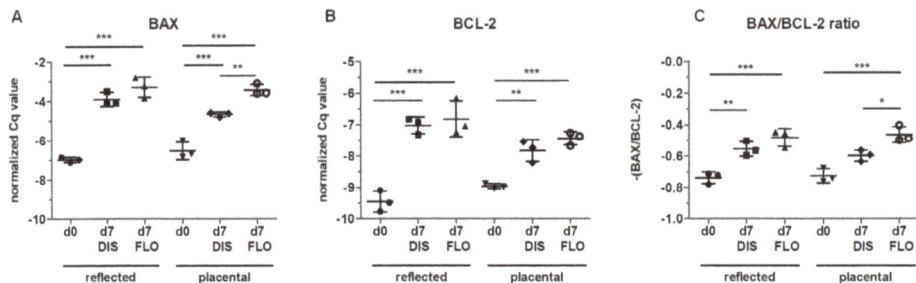

Figure 6. Gene expression of B-cell lymphoma 2-associated X protein (BAX) (**A**) and B-cell lymphoma (BCL)-2 (**B**) was determined by qPCR in fresh biopsies (day 0) and at day 7 in biopsies cultivated while mechanically stretched (DIS) or kept floating (FLO) in reflected and placental amnion. The results were normalized on the geometric mean of 4 different reference genes. The BAX/BCL-2 ratio is shown in (**C**). Mean ± SD, n = 3 (donors). DIS: distended biopsies; FLO: floating biopsies; Cq value: cycle of quantification value. Level of significance is indicated as $*p < 0.05$, $**p < 0.01$, $***p < 0.001$.

4. Limitations of the Study

A limitation of this study is that no specific set of inhibitors was used for this pathway.

5. Conclusions

Our data suggest that there is an unknown tension-driven mitochondrial pathway (TDMP), which may control viability of hAMs via triggering mitochondria-mediated apoptosis. This process starts with loss of tissue tension, followed by activation of TDMP, impairment of mitochondria, the release of mitochondrial apoptotic factors, induction of caspase 3-mediated apoptosis and the loss of viability of hAM cells. The presence of tissue distention prolongs the cellular life span of human amniotic membranes. Further studies are required to obtain a detailed time course of activation of apoptosis and to investigate the TDMP to shed more light on the hAM physiology. This knowledge will support optimization of hAM tissue cultures, as the distended hAM comes closer to the in vivo situation than non-distended samples.

Supplementary Materials: The following are available online at http://www.mdpi.com/2073-4409/8/12/1641/s1, Supplementary Methods 1: Measuring mitochondrial oxygen consumption using high resolution respirometry. 2: ATP measurement using Bioluminescence Assay Kit CLS II. Table S1: Primer sequences used for mRNA reverse-transcription quantitative PCR analysis.

Author Contributions: A.B. and A.W. conceptualized and designed the experiments; L.P., K.S., A.B., A.W. performed experiments; L.P., K.S., A.B., A.W. analyzed data; L.P., A.L., K.S., A.V.K., J.G., S.W., A.B., A.W. interpreted results; L.P., A.B., A.W. drafted the manuscript and figures; L.P., A.L., K.S., A.V.K., J.G., S.W., A.B., A.W. critically read/edited the manuscript; all authors approved the manuscript.

Funding: The study was funded by the Austrian Research Promotion Agency (FFG; grant number 867674).

Acknowledgments: The authors are grateful for the support of Cornelia Schneider and Simone Hennerbichler-Lugscheider (Blutzentrale Linz). We are also thankful for the histological support from Barbara Schädl and the team of the joint LBI Trauma/MUW histology lab. Special thanks to Anton Dobsak from the Karl Donath Laboratory for Hard Tissue and Biomaterial Research at the University Clinic of Dentistry.

Conflicts of Interest: J.G. is the co-founder of Evercyte GmbH and TAmiRNA GmbH. All other authors declare no conflict of interest.

References

1. Stern, M. The Grafting of Preserved Amniotic Membrane to Burned and Ulcerated Surfaces, substituting Skin Grafts. *J. Am. Med. Assoc.* **1912**, *60*, 973–974. [CrossRef]
2. Sabella, N. Use of Fetal Membranes in Skin Grafting. *Med. Rec.* **1913**, *83*, 478–480.
3. Rötth, A. De PLASTIC REPAIR OF CONJUNCTIVAL DEFECTS WITH FETAL MEMBRANES. *Arch. Ophthalmol.* **1940**, *23*, 522–525. [CrossRef]
4. Rohleder, N.H.; Loeffelbein, D.J.; Feistl, W.; Eddicks, M.; Wolff, K.D.; Gulati, A.; Steinstraesser, L.; Kesting, M.R. Repair of oronasal fistulae by interposition of multilayered amniotic membrane allograft. *Plast. Reconstr. Surg.* **2013**, *132*, 172–181. [CrossRef] [PubMed]
5. Silini, A.R.; Cargnoni, A.; Magatti, M.; Pianta, S.; Parolini, O. The Long Path of Human Placenta, and Its Derivatives, in Regenerative Medicine. *Front. Bioeng. Biotechnol.* **2015**, *3*, 162. [CrossRef] [PubMed]
6. Sadler, T.W.; Langman, J. *Langman's Medical Embryology*, 9th ed.; Lippincott Williams & Wilkins: Philadelphia, PA, USA, 2013.
7. Sakuragawa, N.; Enosawa, S.; Ishii, T.; Thangavel, R.; Tashiro, T.; Okuyama, T.; Suzuki, S. Human amniotic epithelial cells are promising transgene carriers for allogeneic cell transplantation into liver. *J. Hum. Genet.* **2000**, *45*, 171–176. [CrossRef]
8. Portmann-Lanz, C.B.; Schoeberlein, A.; Huber, A.; Sager, R.; Malek, A.; Holzgreve, W.; Surbek, D.V. Placental mesenchymal stem cells as potential autologous graft for pre- and perinatal neuroregeneration. *Am. J. Obstet. Gynecol.* **2006**, *194*, 664–673. [CrossRef]
9. Lindenmair, A.; Wolbank, S.; Stadler, G.; Meinl, A.; Peterbauer-Scherb, A.; Eibl, J.; Polin, H.; Gabriel, C.; van Griensven, M.; Redl, H. Human Amniotic Membrane: Osteogenic Differentiation in toto. *Biomaterials* **2010**, *31*, 8659–8665. [CrossRef]
10. Banerjee, A.; Nürnberger, S.; Hennerbichler, S.; Riedl, S.; Schuh, C.M.A.P.; Hacobian, A.; Teuschl, A.; Eibl, J.; Redl, H.; Wolbank, S. In toto differentiation of human amniotic membrane towards the Schwann cell lineage. *Cell Tissue Bank.* **2014**, *15*, 227–239. [CrossRef]

11. Miki, T.; Mitamura, K.; Ross, M.A.; Stolz, D.B.; Strom, S.C. Identification of stem cell marker-positive cells by immunofluorescence in term human amnion. *J. Reprod. Immunol.* **2007**, *75*, 91–96. [CrossRef]
12. Bailo, M.; Soncini, M.; Vertua, E.; Signoroni, P.B.; Sanzone, S.; Lombardi, G.; Arienti, D.; Calamani, F.; Zatti, D.; Paul, P.; et al. Engraftment Potential of Human Amnion and Chorion Cells Derived from Term Placenta. *Transplantation* **2004**, *78*, 1439–1448. [CrossRef] [PubMed]
13. Li, H.; Niederkorn, J.Y.; Neelam, S.; Mayhew, E.; Word, R.A.; McCulley, J.P.; Alizadeh, H. Immunosuppressive factors secreted by human amniotic epithelial cells. *Investig. Ophthalmol. Vis. Sci.* **2005**, *46*, 900–907. [CrossRef] [PubMed]
14. Wolbank, S.; Peterbauer, A.; Fahrner, M.; Hennerbichler, S.; van Griensven, M.; Stadler, G.; Redl, H.; Gabriel, C. Dose-dependent immunomodulatory effect of human stem cells from amniotic membrane: a comparison with human mesenchymal stem cells from adipose tissue. *Tissue Eng.* **2007**, *13*, 1173–1183. [CrossRef] [PubMed]
15. Kronsteiner, B.; Wolbank, S.; Peterbauer, A.; Hackl, C.; Redl, H.; van Griensven, M.; Gabriel, C. Human Mesenchymal Stem Cells from Adipose Tissue and Amnion Influence T-Cells Depending on Stimulation Method and Presence of Other Immune Cells. *Stem Cells Dev.* **2011**, *20*, 2115–2126. [CrossRef] [PubMed]
16. Han, Y.M.; Romero, R.; Kim, J.-S.; Tarca, A.L.; Kim, S.K.; Draghici, S.; Kusanovic, J.P.; Gotsch, F.; Mittal, P.; Hassan, S.S.; et al. Region-Specific Gene Expression Profiling: Novel Evidence for Biological Heterogeneity of the Human Amnion1. *Biol. Reprod.* **2008**, *79*, 954–961. [CrossRef] [PubMed]
17. Kim, S.Y.; Romero, R.; Tarca, A.L.; Bhatti, G.; Lee, J.H.; Chaiworapongsa, T.; Hassan, S.S.; Kim, C.J. MiR-143 regulation of prostaglandin-endoperoxidase synthase 2 in the amnion: Implications for human parturition at term. *PLoS ONE* **2011**, *6*, 1–10. [CrossRef] [PubMed]
18. Banerjee, A.; Weidinger, A.; Hofer, M.; Steinborn, R.; Lindenmair, A.; Hennerbichler-Lugscheider, S.; Eibl, J.; Redl, H.; Kozlov, A.V.; Wolbank, S. Different metabolic activity in placental and reflected regions of the human amniotic membrane. *Placenta* **2015**, *36*, 1329–1332. [CrossRef]
19. Litwiniuk, M.; Radowicka, M.; Krejner, A.; Śladowska, A.; Grzela, T. Amount and distribution of selected biologically active factors in amniotic membrane depends on the part of amnion and mode of childbirth. Can we predict properties of amnion dressing? A proof-of-concept study. *Cent.-Eur. J. Immunol* **2017**, *42*, 1–6. [CrossRef]
20. Islam, M.N.; Das, S.R.; Emin, M.T.; Wei, M.; Sun, L.; Rowlands, D.J.; Quadri, S.K.; Bhattacharya, S. Mitochondrial transfer from bone marrow-derived stromal cells to pulmonary alveoli protects against acute lung injury. *Nat. Med.* **2013**, *18*, 759–765. [CrossRef]
21. Liu, C.-S.; Chang, J.-C.; Kuo, S.-J.; Liu, K.-H.; Lin, T.-T.; Cheng, W.-L.; Chuang, S.-F. Delivering healthy mitochondria for the therapy of mitochondrial diseases and beyond. *Int. J. Biochem. Cell Biol.* **2014**, *53*, 141–146. [CrossRef]
22. Hayakawa, K.; Esposito, E.; Wang, X.; Terasaki, Y.; Liu, Y.; Xing, C.; Ji, X.; Lo, E.H. Transfer of mitochondria from astrocytes to neurons after stroke. *Nature* **2016**, *535*, 551–555. [CrossRef] [PubMed]
23. Kruse, F.E.; Joussen, A.M.; Rohrschneider, K.; You, L.; Sinn, B.; Baumann, J.; Volcker, H.E. Cryopreserved human amniotic membrane for ocular surface reconstruction. *Graefes Arch. Clin. Exp. Ophthalmol.* **2000**, *238*, 68–75. [CrossRef] [PubMed]
24. Lindenmair, A.; Nürnberger, S.; Stadler, G.; Meinl, A.; Hackl, C.; Eibl, J.; Gabriel, C.; Hennerbichler, S.; Redl, H.; Wolbank, S. Intact human amniotic membrane differentiated towards the chondrogenic lineage. *Cell Tissue Bank.* **2014**, *15*, 213–225. [CrossRef] [PubMed]
25. Skinner, S.J.; Campos, G.A.; Liggins, G.C. Collagen content of human amniotic membranes: Effect of gestation length and premature rupture. *Obstet. Gynecol.* **1981**, *57*, 487–489. [PubMed]
26. Parry, S.; Strauss, J.F. Premature Rupture of the Fetal Membranes. *N. Engl. J. Med.* **1998**, *338*, 663–670. [CrossRef] [PubMed]
27. Millar, L.K.; Stollberg, J.; DeBuque, L.; Bryant-Greenwood, G. Fetal membrane distention: Determination of the intrauterine surface area and distention of the fetal membranes preterm and at term. *Am. J. Obstet. Gynecol.* **2000**, *182*, 128–134. [CrossRef]
28. Zorova, L.D.; Popkov, V.A.; Plotnikov, E.Y.; Silachev, D.N.; Pevzner, I.B.; Jankauskas, S.S.; Babenko, V.A.; Zorov, S.D.; Balakireva, A.V.; Juhaszova, M.; et al. Mitochondrial membrane potential. *Anal. Biochem.* **2018**, *552*, 50–59. [CrossRef]

29. Banerjee, A.; Lindenmair, A.; Hennerbichler, S.; Steindorf, P.; Steinborn, R.; Kozlov, A.V.; Redl, H.; Wolbank, S.; Weidinger, A. Cellular and Site-Specific Mitochondrial Characterization of Vital Human Amniotic Membrane. *Cell Transplant.* **2018**, *27*, 3–11. [CrossRef]
30. Banerjee, A.; Lindenmair, A.; Steinborn, R.; Dumitrescu, S.D.; Hennerbichler, S.; Kozlov, A.V.; Redl, H.; Wolbank, S.; Weidinger, A. Oxygen Tension Strongly Influences Metabolic Parameters and the Release of Interleukin-6 of Human Amniotic Mesenchymal Stromal Cells In vitro. *Stem Cells Int.* **2018**, *2018*, 1–11. [CrossRef]
31. Malak, T.M.; Bell, S.C. Structural characteristics of term human fetal membranes: A novel zone of extreme morphological alteration within the rupture site. *Br. J. Obstet. Gynaecol.* **1994**, *101*, 375–386. [CrossRef]
32. Saikumar, P.; Dong, Z.; Patel, Y.; Hall, K.; Hopfer, U.; Weinberg, J.M.; Venkatachalam, M.A. Role of hypoxia-induced Bax translocation and cytochrome c release in reoxygenation injury. *Oncogene* **1998**, *17*, 3401–3415. [CrossRef] [PubMed]
33. Latta, M.; Künstle, G.; Leist, M.; Wendel, A. Metabolic depletion of ATP by fructose inversely controls CD95- and tumor necrosis factor receptor 1-mediated hepatic apoptosis. *J. Exp. Med.* **2000**, *191*, 1975–1985. [CrossRef] [PubMed]
34. Nicholson, D.W.; Ali, A.; Thornberry, N.A.; Vaillancourt, J.P.; Ding, C.K.; Gallant, M.; Gareau, Y.; Griffin, P.R.; Labelle, M.; Lazebnik, Y.A.; et al. Identification and inhibition of the ICE/CED-3 protease necessary for mammalian apoptosis. *Nature* **1995**, *376*, 37–43. [CrossRef] [PubMed]
35. Scorrano, L.; Ashiya, M.; Buttle, K.; Weiler, S.; Oakes, S.A.; Mannella, C.A.; Korsmeyer, S.J. A distinct pathway remodels mitochondrial cristae and mobilizes cytochrome c during apoptosis. *Dev. Cell* **2002**, *2*, 55–67. [CrossRef]
36. Seo, A.Y.; Joseph, A.-M.M.; Dutta, D.; Hwang, J.C.; Aris, J.P.; Leeuwenburgh, C. New insights into the role of mitochondria in aging: mitochondrial dynamics and more. *J. Cell Sci.* **2010**, *123*, 2533–2542. [CrossRef] [PubMed]
37. Fortunato, S.J.; Menon, R.; Bryant, C.; Lombardi, S.J. Programmed cell death (apoptosis) as a possible pathway to metalloproteinase activation and fetal membrane degradation in premature rupture of membranes. *Am. J. Obstet. Gynecol.* **2000**, *182*, 1468–1476. [CrossRef]
38. Shen, Z.Y.; Li, E.M.; Lu, S.Q.; Shen, J.; Cai, Y.M.; Wu, Y.E.; Zheng, R.M.; Tan, L.J.; Xu, L.Y. Autophagic and Apoptotic Cell Death in Amniotic Epithelial Cells. *Placenta* **2008**, *29*, 956–961. [CrossRef]
39. Kendal-Wright, C.E.; Hubbard, D.; Bryant-Greenwood, G.D. Chronic Stretching of Amniotic Epithelial Cells Increases Pre-B Cell Colony-Enhancing Factor (PBEF/Visfatin) Expression and Protects Them from Apoptosis. *Placenta* **2008**, *29*, 255–265. [CrossRef]

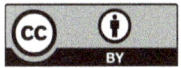

© 2019 by the authors. Licensee MDPI, Basel, Switzerland. This article is an open access article distributed under the terms and conditions of the Creative Commons Attribution (CC BY) license (http://creativecommons.org/licenses/by/4.0/).

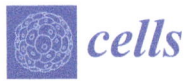

Review

Telomeres and Telomerase in Heart Ontogenesis, Aging and Regeneration

Denis Nalobin [1,*], Svetlana Alipkina [1], Anna Gaidamaka [1], Alexander Glukhov [1,2] and Zaza Khuchua [2,3,4]

1. Faculty of Biology, Lomonosov Moscow State University, 119991 Moscow, Russian;
   svetlana.alipkina@gmail.com (S.A.); stadtrand@yandex.ru (A.G.); aiglukhov1958@gmail.com (A.G.)
2. Department of Biochemistry, Sechenov First Moscow State Medical University,
   119991 Moscow, Russian; zkhuchua@gmail.com
3. Institute of Chemical Biology Ilia State University, 0162 Tbilisi, Georgia
4. Division of Molecular and Cardiovascular Biology, Cincinnati Children's Medical Center,
   Cincinnati, OH 45229, USA
* Correspondence: Denis.Nalobin@gmail.com; Tel.: +7-916-939-0990

Received: 30 November 2019; Accepted: 14 February 2020; Published: 22 February 2020

Abstract: The main purpose of the review article is to assess the contributions of telomere length and telomerase activity to the cardiac function at different stages of development and clarify their role in cardiac disorders. It has been shown that the telomerase complex and telomeres are of great importance in many periods of ontogenesis due to the regulation of the proliferative capacity of heart cells. The review article also discusses the problems of heart regeneration and the identification of possible causes of dysfunction of telomeres and telomerase.

Keywords: cardiomyocytes; telomere length; telomerase activity; development; regeneration; reactive oxygen species

---

1. Introduction

The cardiovascular system plays a vital for the whole organism. It performs many vital functions such as supplying organs and tissues with nutrients, hormones, carrying oxygen to the cells and maintaining physiological temperature.

According to the World Health Organization, diseases of the cardiovascular system are the main cause of lethality worldwide. Every year, more than 7.4 million people die from coronary heart disease worldwide, and these rates continue to grow. Congenital heart defects are also highly prevalent and may be a cause of serious complications in the future. Thus, the search for solutions to the cause and consequences of heart diseases is one of the most serious biomedical problems.

The possibility to regenerate the mammalian heart is still rarely studied; however, studying it would allow finding new ways to restore the heart after severe injuries.

A huge number of factors affect the functioning of the heart. One of them is cell aging, which manifests itself in the form of various disorders. Cellular aging is associated to a greater extent with the loss of telomere length and a decrease in telomerase activity.

Understanding the processes of regulation of telomere length and telomerase activity in the ontogenesis of cardiac tissue can help to understand the causes of heart disease in one or another period of development of the organism.

2. Telomeres and Telomere Complex

In 1961, Leonard Hayflick discovered the limit of somatic cell division in vitro. The limit is named after the scientist—the Hayflick limit. According to Hayflick's observations, human fibroblasts dividing in a cell culture died after approximately 50 divisions. The cells showed signs of aging, stopped dividing and underwent programmed cell death [1].

Ten years after the discovery of the Hayflick limit, Olovnikov hypothesized that DNA polymerase cannot copy a small region at the end of chromosome (telomere), which leads to terminal under-replication of DNA [2] (Figure 1).

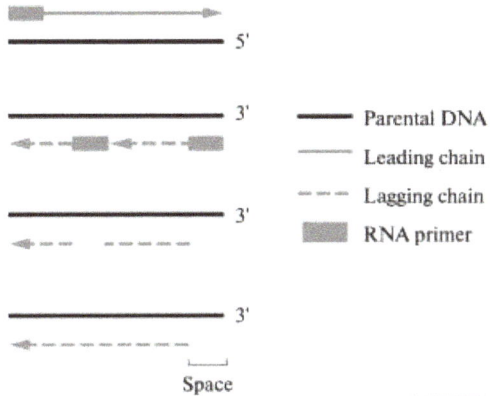

Figure 1. Problems associated with chromosomes' terminal under-replication [2].

Scientists postulated that telomeres undergo shortening with each cell division and assumed that this phenomenon was associated with the cell division limit. This hypothesis was confirmed in 1985, when Greider and Blackburn (1985) identified an enzyme in the ciliate *Tetrahymena thermophila* that prevented the degradation of the ends of chromosomes. The enzyme was named telomerase [2].

Vertebrate telomeres consist of repeating TTAGGG sequences at the ends of chromosomes and maintain their integrity. Since DNA replication is asymmetric at both strands, the sequence at the 3' end would lose 30–200 nucleotides with each cycle of DNA replication and cell division. Telomeres have non-coding recurring sequences at the 3' end to prevent the loss of coding sequences during replication [3]. Moreover, telomeres are covered with Shelterin complex consisting of six proteins: TRF1 (telomere repeat binding factor 1), TRF2 (telomere repeat binding factor 2), TIN2 (TRF1-interacted nuclear protein 2), RAP1 (rif-associated protein), POT1 (protection of telomeres) and TPP1 (telomere protected protein 1). Telomeres end with a single-stranded 3'-end, which has a compact T-loop structure that maintains their stability [4]. Telomeres were proposed as mitotic clocks that show how many times a cell has divided [5].

When telomeres shorten to a critical length, the cell goes into a state of senescence, which initiates a series of changes in gene expression patterns of cell cycle inhibitors, decreases cellular proliferative potential and activates apoptosis [6].

Telomerase is responsible for telomere elongation and consists of an RNA component (TERC) and telomerase reverse transcriptase (TERT), a catalytic component. TERT uses TERC as a template for synthesizing new repeats of telomeric DNA at the single-stranded ends of chromosomes [7]. Most somatic cells lack telomerase activity, but undifferentiated germ cells, stem cells, activated lymphocytes and most tumor cells have a high level of telomerase activity to overcome telomere contraction and maintain limitless cell division. However, differentiated resting cells usually have a low or undetectable level of telomerase activity [8].

3. Embryonic Development of the Heart

The heart begins to function in the early stages of development in both mammals and lower vertebrates such as *Danio rerio* (zebrafish) [9,10]. In mice, the level of proliferation of cardiomyocytes

(CM) is high in early embryogenesis, and then it gradually decreases until the 10th to 12th day of embryonic development (E10–12) when the heart is almost fully formed [9,11]. Similar dynamics are also shown for telomerase: its activity is detected in the heart tissue of the human fetus until the 12th week of embryonic development, which coincides with the histological differentiation of the myoblasts of the heart into cardiomyocytes [12]. This observation is consistent with the fact that, by the sixth month of prenatal development, the morphological appearance of the heart muscle is almost the same as that of an adult [12].

However, a full picture of dynamics of telomerase activity during the cardiac embryonic development is still unclear. It is known that activity is registered during E11.5 [13] and E16.5 in mice [14], as well as on E10 and E20 in rats. Moreover, telomerase activities in developing rat hearts start to decline after E10 [15]. Dynamics of telomerase inactivation in developing hearts of rats and humans appear to have similar patterns since, in rats, the heart becomes a fully formed functional organ by E16 [16].

4. Early Postnatal Heart Development

Proliferation reaches the first minimum point in the heart of newborn mice (i.e., day 0 of postnatal development; P0) [17]. During this period, the system that is responsible for the cell cycle is transformed from embryonic to postnatal mode. Before birth, the number of CMs increases, and after birth, it remains almost unchanged. At the same period, tetraploid and binuclear CMs begin to appear [17]. At P3, the peak of mitotic activity appears again, which correlates with an increased number of binuclear CMs (up to 80%) and a decrease in the number of mononuclear CMs. At the same time, both in binuclear and mononuclear CM populations, there is a transition to the G1 phase and cessation of the cell cycle [17]. After P3 there is a sharp decrease in the number of CMs that have entered mitosis [17,18].

If we take a look at the activity of telomerase in the heart at this stage of development, we find a correlation both with a decrease of proliferation and with the advent of binuclear and polyploid CMs. Therefore, it can be speculated that negative telomerase regulation may be important for permanent stopping of the CM cell cycle [15]. Thus, in newborn mice, gradual suppression of telomerase activity occurs, and by P2 the activity decreases by more than 65% [14]. By the third month of postnatal development, only a very small number of *Tert*-expressing cells remain [19]. A number of studies have shown a sharp decline in telomerase activity in newborn mice relative to the hearts of E11.5, and after P10 it is almost undetectable [13]. *Tert* expression has a similar dynamic, which indicates a possible mechanism for the suppression of telomerase activity through the catalytic subunit of telomerase [13,20].

Similar to previous data, it was found that five days after birth, the activity of telomerase in the rat heart was only 20% of the activity at E10. Telomerase activity was absent in P20 heart and remained below the detection limit up to four months of age [15].

Regarding the distribution of telomerase activity in the heart, *TERT* expression is found in a population of cells, including CM, fibroblasts and endothelial cells [19].

The decrease in proliferation potential of CMs positively correlates with telomere depletion in newborn mice. Rapid reduction of telomere length occurs within the first two weeks after birth. Further, the length of the telomeres does not change, as the CMs leave the cell cycle, which contributes to the conservation of telomere reserves. In the first days after birth, the proliferating CMs have a longer telomere than non-proliferating CMs. However, after P15, these differences are already nullified [13].

There are several possible causes for the sharp drop in telomere length in newborn mice. Telomeres shorten during phase S due to the inability of the DNA replication mechanism to support the ends of linear DNA molecules [5]. Therefore, the absence of telomerase predetermines the loss of telomere reserves in CM during the period of their postnatal DNA replication.

More surprising is the high rate of loss of telomeres, starting with P1, which leads to a significant increase in DNA damage in telomeric sites in a one-week period [13]. In this regard, another cause of damage and further loss of telomeres may be the appearance of reactive oxygen species (ROS) in CM after the metabolic transition from anaerobic glycolysis to mitochondrial oxidative phosphorylation during the first week after birth. So, it was found that the level of ROS increased in newborn mice, which probably leads to an increase in the number of DNA damage foci (replacement of guanine with 8-oxo-7,8-dihydroguanine) between P4 and P7 [21]. Such alterations have a particularly noticeable effect on the promoter regions of genes that have a high GC content [22]. Telomeres also have a high GGG content, which makes them an ideal target for ROS attacks [23]. Due to an increase in the level of oxidizers and disturbances in telomeres, the DNA damage response is activated, which leads to a halt in proliferation through activation of the cell cycle inhibitor p21 [13,21]. However, if the oxygen concentration or the ROS levels are reduced, then the proliferation window of the CMs in the early postembryonic period expands along with the increase in the numbers of mononuclear cells relative to two- and multi-nuclei CMs [21]. ROS can be associated with telomerase inhibition due to telomere DNA damage or deoxynucleotides oxidation that explains a sharp drop of telomerase activity after birth [24].

The mechanism that promotes cell cycle arrest in postnatal CMs can also be associated with the gap-fusion-bridge cycle, which leads to tetraploidization, appearance of binucleated cells and inhibition of proliferation [25]. In the gap-fusion-bridge cycle, chromosomes with nonfunctional telomeres merge with each other, forming bridges during mitosis. These chromosome bridges may eventually collapse under the action of forces emanating from the anaphase poles, and further proliferation is inhibited. In murine CMs, decrease in telomeres is associated with the appearance of chromosomal bridges between the daughter nuclei: eight days after birth, CMs display the presence of chromosomal bridges, which correlates with a decrease in telomere length. A potential genomic imbalance caused by the breakdown of chromosomal bridges in binucleated CMs can be a barrier to proliferation [13].

The knockout for the *Terc* gene confirms the role of telomeres in proliferation. Third-generation *Terc*-null mice have shorter telomeres, anaphase bridges and a lower proliferation level than wild-types (WTs) at P1 [13].

It should be noted that in lower vertebrates, such as *D. rerio*, telomerase activity in many tissues is sufficiently high both during embryonic and postnatal development [26]. This observation is used to study the proliferative potential of CMs in the regenerative process [27]. In addition, it was shown that CMs of *D. rerio* are single-nucleated and diploid [28,29], which may be associated with high telomerase activity capable of maintaining sufficient telomere length for normal proliferation [28,29].

5. Prepubertal Period

CMs of mammals lose their ability to proliferate after birth due to telomere dysfunction and reduced telomerase activity [13]. However, there is evidence of a proliferation surge in the prepubertal period. Thus, from P14 to P15, activation of mitosis with subsequent cytokinesis is observed in both mononucleated or binucleated CMs. Proliferation is accompanied by the expression of cell cycle regulating genes [30]. From this, it can be speculated that there is a molecular mechanism for overcoming the proliferative barrier associated with short telomeres and low telomerase activity. The authors of the study suggest that the wave of synthesis of the hormone triiodothyronine is an impulse for the induction of mitosis [30]. On the other hand, the cause of the activation of proliferation can be telomere elongation due to the start of telomerase expression. This hypothesis is derived from data on increasing the length of telomeres and subsequently the level of proliferation due to the introduction of Tert in the heart of an adult mouse in response to heart damage [20]. At the same time, there is another point of view on this observation: during growth, the size of the heart increases almost exclusively due to hypertrophy, but not hyperplasia. It was shown that the increase in the number of CMs or proliferation rate was not observed between P13 and P100, and that no active DNA synthesis occurred [31]. Similar results were demonstrated for P14–P21 [32].

However, the contribution of hyperplasia to an increase in the size of the heart should not be completely ruled out, although it is probably not as high as was presented in the study of Naqvi et al., 2014 [30]. Indeed, it has been found that proliferating mononuclear cells with increased telomerase activity are present in the hearts of young cats, and they have the physiological properties of immature cells in the form of calcium current in T-type channels [33]. Mitotic activity in human mononuclear CMs is shown during the first 20 years of life (1.9% of the total number of CM), which decreases, but is registered up to the age of 40 [34], as confirmed by earlier works [35]. There is also evidence of an increase in ploidy of CMs and the absence of growth in the number of binuclear cells during the first 20 years of life [35].

6. Heart of Adult Vertebrates

As described above, telomerase activity in mammals drops to a minimum shortly after birth, which causes telomere shortening. However, in the heart of adult animals, as shown in mice, telomerase activity is registered, both in CMs, and in fibroblasts and endothelial cells [19].

CMs of adult mice vary in size: binucleated and multinucleated CMs undergo hypertrophy, and small mononucleated CMs show features of proliferating cells. The length of telomeres in these classes of CMs is inversely related to cell size. In addition, $p16^{CDKN2}$ expression is observed in large binucleated and multinucleated CMs with the shortest telomeres [36]. $P16^{CDKN2}$ specifically binds and inhibits cyclin-dependent kinases CDK4 and CDK6, which act as regulators of the progression of the cell cycle in G1, contribute to the phosphorylation of the retinoblastoma protein (pRB) and induce cell cycle arrest [37].

With a TRF assay, it has been demonstrated that, unlike mammals, telomerase activity in the hearts of *D. rerio* is high throughout life, and telomere length remains almost unchanged [38]. Further studies were conducted on changes in telomere length in fish of different ages using the Q-Fish method. It was shown that in *D. rerio* the activity of telomerase and the length of telomeres in CMs also varied with age, and the aging of fish leads to a decrease of telomere length and telomerase activity [26].

7. Heart Aging

Aging of the heart includes a number of physiological changes that increase the risk of developing diseases and conditions that are hazardous to health. Cardiac diseases are associated with age and have a detrimental impact on the whole organism. However, it remains unclear how cellular aging of heart tissue affects the appearance of heart diseases.

It is known that telomere length decreases with age. For human heart tissue, telomere loss is approximately 20 base pairs per year [39]. In addition to this, it was found that in old rats there was a tendency to reduce the length of terminal restriction fragments (TRF) related to the telomeric and subtelomeric region. Interestingly, only the heart showed a significant decrease in the average length of telomeres compared to the brain, kidney, lung and liver. [40]. A similar state of telomeres was found in coronary artery endothelial cells, where the T/C ratio (ratio of telomere length to centromeres) was reduced depending on the age of the donor [41]. At the same time, the reduction of the end sections of chromosomes is unlikely to be associated with cell division, as described above.

As for the age-dependent diseases, there is a correlation between the length of telomeres and the presence of one or another heart disease. For example, the risks of coronary heart disease are associated with telomeres shorter than 200 base pairs [42]. The mechanism of a possible causal link between short telomeres and ischemic disease has not been fully elucidated, but shorter telomeres are positively associated with the rapid formation of plaques observed in atherosclerosis and marked atherogenesis [42]. Indeed, direct measurement of telomere length in coronary endothelial cells supports the concept that telomere shortening in coronary endothelial cells with aging can contribute to the development of coronary endothelial dysfunction and the development of coronary heart disease in humans [41].

Dilated cardiomyopathy (DC) is characterized by an increase in cardiac ventricular volumes, thinning ventricular wall thickness, hypertrophy and impairment of cardiac function [43,44]. In an aging heart with DC, the forced entry of primitive cells, which express stem cell surface antigen c-kit, into irreversible quiescent state was identified by the expression of cell cycle inhibitor p16^{INK4a} and by very short telomeres [45].

Telomeric shortening in CMs with age can be explained by the launch of miRNA-34a synthesis, the target of which is phosphatase 1 of the nuclear targeting subunit (PNUTS), which is involved in the maintenance of telomeres by interacting with TRF2. TRF2, together with PNUTS, is also involved in regulating the response to DNA damage and inhibiting the phosphorylation of Chk2 (checkpoint kinase), leading to apoptosis. Increased expression of PNUTS inhibits telomere depletion without telomerase involvement [46]. However, there are probably other molecular pathways that result in a reduction in telomere length. They can be associated, for example, with oxidative stress, leading to the accumulation of DNA damage in telomeric regions.

To determine the possible role of telomeres and telomerase in cardiac aging, mice with telomere-induced dysfunction were examined by knockout on telomerase subunit genes. Mice of the fifth generation (G5) with a *Terc* gene knockout (*Terc$^{-/-}$*) suffered from severe left ventricular insufficiency and DC. Compared to WT mice, the masses of the heart and left ventricle were significantly reduced in G5 mice. Despite the decrease in heart weight in G5, hypertrophy was demonstrated, which was accompanied by a decrease in the number of CMs [47]. The phenotype was also characteristic for G4 *Tert$^{-/-}$* mice: a decrease in body weight and endurance and an increase in free fatty acids and mitochondrial dysfunction. Mitochondrial dysfunction manifested as inhibition of PGC-1α and PGC-1β, key metabolic regulators. This led to a decrease of gluconeogenesis, a reduction in ATP synthesis, cardiomyopathy, and increased oxidative stress [48], which is a sign of tissue aging [49].

The tumor suppressor protein p53 is an important mediator of telomere dysfunction. An increase in this protein is observed in *Terc$^{-/-}$* mice when telomeres reach a critically short length. These results are consistent with the notion that telomere loss in mice activates p53, which modulates both apoptosis and growth arrest [47]. In addition to these functions, the p53 protein is a link between telomere length and mitochondrial function: an increase in its synthesis leads to inhibition of the promoters *PGC-1α* and *PGC-1β* [48]. Thus, dysfunction of telomeres leads to premature aging of the heart, which manifests itself in the form of diseases dependent on age.

As described previously [50], premature aging of the cardiovascular system is induced by metabolic stress, obesity, hypertension, insulin resistance and type 2 diabetes [51–54]. Additionally, there is evidence that autophagy is important for longevity and health [55], and a change in autophagy contributes to heart aging [56–58]. Although it has been shown that autophagy inducers have a beneficial effect on life expectancy and slow down the aging of the cardiovascular system [56], there is still a contradiction between the protective and harmful effects of autophagy induction on aging [59]. There are many aging treatment options based on telomerase activation, NO modulation, antioxidants, PARP inhibition, senolytic therapy, plasma membrane redox system (PMRS) activators and stem cell therapy [55,60].

There are reports about the use of telomerase as a therapeutic tissue-specific target for diseases of the cardiovascular system [61,62]. Telomerase can be used to treat coronary heart disease due to protection against ROS [63,64]. With ischemia reperfusion injury, telomerase deficiency leads to heart failure [65]. Telomere depletion is a characteristic sign of cardiac hypertrophy. Shortening of telomeres in CMs is a marker of heart failure in humans, and shorter telomere length in CMs usually correlate with a reduced ejection fraction [66].

8. Heart Regeneration

As we stated above, the regenerative potential of CMs, as well as telomerase activity, decreases in mammalian hearts shortly after birth [13].

In newborn mice (P1), in response to injury, accelerated differentiation of CM occurs [67,68]. Following the P1 period, the regenerative potential is quickly lost, and a similar injury on P7 leads to fibrosis instead of regeneration [67]. Tetraploidy, binucleation, diminished telomerase activity and telomere shortening during this period can be causative of a loss of proliferative potential of

CMs in response to injury [13]. A recent study showed that co-cultivation of mononucleated and bi/multinucleated CMs from adult and newborn animals, respectively, led to the de-differentiation and proliferation of not only mononucleated, but also bi/multinucleated CMs, although to a lesser extent [69].

Telomerase expression in the mammalian heart was investigated using transgenic mice expressing green fluorescence protein (GFP) driven by the promoter for murine telomerase reverse transcriptase (mTert), which is a necessary and rate-limiting component of telomerase [19]. Local proliferation of *mTert-GFP*-expressing cells in the adult heart suggests the existence of a subpopulation of mTERT-positive cells that display a phenotype similar to stem cells. This observation is supported by the expression of the heart-specific transcription factors NKX2.5 and GATA4 in these cells, which are necessary for the differentiation into CM lineage. These factors are described as distinctive features of the native stem cells of the heart. A marked local increase in their number in response to trauma in the adult heart indicates their role in regeneration [19]. A similar increase in the number of stem-like cells with the surface antigen Sca-1 and c- kit and their proliferation was observed during a heart attack, which was accompanied by an increase in telomerase activity [70]. Telomerase delays growth arrest, aging and prevents cell death. It may also be involved in the fight against mechanical and oxidative stress [71], which increases with a concomitant increase in ROS during necrosis and inflammation [72].

Conditions of hypoxia can reduce the oxidative stress after induced myocardial infarction. This leads to an increase in proliferation, which further helps to reduce the area of fibrosis and improves systolic function [73]. In addition to these data, the possibility was found of increasing the regenerative potential of hearts at one week of postnatal development of mice after administration of the antioxidant *N*-acetyl-*L*-cysteine [21].

Cardiac muscle regeneration after an injury is complicated by an "irreversible" exit of CMs from the cell cycle. A forced expression of *Tert* in the cardiac muscle in mice is sufficient to restore telomerase activity and telomere length. This, in turn, can delay the exit from the cell cycle in the cardiac muscle, cause hypertrophy in postmitotic cells and contribute to CM survival [14].

To elucidate a role of telomerase in cardiac regeneration, *Tert* was overexpressed in mouse hearts by adeno-associated viral delivery [14,20]. Mice were subjected to experimental myocardial infarction (MI). Upon MI, *Tert*-expressing hearts showed attenuated cardiac dilation, improved ventricular function and smaller infarct scars concomitant with increased survival by 17% compared with controls. Cardiac transcriptome analysis revealed an increase of epidermal growth factor receptor (EGF) in *Tert*-expressing hearts. Signaling through EGF is cardio-protective, emphasizing defensive function of Tert. Tert therapy also leads to activation of pathways associated with extracellular matrix remodeling (an increase in serum MMP-9 and TGF-b). TGF-b has a pleiotropic effect on almost all cell types involved in the repair and heart remodeling after injury. Long-term activation of these genes may also be a consequence of enhanced heart regeneration, which requires matrix remodeling to integrate new CMs. Indeed, the CM can re-enter the cell cycle after injury. Expression of Ki-67 and the presence of phosphorylated forms of histone H3 (proteins, the maximum expression of which coincides with mitosis) was found to increase the number of proliferating CMs near the infarct zone in the Tert-treated group. According to these results, it is plausible that activation of Tert may assist cardiac regeneration [13].

After injury, sufficient telomere length is required for proliferation. In P1 G3 *Terc*-null newborn mice, the proliferative capacity is lower than that of WT controls. Instead of increasing proliferation, CMs of G3 *Terc*$^{-/-}$ mice grow hypertrophic. The aggravation of telomere shortening after cryogenic damage at P1 in the heart of G3 mice causes an increase of p21 levels compared to WTs, which indicates the activation of the DNA damage response. This leads to the cessation of the cell cycle. A reliable proliferative response was observed in CMs of p21$^{-/-}$ mice that were seven days old. This is the age at which the CMs of WT mice lose the ability to divide after injury. This observation further emphasizes the participation of telomerase inhibition through the expression of p21 in stopping cell cycle and inhibition of the regeneration reaction after injury in the early postnatal period [13].

The proliferative ability is obviously associated with increased telomerase activity relative to mammals; therefore, the *D. rerio* model is interesting from the point of view of the possibility of regeneration of CMs.

In a recent study, it was shown that cryogenic damage to the heart leads to an increase in telomerase activity in WT zebrafish, which was associated with an increase in *tert* gene expression. To determine the role of telomeres in regeneration, damage to the heart was performed with $tert^{-/-}$ and WT *D. rerio*. It was shown that the cardiac output was not restored, and the area of damage did not decrease in $tert^{-/-}$ fish, which indicates the need for telomerase during regeneration. However, the level of the inflammatory response, an important process for regeneration, was the same for WT and $tert^{-/-}$ fish. Similarly, dedifferentiation of CMs in response to an injury occurs normally in the absence of telomerase. The length of telomeres increases only in WT CMs during regeneration, and this is characteristic of both actively proliferating cells and nondividing cells. Therefore, we can conclude that telomere elongation is important for CM regeneration [27].

Induction of polyploidy in the heart of zebrafish leads to a loss of regenerative potential after injury [29]. Consequently, for recovery of the myocardium, diploid CMs are required, the number of which decreases in the mammalian heart with age as a result of telomere depletion [13].

9. Conclusions

Thus, telomerase activity and telomere length are not only markers of cellular aging of CMs, but they also make a significant contribution to the development of age-related diseases. Further study of the influence of various factors on the telomerase complex and telomeric regions of chromosomes can contribute to a better understanding of the processes of telomere length changes that occur in cardiac tissue throughout life.

Studies of the regenerative capacity of the hearts of mammals and other vertebrates can also help in the formation of new approaches in the field of regenerative medicine for the treatment of such serious diseases as, for example, myocardial infarction and heart failure.

Author Contributions: All authors have equal contribution. All authors have read and agreed to the published version of the manuscript.

Funding: This research received no external funding.

Conflicts of Interest: The authors declare no conflicts of interest.

References

1. Hayflick, L.; Moorhead, P.S. The serial cultivation of human diploid cell strains. *Experim. Cell Res.* **1961**, *25*, 585–621. [CrossRef]
2. Nalobin, D.S.; Galiakberova, A.A.; Alipkina, S.I.; Glukhov, A.I. Regulation of Telomerase Activity. *Biol. Bull. Rev.* **2018**, *8*, 142–154. [CrossRef]
3. Blackburn, E.H. Switching and signaling at the telomere. *Cell* **2001**, *10*, 661–673. [CrossRef]
4. Palm, W.; de Lange, T. How shelterin protects mammalian telomeres. *Annu. Rev. Genet.* **2008**, *42*, 301–334. [CrossRef] [PubMed]
5. Harley, C.B. Telomere loss: Mitotic clock or genetic time bomb? *Mutat. Res.* **1991**, *256*, 271–282. [CrossRef]
6. Artandi, S.E.; Attardi, L.D. Pathways connecting telomeres and p53 in senescence, apoptosis, and cancer. *Biochem. Biophys. Res. Commun.* **2005**, *331*, 881–890. [CrossRef] [PubMed]
7. Greider, C.W.; Blackburn, E.H. Identification of a specific telomere terminal transferase activity in Tetrahymena extracts. *Cell* **1985**, *43*, 405–413. [CrossRef]
8. Greider, W. Telomerase activity, cell proliferation, and cancer. *Proc. Natl. Acad. Sci. USA* **1998**, *95*, 90–92. [CrossRef]
9. Sun, C.; Kontaridis, M.I. Physiology of cardiac development: From genetics to signaling to therapeutic strategies. *Curr. Opin. Physiol.* **2018**, *1*, 123–139. [CrossRef]
10. Burggren, W.W.; Dubansky, B.; Bautista, N.M. Cardiovascular development in embryonic and larval fishes. *Fish. Physiol.* **2017**, *36*, 107–184.

11. Erokhina, E.L. Proliferation dynamics of cellular elements in the differentiating mouse myocardium. *Tsitologiia* **1968**, *10*, 1391–1409. [PubMed]
12. Nishimura, H. *Atlas of Human Prenatal Histology*; Igaku-Shoin: Tokyo, Japan, 1983; p. 316.
13. Aix, E.; Gutierrez-Gutierrez, O.; Sanchez-Ferrer, C.; Aguado, T.; Flores, I. Postnatal telomere dysfunction induces cardiomyocyte cell-cycle arrest through p21 activation. *J. Cell Biol.* **2016**, *13*, 571–583. [CrossRef] [PubMed]
14. Oh, H.; Taffet, G.E.; Youker, K.A.; Entman, M.L.; Overbeek, P.A.; Michael, L.H.; Schneider, M.D. Telomerase reverse transcriptase promotes cardiac muscle cell proliferation, hypertrophy, and survival. *Proc. Natl. Acad. Sci. USA* **2001**, *98*, 10308–10313. [CrossRef] [PubMed]
15. Borges, A.; Liew, C. Telomerase activity during cardiac development. *J. Mol. Cell. Cardiol.* **1997**, *29*, 2717–2724. [CrossRef]
16. Marcela, S.G.; Cristina, R.M.; Angel, P.G.; Manuel, A.M.; Sofía, D.-C.; De La Patricia, R.-S.; Bladimir, R.-R.; Concepción, S.G. Chronological and morphological study of heart development in the rat. *Anat. Rec.* **2012**, *295*, 1267–1290. [CrossRef]
17. Ikenishi, A.; Okayama, H.; Iwamoto, N.; Yoshitome, S.; Tane, S.; Nakamura, K.; Obayashi, T.; Hayashi, T.; Takeuchi, T. Cell cycle regulation in mouse heart during embryonic and postnatal stages. *Dev. Growth. Differ.* **2012**, *54*, 731–738. [CrossRef]
18. Soonpaa, M.H.; Kim, K.K.; Pajak, L.; Franklin, M.; Field, L.J. Cardiomyocyte DNA synthesis and binucleation during murine development. *Am. J. Physiol.* **1996**, *271*, 2183–2189. [CrossRef]
19. Richardson, G.D.; Breault, D.; Horrocks, G.; Cormack, S.; Hole, N.; Owens, W.A. Telomerase expression in the mammalian heart. *FASEB J.* **2012**, *26*, 4832–4840. [CrossRef]
20. Bar, C.; Bernardes de Jesus, B.; Serrano, R.; Tejera, A.; Ayuso, E.; Jimenez, V.; Formentini, I.; Bobadilla, M.; Mizrahi, J.; de Martino, A.; et al. Telomerase expression confers cardioprotection in the adult mouse heart after acute myocardial infarction. *Nat. Commun.* **2014**, *5*, 1–14. [CrossRef]
21. Puente, B.N.; Kimura, W.; Muralidhar, S.A.; Moon, J.; Amatruda, J.F.; Phelps, K.L.; Grinsfelder, D.; Rothermel, B.A.; Chen, R.; Garcia, J.A.; et al. The oxygen-rich postnatal environment induces cardiomyocyte cell-cycle arrest through DNA damage response. *Cell* **2014**, *157*, 565–579. [CrossRef]
22. Ghosh, R.; Mitchell, D.L. Effect of oxidative DNA damage in promoter elements on transcription factor binding. *Nucleic Acids Res.* **1999**, *27*, 3213–3218. [CrossRef] [PubMed]
23. Kawanishi, S.; Oikawa, S. Mechanism of telomere shortening by oxidative stress. *Ann. NY. Acad. Sci.* **2004**, *1019*, 278–284. [CrossRef] [PubMed]
24. Fouquerel, E.; Lormand, J.; Bose, A.; Lee, H.T.; Kim, G.S.; Li, J.; Sobol, R.W.; Freudenthal, B.D.; Myong, S.; Opresko, P.L. Oxidative guanine base damage regulates human telomerase activity. *Nat. Struct. Mol. Biol.* **2016**, *23*, 1092–1100. [CrossRef] [PubMed]
25. Pampalona, J.; Frías, C.; Genescà, A.; Tusell, L. Progressive telomere dysfunction causes cytokinesis failure and leads to the accumulation of polyploid cells. *PLoS Genet.* **2012**, *8*, 4. [CrossRef] [PubMed]
26. Anchelin, M.; Murcia, L.; Alcaraz-Pérez, F.; García-Navarro, E.M.; Cayuela, M.L. Behavior of telomere and telomerase during aging and regeneration in zebrafish. *PLoS ONE* **2011**, *6*, 2. [CrossRef] [PubMed]
27. Bednarek, D.; González-Rosa, J.M.; Guzmán-Martínez, G.; Gutiérrez-Gutiérrez, Ó.; Aguado, T.; Sánchez-Ferrer, C.; Marques, I.J.; Galardi-Castilla, M.; de Diego, I.; Gómez, M.J.; et al. Telomerase Is Essential for Zebrafish Heart Regeneration. *Cell Rep.* **2015**, *12*, 1691–1703. [CrossRef]
28. Wills, A.A.; Holdway, J.E.; Major, R.J.; Poss, K.D. Regulated addition of new myocardial and epicardial cells fosters homeostatic cardiac growth and maintenance in adult zebrafish. *Development* **2008**, *135*, 183–192. [CrossRef]
29. Gonzalez-Rosa, J.M.; Sharpe, M.; Field, D.; Soonpaa, M.H.; Field, L.J.; Burns, C.E.; Burns, C.G. Myocardial polyploidization creates a barrier to heart regeneration in zebrafish. *Dev. Cell.* **2018**, *44*, 433–446. [CrossRef]
30. Naqvi, N.; Li, M.; Calvert, J.W.; Tejada, T.; Lambert, J.P.; Wu, J.; Kesteven, S.H.; Holman, S.R.; Matsuda, T.; Lovelock, J.D.; et al. A proliferative burst during preadolescence establishes the final cardiomyocyte number. *Cell* **2014**, *157*, 795–807. [CrossRef]
31. Alkass, K.; Panula, J.; Westman, M.; Wu, T.D.; Guerquin-Kern, J.L.; Bergmann, O. No Evidence for cardiomyocyte number expansion in preadolescent mice. *Cell* **2015**, *163*, 1026–1036. [CrossRef]
32. Soonpaa, M.H.; Zebrowski, D.C.; Platt, C.; Rosenzweig, A.; Engel, F.B.; Field, L.J. Cardiomyocyte Cell-Cycle Activity during Preadolescence. *Cell* **2015**, *163*, 781–782. [CrossRef] [PubMed]

33. Chen, X.; Wilson, R.M.; Kubo, H.; Berretta, R.M.; Harris, D.M.; Zhang, X.; Jaleel, N.; MacDonnell, S.M.; Bearzi, C.; Tillmanns, J.; et al. Adolescent feline heart contains a population of small, proliferative ventricular myocytes with immature physiological properties. *Circ. Res.* **2007**, *100*, 536–544. [CrossRef] [PubMed]
34. Mollova, M.; Bersell, K.; Walsh, S.; Savla, J.; Tanmoy Das, L.; Park, S.-Y.; Silberstein, L.E.; dos Remedios, C.G.; Graham, D.; Colan, S.; et al. Cardiomyocyte proliferation contributes to heart growth in young humans. *Proc. Natl. Acad. Sci. USA* **2013**, *110*, 1446–1451. [CrossRef] [PubMed]
35. Bergmann, O.; Bhardwaj, R.D.; Bernard, S.; Zdunek, S.; Barnabé-Heider, F.; Walsh, S.; Zupicich, J.; Alkass, K.; Buchholz, B.A.; Druid, H.; et al. Evidence for cardiomyocyte renewal in humans. *Science* **2009**, *324*, 98–102. [CrossRef]
36. Rota, M.; Hosoda, T.; De Angelis, A.; Arcarese, M.L.; Esposito, G.; Rizzi, R.; Tillmanns, J.; Tugal, D.; Musso, E.; Rimoldi, O.; et al. The young mouse heart is composed of myocytes heterogeneous in age and function. *Circ. Res.* **2007**, *101*, 387–399. [CrossRef]
37. Hara, E.; Smith, R.; Parry, D.; Tahara, H.; Stone, S.; Peters, G. Regulation of p16CDKN2 expression and its implications for cell immortalization and senescence. *Mol. Cell Biol.* **1996**, *16*, 859–867. [CrossRef]
38. Lund, T.C.; Glass, T.J.; Tolar, J.; Blazar, B.R. Expression of telomerase and telomere length are unaffected by either age or limb regeneration in *Danio rerio*. *PLoS ONE* **2009**, *4*, 11. [CrossRef]
39. Terai, M.; Izumiyama-Shimomura, N.; Aida, J.; Ishikawa, N.; Sawabe, M.; Arai, T.; Fujiwara, M.; Ishii, A.; Nakamura, K.; Takubo, K. Association of telomere shortening in myocardium with heart weight gain and cause of death. *Sci. Rep.* **2013**, *3*, 2401. [CrossRef]
40. Hastings, R.; Li, N.C.; Lacy, P.S.; Patel, H.; Herbert, K.E.; Stanley, A.G.; Williams, B. Rapid telomere attrition in cardiac tissue of the ageing Wistar rat. *Exp. Gerontol.* **2004**, *39*, 855–857. [CrossRef]
41. Ogami, M.; Ikura, Y.; Ohsawa, M.; Matsuo, T.; Kayo, S.; Yoshimi, N.; Hai, E.; Shirai, N.; Ehara, S.; Komatsu, R.; et al. Telomere shortening in human coronary artery diseases. *Arterioscler. Thromb. Vasc. Biol.* **2004**, *24*, 546–550. [CrossRef]
42. Scheller Madrid, A.; Rode, L.; Nordestgaard, B.G.; Bojesen, S.E. Short telomere length and ischemic heart disease: Observational and genetic studies in 290 022 individuals. *Clin. Chem.* **2016**, *62*, 1140–1149. [CrossRef] [PubMed]
43. Lily, L. *Pathophysiology of Diseases of the Cardiovascular System*, 4th ed.; BINOM: Moscow, Russia, 2016; p. 598.
44. McNally, E.M.; Mestroni, L. Dilated Cardiomyopathy: Genetic Determinants and Mechanisms. *Circ. Res.* **2017**, *121*, 731–748. [CrossRef] [PubMed]
45. Chimenti, C.; Kajstura, J.; Torella, D.; Urbanek, K.; Heleniak, H.; Colussi, C.; Di Meglio, F.; Nadal-Ginard, B.; Frustaci, A.; Leri, A.; et al. Senescence and death of primitive cells and myocytes lead to premature cardiac aging and heart failure. *Circ. Res.* **2003**, *93*, 604–613. [CrossRef] [PubMed]
46. Boon, R.A.; Iekushi, K.; Lechner, S.; Seeger, T.; Fischer, A.; Heydt, S.; Kaluza, D.; Tréguer, K.; Carmona, G.; Bonauer, A.; et al. MicroRNA-34a regulates cardiac ageing and function. *Nature* **2013**, *495*, 107–110. [CrossRef] [PubMed]
47. Leri, A.; Franco, S.; Zacheo, A.; Barlucchi, L.; Chimenti, S.; Limana, F.; Nadal-Ginard, B.; Kajstura, J.; Anversa, P.; Blasco, M.A. Ablation of telomerase and telomere loss leads to cardiac dilatation and heart failure associated with p53 upregulation. *EMBO J.* **2003**, *22*, 131–139. [CrossRef] [PubMed]
48. Sahin, E.; Colla, S.; Liesa, M.; Moslehi, J.; Müller, F.L.; Guo, M.; Cooper, M.; Kotton, D.; Fabian, A.J.; Walkey, C.; et al. Telomere dysfunction induces metabolic and mitochondrial compromise. *Nature* **2011**, *470*, 359–365. [CrossRef]
49. Guarente, L. Mitochondria–a nexus for aging, calorie restriction, and sirtuins? *Cell* **2008**, *132*, 171–176. [CrossRef]
50. Ren, J.; Sowers, J.R.; Zhang, Y. Metabolic Stress, Autophagy and Cardiovascular Aging: From Pathophysiology to Therapeutics. *Trends Endocrinol. Metab.* **2018**, *29*, 699–711. [CrossRef]
51. Barton, M.; Husmann, M.; Meyer, M.R. Accelerated Vascular Aging as a Paradigm for Hypertensive Vascular Disease: Prevention and Therapy. *Can. J. Cardiol.* **2016**, *32*, 680–686. [CrossRef]
52. Buford, T.W. Hypertension and aging. *Ageing Res. Rev.* **2016**, *26*, 96–111. [CrossRef]
53. Bertolotti, M.; Lonardo, A.; Mussi, C.; Baldelli, E.; Pellegrini, E.; Ballestri, S.; Romagnoli, D.; Loria, P. Nonalcoholic fatty liver disease and aging: Epidemiology to management. *World J. Gastroenterol.* **2014**, *20*, 14185–14204. [CrossRef] [PubMed]

54. Abel, E.D. Obesity stresses cardiac mitochondria even when you are young. *J. Am. Coll Cardiol.* **2011**, *57*, 586–589. [CrossRef] [PubMed]
55. Ren, J.; Zhang, Y. Targeting Autophagy in Aging and Aging-Related Cardiovascular Diseases. *Trends Pharm. Sci.* **2018**, *39*, 1064–1076. [CrossRef] [PubMed]
56. Nakamura, S.; Yoshimori, T. Autophagy and Longevity. *Mol. Cells* **2018**, *41*, 65–72. [PubMed]
57. Hansen, M.; Rubinsztein, D.C.; Walker, D.W. Autophagy as a promoter of longevity: Insights from model organisms. *Nat. Rev. Mol. Cell Biol.* **2018**, *19*, 579–593. [CrossRef] [PubMed]
58. Cuervo, A.M.; Bergamini, E.; Brunk, U.T.; Dröge, W.; Ffrench, M.; Terman, A. Autophagy and aging: The importance of maintaining "clean" cells. *Autophagy* **2005**, *1*, 131–140. [CrossRef] [PubMed]
59. Schafer, M.J.; Miller, J.D.; LeBrasseur, N.K. Cellular senescence: Implications for metabolic disease. *Mol. Cell Endocrinol.* **2017**, *455*, 93–102. [CrossRef]
60. Alfaras, I.; Di Germanio, C.; Bernier, M.; Csiszar, A.; Ungvari, Z.; Lakatta, E.G.; de Cabo, R. Pharmacological Strategies to Retard Cardiovascular Aging. *Circ. Res.* **2016**, *118*, 1626–1642. [CrossRef]
61. Sonneborn, J.S. Telomerase Biology Associations Offer Keys to Cancer and Aging Therapeutics. *Curr. Aging Sci.* **2019**. [CrossRef]
62. Haendeler, J.; Hoffmann, J.; Brandes, R.P.; Zeiher, A.M.; Dimmeler, S. Hydrogen peroxide triggers nuclear export of telomerase reverse transcriptase via Src kinase family-dependent phosphorylation of tyrosine 707. *Mol. Cell Biol.* **2003**, *23*, 4598–4610. [CrossRef]
63. Ait-Aissa, K.; Ebben, J.D.; Kadlec, A.O.; Beyer, A.M. Friend or foe? Telomerase as a pharmacological target in cancer and cardiovascular disease. *Pharmacol. Res.* **2016**, *111*, 422–433. [CrossRef] [PubMed]
64. Quryshi, N.; Norwood Toro, L.E.; Ait-Aissa, K.; Kong, A.; Beyer, A.M. Chemotherapeutic-Induced Cardiovascular Dysfunction: Physiological Effects, Early Detection-The Role of Telomerase to Counteract Mitochondrial Defects and Oxidative Stress. *Int. J. Mol. Sci* **2018**, *19*, 3. [CrossRef] [PubMed]
65. Ait-Aissa, K.; Heisner, J.S.; Norwood Toro, L.E.; Bruemmer, D.; Doyon, G.; Harmann, L.; Geurts, A.; Camara, A.K.S; Beyer, A.M. Telomerase Deficiency Predisposes to Heart Failure and Ischemia-Reperfusion Injury. *Front. Cardiovasc. Med.* **2019**, *6*, 31. [CrossRef] [PubMed]
66. Sharifi-Sanjani, M.; Oyster, N.M.; Tichy, E.D.; Bedi, K.C. Jr.; Harel, O.; Margulies, K.B.; Mourkioti, F. Cardiomyocyte- Specific Telomere Shortening is a Distinct Signature of Heart Failure in Humans. *J. Am. Heart Assoc.* **2017**, *6*, 9. [CrossRef] [PubMed]
67. Porrello, E.R.; Mahmoud, A.I.; Simpson, E.; Johnson, B.A.; Grinsfelder, D.; Canseco, D.; Mammen, P.P. ' Rothermel, B.A.; Olson, E.N.; Sadek, H.A. Regulation of neonatal and adult mammalian heart regeneration by the miR-15 family. *Proc. Natl. Acad. Sci.USA* **2013**, *110*, 187–192. [CrossRef] [PubMed]
68. Zebrowski, D.C.; Jensen, C.H.; Becker, R.; Ferrazzi, F.; Baun, C.; Hvidsten, S.; Sheikh, S.P.; Polizzotti, B.D.; Andersen, D.C.; Engel, F.B. Cardiac injury of the newborn mammalian heart accelerates cardiomyocyte terminal differentiation. *Sci. Rep.* **2017**, *7*, 8362. [CrossRef]
69. Wang, W.E.; Li, L.; Xia, X.; Fu, W.; Liao, Q.; Lan, C.; Yang, D.; Chen, H.; Yue, R.; Zeng, C.; et al. Dedifferentiation, proliferation, and redifferentiation of adult mammalian cardiomyocytes after ischemic injury. *Circulation* **2017**, *136*, 834–848. [CrossRef]
70. Urbanek, K.; Rota, M.; Cascapera, S.; Bearzi, C.; Nascimbene, A.; De Angelis, A.; Hosoda, T.; Chimenti, S.; Baker, M.; Limana, F.; et al. Cardiac stem cells possess growth factor-receptor systems that after activation regenerate the infarcted myocardium, improving ventricular function and long-term survival. *Circ. Res.* **2005**, *97*, 663–673. [CrossRef]
71. Oh, H.; Wang, S.C.; Prahash, A.; Sano, M.; Moravec, C.S.; Taffet, G.E.; Michael, L.H.; Youker, K.A.; Entman, M.L.; Schneider, M.D. Telomere attrition and Chk2 activation in human heart failure. *Proc. Natl. Acad. Sci. USA* **2003**, *100*, 5378–5383. [CrossRef]

72. Angelos, M.G.; Kutala, V.K.; Torres, C.A.; He, G.; Stoner, J.D.; Mohammad, M.; Kuppusamy, P. Hypoxic reperfusion of the ischemic heart and oxygen radical generation. *Am. J. Physiol. Heart. Circ. Physiol.* **2006**, *290*, 341–347. [CrossRef]
73. Nakada, Y.; Canseco, D.C.; Thet, S.; Abdisalaam, S.; Asaithamby, A.; Santos, C.X.; Shah, A.M.; Zhang, H.; Faber, J.E.; Kinter, M.T.; et al. Hypoxia induces heart regeneration in adult mice. *Nature* **2017**, *541*, 222–227. [CrossRef] [PubMed]

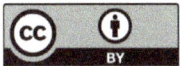

© 2020 by the authors. Licensee MDPI, Basel, Switzerland. This article is an open access article distributed under the terms and conditions of the Creative Commons Attribution (CC BY) license (http://creativecommons.org/licenses/by/4.0/).

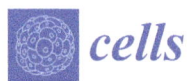

Article

Pravastatin and Gemfibrozil Modulate Differently Hepatic and Colonic Mitochondrial Respiration in Tissue Homogenates from Healthy Rats

Anna Herminghaus *, Eric Laser [†], Jan Schulz, Richard Truse, Christian Vollmer, Inge Bauer and Olaf Picker

Department of Anesthesiology, University Hospital Duesseldorf, Moorenstrasse 5, 40225 Duesseldorf, Germany
* Correspondence: anna.herminghaus@med.uni-duesseldorf.de; Tel: +49-211-81-12195
† In partial fulfillment of the requirements for a doctoral thesis (Eric Laser).

Received: 24 July 2019; Accepted: 24 August 2019; Published: 27 August 2019

Abstract: Statins and fibrates are widely used for the management of hypertriglyceridemia but they also have limitations, mostly due to pharmacokinetic interactions or side effects. It is conceivable that some adverse events like liver dysfunction or gastrointestinal discomfort are caused by mitochondrial dysfunction. Data about the effects of statins and fibrates on mitochondrial function in different organs are inconsistent and partially contradictory. The aim of this study was to investigate the effect of pravastatin (statin) and gemfibrozil (fibrate) on hepatic and colonic mitochondrial respiration in tissue homogenates. Mitochondrial oxygen consumption was determined in colon and liver homogenates from 48 healthy rats after incubation with pravastatin or gemfibrozil (100, 300, 1000 µM). State 2 (substrate dependent respiration) and state 3 (adenosine diphosphate: ADP-dependent respiration) were assessed. RCI (respiratory control index)—an indicator for coupling between electron transport chain system (ETS) and oxidative phosphorylation (OXPHOS) and ADP/O ratio—a parameter for the efficacy of OXPHOS, was calculated. Data were presented as a percentage of control (Kruskal–Wallis + Dunn's correction). In the liver both drugs reduced state 3 and RCI, gemfibrozil-reduced ADP/O (complex I). In the colon both drugs reduced state 3 but enhanced ADP/O. Pravastatin at high concentration (1000 µM) decreased RCI (complex II). Pravastatin and gemfibrozil decrease hepatic but increase colonic mitochondrial respiration in tissue homogenates from healthy rats.

Keywords: pravastatin; gemfibrozil; liver; colon; mitochondrial function

1. Introduction

Statins are among the most widely prescribed drug classes in the world. They are used to lower low density lipoprotein-cholesterol (LDL-C) serum levels in patients for the prevention and treatment of cardiovascular diseases [1]. They exhibit a wide range of effects: additionally to the inhibition of cholesterol synthesis, they modulate inflammatory response, affect coagulation system, induce apoptosis and decrease oxidative stress [2].

If statins are not successful, guidelines recommend peroxisome proliferator-activated receptor alpha (PPARα) agonists (fibrates) for the management of hypertriglyceridemia [3]. Studies have shown that fibrates also have pleiotropic effects like improving endothelial dysfunction [4,5], inhibiting the expression of adhesion molecules and inflammatory cytokines [6] and decreasing oxidative stress and nitric oxide production [5]. Moreover, fibrates can inhibit coagulation [4,7] and improve haemorheologic parameters [8].

However, these agents also have limitations, most importantly due to pharmacokinetic interactions, such as an increased risk of myopathy through a combination of statins and gemfibrozil [9], or side effects, which include digestive disorders, reversible elevation in serum creatinine and liver enzymes [10].

It is conceivable that some of the adverse events like liver dysfunction or gastrointestinal discomfort are caused by mitochondrial dysfunction [11,12]. However, data about effects of statins and fibrates on mitochondrial function in different organs are inconsistent and partially contradictory. Data about effects of these drugs on colonic mitochondria are lacking completely.

Statins can affect skeletal muscle mitochondria in vitro by inhibiting respiratory chain complexes and oxidative capacity [12,13], decreasing mitochondrial membrane potential [13], uncoupling oxidative phosphorylation, inducing mitochondrial swelling and apoptosis [13] and decreasing mitochondrial density [14]. Statins also uncouple state 2 respiration and can inhibit the activity of the complexes of the respiratory chain in liver mitochondria, but the effect is drug-dependent (simvastatin has a strong deteriorating effect, while pravastatin does not seem to affect hepatic mitochondria) [15].

Hydrophilic statins (e.g., pravastatin) are considered as less 'mitotoxic' compared to lipophilic statins such as cerivastatin, fluvastatin, atorvastatin and simvastatin [13]. Even if some authors failed to show any effects of pravastatin on mitochondrial respiration in muscle [13], in the liver [16] and in HL-1 cardiomyocytes [1], cases of drug induced hepatotoxicity are reported [17]. Furthermore, evidence exists for even positive effects of statins on mitochondrial function. Bouitbir et al. showed that statins promote mitochondrial function and mitochondrial biogenesis in human heart muscle [18].

Effects of fibrates on mitochondrial function are also not clearly understood. From one side, in vitro results suggest impaired mitochondrial function, via direct inhibition of mitochondrial respiration (mainly complex I) [19], by membrane depolarization [20] and through increases in uncoupled respiration [15,21]. From the other side, fibrates as PPAR-α agonists can enhance mitogenesis and therefore mitochondrial activity [22]. There are also differences among single fibrates concerning effects on mitochondrial function and gemfibrozil seems to be less mitotoxic than the other drugs from this group [19].

Taken together, the effects of statins and fibrates on mitochondrial function in different organs have been insufficiently examined. Data concerning hepatic mitochondria are inconsistent and about other organs like colon are lacking completely. The aim of this study was therefore to investigate the concentration dependent effect of pravastatin (statin) and gemfibrozil (fibrate) on hepatic and colonic mitochondrial respiration in tissue homogenates from healthy rats.

2. Materials and Methods

2.1. Animals:

The study was approved from the Animal Ethics Committee of the University of Duesseldorf, Germany (project identification code: O27/12), and performed in accordance with the Guide for the Care and Use of Laboratory Animals of the National Institutes of Health. The authors ensured that their research complied with the commonly accepted '3Rs': replacement, reduction and refinement.

Male Wistar rats were purchased from the breeding facilities of the University of Düsseldorf (Düsseldorf Germany) or from Janvier Labs (Le Genest-Saint-Isle, France). They were kept at an artificial 12-h light/dark cycle at constant room temperature and humidity with free access to standard chow and tap water.

Forty eight rats (approximately 3 months old) were sacrificed by decapitation under deep sedation with sodium pentobarbital (90 mg/kg) and liver and colon were harvested.

2.2. Preparation of Liver and Colon Homogenates

Liver and colon homogenates were prepared as described previously [23–25]. Briefly, liver tissue was placed in 4 °C cold isolation buffer, minced into 2–3-mm^3 pieces, rinsed twice in isolation buffer to remove traces of blood, and homogenized (Potter-Elvehjem, Pro Scientific, Swedesboro, NJ, USA, 5 strokes, 2000 rpm). Freshly harvested colon tissue was placed in isolation buffer enriched with 2% bovine serum albumin (BSA, Sigma-Aldrich Corporation, St. Louis, MO, USA), longitudinally opened, and dried with a cotton pad to remove remains of faeces and mucus. After incubation with

0.05% trypsin (Thermo Fisher Scientific, Dreieich, Germany) for 5 min, the tissue was transferred into the isolation buffer containing 2% BSA and protease inhibitors (cOmplete™ Protease Inhibitor Cocktail, Roche Life Science, Mannheim, Germany), minced, and finally homogenized (see above). Protein concentration in the tissue homogenates was determined by the Lowry method [26] with bovine serum albumin as a standard. All procedures were performed on ice, all buffer were kept by 4 °C.

2.3. Measurement of Mitochondrial Respiratory Rates

Mitochondrial oxygen consumption was measured as described previously [23–25]. Briefly, the measurement was performed at 30 °C using a Clark-type electrode (model 782, Strathkelvin instruments, Glasgow, Scotland). Tissue homogenates were suspended in respiration medium to yield a protein concentration of 4 mg/mL or 6 mg/mL for liver and colon, respectively.

2.3.1. Mitochondrial State 2 Respiration

Mitochondrial state 2 respiration was performed in the presence of either complex I substrates glutamate (Fluka, München, Germany) and malate (Serva Electrophoresis GmbH, Heidelberg, Germany) (both 2.5 mM, G–M) or the complex II substrate succinate (Sigma-Aldrich Corporation, St. Louis, MO, USA) (10 mM for liver, 5 mM for colon, S) combined with 0.5 µM rotenone (Sigma-Aldrich Corporation, St. Louis, MO, USA)—the inhibitor of complex I activity. Rotenon was always added before addition of succinate.

2.3.2. Mitochondrial State 3 Respiration

The maximal coupled mitochondrial respiration (state 3) was measured after the addition of adenosine diphosphate—ADP (Sigma-Aldrich Corporation, St. Louis, MO, USA) (250 µM for liver, 50 µM for colon). The respiratory control index (RCI) was calculated (state 3/state 2) to define the coupling between the electron transport system (ETS) and oxidative phosphorylation (OXPHOS). To reflect the efficacy of OXPHOS, the ADP/O ratio was calculated from the amount of ADP added and oxygen consumed in state 3. The average oxygen consumption was calculated as the mean from three technical replicates.

2.3.3. General Conditions

The solubility of oxygen was assumed to be 223 µmol O_2/L at 30 °C according to the Strathkelvin instruments manual. Respiration rates were expressed as nmol/min/mg protein. No correction of the natural drift of the electrode was made since a drift of less than 0.5% over 12 h is neglectable in our experimental setup.

2.3.4. Quality Control for the Preparation Procedure

At the beginning of every experiment mitochondria were checked for leakage by the addition of 2.5 µM cytochrome c (Sigma-Aldrich Corporation, St. Louis, MO, USA) and 0.05 µg/mL oligomycin (Calbiochem by Merck KGaA, Darmstadt, Germany) at the beginning of every experiment. There was no increase in flux after the addition of cytochrome c, indicating integrity of the mitochondrial outer membrane. When ATP synthesis was inhibited by oligomycin, the mitochondria were transferred to state 2, which reflects the respiration rate compensating the proton leak. The lack of difference in O_2 consumption after adding oligomycin compared to state 2 indicates that the inner membrane was intact and mitochondria were not damaged through the preparation procedure.

2.3.5. Experimental Conditions

The assessment of mitochondrial respiration was performed after addition of carrier substance (distilled water)—control, or different concentrations of pravastatin (100 µM, 300 µM and 1000 µM).

For experiments with gemfibrozil (100 µM, 300 µM and 1000 µM), dimethyl sulfoxide (DMSO) (Sigma-Aldrich Corporation, St. Louis, MO, USA) 0.5%, 1.5% and 5% respectively were used as controls. The incubation took place at room temperature (kept at 21 °C) for 3 min. Eight biological and three technical (three separate measurements from a single homogenate) replicates were performed.

2.4. Statistical Analysis

Statistical analysis was performed with GraphPad Prism 8.0 (GraphPad Software, GraphPad Software, San Diego, CA, USA). After checking the data set for normality (Kolmogorov–Smirnov) a Kruskal–Wallis test of variance followed by a post hoc Dunn's correction were performed. Means ± standard deviations (S.D.) were determined. Data are presented as percentage of control values, $P < 0.05$ was considered significant.

3. Results

3.1. Effects of Pravastatin on Hepatic Mitochondrial Respiration

The lowest concentration of pravastatin (100 µM) did not affect the mitochondrial respiration in the liver. Pravastatin in higher concentrations (300 µM and 1000 µM) reduced state 3 (complex I: pravastatin 300 µM: 77.5% ± 3.2%*, pravastatin 1000 µM: 60.7% ± 5.3%*; complex II: pravastatin 300 µM: 84.8% ± 2.4%*, pravastatin 1000 µM: 72.3% ± 6.2%*) (Figure 1A,D) and RCI (complex I: pravastatin 300 µM: 75.3% ± 5.0%*, pravastatin 1000 µM: 66.4% ± 4.2%*, complex II: pravastatin 300 µM: 82.6% ± 6.1%*, pravastatin 1000 µM: 72.2% ± 5.9%*) (Figure 1B,E) for both complexes without changing the ADP/O-ratio (Figure 1C,F).

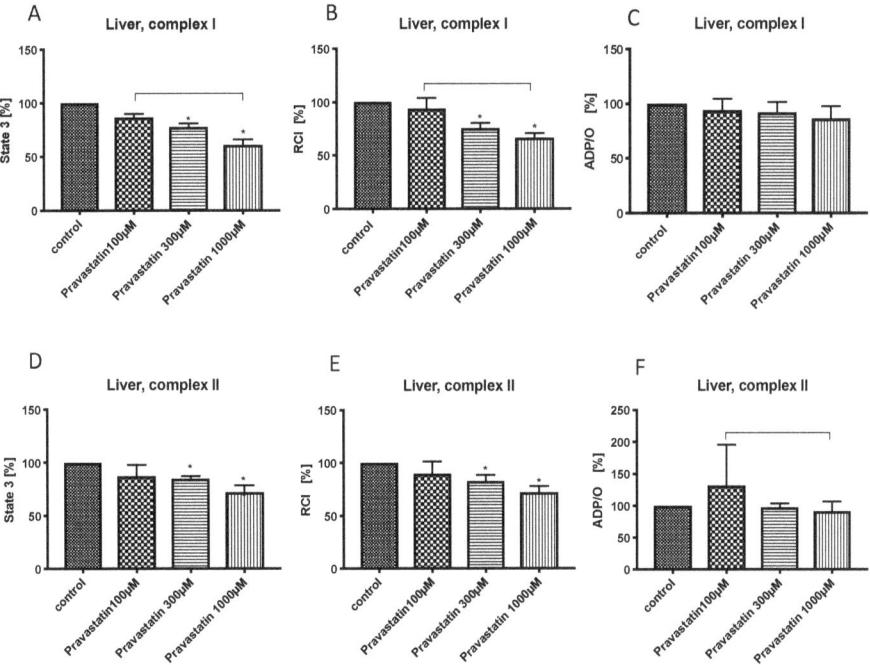

Figure 1. Effect of pravastatin (100 µM, 300 µM and 1000 µM) on hepatic mitochondrial respiration: State 3 for complex I (**A**) and II (**D**), respiratory control index (RCI) for complex I (**B**) und II (**E**) and ADP/O ratio for complex I (**C**) and II (**F**). Data are presented as mean ± standard deviation (S.D.), $n = 7$–8, * $P < 0.05$ vs. control, $P < 0.05$ between groups.

3.2. Effects of Pravastatin on Colonic Mitochondrial Respiration

The lowest concentration of pravastatin (100 µM) did not affect the mitochondrial respiration in the colon. Pravastatin in middle concentration (300 µM) reduced state 3 for complex II (86.1% ± 4.8%*) (Figure 2D) and in high concentration (1000 µm) decreased state 3 for both complexes (complex I: 63.6% ± 8.2%*, complex II: 77.3% ± 4.1%*) (Figure 2A,D).

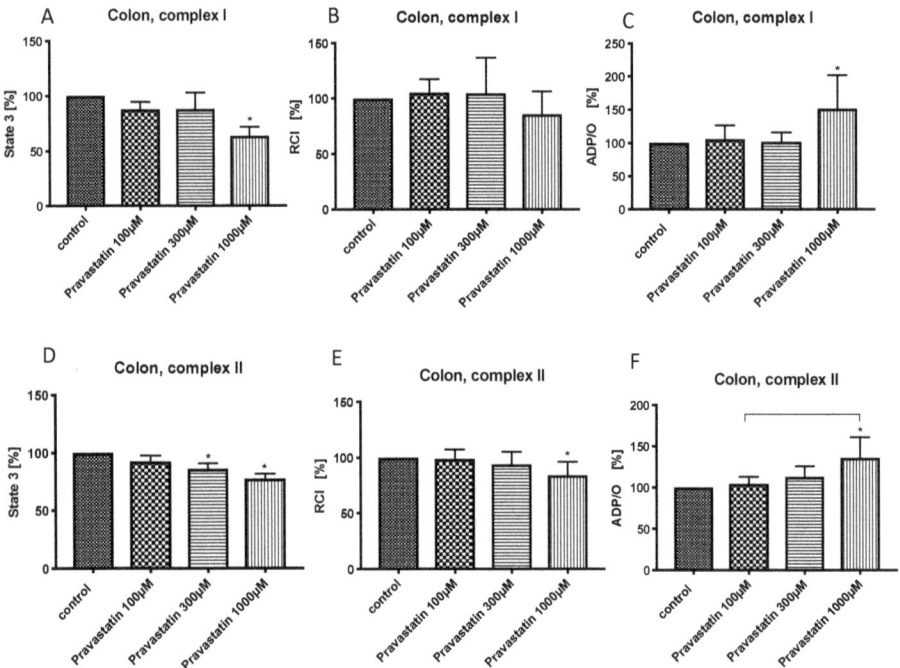

Figure 2. Effect of pravastatin (100 µM, 300 µM and 1000 µM) on colonic mitochondrial respiration: State 3 for complex I (**A**) and II (**D**), respiratory control index (RCI) for complex I (**B**) und II (**E**) and ADP/O ratio for complex I (**C**) and II (**F**). Data are presented as mean ± S.D., $n = 7–8$, * $P < 0.05$ vs. control, $P < 0.05$ between groups.

The RCI in colonic mitochondria was decreased only by pravastatin at the highest concentration (1000 µM) and only for complex II (83.8 ± 12.6%*) (Figure 2E).

Pravastatin in high concentration (1000 µM) increased the ADP/O-ratio for both complexes (complex I: 151.5% ± 50.4%*, complex II: 136.4% ± 24.9%*) (Figure 2C,F).

3.3. Effects of Gemfibrozil on Hepatic Mitochondrial Respiration

Similarly to pravastatin, gemfibrozil in low concentration (100 µM) did not affect the mitochondrial respiration in the liver. Gemfibrozil at higher concentrations (300 µM and 1000 µM) reduced state 3 (complex I: gemfibrozil 300 µM: 56.9% ± 5.5%*, gemfibrozil 1000 µM: 24.4% ± 2.5%*; complex II: gemfibrozil 300 µM: 87.8% ± 18.5%*, gemfibrozil 1000 µM: 50.9% ± 11.4%*) (Figure 3A,D) and RCI (complex I: gemfibrozil 300 µM: 45.1% ± 5.2%*, gemfibrozil 1000 µM: 21.5% ± 2.8%*, complex II: gemfibrozil 300 µM: 70.4% ± 5.5%*, gemfibrozil 1000 µM: 37.8% ± 8.3%*) (Figure 3B,E) for both complexes. Gemfibrozil 300 µM reduced ADP/O for complex I (81.5% ± 7.6%*) (Figure 3C). ADP/O-ratio after treatment with gemfibrozil 1000 µM was significantly higher than ADP/O-ratio in other gemfibrozil-groups.

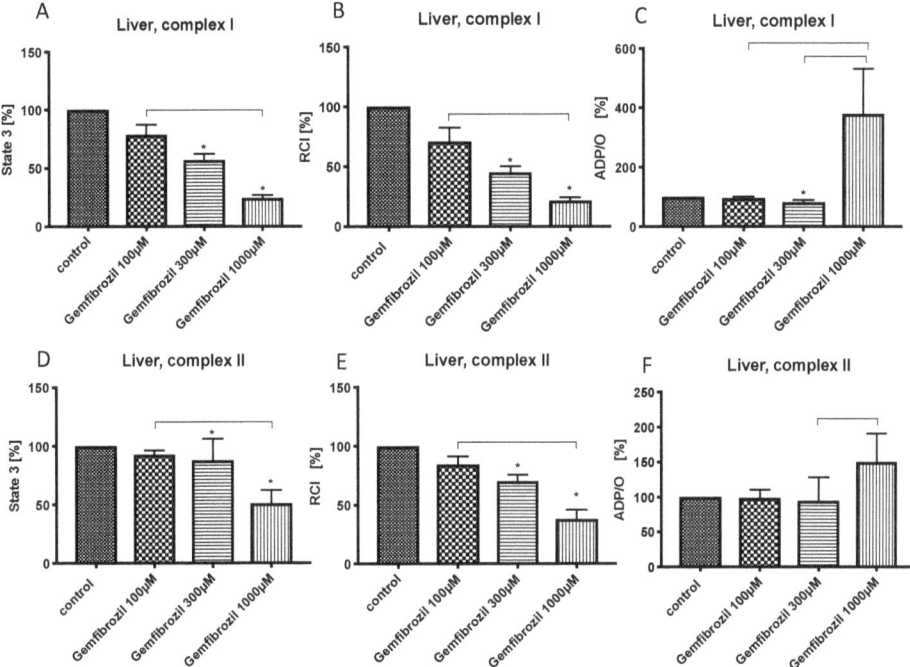

Figure 3. Effect of gemfibrozil (100 μM, 300 μM and 1000 μM) on hepatic mitochondrial respiration: State 3 for complex I (**A**) and II (**D**), respiratory control index (RCI) for complex I (**B**) und II (**E**) and ADP/O ratio for complex I (**C**) and II (**F**). Data are presented as mean ± S.D., $n = 7$–8, * $P < 0.05$ vs. control, $P < 0.05$ between groups.

3.4. Effects of Gemfibrozil on Colonic Mitochondrial Respiration

Gemfibrozil in low concentration (100 μM) reduced state 3 for complex I (89.3% ± 5.5%*). Gemfibrozil at the middle concentration (300 μM) did not show any effect on colonic mitochondrial respiration. Gemfibrozil at high concentration (1000 μM) reduced state 3 for both complexes (complex I: 80.8% ± 6.6*, complex II: 92.5% ± 15.2%*) and increased the ADP/O-ratio for complex I (133.8% ± 33.8%*) without changing the RCI (Figure 4B,E).

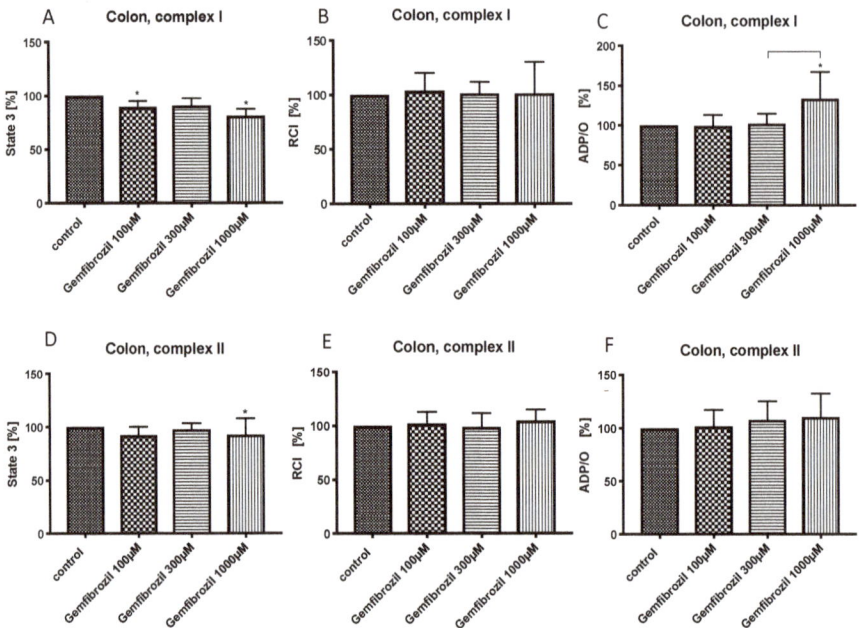

Figure 4. Effect of gemfibrozil (100 μM, 300 μM and 1000 μM) on colonic mitochondrial respiration: State 3 for complex I (**A**) and II (**D**), respiratory control index (RCI) for complex I (**B**) und II (**E**) and ADP/O ratio for complex I (**C**) and II (**F**). Data are presented as mean ± S.D., n = 7–8, * $P < 0.05$ vs. control, $P < 0.05$ between groups.

4. Discussion

The main result of this study is that the effect of pravastatin and gemfibrozil is organ specific and dose dependent. Both drugs seem to have a deteriorating effect on hepatic mitochondria but rather positive influence on colonic mitochondrial respiration.

The chosen experimental setting is based on our previous study [24]. The drug concentrations correspond to the literature describing similar in vitro experiments [13,15,19,27]. The measurements are performed at 30 °C which is a methodological standard [13,15,20], but not a physiological condition. Thus, the data may not reflect full effects of the drugs in vivo. While liver is mainly composed of hepatocytes, colon consists of different cell lines like epithelial cells, smooth muscle cells, adipocytes and many others. Therefore, our results cannot relate to a special cell line.

In hepatic mitochondria, pravastatin dose dependently reduced ADP-induced mitochondrial respiration-state 3, and coupling between electron transport chain (ETS) and oxidative phosphorylation (OXPHOS)-RCI, without changing the efficacy of oxidative phosphorylation-ADP/O.

In colonic mitochondria, pravastatin also reduced state 3 and RCI, however, to a minor extent, mainly at the higher concentration and preferably through complex II. In contrast to hepatic mitochondria, pravastatin increased the efficacy of OXPHOS in the colon for both complexes.

Our results concerning pravastatin and mitochondrial respiration are new findings compared to the results of other authors who mainly could not show any effects of this drug on mitochondrial respiration. Marques et al. examined the effect of pravastatin on hepatic mitochondrial in LDL knockout mice after oral pretreatment with 40 mg/kg pravastatin and did not observe any changes either [16]. Sugiyama et al. tested the effects of pravastatin on age-related changes in mitochondrial function in rats after long-term therapy. They could show that pravastatin significantly accelerated the age-related decline in the activity of complex I of diaphragm mitochondria, whereas the aging effect on mitochondrial respiratory function was not observed on heart muscle and liver. Pravastatin did not significantly affect cardiac and hepatic respiratory function [28]. Kaufmann et al. [13] did not observe any effects of pravastatin on mitochondrial oxygen consumption in isolated muscle mitochondria in vitro using similar pravastatin concentrations (50–400 µM). Godoy et al. [1] tested the influence of atorvastatin and pravastatin (10 µM) on HL-1 cardiomyocyte mitochondrial function and could show, that atorvastatin altered mitochondrial function compared to cardiomyocytes treated with pravastatin. The difference between our results (declined mitochondrial respiration in liver) and the other findings (unchanged mitochondrial respiration) could be caused by many factors like different experimental conditions (in vitro vs. ex vivo, different drug concentrations in in vitro experiments and oral pretreatment), long-term therapy vs. single dose and different tissues (liver, muscle, cardiomyocytes). It is well known, that mitochondrial function varies between organs [29].

The effect of pravastatin on colonic mitochondria was different from that in the liver. The drug moderately reduced state 3 and RCI, mainly in high concentration and preferably through complex II but increased the efficacy of OXPHOS for both complexes. It seems to be a rather positive effect reflected in a higher efficacy of OXPHOS with reduced mitochondrial respiration. In general, an increase in mitochondrial respiration is considered as an improvement and vice versa. However, mitochondria may also dynamically respond to specific conditions, and changes in oxphos capacity or RCI may simply reflect a response rather than an improvement or impairment. Under physiological conditions with sufficient oxygen supply, the impact on cell metabolism is probably of minor relevance. However, this effect might gain a major importance as an adaptive response under compromised conditions associated with e.g., cellular hypoxia. To clarify, whether this observation is favorable for the cell metabolism, the underlying processes like activity of the single complexes of the respiratory chain, mitochondrial membrane potential or tissue ATP-concentration need to be further analyzed.

To our best knowledge, there are no data about influence of pravastatin on mitochondrial function in the colon so we cannot refer our results to those of other authors.

For pravastatin, plasma concentrations after oral administration of 20–40 mg/day are in the range of 0.1–0.229 µM [30] which is considerably lower than those concentrations applied in our in vitro study. The oral bioavailability of pravastatin is low (17%) because of incomplete absorption and a first-pass effect. The drug is rapidly absorbed from the upper part of the small intestine, probably via proton-coupled carrier-mediated transport, and then taken up by the liver by a sodium-independent bile acid transporter [31,32]. The uptake of the drugs into different tissues differs substantially and leads to wide ranges of drug concentrations in the target organs. Yamazaki et al. [33] examined the pharmacokinetic properties of pravastatin after intravenous and portal vein application in rats and could show that the largest clearance was observed for the liver, followed by the kidney whereas other tissues like small intestine exhibited only a minor uptake. Hatanaka et al. showed that pravastatin accumulated in the liver and reached even higher concentrations compared to plasma levels. Interestingly, the pravastatin plasma concentration increased with increasing dose, whereas the contrary was the case in liver and small intestine [34]. We chose relatively high drug concentration according to the similar in vitro experiments described in the literature [13,17]. Nevertheless, our results may be relevant for the in vivo situation since the most adverse events with statins have been described in patients having a drug–drug interaction leading to a higher drug concentration or underlying mitochondrial disease rendering them more sensitive to statins [35,36]. Moreover, many patients suffer from multimorbidity. Renal and/or liver insufficiency can also result in supraclinical or even toxic drug plasma concentrations.

The effects of gemfibrozil on hepatic mitochondrial respiration were similar to pravastatin but seem to be more pronounced. Gemfibrozil reduced dose dependently state 3 and RCI for both complexes and ADP/O-ratio for complex I. However, the increase in ADP/O ratio after treatment with gemfibrozil 1000 µM most likely reflects rather a sign of terminal uncoupling than improvement of efficacy of OXPHOS. To test this hypothesis, we treated hepatic mitochondria with an uncoupler—2-[2-(3-Chlorophenyl)hydrazinylyidene]propanedinitrile (CCCP)—and there was no further enhancement in mitochondrial respiration confirming the terminal uncoupling.

Our results are consistent with those of other authors, who also observed a decrease in mitochondrial respiration and uncoupling effect of gemfibrozil. Nadanaciva et al. [15] showed that gemfibrozil in concentration of 500 nmol/mg mitochondrial proteins (which would correspond to 2000 µM in our experimental setting) lowered state 3 in isolated hepatic rat mitochondria about more than 50%. Zhou et al. [20] examined the effects of different fibrates on mitochondrial bioenergetics and showed that gemfibrozil at 75 µM uncouples isolated hepatic rat mitochondria and reduces the efficacy of the OXPHOS. Zhou et al. suggest that the underlying mechanism of uncoupling could be the induction of mitochondrial permeability transition pores.

In the colon, gemfibrozil decreased slightly ADP-dependent mitochondrial respiration, but did not affect the coupling between ETS and OXPHOS and improved the efficacy of OXPHOS for complex I. Similar to pravastatin, we presume that gemfibrozil could also have a protective effect on colonic mitochondria, allowing an efficient ATP-production by reduced mitochondrial oxygen consumption. Also in this case, this mechanism may be relevant under pathologic conditions like sepsis or hemorrhagic shock, but probably does not play a pivotal role when the oxygen supply is sufficient. Nevertheless, mechanisms compensating a lack of oxygen are substantially important in organs like the colon. When circulation becomes unstable, e.g., in septic shock, blood flow is redistributed to maintain the oxygenation of vital organs as heart or brain, while microcirculation in less essential organs like the splanchnic region, kidney and liver is critically reduced [37]. We are the first to analyze the effects of gemfibrozil on colonic mitochondrial function, so no comparison with other results can be made.

As described above, we used in our experiment higher gemfibrozil concentrations than clinically occur. After the standard oral administration of 1200 mg/day, the plasma concentration of gemfibrozil reaches 10–20 mg/L (40–80 µM) [38,39]. Also in this case we consider our result as clinically relevant, because fibrates are often combined with other lipid-lowering drugs like statins or thiazolidinediones and the combination can lead to higher plasma levels. Moreover, the clinically used drug combinations, like statins plus fibrates, show different effects to the single application. In our experiments, pravastatin and gemfibrozil showed similar negative effects on mitochondrial respiration in liver and positive influence on the colonic mitochondria. So it is conceivable, that additive effects are observed with co-incubation. Nadanaciva et al. showed that gemfibrozil at 62 nmol/mg protein (which would correspond to 248 µM in our experimental setting) did not affect mitochondrial function, but in combination with cerivastatin depressed the mitochondrial respiration significantly [15].

5. Conclusions

Taken together, we show new findings about organ-specific and concentration-dependent effects of two clinically important and widely used drugs, pravastatin and gemfibrozil, on hepatic and colonic mitochondrial respiration. Results from this study reveal a rather negative effect of both drugs on hepatic mitochondrial respiration. This could possibly be one of the mechanisms contributing to elevated liver enzymes during the therapy with these drugs. This hypothesis must be considered very carefully because we examined the mitochondrial oxygen consumption, which depicts only one aspect of the complex mitochondrial function within a cell. Furthermore, our experiments are conducted in vitro with animal tissues and these adverse effects are not fully understood and are complex processes including many factors like preexisting organ damage and co-medication.

The positive effects of pravastatin and gemfibrozil on colonic mitochondria could contribute to adaptive cell mechanisms under pathological conditions like sepsis or hemorrhagic shock, where tissue hypoxia may occur, allowing better oxygen utilization. Also in this case, the results must be interpreted very cautiously and further research in this field is needed. Our data extend our knowledge about a possible mode of action of both drugs and offer a new insight into conceivable mechanisms of their side effects.

Author Contributions: Conceptualization: A.H., I.B. and O.P.; Methodology: A.H. and E.L.; Software: A.H. and E.L.; Validation: A.H., E.L., J.S. and R.T.; Formal Analysis: A.H, I.B. and O.P.; Investigation: A.H. and E.L.; Resources: I.B. and O.P.; Data Curation: A.H. and E.L.; Writing—Original Draft Preparation: A.H.; Writing—Review and Editing: A.H., J.S., R.T., C.V., I.B. and O.P.; Visualization: A.H.; Supervision: C.V., I.B. and O.P.; Project Administration: A.H., I.B., O.P.

Funding: This research received no external funding.

Acknowledgments: The authors would like to thank Adelheid Weidinger for scientific and Birgitt Berke and Claudia Dohle for technical support.

Conflicts of Interest: The authors declare no conflict of interest.

References

1. Godoy, J.C.; Niesman, I.R.; Busija, A.R.; Kassan, A.; Schilling, J.M.; Schwarz, A.; Alvarez, E.A.; Dalton, N.D.; Drummond, J.C.; Roth, D.M.; et al. Atorvastatin, but not pravastatin, inhibits cardiac Akt/mTOR signaling and disturbs mitochondrial ultrastructure in cardiac myocytes. *FASEB J. Off. Publ. Fed. Am. Soc. Exp. Biol.* **2019**, *33*, 1209–1225. [CrossRef]
2. Terblanche, M.; Almog, Y.; Rosenson, R.S.; Smith, T.S.; Hackam, D.G. Statins and sepsis: Multiple modifications at multiple levels. *Lancet Infect. Dis.* **2007**, *7*, 358–368. [CrossRef]
3. Piepoli, M.F.; Hoes, A.W.; Agewall, S.; Albus, C.; Brotons, C.; Catapano, A.L.; Cooney, M.-T.; Corrà, U.; Cosyns, B.; Deaton, C.; et al. 2016 European Guidelines on cardiovascular disease prevention in clinical practice: The Sixth Joint Task Force of the European Society of Cardiology and Other Societies on Cardiovascular Disease Prevention in Clinical Practice (constituted by representatives of 10 societies and by invited experts) Developed with the special contribution of the European Association for Cardiovascular Prevention & Rehabilitation (EACPR). *Eur. Heart J.* **2016**, *37*, 2315–2381. [PubMed]
4. Wiel, E.; Lebuffe, G.; Robin, E.; Gasan, G.; Corseaux, D.; Tavernier, B.; Jude, B.; Bordet, R.; Vallet, B. Pretreatment with peroxysome proliferator-activated receptor alpha agonist fenofibrate protects endothelium in rabbit Escherichia coli endotoxin-induced shock. *Intensive Care Med.* **2005**, *31*, 1269–1279. [CrossRef] [PubMed]
5. Goya, K.; Sumitani, S.; Xu, X.; Kitamura, T.; Yamamoto, H.; Kurebayashi, S.; Saito, H.; Kouhara, H.; Kasayama, S.; Kawase, I. Peroxisome proliferator-activated receptor alpha agonists increase nitric oxide synthase expression in vascular endothelial cells. *Arterioscler. Thromb. Vasc. Biol.* **2004**, *24*, 658–663. [CrossRef] [PubMed]
6. Jiang, C.; Ting, A.T.; Seed, B. PPAR-gamma agonists inhibit production of monocyte inflammatory cytokines. *Nature* **1998**, *391*, 82–86. [CrossRef] [PubMed]
7. Nilsson, L.; Takemura, T.; Eriksson, P.; Hamsten, A. Effects of Fibrate Compounds on Expression of Plasminogen Activator Inhibitor-1 by Cultured Endothelial Cells. *Arterioscler. Thromb. Vasc. Biol.* **1999**, *19*, 1577–1581. [CrossRef]
8. Frost, R.J.; Otto, C.; Geiss, H.C.; Schwandt, P.; Parhofer, K.G. Effects of atorvastatin versus fenofibrate on lipoprotein profiles, low-density lipoprotein subfraction distribution, and hemorheologic parameters in type 2 diabetes mellitus with mixed hyperlipoproteinemia. *Am. J. Cardiol.* **2001**, *87*, 44–48. [CrossRef]
9. Davidson, M.H. Statin/fibrate combination in patients with metabolic syndrome or diabetes: Evaluating the risks of pharmacokinetic drug interactions. *Expert Opin. Drug Saf.* **2006**, *5*, 145–156. [CrossRef] [PubMed]
10. Hedrington, M.S.; Davis, S.N. Peroxisome proliferator-activated receptor alpha-mediated drug toxicity in the liver. *Expert Opin. Drug Metab. Toxicol.* **2018**, *14*, 671–677. [CrossRef]
11. Scatena, R.; Bottoni, P.; Vincenzoni, F.; Messana, I.; Martorana, G.E.; Nocca, G.; De Sole, P.; Maggiano, N.; Castagnola, M.; Giardina, B. Bezafibrate Induces a Mitochondrial Derangement in Human Cell Lines: A PPAR-Independent Mechanism for a Peroxisome Proliferator. *Chem. Res. Toxicol.* **2003**, *16*, 1440–1447. [CrossRef] [PubMed]
12. Mullen, P.J.; Zahno, A.; Lindinger, P.; Maseneni, S.; Felser, A.; Krähenbühl, S.; Brecht, K. Susceptibility to simvastatin-induced toxicity is partly determined by mitochondrial respiration and phosphorylation state of Akt. *Biochim. Biophys. Acta* **2011**, *1813*, 2079–2087. [CrossRef] [PubMed]
13. Kaufmann, P.; Török, M.; Zahno, A.; Waldhauser, K.M.; Brecht, K.; Krähenbühl, S. Toxicity of statins on rat skeletal muscle mitochondria. *Cell. Mol. Life Sci. CMLS* **2006**, *63*, 2415–2425. [CrossRef] [PubMed]

14. Päivä, H.; Thelen, K.M.; Van Coster, R.; Smet, J.; De Paepe, B.; Mattila, K.M.; Laakso, J.; Lehtimäki, T.; von Bergmann, K.; Lütjohann, D.; et al. High-dose statins and skeletal muscle metabolism in humans: A randomized, controlled trial. *Clin. Pharmacol. Ther.* **2005**, *78*, 60–68. [CrossRef] [PubMed]
15. Nadanaciva, S.; Rana, P.; Beeson, G.C.; Chen, D.; Ferrick, D.A.; Beeson, C.C.; Will, Y. Assessment of drug-induced mitochondrial dysfunction via altered cellular respiration and acidification measured in a 96-well platform. *J. Bioenerg. Biomembr.* **2012**, *44*, 421–437. [CrossRef] [PubMed]
16. Marques, A.C.; Busanello, E.N.B.; de Oliveira, D.N.; Catharino, R.R.; Oliveira, H.C.F.; Vercesi, A.E. Coenzyme Q10 or Creatine Counteract Pravastatin-Induced Liver Redox Changes in Hypercholesterolemic Mice. *Front. Pharmacol.* **2018**, *9*, 685. [CrossRef] [PubMed]
17. Bhardwaj, S.S.; Chalasani, N. Lipid-lowering agents that cause drug-induced hepatotoxicity. *Clin. Liver Dis.* **2007**, *11*, 597–613. [CrossRef]
18. Bouitbir, J.; Charles, A.-L.; Echaniz-Laguna, A.; Kindo, M.; Daussin, F.; Auwerx, J.; Piquard, F.; Geny, B.; Zoll, J. Opposite effects of statins on mitochondria of cardiac and skeletal muscles: A "mitohormesis" mechanism involving reactive oxygen species and PGC-1. *Eur. Heart. J.* **2012**, *33*, 1397–1407. [CrossRef]
19. Brunmair, B.; Lest, A.; Staniek, K.; Gras, F.; Scharf, N.; Roden, M.; Nohl, H.; Waldhäusl, W.; Fürnsinn, C. Fenofibrate impairs rat mitochondrial function by inhibition of respiratory complex I. *J. Pharmacol. Exp. Ther.* **2004**, *311*, 109–114. [CrossRef]
20. Zhou, S.; Wallace, K.B. The effect of peroxisome proliferators on mitochondrial bioenergetics. *Toxicol. Sci. Off. J. Soc. Toxicol.* **1999**, *48*, 82–89. [CrossRef]
21. Zungu, M.; Young, M.E.; Stanley, W.C.; Essop, M.F. Chronic treatment with the peroxisome proliferator-activated receptor alpha agonist Wy-14,643 attenuates myocardial respiratory capacity and contractile function. *Mol. Cell. Biochem.* **2009**, *330*, 55–62. [CrossRef] [PubMed]
22. Andreux, P.A.; Houtkooper, R.H.; Auwerx, J. Pharmacological approaches to restore mitochondrial function. *Nat. Rev. Drug Discov.* **2013**, *12*, 465–483. [CrossRef] [PubMed]
23. Herminghaus, A.; Eberhardt, R.; Truse, R.; Schulz, J.; Bauer, I.; Picker, O.; Vollmer, C. Nitroglycerin and Iloprost Improve Mitochondrial Function in Colon Homogenate Without Altering the Barrier Integrity of Caco-2 Monolayers. *Front. Med.* **2018**, *5*, 291. [CrossRef] [PubMed]
24. Herminghaus, A.; Buitenhuis, A.J.; Schulz, J.; Vollmer, C.; Scheeren, T.W.L.; Bauer, I.; Picker, O.; Truse, R. Propofol improves colonic but impairs hepatic mitochondrial function in tissue homogenates from healthy rats. *Eur. J. Pharmacol.* **2019**, *853*, 364–370. [CrossRef] [PubMed]
25. Herminghaus, A.; Papenbrock, H.; Eberhardt, R.; Vollmer, C.; Truse, R.; Schulz, J.; Bauer, I.; Weidinger, A.; Kozlov, A.V.; Stiban, J.; et al. Time-related changes in hepatic and colonic mitochondrial oxygen consumption after abdominal infection in rats. *Intensive Care Med. Exp.* **2019**, *7*, 4. [CrossRef] [PubMed]
26. Lowry, O.H.; Rosebrough, N.J.; Farr, A.L.; Randall, R.J. Protein Measurement with the Folin Phenol Reagent. *J. Biol. Chem.* **1951**, *193*, 265–275. [PubMed]
27. Cámara-Lemarroy, C.R.; Guzman-DE LA Garza, F.J.; Cordero-Perez, P.; Ibarra-Hernandez, J.M.; Muñoz-Espinosa, L.E.; Fernandez-Garza, N.E. Gemfibrozil attenuates the inflammatory response and protects rats from abdominal sepsis. *Exp. Ther. Med.* **2015**, *9*, 1018–1022. [CrossRef] [PubMed]
28. Sugiyama, S. HMG CoA reductase inhibitor accelerates aging effect on diaphragm mitochondrial respiratory function in rats. *Biochem. Mol. Biol. Int.* **1998**, *46*, 923–931.
29. Jeger, V.; Djafarzadeh, S.; Jakob, S.M.; Takala, J. Mitochondrial function in sepsis. *Eur. J. Clin. Invest.* **2013**, *43*, 532–542. [CrossRef]
30. Siekmeier, R.; Gross, W.; März, W. Determination of pravastatin by high performance liquid chromatography. *Int. J. Clin. Pharmacol. Ther.* **2000**, *38*, 419–425. [CrossRef]
31. McTavish, D.; Sorkin, E.M. Pravastatin. A review of its pharmacological properties and therapeutic potential in hypercholesterolaemia. *Drugs* **1991**, *42*, 65–89. [CrossRef]
32. Hatanaka, T. Clinical pharmacokinetics of pravastatin: Mechanisms of pharmacokinetic events. *Clin. Pharmacokinet.* **2000**, *39*, 397–412. [CrossRef]
33. Yamazaki, M.; Tokui, T.; Ishigami, M.; Sugiyama, Y. Tissue-selective uptake of pravastatin in rats: Contribution of a specific carrier-mediated uptake system. *Biopharm. Drug Dispos.* **1996**, *17*, 775–789. [CrossRef]
34. Hatanaka, T.; Honda, S.; Sasaki, S.; Katayama, K.; Koizumi, T. Pharmacokinetic and pharmacodynamic evaluation for tissue-selective inhibition of cholesterol synthesis by pravastatin. *J. Pharmacokinet. Biopharm.* **1998**, *26*, 329–347. [CrossRef]

35. Omar, M.A.; Wilson, J.P. FDA adverse event reports on statin-associated rhabdomyolysis. *Ann. Pharmacother.* **2002**, *36*, 288–295. [CrossRef]
36. Vladutiu, G.D.; Simmons, Z.; Isackson, P.J.; Tarnopolsky, M.; Peltier, W.L.; Barboi, A.C.; Sripathi, N.; Wortmann, R.L.; Phillips, P.S. Genetic risk factors associated with lipid-lowering drug-induced myopathies. *Muscle Nerve* **2006**, *34*, 153–162. [CrossRef]
37. Herminghaus, A.; Barthel, F.; Heinen, A.; Beck, C.; Vollmer, C.; Bauer, I.; Weidinger, A.; Kozlov, A.V.; Picker, O. Severity of polymicrobial sepsis modulates mitochondrial function in rat liver. *Mitochondrion* **2015**, *24*, 122–128. [CrossRef]
38. Evans, J.R.; Forland, S.C.; Cutler, R.E. The effect of renal function on the pharmacokinetics of gemfibrozil. *J. Clin. Pharmacol.* **1987**, *27*, 994–1000. [CrossRef]
39. Busse, K.H.; Hadigan, C.; Chairez, C.; Alfaro, R.M.; Formentini, E.; Kovacs, J.A.; Penzak, S.R. Gemfibrozil concentrations are significantly decreased in the presence of lopinavir-ritonavir. *J. Acquir. Immune Defic. Syndr.* **2009**, *52*, 235–239. [CrossRef]

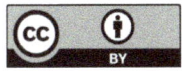

© 2019 by the authors. Licensee MDPI, Basel, Switzerland. This article is an open access article distributed under the terms and conditions of the Creative Commons Attribution (CC BY) license (http://creativecommons.org/licenses/by/4.0/).

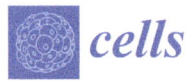

Article

Mitochondria in the Nuclei of Rat Myocardial Cells

Chupalav M. Eldarov [1], Irina M. Vangely [1], Valeriya B. Vays [1], Eugene V. Sheval [1], Susanne Holtze [2], Thomas B. Hildebrandt [2], Natalia G. Kolosova [3], Vasily A. Popkov [1], Egor Y. Plotnikov [1], Dmitry B. Zorov [1], Lora E. Bakeeva [1] and Vladimir P. Skulachev [1,4,*]

[1] A.N. Belozersky Institute of Physico-Chemical Biology, Lomonosov Moscow State University, 119991 Moscow, Russia; chupalav@protonmail.ch (C.M.E.); sim870@mail.ru (I.M.V.); valeriya.vays@yandex.ru (V.B.V.); sheval_e@belozersky.msu.su (E.V.S.); popkov.vas@gmail.com (V.A.P.); plotnikov@belozersky.msu.ru (E.Y.P.); zorov@belozersky.msu.ru (D.B.Z.); bakeeva@belozersky.msu.ru (L.E.B.)
[2] Department of Reproduction Management, Leibniz-Institute for Zoo and Wildlife Research, Alfred-Kowalke-Str. 17, 10315 Berlin, Germany; holtze@izw-berlin.de (S.H.); hildebrandt@izw-berlin.de (T.B.H.)
[3] Institute of Cytology and Genetics, Siberian Branch of Russian Academy of Sciences, Novosibirsk 630090, Russia; kolosova@bionet.nsc.ru
[4] Faculty of Bioengineering and Bioinformatics, Lomonosov Moscow State University, 119992 Moscow, Russia
* Correspondence: skulach@belozersky.msu.ru; Tel.: +7-495-939-55-30

Received: 12 December 2019; Accepted: 5 March 2020; Published: 14 March 2020

Abstract: Electron microscopic study of cardiomyocytes taken from healthy Wistar and OXYS rats and naked mole rats (*Heterocephalus glaber*) revealed mitochondria in nuclei that lacked part of the nuclear envelope. The direct interaction of mitochondria with nucleoplasm is shown. The statistical analysis of the occurrence of mitochondria in cardiomyocyte nuclei showed that the percentage of nuclei with mitochondria was roughly around 1%, and did not show age and species dependency. Confocal microscopy of normal rat cardiac myocytes revealed a branched mitochondrial network in the vicinity of nuclei with an organization different than that of interfibrillar mitochondria. This mitochondrial network was energetically functional because it carried the membrane potential that responded by oscillatory mode after photodynamic challenge. We suggest that the presence of functional mitochondria in the nucleus is not only a consequence of certain pathologies but rather represents a normal biological phenomenon involved in mitochondrial/nuclear interactions.

Keywords: intranuclear mitochondria; healthy cells; electron and confocal microscopy; heart

1. Introduction

In 1958, Australian electron microscopists H. Hoffman and G. W. Grigg, when analyzing ultrathin sections of lymph nodes of adult mice found clustering of mitochondria around the concavities in the nuclear membrane, some lying in very close juxtaposition to the membrane [1]. They even suggested the presence of mitochondria inside of the nucleus but given that the quality of electron microscopic images was not perfect, this suggestion stayed hypothetical. However, in 1960, H. Mori described mitochondria in nuclei of cells from four types of ascites cancer, as well as of tongue cancer, pancreatic cancer, and in regenerating hepatocytes of newts [2]. Later, this phenomenon was reproduced by D. Brandes et al., who published in 1965 in *Science* a brief article entitled "Nuclear Mitochondria?" In their study, similar to that of Mori, cancer (leukemic) cells were used [3]. Since then, mitochondria in nuclei have been found in white blood cells [4,5], lymph nodes of patients with Hodgkin's disease [6], leukemic myoblasts [7], in cardiomyocytes of a patient with rheumatic heart disease [8], and certain other cardiac pathologies [9–12]. Given that the presence of intranuclear mitochondria has been exclusively proven in abnormal cells, these facts were attributed to the manifestation of the pathology.

Two main issues elicit discussion: how do mitochondria get into the nucleus and what advantages or disadvantages arise as a result of such organelle interaction? Several explanations of such observations have been suggested. Most frequently, the appearance of mitochondria inside nucleus was assigned to the improper execution of mitosis. Using immunofluorescence techniques, it has been shown that a brief opening of the nuclear membrane can occur in the interphase nucleus. Nuclear membrane remodeling was found during viral infections [13–15], laminopathy [16–18], muscular dystrophy, cardiomyopathy, lipodystrophy [19,20], Hutchinson–Gilford progeria syndrome [21], and cancerogenesis [18,22–25]. However, it may be premature to consider this phenomenon as specific for pathological processes only. For example, mitochondria in nuclei were observed by Zhao et al. at the final stage of erythropoiesis in mice [26]. Immunofluorescence assays as well as focused-beam and scanning electron microscopy methods have shown that erythroblast nuclei can be in the opened and fragmented state for 3–5 min. The opening is followed by relatively stable periods of closure lasting about an hour with caspase-3 to be essential for this cyclic process. Loss of caspase-3 blocks not only the opening but also erythroid differentiation, leading to hematologic disorders.

There is no doubt that in terms of energy, nucleus function is quite costly in using, for many processes, cytosolic ATP, which is mostly generated by mitochondria. Limiting diffusion distance for intracellular ATP transport to the site of its use may be an issue to facilitate ATP transport directly to the site of priority use. On the other hand, mitochondria and the nucleus possess genomes of different nature and properties, and numerous data have reported on their interaction and cross-talk. A common opinion is that the transfer of mitochondrial DNA to the nucleus has contributed to the evolution of eukaryotic genomes [27–29]. Mitochondrial DNA transfer to the nucleus is an established fact, possibly playing both normal [30] and pathological [31,32] roles. Vice versa, anterograde signaling (from nucleus to mitochondria) includes numerous regulatory factors coordinating the function of subcellular organelles and integrating cellular and environmental signals, such as nuclear respiratory factor 1 (NRF1) [33], nuclear factor erythroid 2-like 2 [34] (NFE2L2 or NRF2), peroxisome proliferator-activated receptors (PPARs), and estrogen-related receptors (ERRs) [35], as well as many others that regulate mitochondrial-specific activities.

It is reasonable to consider that increasing nuclear membrane surface would facilitate the exchange rate between nucleoplasm and cytosol. Indeed, numerous deep and branching invaginations of the nuclear envelope [36,37], especially in cancer cells [38], were found.

Unlike nuclear envelope invaginations possibly serving as mechanism for importing cytosolic components to the nucleoplasm, envelope herniations may serve the opposite role through exporting nuclear content to cytosol [25,39]. Recently found mitochondria-derived vesicles [40,41] may play a role as a vehicle providing transport of genetic material to the nucleus.

In this study, we made an attempt to analyze the appearance of mitochondria in the nucleus, comparing the heart cells of two species of animals, radically different in life expectancy: rats and naked mole-rats (*Heterocephalus glaber*), as well as the line of rats named by the breeder as OXYS, characterized by accelerated aging. To analyze the structure of the mitochondrial network and its relationship with the nucleus, two microscopic techniques were used: confocal and electron microscopy. Confocal microscopy by itself is not able to resolve mitochondria in nuclear membrane invaginations of those residing in the nucleoplasm. A combination of confocal and electron microscopy may become not only the instrument to address this question but also it would help to address the functionality of nuclear mitochondria.

Indeed, our analysis using confocal microscopy revealed a specially organized functional mitochondrial network in the vicinity of the nuclei in normal cardiac myocytes, whereas electron microscopic images convincingly demonstrated the absence of nuclear membrane over relatively large areas of the nucleus. Regardless of the disruption of the nuclear membrane integrity, the content of the nucleus preserved its specific morphology. Here, we present the ultrastructure of open nuclei containing mitochondria in normal cardiomyocytes of Wistar and OXYS rats, as well as naked mole-rat (*Heterocephalus glaber*). The latter species is of particular interest because it is very long-lived and is resistant to many pathologies inherent in other species. Therefore, it can be an example of a mammal that has succeeded in maintaining a long and healthy life.

2. Results

Confocal microscopy of a normal Wistar rat cardiac mitochondrial architecture in the vicinity of nuclei revealed a very complicated mitochondrial network organized by tiny branched mitochondrial filaments. Practically all cardiac nuclei were surrounded by a mitochondrial web, deeply penetrating the body of the nucleus (Figure 1, Supplementary Video S1). These visually observed structures were identified with a variety of mitochondrial dyes, at least one of these being potential-dependent tetramethyl rhodamine methyl ester (TMRM). Mitochondrial dye nonyl acridine orange (NAO), apparently interacting with mitochondrial cardiolipin independently of the existence of the membrane potential (Supplementary Video S4), as well as Mitotracker Deep Red (not shown), revealed the same peri(intra) nuclear mitochondrial network suggesting that these nuclear mitochondria are fully functional. To exclude that these structures belong to sarcoplasmic reticulum non-specifically stained with mitochondrial dyes, we used an approach of photo-induced oscillations of the mitochondrial membrane potential [42]. Observed oscillations of a different part of the mitochondrial reticulum including the peri(intra)nuclear part confirmed that these structures were mitochondria with maintained membrane potential (Figure 2, Supplementary Video S2). However, in spite of obvious very deep penetration of mitochondrial fluorescence images into the space occupied by the nucleus, the light microscopic level approach did not allow us to discriminate mitochondria deeply invaginated in the nucleus from those residing in the nucleoplasm. Subsequent electron microscopic study of the normal cardiac myocyte was designed to resolve this question.

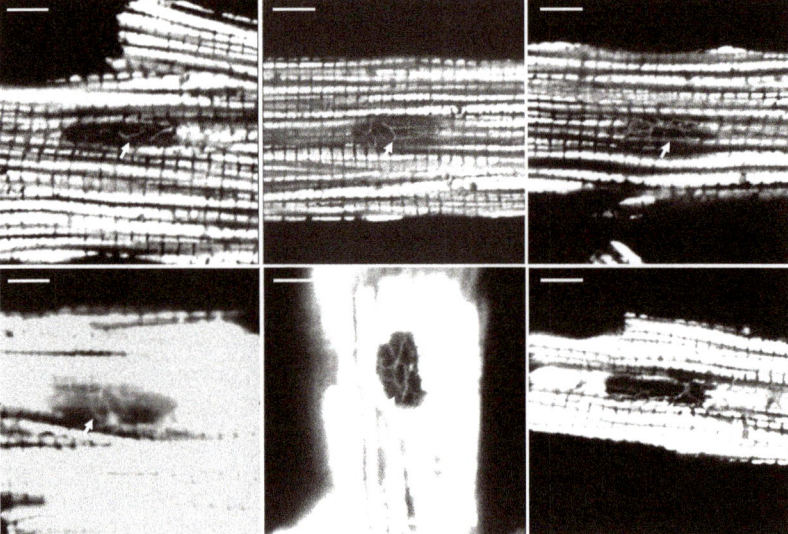

Figure 1. Variability of the mitochondrial architecture in the vicinity of nuclei in normal rat ventricular cardiac myocyte was stained with the mitochondria-targeted probe tetramethyl rhodamine methyl ester (TMRM; 200 nM). Confocal microscopy. Bright images represent energized mitochondria along myofilaments of the heart cell. We used a pinhole of 150 mµ allowing one to observe tilted mitochondrial chains spanning the cell, thus making an impression of the appearance and disappearance of these chains. In some images, in order to reveal the peri(intra)nuclear mitochondrial network (arrows), the detector gain was artificially enhanced, making the fluorescence of interfibrillar mitochondria saturated. Scale: 5 mµ.

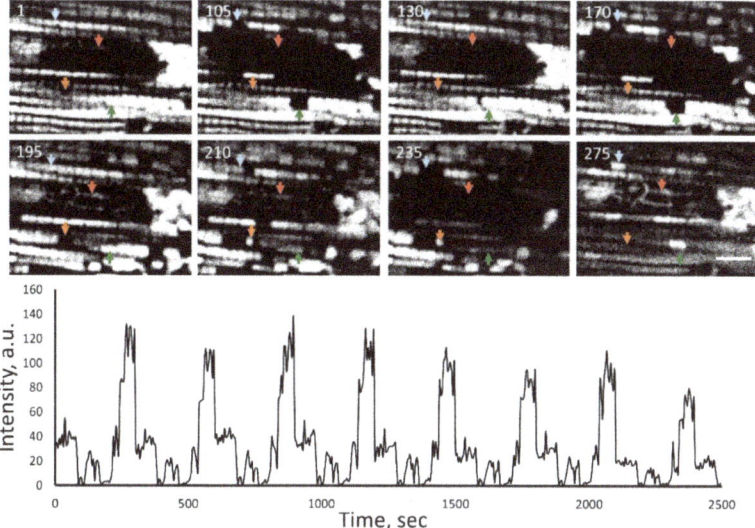

Figure 2. Photo-induced oscillations of the membrane potential in mitochondrial clusters within cardiac myocytes loaded with 200 nM TMRM. Colored arrows show some oscillatory elements at different time intervals indicated in the upper-left corner (in seconds) of each confocal scan. The example at the bottom shows periodic changes of the fluorescence intensity of TMRM in the region shown by the red arrow. Scale: 5 mμ. Full-time series of this sample is presented in Supplementary Video S2.

Figure 3A–C represents three consecutive ultrathin sections of cardiac myocytes of a 3-month-old Wistar rat. As shown in Figure 3A, three mitochondria were clearly visible inside the nucleus. The mitochondria were not separated from the contents of the nucleus by the nuclear membrane, that is, they, in fact, were located in the nucleoplasm. In the subsequent sections of this nucleus, the number of mitochondria inside the nucleus was increased. In Figure 3B,C, the contents of the nucleus were in direct contact with a mitochondrial cluster due to the partial absence of the nuclear membrane. It should be noted that in Figure 3A,B, the nuclear area directly surrounding the mitochondria had a fine fibrillar structure differing greatly from the granular structure in the main part of the nucleoplasm. In this case, a fragment of cytoplasm containing mitochondria was supposed to enter the nucleus through the open aperture in the nuclear membrane. Figure 4A,B show direct contact between a mitochondrial cluster and nuclear structures in a cardiomyocyte of a 24-month-old OXYS rat. Furthermore, using heart samples from a 3-month-old Wistar rat, we performed a three-dimensional reconstruction of a part of the nucleus with the mitochondria present inside, showing the architecture of the chromatin and nuclear membrane on the basis of the analysis of a sequential series of ultrathin sections for electron microscopy (Figure 5 and Supplementary Movie 3).

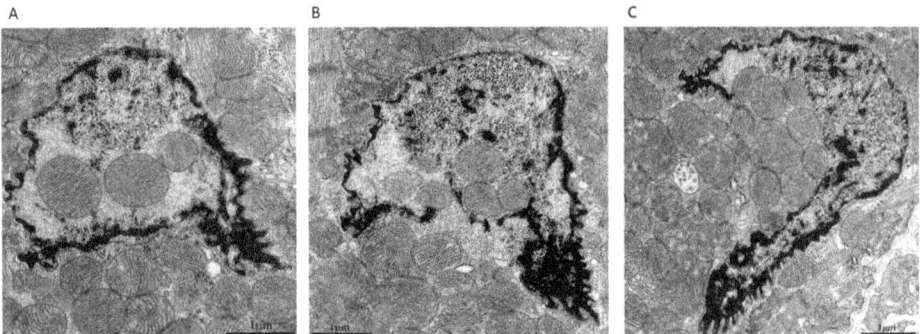

Figure 3. (**A**–**C**) Consecutive ultrathin sections from serial sections of a cardiomyocyte nucleus of a 3-month-old Wistar rat. Electron microscopy.

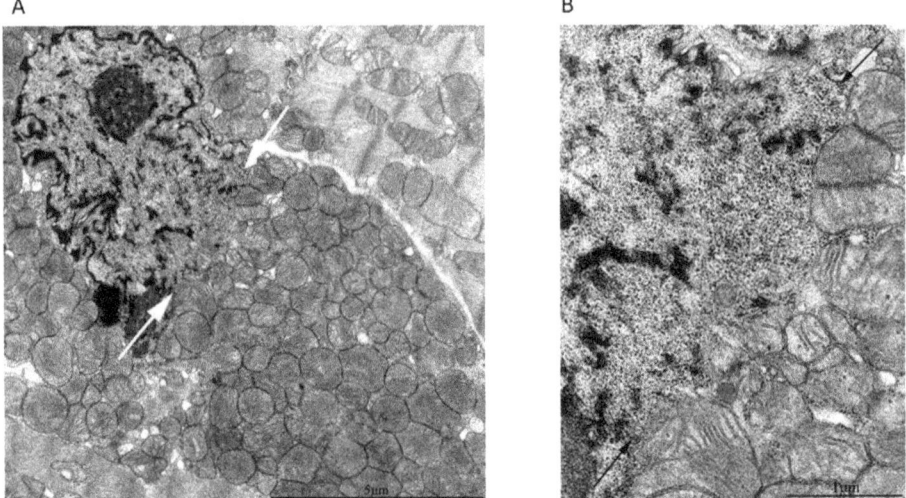

Figure 4. (**A**) Direct contact of a mitochondrial cluster with nuclear structures in a cardiomyocyte from a 24-month-old OXYS rat. The area of contact is indicated by an arrow. (**B**) The local fragment of the nucleus indicated by the arrows in Figure 4A. The nuclear membrane was absent, and individual mitochondria were directly adjacent to the nucleoplasm.

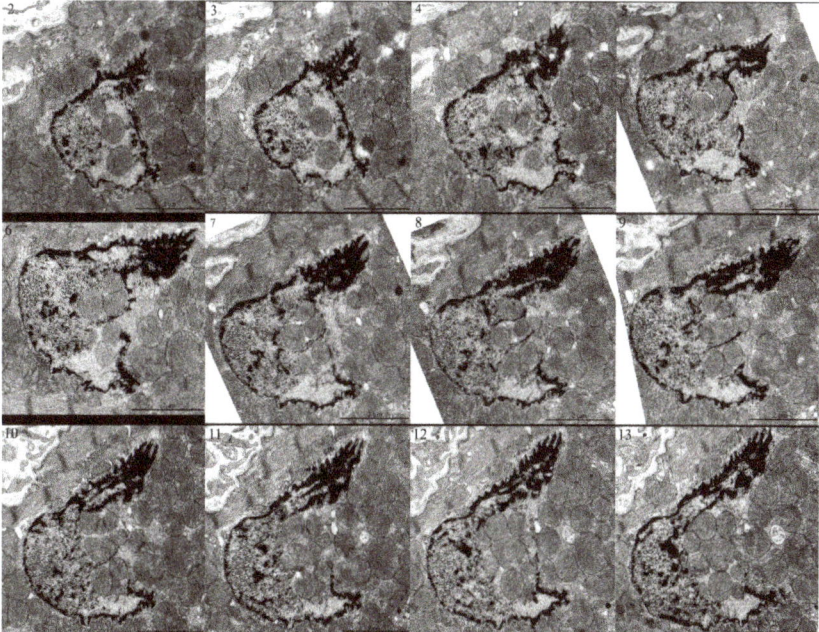

Figure 5. Serial micrographs of 12 sections over the nucleus of the cardiomyocyte of a 3-month-old Wistar rat with mitochondria embedded in the nucleoplasm.

The main and very important argument is that this particular examined cell with the intranuclear mitochondria was abnormal. However, this was not confirmed by the ultramicroscopic characteristics of the nucleus and the cytoplasm surrounding this nucleus. We compared the ultrastructure of these cells containing the obvious intranuclear mitochondria with ultrastructure of cells where intranuclear mitochondria were missing and found no significant alterations indicating cell damage (Figure 6).

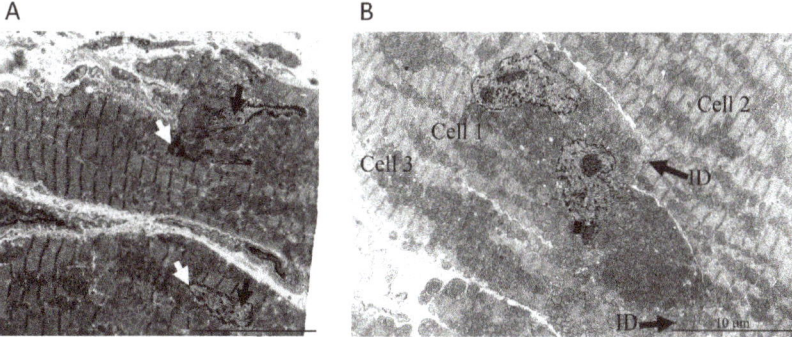

Figure 6. Ultrastructures of nuclei and cytosols of the rat heart tissue with cells, one of which contained intranuclear mitochondria while the others did not. (**A**) Ultrastructure of cardiomyocytes from a 3-month-old Wistar rat with mitochondria in the nucleus (upper cell) and without them (lower cell). White arrows indicate condensed chromatin and black arrows indicate decondensed chromatin. (**B**) Cytosolic ultrastructure of the 24-month-old OXYS rat cell with intra-nuclear mitochondria (cell 1) and adjacent cells (cell 2 and cell 3), connected by intercalated discs (ID). Note that (**B**) is a low zoom of the cardiac tissue containing the region depicted in Figure 4A,B in the manuscript.

In the nuclei of cardiomyocytes with nuclear ruptures, chromatin was preferentially decondensed, and the condensed chromatin was visible at nuclear periphery in close contact with the nuclear envelope, around the nucleoli (perinucleolar chromatin), and inside the nucleoplasm. The blocks of condensed chromatin in the nucleoplasm adjusting the nuclear envelope ruptures had elongated shape, probably due to mechanical tension. The similar localization of condensed chromatin was detected in the nuclei without nuclear envelope ruptures. This apparently mechanical deformation of chromatin complexes was visible near nuclear envelope ruptures, indicating that nuclei were under a strong pulling force action, which potentially could induce these ruptures. Decondensed chromatin was not substantially modified, even in regions that were in direct contact with the mitochondria. Thus, in the nuclear regions adjacent to broken nuclear membrane, the changes in chromatin were minimal, whereas on the nuclear periphery far from these regions, the chromatin configuration was not distinguished in both types of cells (Figure 6A).

As for the cytosolic ultrastructure of the cell with intranuclear mitochondria (Figure 6B), the ultrastructure of myofibrils was conventional with regular position of isotropic and anisotropic regions separated by a Z-line. Myofibrils are longitudinally oriented and densely packed. Sarcomeres have a conventional size of 2–3 microns in length. Intercalated disks are not damaged with a typical structure. The sarcoplasma is not swollen with mitochondria having a normal orthodox structure.

A more striking picture of a direct contact between mitochondria and structures of the nucleus was found in a cardiomyocyte of a 5-year-old naked mole rat (Figure 7A,B). In this case, the sections were made in such a way that the absence of the nuclear membrane was revealed along the entire perimeter of the nucleus. The specific morphology of the nucleus was preserved despite the vast area lacking the nuclear membrane. Figure 7B at higher magnification the mitochondrial group indicated by arrows in Figure 7A. It is clearly seen that the mitochondria were in direct contact with the intranuclear structures. The analysis of serial sections of this nucleus (Figure 8) revealed that mitochondria did not form a continuous layer contacting the contents of the nucleus. There were some nuclear areas directly adjacent to myofibrils (indicated by the arrow, Figure 8, section h).

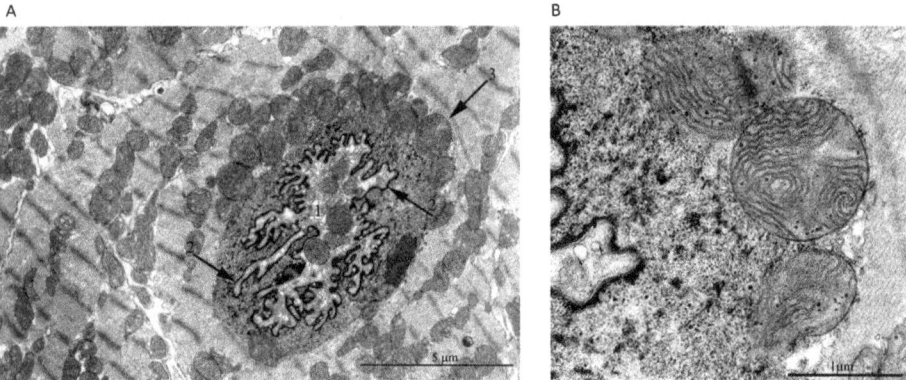

Figure 7. (**A**) Direct contact of mitochondria with nuclear structures in a cardiomyocyte from a 5-year-old naked mole-rat. In this section, the nuclear membrane was absent along the entire perimeter of the nucleus. Arrow 1 shows the cytoplasm with organelles including mitochondria was located inside the nuclear invagination. Arrow 2 shows the nuclear membrane of the nucleus invagination. (**B**) A group of mitochondria shown by arrow 3 in Figure 7A at high magnification. Mitochondria were in direct contact with nuclear structures and were submerged in the nucleoplasm.

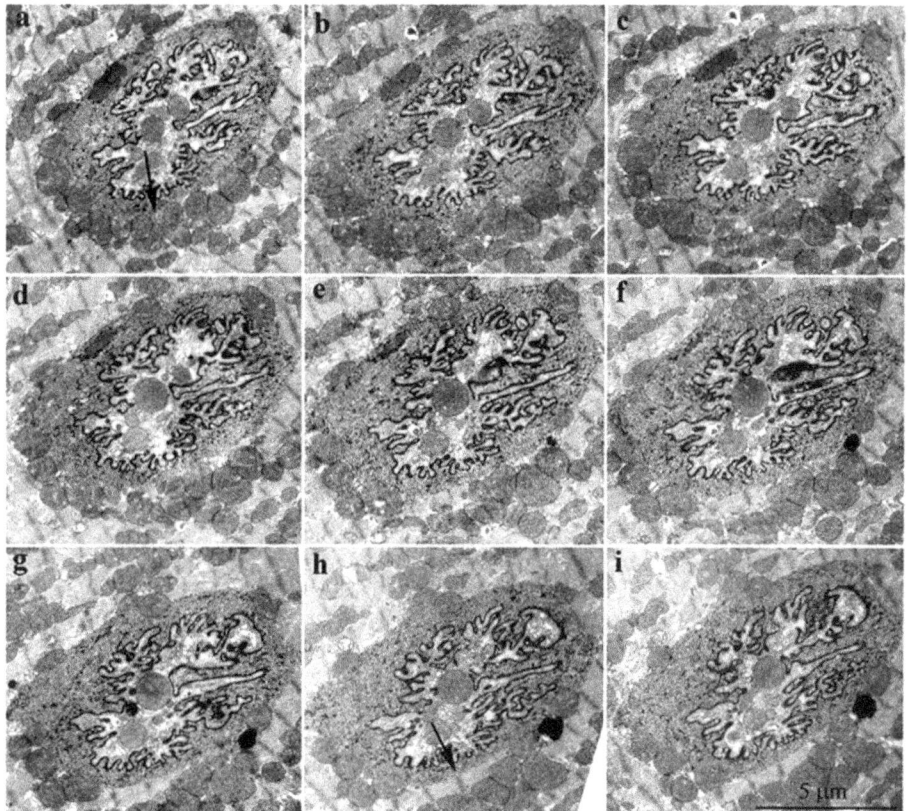

Figure 8. Serial of consecutive sections of the nucleus of a cardiomyocyte (from **a** to **i** with the thickness of each section ~500 Å) from the 5-year-old naked mole-rat presented in Figure 7A. Arrows in sections **a** and **h** point to the same area of the nucleus, proving that mitochondria did not form a continuous layer contacting the nuclear contents. In section **a**, the mitochondria were in direct contact with nuclear structures, whereas in section **h**, there was direct contact of nuclear content with adjacent myofibrils.

The statistical analysis of the occurrence of mitochondria in cardiomyocyte nuclei showed that, on average, the percentage of nuclei with mitochondria was roughly around 1%, and it did not show age and species dependency (see Supplementary Table S1).

3. Discussion

The presence of mitochondria in the nuclei was claimed more than 50 years ago [1–3], but the objects used for these studies belonged to pathological tissues. This was the reason to assign such a feature to a pathological symptom. In addition, these data were criticized due to the poor quality of the sample and the possibility of artifacts caused by improper treatment of the sample as part of the electron microscopic technique. Penetration of mitochondria into the nucleus as a result of mechanical tissue damage occurring during fixation was discussed by Takemura et al. [10], who found mitochondria in nuclei of myocardial cells taken from patients with various cardiac diseases. However, mitochondria were found in the nucleus of cultured cells, where, due to specific fixation techniques, mechanical damage did not occur.

A reasonable explanation of the presence of mitochondria inside a nucleus was improper execution of mitosis. However, this explanation was not suitable for cardiac myocytes, which belong to postmitotic cells. Several other observations have recently been made that disprove the assertion that invasion of mitochondria to the nucleus occurs when the nuclear membrane is disassembled during mitosis [23–26].

Confocal microscopy revealed mitochondrial organization in the vicinity of a nucleus, which was different from the well-known interfibrillar and subsarcolemmal mitochondrial population. Mitochondrial web consisting of thin branched filaments covering all peri(intra)nuclear space was typical for all explored normal nuclei of isolated rat ventricular cardiac myocytes. 3D reconstruction of the space occupied by a nucleus demonstrated deep sprouting of mitochondrial filaments into this space (see Supplementary Movie 1). All mitochondrial filaments were fully functional because they were stained with membrane potential sensitive dye and specific mitochondrial marker cardiolipin, and responded to photoexcitation by the partially reversible oscillations of the mitochondrial membrane potential (see Supplementary Movie 2).

Using electron microscopy, we concluded that there was direct contact between mitochondrial clusters and nucleoplasm in cardiomyocytes of the healthy rodents: 3-month-old Wistar rat, 24-month-old OXYS rat, and 5-year-old naked mole rat. Serial ultrathin sections of the same nucleus showed that, depending on the section level, it was possible to observe mitochondria either inside of the closed nucleus or inside of the open nucleus partially devoid of the nuclear membrane. Statistics showed that 1–2% of nuclei present on ultrathin sections of cardiomyocytes contained mitochondria. Our findings are in line with the findings of a Norwegian research group who reported mitochondria in 2–3% of cardiomyocyte nuclei in a patient with rheumatic heart disease [8]. The observations, first made already in the middle of the 20th century of mitochondria inside a nucleus, are no longer considered an artifact of electron microscopy technique [42]. On the basis of a great number of immunofluorescence assays in which brief disruption of the nuclear membrane in interphase nuclei was observed in association with various diseases and abnormal conditions [18,22–25] as well as in healthy cells [26,43], the presence of mitochondria in the nucleoplasm is usually considered as a result of catastrophic loss of the barrier function of the nuclear membrane that might be a contributing factor of disease progression [44]. In some reports, the penetration of mitochondria into the nucleus was believed to occur due only to a mechanical process [12,44]. It was suggested that the constant contractile function in cardiomyocytes contributes to the penetration of mitochondria into the nucleus through a pathology-weakened nuclear membrane. However, in this study, we showed that mitochondria appeared in the nucleus of normal cardiomyocytes. On the basis of the 3D reconstruction of a part of the cardiomyocyte with nuclei-containing mitochondria, we conclude that the nuclear membrane could be absent in the extensive nuclear region and that it is represented by patches. In all our cases, we describe the presence of mitochondria in nuclei having open configuration without nuclear membrane resealed.

We were unable to answer the question of how specific this discovered phenomenon is for cardiomyocytes. There is evidence that the nuclear membrane undergoes structural changes during mechanical action, which are expressed in local loss of the nuclear envelope integrity [45,46]. This was especially well-observed in the example of migration of cancer cells through narrow holes that led to deformation of the nuclei combined with local breaks of the nuclear membrane [25], which allowed simulating the situation by direct physical actions on the cell [47,48]. Thus, chronic mechanical effects on the cell nucleus [49], associated with contractile activity of the heart, could be the cause of similar changes in the structure of the nucleus, leading to local damage/elimination of the nuclear envelope. Cardiomyocytes are cells chronically exposed to a deforming challenge, with mitochondria changing their shape under a normal cardiomyocyte twitch, caused by the dynamic force-balance inside cardiomyocytes and by changes in the spatial stiffness characteristics [50]. A similar mechanotransduction at the nuclear level was observed in endothelial cells a priori exposed to a chronic shear stress [51].

In 2016, Zhao et al. were the first to study the functional significance of nuclear membrane remodeling in interphase nuclei during erythropoiesis in mice [26]. They showed that this process is not accompanied by a dramatic release of nuclear components into the cytoplasm leading to the loss of cell functions and cell viability, as previously supposed [44]. They showed that the dynamic nature and cyclic repetition of nuclear opening are essential for normal differentiation, ensuring the release of nuclear histones into the cytoplasm for chromatin to be condensed during terminal erythropoiesis. They showed that the release of histones into the cytoplasm is a selective process, and that non-histone nuclear proteins stay inside the nucleus. The released nuclear histones accumulate around the open fragment of the nucleus, performing a protective function, blocking the release of non-histone nuclear proteins, and supporting nuclear/cytoplasmic compartmentalization.

We suppose that local nuclear membrane disassembling, which we observed in cardiomyocytes, as well as subsequent contact between mitochondria and nuclear contents, are of functional significance. Unfortunately, at present, it is impossible to trace the fate of such nuclei and cardiomyocytes containing them. However, during terminal erythropoiesis, Zhao et al. [26] proposed the necessity of the nuclear opening process. As follows from the ultrastructural picture of open nuclei in erythroblasts presented by those authors, the contact between nuclear and cytoplasm components along relatively large areas of the nucleus lacking the nuclear membrane does not lead to cell pathology or apoptosis. In this connection, it is important to mention reports in which authors discovered the direct contact of mitochondria with nuclear components in *Ciona internalis* oocytes [52], as well as with nucleus-like bodies in *Rana pipiens* oocytes [53], and authors have even described special filaments mediating the association of mitochondria with nuclear structures.

It seems that so-called open nuclei, as well as the presence of mitochondria inside nuclei, are a natural and common biological phenomenon related to mitochondrial/nuclear interactions. In eukaryotic cells, mitochondria take part in intracellular regulations mediated by cross-talk between mitochondria and the nucleus. This interaction is represented by anterograde (nucleus–mitochondrion) and retrograde (mitochondrion–nucleus) signaling [32]. This cross-talk includes exchange by ATP/ADP, regulatory proteins and genetic material going in both directions. Bidirectional transport of genetic material is of primary interest for molecular biologists due to its high relevance to the evolution of eukaryotic genomes [27–29] and the occurrence of diseases through regulation of gene expression, possibly by non-coding RNAs originating both from mitochondria [32] and nuclei [31–34,54–57]. The so-called "escape" of nucleic acids from nuclei and mitochondria [58] seems to be part of a well-designed strategy of communication of genomes rather than being an occasional stochastic process. Shortening the distance between genomes will not only facilitate their interaction but also reduce the probability of degradation; in particular, cytosolic nucleases and penetration of mitochondria in the nucleus might serve this strategy.

4. Materials and Methods

Animals: 3- and 24-month-old male senescence-accelerated OXYS and Wistar rats were obtained from the Shared Center for Genetic Resources of the Institute of Cytology and Genetics (ICG), Siberian Branch of the Russian Academy of Sciences (Novosibirsk, Russia). The OXYS rat strain was established on the basis of the Wistar rat strain at the Institute of Cytology and Genetics, as described earlier [59], and registered in the Rat Genome Database (http://rgd.mcw.edu/). At the age of 4 weeks, the pups were taken from their mothers, housed in groups of five animals per cage (57 × 36 × 20 cm), and kept under standard laboratory conditions (at 22 ± 2 °C, 60% relative humidity, and natural light), provided with standard rodent food, PK-120-1, Ltd. (Laboratorsnab, Russia). Naked mole rat colonies were maintained at the Leibniz Institute for Zoo and Wildlife Research, Berlin, Germany, in an artificial burrow system with plexiglass tunnels and boxes. The system was heated to 26–29 °C with constant humidity of 60–80%. The chambers contained wood bedding, twigs, and unbleached paper tissue. Fresh food was given daily ad libitum. It included sweet potatoes, carrots, fennel, apples, a cereal supplement containing vitamins and minerals, and oat flakes. The local ethics committee of the "Landesamt für Gesundheit und Soziales", Berlin, Germany (#ZH 156), approved sampling.

4.1. Cardiac Myocytes Isolation

Ventricular cardiac myocytes used in the study were isolated from adult Wistar rats (2–4 mo old) by a standard enzymatic technique [60] through initial perfusion of hanged isolated heart with the medium containing collagenase type II and subsequent breakage of digested heart pieces by a gentle pipetting and transfer to media with growing Ca^{2+} content. Final HEPES-buffered solution contained (in millimoles per liter) 137 NaCl, 4.9 KCl, 1.2 $MgSO_4$, 1.2 NaH_2PO_4, 15 glucose, 20 HEPES, and 1.0 $CaCl_2$, pH 7.4.

4.2. Confocal Microscopy

Myocytes were loaded with dyes for >20 min on a glass-bottom Petri dishes, incubated in HEPES-buffered solution (same composition as the storage solution) at 23 °C, and imaged with a LSM-510 inverted confocal microscope using a Plan-Neofluar 63 ×/1.25N.A. oil immersion lens (Carl Zeiss Inc., Jena, Germany). Scans were recorded in a single channel mode with excitation at 543 nm (for tetramethyl rhodamine methyl ester (TMRM; Molecular Probes, Inc., Eugene, OR, USA), nonyl acridine orange (NAO; Sigma-Aldrich, St. Louis, MI, USA), and mitotracker Deep Red (MTDR; ThermoFisher Scientific, Waldham, MA, USA)), collecting simultaneous fluorescence emission with LP560, LP 505, and LP650 nm, respectively. The confocal pinhole was set to obtain spatial resolutions of 0.4 μm in the horizontal plane and 1.0 μm in the axial dimension. Image processing was performed using Fiji software (U.S. National Institutes of Health, Bethesda, MD, USA). Frame scan along z-direction was performed to cover the entire space occupied with nuclei, which was identified as space of a spheroid shape (usually two per cell) poor in mitochondria. Time series mode along a single x–y plane was performed with 5 s intervals between scans.

4.3. Electron Microscopy

For electron microscopic investigation, samples were fixed with 3% glutaraldehyde solution (pH 7.4) for 2 h at 4 °C, over-fixed with 1% osmium tetraoxide solution for 1.5 h, and then dehydrated in alcohol series with increasing alcohol concentrations (70% alcohol was saturated with uranyl acetate). The samples were embedded in Epon-812 epoxy resin. Serial ultrathin sections were made with a Leica ULTRACUT UCT microtome and stained by lead according to Reynolds [61]. The resulting preparations were scanned and photographed using a JEM-1400 electron microscope (JEOL, Japan).

Supplementary Materials: The following are available online at http://www.mdpi.com/2073-4409/9/3/712/s1: Video S1. 3D reconstruction of the mitochondrial network from rat ventricular cardiac myocyte stained with the tetramethyl rhodamine methyl ester (TMRM). Video S2. Timeseries of the mitochondrial network from rat ventricular cardiac myocyte stained with tetramethyl rhodamine methyl ester (TMRM). Video S3. 3D reconstruction of the mitochondria from ultrathin sections from serial sections of a cardiomyocyte nucleus of a 3-month-old Wistar rat. Video S4. 3D reconstruction of the mitochondrial network from rat ventricular cardiac myocyte stained TMRM. Table S1. The frequency of mitochondrial appearance in nuclei of cardiomyocytes of Wistar, Oxys and naked mole rats of different ages.

Author Contributions: C.M.E., I.M.V., V.B.V., L.E.B., and D.B.Z. designed the experiments; S.H., T.B.H., and N.G.K. provided the animals for the experiments; I.M.V., V.B.V., and L.E.B. prepared the samples for electron microscopy; C.M.E., I.M.V., V.B.V., and L.E.B. obtained electron-microscopic images; D.B.Z. ran experiments using confocal microscope; C.M.E., I.M.V., V.B.V., E.V.S., V.A.P., E.Y.P., and L.E.B. analyzed the data; L.E.B., D.B.Z., and V.P.S. wrote the manuscript. All authors have read and agreed to the published version of the manuscript.

Funding: This study was supported by the Russian Science Foundation grant 19-14-00173 (confocal microscopy) and the Russian Foundation of Basic Research grant 19-04-00578 (electron microscopy).

Acknowledgments: The authors thank Dagmar Viertel of the laboratory of electron microscopy and her supervisors Alex Greenwood and Gudrun Wibbelt for their kind support by providing reagents and laboratory space.

Conflicts of Interest: The authors declare that they have no competing interests.

Data Availability: Typical results of this study are included in this published article.

References

1. Hoffman, H.; Grigg, G.W. An electron microscopic study of mitochondria formation. *Exp. Cell Res.* **1958**, *15*, 118–131. [CrossRef]
2. Mori, H. Electron Microscopic studies of the ascites tumor cells. *Fukushima J. Med. Sci.* **1960**, *7*, 21–33.
3. Brandes, D.; Schofield, B.H.H.; Anton, E. Nuclear mitochondria? *Science (80-.)* **1965**, *149*, 1373–1374. [CrossRef] [PubMed]
4. Klug, H. On the occurrence of mitochondria in the cell nucleus. *Naturwissenschaften* **1966**, *53*, 339. [CrossRef] [PubMed]
5. Bloom, G.D. A nucleus with cytoplasmic features. *J. Cell Biol.* **1967**, *35*, 266–268. [CrossRef] [PubMed]
6. Oliva, H.; Valle, A.; Flores, L.D.; Rivas, M.C. Intranuclear mitochondriae in Hodgkin's disease. *Virchows Arch. B Cell Pathol. Zell Pathol.* **1972**, *12*, 189–194.
7. Schumacher, H.R.; Szekely, I.E.; Patel, S.B.; Fisher, D.R. Leukemic Mitochondria. *Am. J. Pathol.* **1973**, *74*, 71–82.
8. Jensen, H.; Engedal, H.; Saetersdal, T.S. Uhrastructure of mitochondria-containing nuclei in human myocardial cells. *Virchows Arch. B Cell Pathol.* **1976**, *21*, 1–12.
9. Tsyplenkova, V.G.; Beskrovnykh, N.N. Comparative morphological and morphometric characteristisation of myocardium in patients with clinically diagnosed hypertrophyc cardiomyopathy. *Arkhiv Patol.* **1993**, *55*, 26–29.
10. Takemura, G.; Takatsu, Y.; Sakaguchi, H.; Fujiwara, H. Intranuclear mitochondria in human myocardial cells. *Pathol. Res. Pract.* **1997**, *193*, 305–311. [CrossRef]
11. Bakeeva, L.E.; Skulachev, V.P.; Sudarikova, Y.V.; Tsyplenkova, V.G. Mitochondria enter the nucleus (One further problem in chronic alcoholism). *Biochemistry (Moscow)* **2001**, *66*, 1335–1341. [CrossRef] [PubMed]
12. Fidzianska, A.; Bilinska, Z.T.; Tesson, F.; Wagner, T.; Walski, M.; Grzybowski, J.; Ruzyllo, W.; Hausmanowa-Petrusewicz, I. Obliteration of cardiomyocyte nuclear architecture in a patient with LMNA gene mutation. *J. Neurol. Sci.* **2008**, *271*, 91–96. [CrossRef] [PubMed]
13. de Noronha, C.M.C. Dynamic Disruptions in Nuclear Envelope Architecture and Integrity Induced by HIV-1 Vpr. *Science (80-.)* **2001**, *294*, 1105–1108. [CrossRef]
14. Klupp, B.G.; Granzow, H.; Fuchs, W.; Keil, G.M.; Finke, S.; Mettenleiter, T.C. Vesicle formation from the nuclear membrane is induced by coexpression of two conserved herpesvirus proteins. *Proc. Natl. Acad. Sci. USA* **2007**, *104*, 7241–7246. [CrossRef]
15. Cohen, S.; Marr, A.K.; Garcin, P.; Panté, N. Nuclear envelope disruption involving host caspases plays a role in the parvovirus replication cycle. *J. Virol.* **2011**, *85*, 4863–4874. [CrossRef]
16. De Vos, W.H.; Houben, F.; Kamps, M.; Malhas, A.; Verheyen, F.; Cox, J.; Manders, E.M.M.; Verstraeten, V.L.R.M.; van Steensel, M.A.M.; Marcelis, C.L.M.; et al. Repetitive disruptions of the nuclear envelope invoke temporary loss of cellular compartmentalization in laminopathies. *Hum. Mol. Genet.* **2011**, *20*, 4175–4186. [CrossRef]
17. Robijns, J.; Molenberghs, F.; Sieprath, T.; Corne, T.D.J.; Verschuuren, M.; De Vos, W.H. In silico synchronization reveals regulators of nuclear ruptures in lamin A/C deficient model cells. *Sci. Rep.* **2016**, *6*, 30325. [CrossRef]
18. Hatch, E.M.; Hetzer, M.W. Nuclear envelope rupture is induced by actin-based nucleus confinement. *J. Cell Biol.* **2016**, *215*, 27–36. [CrossRef]
19. Vigouroux, C.; Auclair, M.; Dubosclard, E.; Pouchelet, M.; Capeau, J.; Courvalin, J.C.; Buendia, B. Nuclear envelope disorganization in fibroblasts from lipodystrophic patients with heterozygous R482Q/W mutations in the lamin A/C gene. *J. Cell Sci.* **2001**, *114*, 4459–4468.
20. Muchir, A.; Medioni, J.; Laluc, M.; Massart, C.; Arimura, T.; van der Kooi, A.J.; Desguerre, I.; Mayer, M.; Ferrer, X.; Briault, S.; et al. Nuclear envelope alterations in fibroblasts from patients with muscular dystrophy, cardiomyopathy, and partial lipodystrophy carrying lamin A/C gene mutations. *Muscle Nerve* **2004**, *30*, 444–450. [CrossRef]
21. Goldman, R.D.; Shumaker, D.K.; Erdos, M.R.; Eriksson, M.; Goldman, A.E.; Gordon, L.B.; Gruenbaum, Y.; Khuon, S.; Mendez, M.; Varga, R.; et al. Accumulation of mutant lamin A causes progressive changes in nuclear architecture in Hutchinson-Gilford progeria syndrome. *Proc. Natl. Acad. Sci. USA* **2004**, *101*, 8963–8968. [CrossRef]

22. Zwerger, M.; Kolb, T.; Richter, K.; Karakesisoglou, I.; Herrmann, H. Induction of a massive endoplasmic reticulum and perinuclear space expansion by expression of lamin B receptor mutants and the related sterol reductases TM7SF2 and DHCR7. *Mol. Biol. Cell* **2010**, *21*, 354–368. [CrossRef]
23. Vargas, J.D.; Hatch, E.M.; Anderson, D.J.; Hetzer, M.W. Transient nuclear envelope rupturing during interphase in human cancer cells. *Nucleus* **2012**, *3*, 88–100. [CrossRef]
24. Lim, S.; Quinton, R.J.; Ganem, N.J. Nuclear envelope rupture drives genome instability in cancer. *Mol. Biol. Cell* **2016**, *27*, 3210–3213. [CrossRef]
25. Denais, C.M.; Gilbert, R.M.; Isermann, P.; McGregor, A.L.; te Lindert, M.; Weigelin, B.; Davidson, P.M.; Friedl, P.; Wolf, K.; Lammerding, J. Nuclear envelope rupture and repair during cancer cell migration. *Science (80-.)* **2016**, *352*, 353–358. [CrossRef]
26. Zhao, B.; Mei, Y.; Schipma, M.J.J.; Roth, E.W.W.; Bleher, R.; Rappoport, J.Z.Z.; Wickrema, A.; Yang, J.; Ji, P. Nuclear Condensation during Mouse Erythropoiesis Requires Caspase-3-Mediated Nuclear Opening. *Dev. Cell* **2016**, *36*, 498–510. [CrossRef]
27. Timmis, J.N.; Ayliffe, M.A.; Huang, C.Y.; Martin, W. Endosymbiotic gene transfer: Organelle genomes forge eukaryotic chromosomes. *Nat. Rev. Genet.* **2004**, *5*, 123–135. [CrossRef]
28. Leister, D. Origin, evolution and genetic effects of nuclear insertions of organelle DNA. *Trends Genet.* **2005**, *21*, 655–663. [CrossRef]
29. Szafranski, P. Intercompartmental Piecewise Gene Transfer. *Genes* **2017**, *8*, 260. [CrossRef]
30. Schneider, J.S.; Cheng, X.; Zhao, Q.; Underbayev, C.; Gonzalez, J.P.; Raveche, E.S.; Fraidenraich, D.; Ivessa, A.S. Reversible mitochondrial DNA accumulation in nuclei of pluripotent stem cells. *Stem Cells Dev.* **2014**, *23*, 2712–2719. [CrossRef]
31. Shay, J.W.; Werbin, H. New evidence for the insertion of mitochondrial DNA into the human genome: Significance for cancer and aging. *Mutat. Res. DNAging* **1992**, *275*, 227–235. [CrossRef]
32. Singh, B.; Modica-Napolitano, J.S.; Singh, K.K. Defining the momiome: Promiscuous information transfer by mobile mitochondria and the mitochondrial genome. *Semin. Cancer Biol.* **2017**, *47*, 1–17. [CrossRef]
33. Scarpulla, R.C.; Vega, R.B.; Kelly, D.P. Transcriptional integration of mitochondrial biogenesis. *Trends Endocrinol. Metab.* **2012**, *23*, 459–466. [CrossRef]
34. Dinkova-Kostova, A.T.; Abramov, A.Y. The emerging role of Nrf2 in mitochondrial function. *Free Radic. Biol. Med.* **2015**, *88*, 179–188. [CrossRef]
35. Fan, W.; Evans, R. PPARs and ERRs: Molecular mediators of mitochondrial metabolism. *Curr. Opin. Cell Biol.* **2015**, *33*, 49–54. [CrossRef]
36. Malhas, A.; Goulbourne, C.; Vaux, D.J. The nucleoplasmic reticulum: Form and function. *Trends Cell Biol.* **2011**, *21*, 362–373. [CrossRef]
37. Lee, S.-H.; Hadipour-Lakmehsari, S.; Miyake, T.; Gramolini, A.O. Three-dimensional imaging reveals endo(sarco)plasmic reticulum-containing invaginations within the nucleoplasm of muscle. *Am. J. Physiol. Cell Physiol.* **2018**, *314*, C257–C267. [CrossRef]
38. Malhas, A.N.; Vaux, D.J. Nuclear envelope invaginations and cancer. *Adv. Exp. Med. Biol.* **2014**, *773*, 523–535.
39. Raab, M.; Gentili, M.; De Belly, H.; Thiam, H.R.; Vargas, P.; Jimenez, A.J.; Lautenschlaeger, F.; Voituriez, R.; Lennon-Duménil, A.M.; Manel, N.; et al. ESCRT III repairs nuclear envelope ruptures during cell migration to limit DNA damage and cell death. *Science (80-.)* **2016**, *352*, 359–362. [CrossRef]
40. Soubannier, V.; McLelland, G.-L.; Zunino, R.; Braschi, E.; Rippstein, P.; Fon, E.A.; McBride, H.M. A vesicular transport pathway shuttles cargo from mitochondria to lysosomes. *Curr. Biol.* **2012**, *22*, 135–141. [CrossRef]
41. Abuaita, B.H.; Schultz, T.L.; O'Riordan, M.X. Mitochondria-Derived Vesicles Deliver Antimicrobial Reactive Oxygen Species to Control Phagosome-Localized Staphylococcus aureus. *Cell Host Microbe* **2018**, *24*, 625–636.e5. [CrossRef]
42. Zorov, D.B.; Filburn, C.R.; Klotz, L.O.; Zweier, J.L.; Sollott, S.J. Reactive oxygen species (ROS)-induced ROS release: A new phenomenon accompanying induction of the mitochondrial permeability transition in cardiac myocytes. *J. Exp. Med.* **2000**, *192*, 1001–1014. [CrossRef]
43. Ventimiglia, L.N.; Martin-Serrano, J. ESCRT machinery: Damage control at the nuclear membrane. *Cell Res.* **2016**, *26*, 641–642. [CrossRef]
44. Hatch, E.; Hetzer, M. Breaching the nuclear envelope in development and disease. *J Cell Biol.* **2014**, *205*, 133–141. [CrossRef]

45. Singh, V.R.; Yang, Y.A.; Yu, H.; Kamm, R.D.; Yaqoob, Z.; So, P.T.C. Studying nucleic envelope and plasma membrane mechanics of eukaryotic cells using confocal reflectance interferometric microscopy. *Nat. Commun.* **2019**, *10*, 3652. [CrossRef]
46. Dahl, K.N.; Ribeiro, A.J.S.; Lammerding, J. Nuclear shape, mechanics, and mechanotransduction. *Circ. Res.* **2008**, *102*, 1307–1318. [CrossRef]
47. Zhang, Q.; Tamashunas, A.C.; Agrawal, A.; Torbati, M.; Katiyar, A.; Dickinson, R.B.; Lammerding, J.; Lele, T.P. Local, transient tensile stress on the nuclear membrane causes membrane rupture. *Mol. Biol. Cell* **2019**, *30*, 899–906. [CrossRef]
48. Wolf, K.; te Lindert, M.; Krause, M.; Alexander, S.; te Riet, J.; Willis, A.L.; Hoffman, R.M.; Figdor, C.G.; Weiss, S.J.; Friedl, P. Physical limits of cell migration: Control by ECM space and nuclear deformation and tuning by proteolysis and traction force. *J. Cell Biol.* **2013**, *201*, 1069–1084. [CrossRef]
49. Vaziri, A.; Lee, H.; Kaazempur, M.R. Deformation of the cell nucleus under indentation: Mechanics and mechanisms. *J. Mater. Res.* **2006**, *21*, 2126–2135. [CrossRef]
50. Yaniv, Y.; Juhaszova, M.; Wang, S.; Fishbein, K.W.; Zorov, D.B.; Sollott, S.J. Analysis of mitochondrial 3D-deformation in cardiomyocytes during active contraction reveals passive structural anisotropy of orthogonal short axes. *PLoS ONE* **2011**, *6*, e21985. [CrossRef]
51. Ji, J.Y. Endothelial nuclear lamina in mechanotransduction under shear stress. In *Advances in Experimental Medicine and Biology*; Springer New York LLC: New York, NY, USA, 2018; Volume 1097, pp. 83–104.
52. Kessel, R.G. An electron microscope study of nuclear-cytoplasmic exchange in oocytes of Ciona intestinalis. *J. Ultrastruct. Res.* **1966**, *15*, 181–196. [CrossRef]
53. Kessel, R.G. Cytodifferentiation in the Rana pipiens oocyte. I. Association between mitochondria and nucleolus-like bodies in young oocytes. *J. Ultrastruct. Res.* **1969**, *28*, 61–77. [CrossRef]
54. Dietrich, A.; Wallet, C.; Iqbal, R.K.; Gualberto, J.M.; Lotfi, F. Organellar non-coding RNAs: Emerging regulation mechanisms. *Biochimie* **2015**, *117*, 48–62. [CrossRef]
55. Mercer, T.R.; Neph, S.; Dinger, M.E.; Crawford, J.; Smith, M.A.; Shearwood, A.-M.J.; Haugen, E.; Bracken, C.P.; Rackham, O.; Stamatoyannopoulos, J.A.; et al. The Human Mitochondrial Transcriptome. *Cell* **2011**, *146*, 645–658. [CrossRef]
56. Dorn, G.W. LIPCAR: A mitochondrial lnc in the noncoding RNA chain? *Circ. Res.* **2014**, *114*, 1548–1550. [CrossRef]
57. Dong, Y.; Yoshitomi, T.; Hu, J.-F.; Cui, J. Long noncoding RNAs coordinate functions between mitochondria and the nucleus. *Epigenet. Chromatin* **2017**, *10*, 41. [CrossRef]
58. Thorsness, P.E.; Weber, E.R. Escape and migration of nucleic acids between chloroplasts, mitochondria, and the nucleus. *Int. Rev. Cytol.* **1996**, *165*, 207–234.
59. Kolosova, N.G.; Stefanova, N.A.; Korbolina, E.E.; Fursova, A.Z.; Kozhevnikova, O.S. Senescence-accelerated OXYS rats: A genetic model of premature aging and age-related diseases. *Adv. Gerontol.* **2014**, *4*, 294–298. [CrossRef]
60. Capogrossi, M.C.; Kort, A.A.; Spurgeon, H.A.; Lakatta, E.G. Single adult rabbit and rat cardiac myocytes retain the Ca^{2+}- and species-dependent systolic and diastolic contractile properties of intact muscle. *J. Gen. Physiol.* **1986**, *88*, 589–613. [CrossRef]
61. Reynolds, E.S. The use of lead citrate at high pH as an electron-opaque stain in electron microscopy. *J. Cell Biol.* **1963**, *17*, 208–212. [CrossRef]

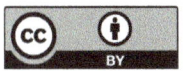

© 2020 by the authors. Licensee MDPI, Basel, Switzerland. This article is an open access article distributed under the terms and conditions of the Creative Commons Attribution (CC BY) license (http://creativecommons.org/licenses/by/4.0/).

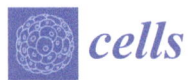

Review

Crosstalk between Mitochondria and Cytoskeleton in Cardiac Cells

Andrey V. Kuznetsov [1,2,*], Sabzali Javadov [3], Michael Grimm [1], Raimund Margreiter [4], Michael J. Ausserlechner [2] and Judith Hagenbuchner [5,*]

1. Cardiac Surgery Research Laboratory, Department of Cardiac Surgery, Innsbruck Medical University, 6020 Innsbruck, Austria; michael.grimm@tirol-kliniken.at
2. Department of Paediatrics I, Medical University of Innsbruck, 6020 Innsbruck, Austria; michael.j.ausserlechner@i-med.ac.at
3. Department of Physiology, School of Medicine, University of Puerto Rico, San Juan, PR 00936-5067, USA; sabzali.javadov@upr.edu
4. Department of Visceral, Transplant and Thoracic Surgery, Medical University of Innsbruck, 6020 Innsbruck, Austria; raimund.margreiter@tirol-kliniken.at
5. Department of Paediatrics II, Medical University of Innsbruck, 6020 Innsbruck, Austria
* Correspondence: andrey.kuznetsov@tirol-kliniken.at (A.V.K.); judith.hagenbuchner@i-med.ac.at (J.H.); Tel.: +43-512-504-27815 (A.V.K.); +43-512-504-81578 (J.H.)

Received: 3 December 2019; Accepted: 13 January 2020; Published: 16 January 2020

Abstract: Elucidation of the mitochondrial regulatory mechanisms for the understanding of muscle bioenergetics and the role of mitochondria is a fundamental problem in cellular physiology and pathophysiology. The cytoskeleton (microtubules, intermediate filaments, microfilaments) plays a central role in the maintenance of mitochondrial shape, location, and motility. In addition, numerous interactions between cytoskeletal proteins and mitochondria can actively participate in the regulation of mitochondrial respiration and oxidative phosphorylation. In cardiac and skeletal muscles, mitochondrial positions are tightly fixed, providing their regular arrangement and numerous interactions with other cellular structures such as sarcoplasmic reticulum and cytoskeleton. This can involve association of cytoskeletal proteins with voltage-dependent anion channel (VDAC), thereby, governing the permeability of the outer mitochondrial membrane (OMM) to metabolites, and regulating cell energy metabolism. Cardiomyocytes and myocardial fibers demonstrate regular arrangement of tubulin beta-II isoform entirely co-localized with mitochondria, in contrast to other isoforms of tubulin. This observation suggests the participation of tubulin beta-II in the regulation of OMM permeability through interaction with VDAC. The OMM permeability is also regulated by the specific isoform of cytolinker protein plectin. This review summarizes and discusses previous studies on the role of cytoskeletal proteins in the regulation of energy metabolism and mitochondrial function, adenosine triphosphate (ATP) production, and energy transfer.

Keywords: heart; cytoskeletal proteins; mitochondria; energy metabolism; mitochondrial interactions; plectin; tubulin beta; signaling

1. Introduction

Cells are highly organized units with multifaceted functional and structural interactions between various subcellular systems. A large number of studies provides strong evidence that elucidating individual organelles alone is not sufficient, and only systemic approaches must be applied for understanding intracellular signaling pathways and crosstalk between subcellular organelles. This may involve a "systems biology" approach and combinations of several most modern technologies such as genetic manipulations, live cell imaging, mathematical modelling, etc. In high oxygen consuming organs like the heart, energy supply (ATP) is provided by mitochondria in the reactions of oxidative phosphorylation (OXPHOS). Notably, mitochondria actively interact with other subcellular organelles and systems like cytoskeleton and sarcoplasmic reticulum (SR) [1–12]. Many cytoskeletal elements play a vital role in the structural and functional organization of mitochondria, including mitochondrial shape and morphology, dynamics, motility, and mitosis [13–17]. Most importantly, the interaction of mitochondria with some cytoskeletal proteins and their connections to voltage dependent anion channel (VDAC) can be involved in the coordination of mitochondrial function [18–23] (Figure 1). In the heart, mitochondrial bioenergetics and oxygen consumption are linearly dependent on the cardiac contractile activity [24,25] at rather stable concentration of the main mitochondrial regulator adenosine diphosphate (ADP), which is a central element in mitochondrial physiology. The exact mechanisms of how mitochondria precisely respond to the heart energy demand remained unknown for a long time and require further investigations. A growing body of evidence shows that the cells contain intracellular metabolic micro-compartments provided by multidirectional mitochondrial interactions with other subcellular organelles and macromolecules, in particular, specific cytoskeletal proteins [26–34]. In this review, we summarize and discuss previous studies that provide strong evidence for the role of cytoskeletal proteins, in particular, tubulin beta-II and plectin 1b, in the regulation of mitochondrial bioenergetics and energy fluxes via the energy-transferring supercomplex VDAC-mitochondrial creatine kinase (MitCK)-ATP-ADP translocase (ANT) under physiological and pathological conditions.

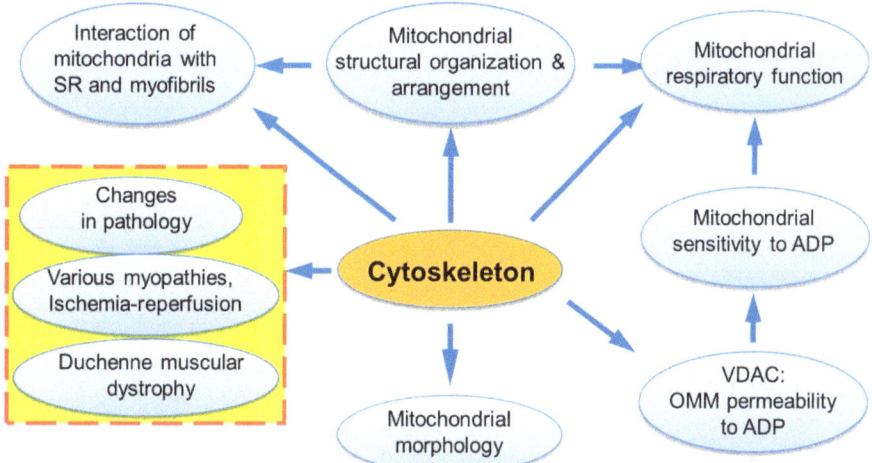

Figure 1. The central roles of cytoskeleton and its interactions in mitochondrial and entire cell physiology.

2. Historical Retrospective

The heart is a high oxygen consuming and ATP demanding organ with a large number of mitochondria that occupy ~30% of cardiac cell volume. Besides supplying the cardiac tissue with ATP, mitochondria play an important role in cell signaling, differentiation and growth, as well as in the maintenance of the cellular redox system, ion homeostasis, and cell death, actively communicating with other cellular systems like SR and cytoskeleton. The presence of micro-compartmentation of ATP and ADP (i.e., their high local concentrations at mitochondria and close to myofibrils) was evident from the observations that cellular bulk concentrations of ATP and ADP are relatively constant, independently of changes in heart workload. Interestingly, the total ischemia or anoxia quickly stops heart contractility while cellular bulk ATP concentration decreases by only ~5% under these conditions. Furthermore, the free cellular concentration of ADP in the heart (usually ~20 µM) cannot be higher than 50 µM, otherwise it will eventually lead to the increased left ventricular end diastolic pressure and thus, to the cardiac rigor super-contracture. On the other hand, the full activation of mitochondrial respiration requires at least 250–300 µM of ADP in isolated mitochondrial preparations. The detailed mechanisms of precise matches and synchronizations of mitochondrial respiratory function and heart contractility (excellently tuned cellular energy production and demand) still remain unclear and are under active investigation by several groups [27,28,30–34]. Apparently, mitochondria–cytoskeleton interactions play a certain role in these crosstalk mechanisms.

The pioneering work of Denton and McCormack in the 1980s [35] followed by other studies [36] proposed that intramitochondrial Ca^{2+} can activate the dehydrogenases involved in the tricarboxylic acid cycle and lead to upregulation of electron transfer chain (ETC) and OXPHOS, associated with high ATP production [35,36]. This metabolic regulation of mitochondrial bioenergetics by Ca^{2+} is known as a "parallel activation model" in the heart. According to this theory, increased cardiac contractile function and energy demands both are achieved by the increased cytosolic and mitochondrial Ca^{2+} with the involvement of several Ca^{2+} carriers. As a result, increased matrix Ca^{2+} stimulates mitochondrial dehydrogenases, mitochondrial function, and ATP production to match the increased energy consumption by myofibrils. Notably, these processes are shown to be strongly tissue specific [36].

For a long period of time, mitochondrial function was investigated mostly using isolated mitochondria in vitro. The apparent Michaelis constant (appKm) for the main mitochondrial substrate ADP in Michaelis–Menten equation is an important parameter of mitochondrial respiratory function, which can be obtained from the respiratory ADP kinetics. This parameter reflects the affinity of mitochondrial respiration to ADP and the permeability of the outer mitochondrial membrane (OMM). For many types of isolated mitochondria, this parameter was in a range of 10–30 µM [37,38]. These types of studies, however, resulted in the loss of the mitochondria-cytoskeleton interactions that are important for the control of metabolites transport in mitochondria, and for the regulation of the mitochondrial respiratory function. In vivo or in situ measurements of mitochondrial respiration (e.g., in permeabilized cells) could also be essential [39,40].

Kummel [41] and several other researchers [42–45] discovered the functional differences between isolated mitochondria in vitro and non-isolated mitochondria in situ (in permeabilized cardiac cells or muscle fibers). It has been found that appKm for external ADP, which is important for regulation of mitochondrial respiratory function, is significantly different in vitro and in situ mitochondria [42,44,45]. Therefore, instead of isolated mitochondria, myocardial fibers or cardiac cells permeabilized by digitonin or saponin were effectively used for the characterization of mitochondrial energetics in studies from the Saks group among others [42–45]. This approach allows avoiding mitochondrial isolation, and therefore has a number of serious advantages, most importantly, preserving mitochondrial contacts with other subcellular structures and systems, including the cytoskeleton [39]. Surprisingly, the appKm for ADP for mitochondria in situ was found to be about 300–400 µM [43–46], which is very different compared to isolated mitochondria. Importantly, the mild proteolytic treatment, e.g., with trypsin, significantly decreased appKm for ADP in permeabilized preparations almost to the value of in vitro, isolated mitochondria [26].

All these observations pointed to the involvement of cytoskeletal proteins as primary candidates in the control of mitochondrial respiratory function. Imaging analysis (fluorescence and immunofluorescence confocal microscopy) of cardiac cells and muscle fibers by using specific mitochondrial markers and various antibodies revealed full colocalization of mitochondria with cytoskeletal protein tubulin beta-II, suggesting its structural and functional interactions with mitochondrial VDAC [22,32,46,47]. Notably, in HL-1 cardiac cells that are devoid of tubulin beta-II, mitochondrial respiratory behavior and sensitivity to ADP (appKm) were similar to that of isolated mitochondria [47]. More recently, respirometrical and imaging analyses demonstrated that plectin 1b isoform is associated with mitochondria [48], which like tubulin beta-II, can also control the permeability of the OMM and thereby, modulate mitochondrial function. In favor of this, cardiac and muscle tissues from plectin 1b knockout mice showed severe mitochondrial changes and reversed sensitivity to ADP as evidenced by decreased appKm [48].

3. The Role of Cytoskeleton in the Mitochondrial Intracellular Organization, Shape Morphology and Dynamics

In various cells, mitochondria are associated with the three major cytoskeletal structures microtubules, intermediate filaments (IFs) and microfilaments [49–55]. It is known that specific cytoskeletal proteins are central for the mitochondrial morphology, dynamics, motility, intracellular traffic and mitosis [2,6]. Mitochondria can be associated with the actin-network and could be either anchored on cytoskeletal filaments or shaped by the forces (mechanical factors) generated by actin (see references in Section 8 "Cytoskeletal-Mitochondria Interactions in Pathology"). Microtubules are considered to be primary tools for mitochondrial transport [55,56]. However, actin is also required for short-distance mitochondrial activities as well as for the immobilization (anchorage) of mitochondria that may be important for holding these organelles at sites of higher energy demands. Moreover, some mutations in actin or actin-binding proteins may affect mitochondrial mechanisms leading to cell death [53]. Actually, mitochondria-actin interactions have been shown to be involved in apoptosis.

In cardiomyocytes, accumulation of intermyofibrillar mitochondria is observed at the vicinity of t-tubular network and separated by sarcomeric Z-lines in sarcomeres, that can be labeled by α-actinin immunofluorescent staining (Figure 2A–C) [32,33,48]. Many specific proteins that regulate mitochondrial intracellular localization, organization, shape/morphology, dynamics, and motility have been discovered [13–17,57]. Mitochondrial shape under physiological conditions usually needs the attachment of the organelles to cytoskeleton elements as the internal scaffolding system. Various mitochondria-shaping proteins have been identified and significant alterations in mitochondrial morphology and/or intracellular organization were observed in specific mutants [53]. Several special proteins can be responsible for the control of the mitochondrial shape through interactions of mitochondria to the cytoskeleton, while others can be responsible for the formation of connections between the OMM and inner mitochondrial membrane (IMM). The formation of the regular tubular shape of mitochondria normally needs several OMM proteins such as Mmm1p, Mmm2p, Mdm10p and Mdm12p as well as the IMM proteins Mdm31p and Mdm32p [57–62]. In mutants lacking any of these proteins, mitochondrial tabulation and elongated and branched shapes of tubules may disappear, and mitochondria can be then organized into big clusters of spherical shape. It has been shown that Mmm1p, Mdm10p, and Mdm12p can form the specific MMM complex, which, in cooperation with Mmm2p, Mdm31p, and Mdm32p proteins, stimulates formation of tubular mitochondria. This complex can be involved in the attachment of mitochondria to actin, interacting also with other cytoskeletal scaffolding systems. Mitochondrial morphology, the IMM and cristae shapes of mitochondria can also be regulated by Mdm33p, Gem1p, mitofilin [63,64], and ATP synthase [65].

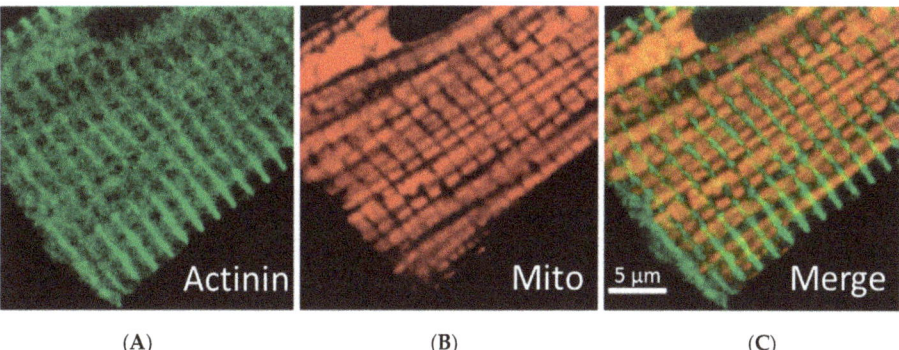

Figure 2. Simultaneous fluorescent and immunofluorescent confocal imaging analysis of mitochondria and sarcomeric Z-line (actinin) tubulin beta-II in rat cardiomyocyte. (**A**): Z-line (actinin); (**B**): Mitochondria; (**C**): Merge image. Scale bar, 5 µm.

In many cell types (mammals, yeast, etc.), the two opposing mitochondrial fission and fusion processes are regulated by various specific proteins [17,66–75]. Mitochondrial fusion and fission are regulated by the dynamin family GTPases [17]. Dynamin-related protein 1 (Drp1 or DLP1) [70,71] and mitochondrial fission 1 protein (Fis1/hFis1) participate in mitochondrial fission [72], whereas mitofusin 1 (Mfn1) and 2 (Mfn2), and optic atrophy protein 1 (OPA1) in mammalian cells regulate mitochondrial fusion [66–69,74]. Importantly, both cytoskeletal microfilaments and microtubules can be involved in the recruitment of Drp1 to mitochondria [70]. Fission–fusion shifts can frequently occur under various stressful conditions (oxidative stress, ischemia-reperfusion injury, etc.) [69,75–79], representing also an early event in the mitochondria-dependent programmed cell death (apoptosis) [80–82]. Cardiac ischemia-reperfusion injury (IRI) and post-infarction heart failure has been shown to increase mitochondrial fragmentation due to alterations in the expression and post-translational modifications of mitochondrial fission-fusion proteins [77,79]. The interactions of mitochondria with the cytoskeleton can be critical for the accumulation of mitochondria in specific cellular regions and mitochondrial movement can provide a local energy production at sites of higher ATP demands [83–86]. Mitochondrial movement (transport along microtubules), well known in neurons, is based on the several specific motor proteins such as the kinesin family of mitochondria-bound proteins and on the interactions with other cytoskeletal microtubules-dependent proteins [84–87]. In contrast, in cardiac cells, mitochondria are strongly fixed between myofibrils (intermyofibrillar mitochondrial subpopulation), which is absolutely obligatory for the normal organ contractile function.

Myosin V additionally contributes to organelle transport along actin networks. It has been shown that several protein kinases as well as the phosphorylation of certain proteins of microtubules can be involved in mitochondria-cytoskeleton crosstalk through interactions with mitochondrial membranes. In addition, phosphatidylinositol 3-kinase signaling pathways are also important for motility of mitochondria [85,88]. The proteins that arrange a link such as motor molecules-mitochondria, motor-independent motilities, and anchorage of mitochondria at cortical sites provide a connection between mitochondria-cytoskeleton interactions and mitochondrial flexibility [88]. The proper coordination of the mitochondrial dynamics is important for normal functioning of mitochondria, and mutations in the proteins that control the mitochondrial dynamics result in human diseases [69,79]. Notably, mitochondrial morphology, intracellular arrangement, and specific proteins involved in the mitochondrial dynamics are extremely cell-tissue specific [89]. Finally, mitochondrial interactions with the cytoskeleton network are shown to be important not only for the control of their morphology, dynamics, and organization, but also for the regulation of the entire energy metabolism [90] and OMM permeability to metabolites [2], as well as overall mitochondrial physiology [91]. The entire cytoskeleton and specific cytoskeletal proteins can contact mitochondria to control the OMM permeability to ADP and regulate OXPHOS, the main function of mitochondria.

4. Cytoskeleton and Mitochondria-SR Interactions

Mitochondria play a central role in cell life and cell death and mediate a myriad of intracellular pro-survival and pro-death signaling pathways [92]. Several physiological mechanisms need precise interactions between various subcellular organelles, like plasma membrane, nucleus, mitochondria and SR. In myocardium, Ca^{2+} released from SR and Ca^{2+} cycling plays a fundamental role in the excitation–contraction coupling, as well as in the interactions of different cytoskeletal elements with mitochondria. Overall, the function of the heart, Ca^{2+} homeostasis, and excitation–contraction coupling vitally depend on the ATP production by mitochondrial OXPHOS. On the other hand, mitochondrial Ca^{2+} overloading can damage mitochondria, reducing ATP production, leading to ROS generation, oxidative stress and various cardiac injuries (for more details, see Section 8).

Some dense structures were frequently observed between the OMM and SR or T-tubules that can link these systems [3,93]. The communications and interactions of subcellular organelles are based on the vesicular trafficking and membrane contact sites important in Ca^{2+} homeostasis and lipid metabolism. These tight interactions and contacts permit cells and their specific compartments to adapt them to the different conditions [3]. It has been proposed that such contacts are essential for the transport of lipids (phospholipids) as well as for the overall cellular Ca^{2+} homeostasis via the complex formed by VDAC and inositol 1,4,5-trisphophate receptors, managing vital cellular processes like contraction, secretion, cell growth, proliferation, apoptosis, etc. [94]. Specific elements of cytoskeleton can be associated with L-type Ca^{2+} channel, and regulate its activity and mitochondrial function, mediating mitochondrial membrane potential [95].

It has been demonstrated that the distances between membranes of organelles assessed by electron microscopy are relatively small, and allow to create structural contacts between proteins of these membranes. This regulates organelle–organelle interactions, restructuring the mitochondrial morphology and network together with Ca^{2+} handling under physiological conditions. The membrane contact sites (mitochondria-associated membranes) occur in response to various mitochondrial or SR stresses (autophagy, apoptosis, inflammation) [96–98], as well as in several diseases associated with changes in mitochondrial dynamics machinery [99]. They may also play an important role in various diseases such as neurodegenerative diseases, diabetes, infection diseases and cancer [100]. Mitochondria-SR contacts have been shown to be involved in the mitochondria–cytoskeleton interactions, regulating mitochondrial dynamics, including mitochondrial fusion and fission processes [96]. On the electron micrographs, such contacts look like SR tubules closely faced to mitochondria.

5. Possible Role of the Intermediate Filaments Proteins Desmin and Vimentin in the Regulation of Mitochondrial Bioenergetics

Cardiac and skeletal muscle cells contain intracellular network that tightly regulates myofibrillar activity and maintains muscle contraction/relaxation. The synchronization of the basic contractile element, sarcomere, involves well-organized filament structures that include myosin (thick structure), actin (thin structure), nebulin, and titin [101]. It is connected to other subcellular organelles such as the nucleus and mitochondria. As a result, the multiorganelle network operates as a platform for general cellular integrity/stability, also governing mitochondrial function, shape, and intracellular organization. The contractile machinery represents a complex network, all three members of which (microtubules, IFs and microfilaments) are associated with mitochondria [49–54]. IFs are considered as the main protectors against various stresses such as oxidative stress, toxic injury, apoptotic stimuli, etc. [91]. They also play an important role in cell growth/differentiation, bioenergetics, cellular signaling and cells relocation. IFs have the ability to be polymerized and their mechanical properties and richness can change in response to pathological stimuli. IFs maintain the cell integrity and thus play an important role in protein targeting and inter-organellar interaction. Mitochondrial function and subcellular organization may be regulated by IFs proteins as shown for IFs desmin, vimentin and some other proteins [30,34,102,103]. Also, intracellular locations of Golgi can be regulated by IFs.

In the cell, the desmin cytoskeleton is responsible for the proper mitochondrial positioning and shape. It may also regulate the formation and stabilization of mitochondrial contact sites. Desmin is present in cardiac, skeletal and smooth muscle cells, in particular, in dense bodies, nearby the nuclei, close to the Z-line and costameres. It can be upregulated during muscle adaptations as well as in myopathies, muscle degeneration, and drug treatments [102]. Desmin has been suggested to participate in the regulation of myofibrillogenesis, mechanical support of the muscle cells, mitochondrial localization, gene expression and intracellular signaling. It can interact with actin, tubulin, plectin (cytolinker protein) and dynein (motor protein). IFs, like microtubules (see above), were suggested to have a significant impact on mitochondrial morphology, as well as cellular organization and functions in different mammalian cell types. Changes in their interactions can lead to various human diseases [104,105]. Several studies with desmin-deficient (desmin-null) mice [30,34,102] have demonstrated the importance of desmin in subcellular distribution and respiratory function of mitochondria. Ultrastructural studies of cardiomyocytes from desmin-null models showed mitochondrial proliferation that was elevated in response to increased workload. Cardiac and skeletal muscles of desmin-null mice exhibited significant changes in the morphology and intracellular organization of mitochondria [30,34].

Mitochondrial alterations in desmin-null muscles were associated with decreased maximal rate of respiration (ADP-stimulated rate of oxygen consumption). Also, the lack of the coupling between MitCK and ANT observed in desmin-null models [22,31,33,106–108] indicates alteration of intracellular energy transfer [22,31,33,92]. In addition, the decrease in mitochondrial respiration was associated with the decline of the appKm for ADP in permeabilized cardiac fibers of desmin-null mice. These data show that desmin can participate in the regulation of the mitochondrial VDAC, directly or via a desmin-associated cytolinker protein plectin. In contrast, mitochondrial function and appKm for ADP in permeabilized fibers from skeletal glycolytic muscles were not seriously affected in the absence of desmin [30]. Proteomic analysis of cardiac mitochondria isolated from desmin knockout mice has demonstrated alterations in various metabolic processes such as apoptic pathways and Ca^{2+} cycling. The changes in VDAC expression suggested a connection between the desmin-determined cellular organization and mitochondrial energy metabolism [30,34]. Cardiac and skeletal muscles of aggregation-prone desmin mutant L345P mice exhibited significant changes in morphology of mitochondria and Ca^{2+} handling. Al these studies proposed that desmin directly or indirectly can participate in the regulation of mitochondrial function.

Several studies suggested that the cytoskeletal IF protein vimentin, like dismin, can also regulate mitochondrial bioenergetics [103]. Like desmin, vimentin can interact with mitochondria [103,109,110] and modulate their shape/morphology, intracellular organization and dynamics [103]. Vimentin-null cells displayed lower mitochondrial membrane potential, which was recovered by adding of external vimentin [110]. The cytolinker protein, plectin, which is expressed ubiquitously, participates in mitochondria–vimentin interaction [109]. Its specific mitochondrial isoform plectin-1b has been suggested to bind vimentin to mitochondria. Thus, desmin, vimentin, and plectin-1b are critical for functional and structural interactions between the cytoskeleton and mitochondria that regulate mitochondrial function. It should be noted that the direct involvement of desmin and vimentin in mitochondrial bioenergetics and physiology is still debated.

6. The Role of Tubulin in the Regulation of Mitochondrial Bioenergetics and Metabolism

In oxidative muscles, mitochondria are organized into functional complexes with myofibrils and SR, and create specific intracellular energetic units [32,33,111,112]. Energy crosstalk within these units provides facilitated diffusion of ADP, metabolic micro-compartmentation and channelling by the local energy transfer network [31,33] which includes creatine kinase and adenylate kinase. The microtubules are mostly composed of tubulin; their assembly and function are regulated by the microtubule associated proteins kinesin and dynein. In many cell types and tissues, mitochondria typically show an intracellular distribution matching the microtubular organization [32,113].

In the heart, tubulins form a network which, together with plectin, desmin, and microfilament proteins (actin), creates a precise structural organization of cardiac cells. This organization is essential to sustain the cardiac contractile function, as well as for the regulation of energy supply and demand [19,21–23,101,113–115]. It is known that tubulin in vivo is dynamic, undergoing assembly/disassembly processes due to interchanges between its subunits. The microtubule units are formed by alpha and beta tubulin heterodimers [116]. In cardiomyocytes, about 70% of total tubulin is present in the polymerized form as microtubules, whereas 30% occurs as a non-polymerized cytosolic heterodimeric protein [117–119]. Many chemical agents that depolymerize microtubules can significantly change mitochondrial intracellular organization [53,113]. Similar alterations in mitochondrial localization and motility were also found in cases of actin-encoding gene mutations demonstrating a possible role of the actin cytoskeleton [55,56]. Interestingly, after the complete dissociation of the microtubular system by colchicine, tubulin is still present in permeabilized cardiomyocytes, possibly due to the association with other cytoskeletal elements [2,120]. In 1990, Saetersdal et al. [114], for the first time, reported a possible connection of β-tubulin isotype to the OMM using microscopy and immunogold labelling of cardiac muscle cells. Furthermore, immunoprecipitation analysis has demonstrated direct association of tubulin with mitochondrial VDAC [121], confirming earlier suggestion of direct interconnections between microtubules and OMM [21]. Moreover, it was found that the addition of isolated dimeric tubulin induces closed state of VDAC, restoring the low permeability of the OMM, thereby, increasing appKm for ADP [19,20,121–124].

The ANT is less accessible to externally added ADP in permeabilized cardiac cells or oxidative muscle fibers than that in isolated mitochondria [40–43] (see Section 2). Regulation of the OMM permeability by VDAC channelling has two major functions. First, it controls mitochondrial respiration and energy transfer from energy source (mitochondria) to different sites of energy utilization in the cytoplasm. Numerous metabolites, such as respiratory substrates, ADP, and Pi, enter mitochondria only through VDAC. On the other side, high-energy phosphates, mostly ATP and phosphocreatine are channelled out through the VDAC to drive cellular energy transfer. Control of energy fluxes through VDAC is regulated by tubulin beta-II bound to VDAC (Figure 3). Second, VDAC becomes a channel for release of pro-apoptotic factors from mitochondria to the cytoplasm in response to apoptotic stimuli. Both tubulin beta-II and plectin can control VDAC permeability and therefore energy and metabolic fluxes of ATP, ADP, creatine (Cr) and phosphocreatine (PCr) (see Figure 3).

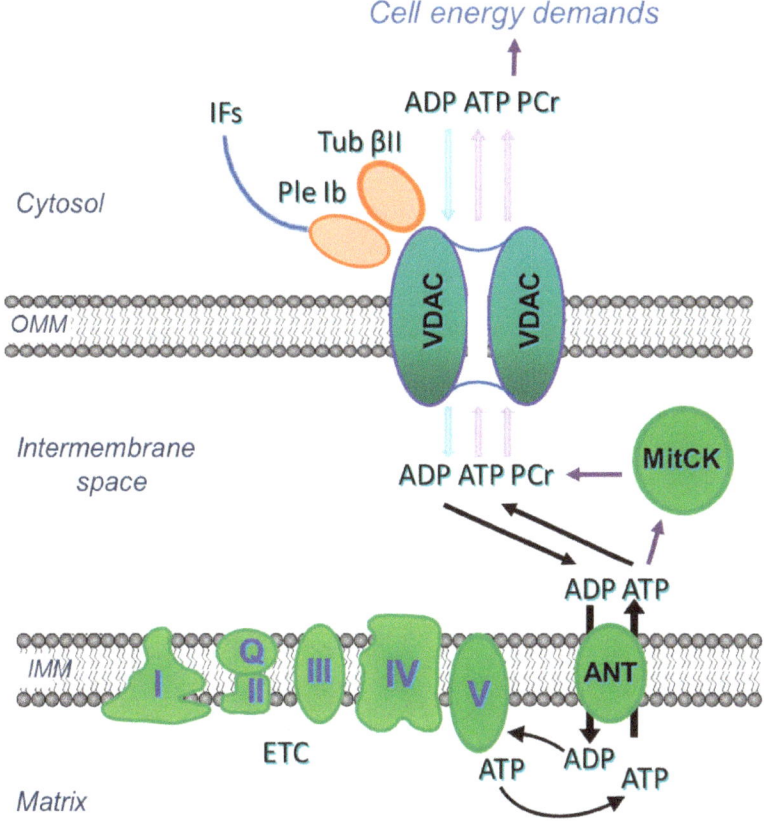

Figure 3. Possible interactions of VDAC of the OMM with tubulin beta-II (Tub βII), plectin 1b (Ple 1b), mitochondrial creatine kinase (MitCK) and ADP-ATP translocase (ANT) in cardiac cells.

The significant role of tubulin in the modulation of mitochondrial VDAC has been extensively analysed during the last two decades [18–20,23,123–125]. It was found that the addition of αβ-tubulin to isolated cardiac mitochondria in vitro, at concentrations below the value critical for the tubulin polymerization, significantly increased appKm for ADP in ADP kinetics of mitochondrial respiration to the value of in situ mitochondria, discovered in the permeabilized preparations, thus demonstrating restricted (decreased) ADP availability to ANT [19,124]. It was also shown that the addition of αβ-heterodimeric tubulin to reconstituted, purified VDAC (three isoforms of VDAC 1, 2, and 3) provoked reversible transition to its closed state, limiting mitochondrial ADP or ATP fluxes [18–20,122]. These findings suggest a mechanism of regulation of mitochondrial energetics, governed by VDAC and tubulin at the mitochondria-cytosol interface. Depending on the applied voltage and phosphorylation state of VDAC, the low concentrations of dimeric tubulin may activate reversible obstruction of VDAC incorporated in the artificial phospholipid membrane. Analysis of the tubulin-closed state demonstrated that it can carry small ions, but is impermeable to ATP, ADP and other mitochondrial metabolites. All these observations were then confirmed in isolated mitochondria or human hepatoma cells. Tubulin–VDAC interactions require a specific structure of the anionic C-terminal tail of tubulin.

Altogether, the results of previous studies suggest cytoskeletal protein tubulin as an important player in the regulation of VDAC states and OMM permeability (permeability restrictions created by interactions of VDAC in OMM with tubulin) in the mechanisms of mitochondrial energetics regulations [19,31,47]. The functional VDAC–tubulin interactions can be either direct or indirect, via cytoskeleton proteins such as specific isoforms of plectin. The interaction between VDAC and tubulin can be affected by isoform patterns of both tubulin and VDAC, as well as by their post-translational modification (e.g., phosphorylation). The main differences between distinct isotypes of tubulin are located in the C-terminal residues (called also isotype defining region). The C-terminus can be a target for various microtubule associated proteins (MAPs) [125–127] and the differences between multiple interactions of tubulin with various cellular systems can be determined by the composition of the C-terminus. In addition, MitCK, which has been shown to tightly interact with VDAC, can act as an important regulating factor in these interactions. Notably, the ANT-MitCK pathway (phosphocreatine shuttle) can be active in oxidative but not in glycolytic muscles and cancer cells [47,128]. It was suggested that tubulin beta-VDAC interactions participate in the modulation of cellular energy metabolism in cancer switching it from the oxidative phosphorylation mode to more glycolytic phenotype known as the Warburg effect [129]. This phenomenon has recently received renewed interest [130–132].

Fluorescent confocal imaging can not only visualize mitochondrial intracellular arrangement, morphology, dynamics, networks, and heterogeneity, but also quantitatively analyze mitochondrial functional parameters, like redox state, membrane potentials and Ca^{2+} levels [133–135]. Moreover, the combination of live mitochondrial imaging in cells or muscle fibers, together with immunofluorescence visualization and immunoblotting of cytoskeletal proteins allows to analyze structural relationships between these structures. The imaging analysis of the intracellular distribution of tubulin isoforms in cardiac cells by immunofluorescence confocal microscopy has discovered a regular arrangement of tubulin beta-II (Figure 4). Most importantly, double imaging analyses by fluorescence and immunofluorescence microscopy demonstrated clear co-localization of tubulin beta-II with cardiac intermyofibrillar mitochondria [8]. Tubulin beta-IV demonstrated an organization in branched network while tubulin beta-III was localized close to Z-lines, and tubulin beta-I was diffusely distributed [8]. The colocalization of tubulin beta-II with mitochondria suggested its functional and structural interaction with mitochondrial VDAC [8,22,32]. Interestingly, permeabilized HL-1 cells with cardiac phenotype demonstrated mitochondrial parameters and appKm for ADP very similar to that of isolated mitochondria that indicates a high open state of VDAC. This parameter was very different from that found in adult cardiomyocytes or H9c2 cardioblastic cells [136,137]. The absence of tubulin beta-II in HL-1 cells shows the importance of tubulin beta-II in the control of the OMM permeability and mitochondrial function through regulations of VDAC open-close states [22,32]. The absence of tubulin beta-II and the presence of only β-IV-tubulin, β tubulin I and III can be explained by cancerous phenotype of these cells. HL-1 cells originate from mouse atrial cardiomyocytes and, apparently, are more dependent on glycolytic rather than mitochondrial energy production. Another important characteristic of HL-1 cells is the lack of MitCK, and therefore phosphocreatine-mediated energy transfer [47]. Accordingly, functional analysis of permeabilized cardiomyocytes and HL-1 cells such as ADP-kinetics, and stimulatory effects of creatine and glucose on mitochondrial respiration rates revealed dramatic differences. In HL-1 cells, the appKm for ADP was the same (~20 µM) as for isolated in vitro mitochondria [136]. All these findings show associative link between the structural (presence or absence of tubulin beta-II and MitCK) and functional (e.g., appKm for ADP) features in different primary cells and cell lines.

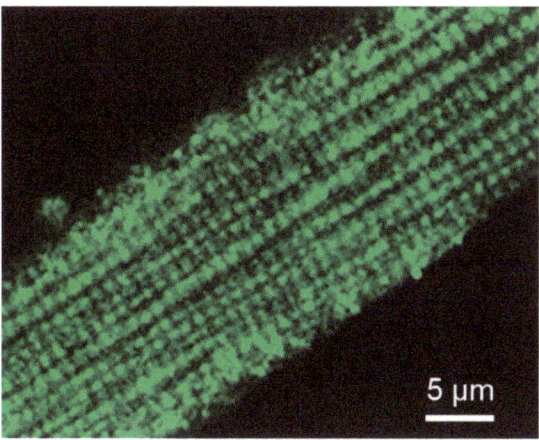

Figure 4. Cellular distribution of tubulin beta-II in adult rat cardiomyocyte. Tubulin beta-II was visualized by immunofluorescent confocal microscopy using specific antibodies. Scale bar 5 µm.

The association of tubulin beta-II with the OMM, when co-expressed with MitCK, may specifically limit the permeability of VDAC for adenine nucleotides, resulting in the formation of adenine nucleotides (ADP, ATP) micro-compartmentation in the mitochondrial intermembrane space. Thus, tubulin beta-II can participate in the control of VDAC, permeability of the OMM, and in the control of metabolic energy and metabolic fluxes (ATP, ADP, PCr, Cr, Pi) via the VDAC-MitCK-ANT supercomplex (Figure 3), thereby controlling cellular energy production and energy transfer in cardiac and oxidative muscle cells (Figures 3 and 5A). This supercomplex, localized at contact sites of two mitochondrial membranes, is a key structure of a specific pathway for the effective energy transport from mitochondria to cytoplasm, as well as for the local regeneration of ATP at sites of energy utilization including myofibrils, SR, anabolic processes, and active transport (via various pumps) across the sarcolemma membrane [32,33,111,112].

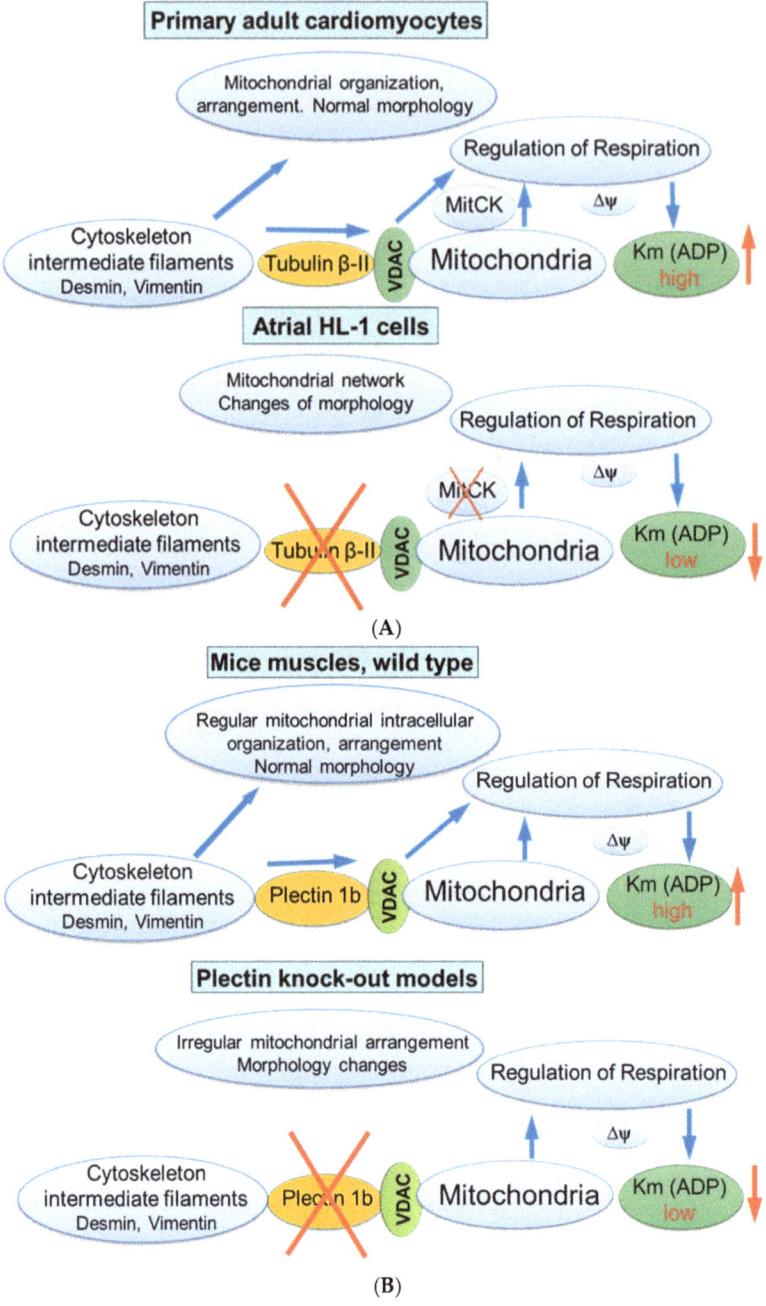

Figure 5. Possible role of cytoskeletal proteins tubulin beta-II (**A**) and plectin 1b (**B**) interactions with mitochondria. Scheme summarizing hypotheses regarding the control of mitochondrial respiratory function by tubulin beta-II and plectin 1b via their connections with VDAC. Km (ADP), apparent Michaelis constant for ADP; MitCK, mitochondrial creatine kinase; $\Delta\Psi m$, the inner mitochondrial membrane potential.

7. Possible Role of Plectin in the Control of Mitochondrial Intracellular Organization and Function

Previous studies demonstrated that the proper cell architecture and subcellular organization in cardiac cells are strongly dependent on plectin and desmin, and proposed that plectin can use desmin in cellular signaling [138]. In muscles, four isoforms of plectin were found that possess different cellular anchoring functions: they control the structure, organization, and stability of the cells [138,139]. Plectin 1f connects desmin to the sarcolemma whereas plectin 1 binds desmin to the nucleus. Plectin 1d connects desmin IFs to the Z-disk in cultured myotubes and plectin 1b, a mitochondrial isoform of plectin can directly interact with VDAC [115,140,141]. Plectin 1b was shown to be inserted into the OMM with the exon 1b encoded N-terminal sequence, which operates as an anchoring and mitochondria-targeting indicator. The disruption of Z-disks and costameres connections leads to the development of muscular dystrophies [142]. Plectin 1b (P1b) was shown to be associated with mitochondria even after the fractionation of cells. Due to their localization [138,139], plectin isoforms 1b and 1d were proposed to be the most plausible candidates for the participation and control of desmin interconnections between IFs and OMM.

Plectin deficiency resulted in progressive degenerative changes in striated muscle, with a significant aggregation and partial loss of IFs, separation of the contractile system from sarcolemma, and alterations in the architecture of costameres. The decreased mitochondrial content was supported by lowered activity of mitochondrial matrix enzyme citrate synthase, frequently used as a mitochondrial marker [48]. Notably, mitochondria-rich oxidative muscles, like the heart and soleus, were most intensely influenced by plectin deficiency. Also, plectin 1b knockout models exhibited changes in mitochondrial shapes, without substantial alterations of mitochondrial motility [48]. In addition to muscles, in primary fibroblasts or myoblasts obtained from plectin-deficient mice, detachment of desmin IFs from Z-disks, costameres, mitochondria and nuclei, and formation of desmin aggregates were observed [140]. At the same time, the initial mitochondrial morphology can be partially restored by the overexpression of isoform-specific P1b in plectin-deficient muscles or in plectin-null cells. Furthermore, it has been demonstrated that some mutations of the plectin genes, or disturbance and pathological changes of the IFs, can be correlated with severe dysfunction of mitochondria [141–143]. Therefore, the effects observed earlier in desmin-deficient models (desmin-null cardiac and soleus muscles) can be explained by the specific participation of a mitochondrial isoform of the cytolinker protein plectin, connecting desmin to mitochondria. Depletion of plectin isoforms (P1b or P1d) significantly changed mitochondrial intracellular organization and respiratory function in conditional plectin knockout mice (MCK-Cre/cKO) [48]. Notably, morphological changes of mitochondria were associated with high levels of Mfn-2, a mitochondrial fusion protein. High resolution respirometry of permeabilized fibers from cardiac and skeletal muscles of conditional plectin knockout mice showed a reduction of maximal rates of respiration and significant decrease in the appKm for ADP, reflecting changed permeability of the OMM (the more open VDAC state) [48].

Taken together, these studies suggest the mitochondrial isoform of plectin 1b as a reliable candidate (similar to tubulin beta-II) for the regulation of mitochondrial respiratory function via its control of VDAC (Figure 5B).

8. Cytoskeletal-Mitochondria Interactions in Pathology

Injured mitochondria play important role in the mechanisms of a variety of pathological conditions, including muscular dystrophy, IRI and various cardiomyopathies. Functional disturbances of several cytoskeletal proteins, namely tubulin, plectin, desmin, and vimentin, can lead to various diseases, associated with the dysfunction of mitochondria and mitochondria-cytoskeleton connections/interactions [92].

Many mechanical interactions can be observed in the cell. Various mechanical forces are transmitted via the cytoskeleton to the different intracellular organelles like mitochondria, affecting their function and morphology. In cardiac cells, mitochondria may possess an evident mechano-sensitivity, serving as subcellular mechano-sensors and showing stretch-induced changes in their function (OXPHOS), $\Delta\psi m$, ROS and Ca^{2+} signaling. Such mechano-sensitivity of mitochondria may contribute to the mechanisms of several pathologies (heart failure, cardiomyopathies, arrhythmias, hypertension) including aging [144–147]. On the other hand, it has been shown that mitochondrial volume changes (e.g., swelling) may be mechanically transduced to the other cellular organelles like myofibrils and nuclei, altering their morphology and function [148].

The common and serious human genetic disease Duchenne muscular dystrophy (DMD) occurs due to the low expression of dystrophin [149]. Dystrophin is an important, tubulin binding, cytoskeletal protein, serving as cellular cytolinker and stabilizer of microtubules [150]. It is associated with glycoproteins of sarcolemma, connecting subsarcolemmal cytoskeleton with the extracellular matrix [151]. Dystrophin-deficient muscles demonstrated serious changes in mitochondrial physiology and function [152]. Mdx mice are frequently used as an animal model for DMD. It has been observed that, instead of well-organized microtubule lattice, DMD skeletal muscles showed largely disarranged microtubules. This was associated with the overexpression of the specific isoform of tubulin (beta 6 class V β-tubulin) pointing to the possible important role of this overexpression in DMD [153]. The study of mitochondrial bioenergetics demonstrated that, in permeabilized skeletal muscle fibers from mdx mice, the maximal rates of mitochondrial respiration were about twice lower than those of controls and similar changes were observed in skeletal muscle biopsies from DMD patients. It has been found that mitochondrial injuries were related to the damage to complex I of the respiratory chain, low creatine-stimulated respiration due to damage in MitCK, and therefore impairment of phosphocreatine shuttle, leading to a less efficient intracellular energy transfer. These findings show that the dysfunction of muscle mitochondria can be the beginning of cardiomyopathy observed in mdx mice [152]. Therefore, mitochondria can represent a target for the treatment of DMD-associated cardiomyopathies and the recovery of mitochondrial bioenergetics can be considered for DMD treatment in patients.

The cytoskeleton of cardiac cells represents a highly organized structure to transmit mechanical forces and maintain proper organization of cellular organelles. Significant concomitant changes in the cytoskeleton, mitochondria, and in their interrelations were observed in IRI. During ischemia, the disruption of the cytoskeleton and its components induces damage of the integrity of myocytes resulting in their destruction and loss [154–157]. Mitochondrial respiratory function and energy transfer via MitCK and PCr pathway also decreased in various cardiomyopathies, heart failure and after IRI [158–161]. Also, ischemia-associated cardiomyopathies may occur due to alterations in the expression and subcellular reorganization of various cytoskeletal proteins [162–165]. Notably, intracellular rearrangement and changes in the location of tubulin beta-II which, under normal conditions, is finely colocalized with mitochondria (see above), was observed after IRI in the Langendorff perfused rat heart model [155]. These changes were concomitant with the increased affinity for ADP in mitochondrial respiration and oxidative phosphorylation (decreased appKm for ADP) and accompanied by decreased functional coupling of these processes with MitCK [155]. The decrease of appKm for ADP in mitochondrial respiration was frequently found in cardiac IRI [166,167], demonstrating a reduction of micro-compartmentation effects and energy fluxes via coupled CK systems. Using this model, it was found that appKm for ADP in the control group and after IRI inversely correlated with left-ventricular end-diastolic pressure [155].

Tubulin beta-II can modulate mitochondrial permeability transition pore (PTP) opening during IRI. The PTP opening in a low conductance increases permeability to solutes $\leq$ 300 Da, mostly ions, and induces negligible matrix swelling which, in turn, stimulates ETC activity, OXPHOS, ATP production, fatty acid oxidation, and other metabolic processes [168,169]. However, a high-conductance PTP opening which occurs in response to oxidative stress such as cardiac IRI enhances unrestricted bi-directional movements of water and solutes $\leq$ 1500 Da across the IMM. As a result, excessive matrix swelling causes IMM depolarization, ATP depletion, and rupture of the OMM, leading to cell death (Reviewed in [170–172]). Several mitochondrial proteins such as cyclophilin D,

VDAC, ANT, phosphate carrier, ETC complex I, and Bcl-2 proteins participate in the regulation of the PTP opening [173–176]. The interaction of tubulin beta-II with VDAC can change the PTP activity under physiological and pathological conditions. In favour of this, disrupting microtubule architecture in permeabilized muscle fibers that demonstrated direct interaction between α-tubulin and tubulin beta-II and VDAC2 decreased Ca^{2+} retention capacity due to increased PTP opening [177].

In the heart, Ca^{2+} is a main player in the control of excitation–contraction coupling, also playing an important role in mitochondrial bioenergetics and cytoskeleton functionality [178–180]. However, increased mitochondrial and cytosolic Ca^{2+} may lead to various pathologies and diseases, such as IRI, hypoxia-reoxygenation, arrhythmias, hypertension, heart failure, and metabolic syndrome, etc. [179,181–184]. This can be tightly associated with multiple Ca^{2+}-modulated processes, such as: mitochondria/cell swelling, changes in the interactions between cytoskeleton, mitochondria, and SR, decline of $\Delta\Psi m$, diminished mitochondrial respiratory capacity and consequent decreased cellular ATP content (energy stress), altered mitochondrial dynamics (fission-fusion balance, Drp1 signaling), increased ROS (oxidative stress), and induction of apoptosis [179,183,185]. It has been shown that a component of the cell-cell interactions (adhesion) machinery may be involved in the control of calcium cycling and homeostasis, and its deficiency may lead to the heart arrhythmia [182].

Interestingly, a heterogeneous value of appKm for ADP was found after relatively short periods of ischemia, revealing at least two populations of mitochondria with normal and low appKm for ADP [155]. Likewise, fluorescence confocal microscopy imaging revealed a heterogeneous response and damage of cardiac mitochondria in response to cold ischemia (organ cold storage, preservation) and reperfusion [186]. This can be due to the absence of electrical continuity of intermyofibrillar mitochondria that may prevent breakdown of the entire bioenergetics in the cell [187]. Furthermore, tubulin beta-II mitochondrial dislocation during IRI was comparable to that found in volume overload cardiac hypertrophy [188]. This dislocation might be due to protein degradation. A remodeling of the cytoskeleton (in particular the microtubular system) was discovered also in cardiac chronic hypertrophy [2,119], associated with increased beta-tubulin expression and tubulin C-terminus post-translational modifications [189–192], in heart failure and various cardiomyopathies [117,118,193].

9. Conclusions

Many structural and functional interactions were found to be involved in the integration of mitochondria with other cellular systems like the SR and cytoskeleton, connecting mitochondrial function, dynamics, and regulation with the entire cell physiology, in particular in the most energy consuming organ, the heart. Overall, existing studies provide strong evidence that cytoskeletal proteins such as tubulin beta-II and plectin 1b interact with mitochondria. The interaction regulates metabolic fluxes via the energy transferring supercomplex VDAC-MitCK-ANT which, in turn, coordinates mitochondrial respiration and OXPHOS and the entire cellular physiology. The detailed characterization of molecular mechanisms implicated in mitochondrial–cytoskeleton interactions under normal and pathological conditions can be helpful for the development of new therapeutic approaches.

It should be pointed out that many structural and functional aspects of mitochondria–cytoskeletal proteins interactions, as well as detailed molecular mechanisms of their formation, are not yet known, and the interactions of tubulin beta-II or plectin 1b with mitochondria (mitochondrial VDAC) have to be shown more directly, using the most modern methodologies, for example, by using: (i) imaging approaches with a higher levels of spatial and temporal resolutions, (ii) application of mitochondrial green fluorescent proteins (GFPs) specifically targeted to mitochondria, (iii) use of fluorescence resonance energy transfer (FRET) method to directly analyze possible protein-protein interactions and proximities, (iv) reconstruction or reconstitution experiments using tubulin β-II transfection and specific fragments of plectin, and (v) advancement of recombinant α- and β-tubulin isoforms with modifications of the C-terminal tail.

Author Contributions: Conceptualization, A.V.K., M.J.A. and S.J.; validation, S.J., M.J.A. and R.M.; resources, M.G. and R.M.; data curation, S.J. and M.G.; writing—original draft preparation, A.V.K. and S.J.; writing—review and editing, A.V.K., J.H. and S.J.; supervision, M.J.A., M.G. and R.M.; project administration, M.J.A., M.G. and R.M.; funding acquisition, J.H. and M.J.A. All authors have read and agreed to the published version of the manuscript.

Funding: This research was funded by MFF-Tirol (Project 291), "Tiroler Wissenschaftsförderung", the Austrian Science Fund (FWF Project I3089-B28), the "Tirol-Kliniken GmbH", and the National Institute of General Medical Sciences of the National Institutes of Health (NIH Grant SC1GM128210 to S.J.).

Conflicts of Interest: The authors declare no conflict of interest.

References

1. Appaix, F.; Kuznetsov, A.V.; Usson, Y.; Kay, L.; Andrienko, T.; Olivares, J.; Kaambre, T.; Sikk, P.; Margreiter, R.; Saks, V. Possible role of cytoskeleton in intracellular arrangement and regulation of mitochondria. *Exp. Physiol.* **2003**, *88*, 175–190. [CrossRef] [PubMed]
2. Rappaport, L.; Oliviero, P.; Samuel, J.L. Cytoskeleton and mitochondrial morphology and function. *Mol. Cell. Biochem.* **1998**, *184*, 101–105. [CrossRef] [PubMed]
3. Cohen, S.; Valm, A.M.; Lippincott-Schwartz, J. Interacting organelles. *Curr. Opin. Cell Biol.* **2018**, *53*, 84–91. [CrossRef] [PubMed]
4. Andrienko, T.; Kuznetsov, A.V.; Kaambre, T.; Usson, Y.; Orosco, A.; Appaix, F.; Tiivel, T.; Sikk, P.; Vendelin, M.; Margreiter, R.; et al. Metabolic consequences of functional complexes of mitochondria; myofibrils and sarcoplasmic reticulum in muscle cells. *J. Exp. Biol.* **2003**, *206*, 2059–2072. [CrossRef]
5. Kaasik, A.; Veksler, V.; Boehm, E.; Novotova, M.; Minajeva, A.; Ventura-Clapier, R. Energetic crosstalk between organelles: Architectural integration of energy production and utilization. *Circ. Res.* **2001**, *89*, 153–159. [CrossRef]
6. Anesti, V.; Scorrano, L. The relationship between mitochondrial shape and function and the cytoskeleton. *Biochim. Biophys. Acta* **2006**, *1757*, 692–699. [CrossRef]
7. Kay, L.; Li, Z.; Mericskay, M.; Olivares, J.; Tranqui, L.; Fontaine, E.; Tiivel, T.; Sikk, P.; Kaambre, T.; Samuel, J.L.; et al. Study of regulation of mitochondrial respiration in vivo. An analysis of influence of ADP diffusion and possible role of cytoskeleton. *Biochim. Biophys. Acta* **1997**, *1322*, 41–59. [CrossRef]
8. Kuznetsov, A.V.; Javadov, S.; Guzun, R.; Grimm, M.; Saks, V.A. Cytoskeleton and regulation of mitochondrial function: The role of beta-tubulin II. *Front. Physiol.* **2013**, *4*, 82. [CrossRef]
9. Rizzuto, R.; Pinton, P.; Carrington, W.; Fay, F.S.; Fogarty, K.E.; Lifshitz, L.M.; Tuft, R.A.; Pozzan, T. Close Contacts with the Endoplasmic Reticulum as Determinants of Mitochondrial Ca^{2+} Responses. *Science* **1998**, *280*, 1763–1766. [CrossRef]
10. Csordás, G.; Renken, C.; Varnai, P.; Walter, L.; Weaver, D.; Buttle, K.F.; Balla, T.; Mannella, C.A.; Hajnóczky, G. Structural and functional features and significance of the physical linkage between ER and mitochondria. *J. Cell Biol.* **2006**, *174*, 915–921. [CrossRef]
11. Lawrie, A.M.; Rizzuto, R.; Pozzan, T.; Simpson, A.W. A role for calcium influx in the regulation of mitochondrial calcium in endothelial cells. *J. Biol. Chem.* **1996**, *271*, 10753–10759. [CrossRef] [PubMed]
12. Csordas, G.; Thomas, A.P.; Hajnoczky, G. Quasi-synaptic calcium signal transmission between endoplasmic reticulum and mitochondria. *EMBO J.* **1999**, *18*, 96–101. [CrossRef] [PubMed]
13. Pereira, A.J.; Dalby, B.; Stewart, R.J.; Doxsey, S.J.; Goldstein, L.S. Mitochondrial association of a plus end-directed microtubule motor expressed during mitosis in Drosophila. *J. Cell Biol.* **1997**, *136*, 1081–1090. [CrossRef] [PubMed]
14. Chan, D.C. Mitochondria: Dynamic organelles in disease, aging, and development. *Cell* **2006**, *125*, 1241–1252. [CrossRef] [PubMed]
15. Yaffe, M.P. Dynamic mitochondria. *Nat. Cell Biol.* **1999**, *1*, e149–e150. [CrossRef]
16. Knowles, M.K.; Guenza, M.G.; Capaldi, R.A.; Marcus, A.H. Cytoskeletal-assisted dynamics of the mitochondrial reticulum in living cells. *Proc. Natl. Acad. Sci. USA* **2002**, *99*, 14772–14777. [CrossRef]
17. Thomson, M. The regulation of mitochondrial physiology by organelle-associated GTP-binding proteins. *Cell Biochem. Funct.* **2002**, *20*, 273–278. [CrossRef]
18. Noskov, S.Y.; Rostovtseva, T.K.; Bezrukov, S.M. ATP transport through VDAC and the VDAC-tubulin complex probed by equilibrium and nonequilibrium MD simulations. *Biochemistry* **2013**, *52*, 9246–9256. [CrossRef]

19. Rostovtseva, T.K.; Sheldon, K.L.; Hassanzadeh, E.; Monge, C.; Saks, V.; Bezrukov, S.M.; Sackett, D.L. Tubulin binding blocks mitochondrial voltage-dependent anion channel and regulates respiration. *Proc. Natl. Acad. Sci. USA* **2008**, *105*, 18746–18751. [CrossRef]
20. Rostovtseva, T.K.; Gurnev, P.A.; Chen, M.-Y.; Bezrukov, S.M. Membrane lipid composition regulates tubulin interaction with mitochondrial voltage-dependent anion channel. *J. Biol. Chem.* **2012**, *287*, 29589–29598. [CrossRef]
21. Puurand, M.; Tepp, K.; Timohhina, N.; Aid, J.; Shevchuk, I.; Chekulayev, V.; Kaambre, T. Tubulin βII and βIII Isoforms as the Regulators of VDAC Channel Permeability in Health and Disease. *Cells* **2019**, *8*, 239. [CrossRef]
22. Guzun, R.; Gonzalez-Granillo, M.; Karu-Varikmaa, M.; Grichine, A.; Usson, Y.; Kaambre, T.; Guerrero-Roesch, K.; Kuznetsov, A.; Schlattner, U.; Saks, V. Regulation of respiration in muscle cells in vivo by VDAC through interaction with the cytoskeleton and MtCK within Mitochondrial Interactosome. *Biochim. Biophys. Acta* **2012**, *1818*, 1545–1554. [CrossRef] [PubMed]
23. Rostovtseva, T.K.; Bezrukov, S.M. VDAC inhibition by tubulin and its physiological implications. *Biochim. Biophys. Acta* **2012**, *1818*, 1526–1535. [CrossRef] [PubMed]
24. Williamson, J.R. Mitochondrial function in the heart. *Annu. Rev. Physiol.* **1979**, *41*, 485–506. [CrossRef] [PubMed]
25. Balaban, R.S. Regulation of oxidative phosphorylation in the mammalian cell. *Am. J. Physiol.* **1990**, *258*, C377–C389. [CrossRef] [PubMed]
26. Saks, V.A.; Kupriyanov, V.V.; Kuznetsov, A.V.; Kapelko, V.I.; Sharov, V.G.; Veksler, V.I.; Javadov, S.A. Quantitative evaluation of relationship between cardiac energy metabolism and post-ischemic recovery of contractile function. *J. Mol. Cell. Cardiol.* **1989**, *21*, 67–78. [CrossRef]
27. Saks, V.; Kuznetsov, A.; Andrienko, T.; Usson, Y.; Appaix, F.; Guerrero, K.; Kaambre, T.; Sikk, P.; Lemba, M.; Vendelin, M. Heterogeneity of ADP diffusion and regulation of respiration in cardiac cells. *Biophys. J.* **2003**, *84*, 3436–3456. [CrossRef]
28. Saks, V.; Dzeja, P.; Schlattner, U.; Vendelin, M.; Terzic, A.; Wallimann, T. Cardiac system bioenergetics: Metabolic basis of the Frank-Starling law. *J. Physiol.* **2006**, *571*, 253–273. [CrossRef]
29. Reipert, S.; Steinböck, F.; Fischer, I.; Bittner, R.E.; Zeöld, A.; Wiche, G. Association of mitochondria with plectin and desmin intermediate filaments in striated muscle. *Exp. Cell Res.* **1999**, *252*, 479–491. [CrossRef]
30. Milner, D.J.; Mavroidis, M.; Weisleder, N.; Capetanaki, Y. Desmin cytoskeleton linked to muscle mitochondrial distribution and respiratory function. *J. Cell Biol.* **2000**, *150*, 1283–1298. [CrossRef]
31. Timohhina, N.; Guzun, R.; Tepp, K.; Monge, C.; Varikmaa, M.; Vija, H.; Sikk, P.; Kaambre, T.; Sackett, D.; Saks, V. Direct measurement of energy fluxes from mitochondria into cytoplasm in permeabilized cardiac cells in situ: Some evidence for Mitochondrial Interactosome. *J. Bioenerg. Biomembr.* **2009**, *41*, 259–275. [CrossRef] [PubMed]
32. Gonzalez-Granillo, M.; Grichine, A.; Guzun, R.; Usson, Y.; Tepp, K.; Chekulayev, V.; Shevchuk, I.; Karu-Varikmaa, M.; Kuznetsov, A.V.; Grimm, M.; et al. Studies of the role of tubulin beta II isotype in regulation of mitochondrial respiration in intracellular energetic units in cardiac cells. *J. Mol. Cell. Cardiol.* **2012**, *52*, 437–447. [CrossRef] [PubMed]
33. Guzun, R.; Kaambre, T.; Bagur, R.; Grichine, A.; Usson, Y.; Varikmaa, M.; Anmann, T.; Tepp, K.; Timohhina, N.; Shevchuk, I.; et al. Modular organization of cardiac energy metabolism: Energy conversion; transfer and feedback regulation. *Acta Physiol.* **2015**, *213*, 84–106. [CrossRef] [PubMed]
34. Capetanaki, Y. Desmin cytoskeleton: A potential regulator of muscle mitochondrial behavior and function. *Trends Cardiovasc. Med.* **2002**, *12*, 339–348. [CrossRef]
35. McCormack, J.G.; Denton, R.M. The role of Ca^{2+} in the regulation of intramitochondrial energy production in heart. *Biomed. Biochim. Acta* **1987**, *46*, S487–S492.
36. Griffiths, E.J.; Rutter, G.A. Mitochondrial calcium as a key regulator of mitochondrial ATP production in mammalian cells. *Biochim Biophys Acta* **2009**, *1787*, 1324–1333. [CrossRef]
37. Clark, J.F.; Kuznetsov, A.V.; Radda, G.K. ADP-regenerating enzyme systems in mitochondria of guinea pig myometrium and heart. *Am. J. Physiol.* **1997**, *272 Pt 1*, C399–C404. [CrossRef]
38. Brdiczka, D. Function of the outer mitochondrial compartment in regulation of energy metabolism. *Biochim. Biophys. Acta* **1994**, *1187*, 264–269. [CrossRef]

39. Kuznetsov, A.V.; Veksler, V.; Gellerich, F.N.; Saks, V.; Margreiter, R.; Kunz, W.S. Analysis of mitochondrial function in situ in permeabilized muscle fibers; tissues and cells. *Nat. Protoc.* **2008**, *3*, 965–976. [CrossRef]
40. Villani, G.; Attardi, G. In vivo control of respiration by cytochrome c oxidase in human cells. *Free Radic. Biol. Med.* **2000**, *29*, 202–210. [CrossRef]
41. Kummel, L. Ca, Mg-ATPase activity of permeabilised rat heart cells and its functional coupling to oxidative phosphorylation of the cells. *Cardiovasc. Res.* **1988**, *22*, 359–367. [CrossRef] [PubMed]
42. Veksler, V.I.; Kuznetsov, A.V.; Sharov, V.G.; Kapelko, V.I.; Saks, V.A. Mitochondrial respiratory parameters in cardiac tissue: A novel method of assessment by using saponin-skinned fibers. *Biochim. Biophys. Acta* **1987**, *892*, 191–196. [CrossRef]
43. Saks, V.A.; Veksler, V.I.; Kuznetsov, A.V.; Kay, L.; Sikk, P.; Tiivel, T.; Tranqui, L.; Olivares, J.; Winkler, K.; Wiedemann, F.; et al. Permeabilized cell and skinned fiber techniques in studies of mitochondrial function in vivo. *Mol. Cell. Biochem.* **1998**, *184*, 81–100. [CrossRef] [PubMed]
44. Saks, V.A.; Belikova, Y.O.; Kuznetsov, A.V. In vivo regulation of mitochondrial respiration in cardiomyocytes: Specific restrictions for intracellular diffusion of ADP. *Biochim. Biophys. Acta* **1991**, *1074*, 302–311. [CrossRef]
45. Saks, V.A.; Vasil'eva, E.; Belikova, Y.O.; Kuznetsov, A.V.; Lyapina, S.; Petrova, L.; Perov, N.A. Retarded diffusion of ADP in cardiomyocytes: Possible role of mitochondrial outer membrane and creatine kinase in cellular regulation of oxidative phosphorylation. *Biochim. Biophys. Acta* **1993**, *1144*, 134–148. [CrossRef]
46. Varikmaa, M.; Bagur, R.; Kaambre, T.; Grichine, A.; Timohhina, N.; Tepp, K.; Shevchuk, I.; Chekulayev, V.; Metsis, M.; Boucher, F.; et al. Role of mitochondria-cytoskeleton interactions in respiration regulation and mitochondrial organization in striated muscles. *Biochim. Biophys. Acta* **2014**, *1837*, 232–245. [CrossRef]
47. Guzun, R.; Karu-Varikmaa, M.; Gonzalez-Granillo, M.; Kuznetsov, A.V.; Michel, L.; Cottet-Rousselle, C.; Saaremäe, M.; Kaambre, T.; Metsis, M.; Grimm, M.; et al. Mitochondria-cytoskeleton interaction: Distribution of β-tubulins in cardiomyocytes and HL-1 cells. *Biochim. Biophys. Acta* **2011**, *1807*, 458–469. [CrossRef]
48. Winter, L.; Kuznetsov, A.V.; Grimm, M.; Zeöld, A.; Fischer, I.; Wiche, G. Plectin isoform P1b and P1d deficiencies differentially affect mitochondrial morphology and function in skeletal muscle. *Hum. Mol. Genet.* **2015**, *24*, 4530–4544. [CrossRef]
49. Ball, E.H.; Singer, S.J. Mitochondria are associated with microtubules and not with intermediate filaments in cultured fibroblasts. *Proc. Natl. Acad. Sci. USA* **1982**, *79*, 123–126. [CrossRef]
50. Mose-Larsen, P.; Bravo, R.; Fey, S.J.; Small, J.V.; Celis, J.E. Putative association of mitochondria with a subpopulation of intermediate-sized filaments in cultured human skin fibroblasts. *Cell* **1982**, *31*, 681–692. [CrossRef]
51. Hirokawa, N. Cross-linker system between neurofilaments, microtubules and membranous organelles in frog axons revealed by quick-freeze, deep etching method. *J. Cell Biol.* **1982**, *94*, 129–142. [CrossRef] [PubMed]
52. Heggeness, M.H.; Simon, M.; Singer, S.J. Association of mitochondria with microtubules in cultured cells. *Proc. Natl. Acad. Sci. USA* **1978**, *75*, 3863–3866. [CrossRef] [PubMed]
53. Smith, M.G.; Simon, V.R.; O'Sullivan, H.; Pon, L.A. Organelle-cytoskeletal interactions: Actin mutations inhibit meiosis-dependent mitochondrial rearrangement in the budding yeast Saccharomyces Cerevisiae. *Mol. Biol. Cell.* **1995**, *6*, 1381–1396. [CrossRef] [PubMed]
54. Boldogh, I.R.; Pon, L.A. Interactions of mitochondria with the actin cytoskeleton. *Biochim. Biophys. Acta* **2006**, *1763*, 450–462. [CrossRef]
55. Morris, R.L.; Hollenbeck, P.J. Axonal transport of mitochondria along microtubules and F-actin in living vertebrate neurons. *J. Cell. Biol.* **1995**, *131*, 1315–1326. [CrossRef]
56. Boldogh, I.R.; Yang, H.C.; Nowakowski, W.D.; Karmon, S.L.; Hays, L.G.; Yates, J.R., 3rd; Pon, L.A. Arp2/3 complex and actin dynamics are required for actin-based mitochondrial motility in yeast. *Proc. Natl. Acad. Sci. USA* **2001**, *98*, 3162–3167.
57. Jensen, R.E. Control of mitochondrial shape. *Curr. Opin. Cell Biol.* **2005**, *17*, 384–388. [CrossRef]
58. Burgess, S.M.; Delannoy, M.; Jensen, R.E. MMM1 encodes a mitochondrial outer membrane protein essential for establishing and maintaining the structure of yeast mitochondria. *J. Cell Biol.* **1994**, *126*, 1375–1391. [CrossRef]
59. Berger, K.H.; Sogo, L.F.; Yaffe, M.P. Mdm12p, a component required for mitochondrial inheritance that is conserved between budding and fission yeast. *J. Cell Biol.* **1997**, *136*, 545–553. [CrossRef]

60. Dimmer, K.S.; Jakobs, S.; Vogel, F.; Altmann, K.; Westermann, B. Mdm31 and Mdm32 are inner membrane proteins required for maintenance of mitochondrial shape and stability of mitochondrial DNA nucleoids in yeast. *J. Cell Biol.* **2005**, *168*, 103–115. [CrossRef]
61. Sogo, L.F.; Yaffe, M.P. Regulation of mitochondrial morphology and inheritance by Mdm10p, a protein of the mitochondrial outer membrane. *J. Cell Biol.* **1994**, *126*, 1361–1373. [CrossRef] [PubMed]
62. Youngman, M.J.; Hobbs, A.E.; Burgess, S.M.; Srinivasan, M.; Jensen, R.E. Mmm2p, a mitochondrial outer membrane protein required for yeast mitochondrial shape and maintenance of mtDNA nucleoids. *J. Cell Biol.* **2004**, *164*, 677–688. [CrossRef] [PubMed]
63. John, G.B.; Shang, Y.; Li, L.; Renken, C.; Mannella, C.A.; Selker, J.M.; Rangell, L.; Bennett, M.J.; Zha, J. The mitochondrial inner membrane protein mitofilin controls cristae morphology. *Mol. Biol. Cell* **2005**, *16*, 1543–1554. [CrossRef] [PubMed]
64. Frederick, R.L.; McCaffery, J.M.; Cunningham, K.W.; Okamoto, K.; Shaw, J.M. Yeast Miro GTPase, Gem1p, regulates mitochondrial morphology via a novel pathway. *J. Cell Biol.* **2004**, *167*, 87–98. [CrossRef] [PubMed]
65. Paumard, P.; Vaillier, J.; Coulary, B.; Schaeffer, J.; Soubannier, V.; Mueller, D.M.; Brethes, D.; Di Rago, J.P.; Velours, J. The ATP synthase is involved in generating mitochondrial cristae morphology. *EMBO J.* **2002**, *21*, 221–230. [CrossRef] [PubMed]
66. Chen, H.; Detmer, S.A.; Ewald, A.J.; Griffin, E.E.; Fraser, S.E.; Chan, D.C. Mitofusins Mfn1 and Mfn2 coordinately regulate mitochondrial fusion and are essential for embryonic development. *J. Cell Biol.* **2003**, *160*, 189–200. [CrossRef]
67. Sesaki, H.; Jensen, R.E. Division versus fusion: Dnm1p and Fzo1p antagonistically regulate mitochondrial shape. *J. Cell Biol.* **1999**, *147*, 699–706. [CrossRef]
68. Griparic, L.; Van der Wel, N.N.; Orozco, I.J.; Peters, P.J.; Van der Bliek, A.M. Loss of the intermembrane space protein Mgm1/OPA1 induces swelling and localized constrictions along the lengths of mitochondria. *J. Biol. Chem.* **2004**, *279*, 18792–18798. [CrossRef]
69. Chen, H.; Chan, D.C. Emerging functions of mammalian mitochondrial fusion and fission. *Hum. Mol. Genet.* **2005**, *14*, R283–R289. [CrossRef]
70. Smirnova, E.; Griparic, L.; Shurland, D.L.; Van der Bliek, A.M. Dynamin-related protein Drp1 is required for mitochondrial division in mammalian cells. *Mol. Biol. Cell* **2001**, *12*, 2245–2256. [CrossRef]
71. Bleazard, W.; McCaffery, J.M.; King, E.J.; Bale, S.; Mozdy, A.; Tieu, Q.; Nunnari, J.; Shaw, J.M. The dynamin-related GTPase Dnm1 regulates mitochondrial fission in yeast. *Nat. Cell Biol.* **1999**, *1*, 298. [CrossRef]
72. James, D.I.; Parone, P.A.; Mattenberger, Y.; Martinou, J.C. hFis1, a novel component of the mammalian mitochondrial fission machinery. *J. Biol. Chem.* **2003**, *278*, 36373–36379. [CrossRef] [PubMed]
73. Cipolat, S.; Martins de Brito, O.; Dal Zilio, B.; Scorrano, L. OPA1 requires mitofusin 1 to promote mitochondrial fusion. *Proc. Natl. Acad. Sci. USA* **2004**, *101*, 15927–15932. [CrossRef] [PubMed]
74. Hermann, G.J.; Thatcher, J.W.; Mills, J.P.; Hales, K.G.; Fuller, M.T.; Nunnari, J.; Shaw, J.M. Mitochondrial fusion in yeast requires the transmembrane GTPase Fzo1p. *J. Cell Biol.* **1998**, *143*, 359–373. [CrossRef] [PubMed]
75. Cereghetti, G.M.; Scorrano, L. The many shapes of mitochondrial death. *Oncogene* **2006**, *25*, 4717–4724. [CrossRef] [PubMed]
76. Chen, L.; Gong, Q.; Stice, J.P.; Knowlton, A.A. Mitochondrial OPA1, apoptosis, and heart failure. *Cardiovasc. Res.* **2009**, *84*, 91–99. [CrossRef] [PubMed]
77. Javadov, S.; Rajapurohitam, V.; Kilić, A.; Hunter, J.C.; Zeidan, A.; Said Faruq, N.; Escobales, N.; Karmazyn, M. Expression of mitochondrial fusion-fission proteins during post-infarction remodeling: The effect of NHE-1 inhibition. *Basic Res. Cardiol.* **2011**, *106*, 99–109. [CrossRef] [PubMed]
78. Adaniya, S.M.; O-Uchi, J.; Cypress, M.W.; Kusakari, Y.; Jhun, B.S. Posttranslational modifications of mitochondrial fission and fusion proteins in cardiac physiology and pathophysiology. *Am. J. Physiol. Cell Physiol.* **2019**, *316*, C583–C604. [CrossRef]
79. Olichon, A.; Guillou, E.; Delettre, C.; Landes, T.; Arnaune-Pelloquin, L.; Emorine, L.J.; Mils, V.; Daloyau, M.; Hamel, C.; Amati-Bonneau, P.; et al. Mitochondrial dynamics and disease. *Biochim. Biophys. Acta* **2006**, *1763*, 500–509. [CrossRef]
80. Karbowski, M.; Norris, K.L.; Cleland, M.M.; Jeong, S.Y.; Youle, R.J. Role of Bax and Bak in mitochondrial morphogenesis. *Nature* **2006**, *443*, 658–662. [CrossRef]

81. Karbowski, M.; Youle, R.J. Dynamics of mitochondrial morphology in healthy cells and during apoptosis. *Cell Death Differ.* **2003**, *10*, 870–880. [CrossRef] [PubMed]
82. Perfettini, J.L.; Roumier, T.; Kroemer, G. Mitochondrial fusion and fission in the control of apoptosis. *Trends Cell Biol.* **2005**, *15*, 179–183. [CrossRef] [PubMed]
83. Vale, R.D.; Funatsu, T.; Pierce, D.W.; Romberg, L.; Harada, Y.; Yanagida, T. Direct observation of single kinesin molecules moving along microtubules. *Nature* **1996**, *380*, 451–453. [CrossRef] [PubMed]
84. Vale, R.D. The molecular motor toolbox for intracellular transport. *Cell* **2003**, *112*, 467–480. [CrossRef]
85. Hollenbeck, P.J.; Saxton, W.M. The axonal transport of mitochondria. *J. Cell Sci.* **2005**, *118*, 5411–5419. [CrossRef] [PubMed]
86. Li, Y.C.; Zhai, X.Y.; Ohsato, K.; Futamata, H.; Shimada, O.; Atsumi, S. Mitochondrial accumulation in the distal part of the initial segment of chicken spinal motoneurons. *Brain Res.* **2004**, *1026*, 235–243. [CrossRef] [PubMed]
87. Chada, S.R.; Hollenbeck, P.J. Mitochondrial movement and positioning in axons: The role of growth factor signaling. *J. Exp. Biol.* **2003**, *206*, 1985–1992. [CrossRef]
88. Boldogh, I.R.; Pon, L.A. Mitochondria on the move. *Trends Cell Biol.* **2007**, *17*, 502–510. [CrossRef]
89. Kuznetsov, A.V.; Hermann, M.; Saks, V.; Hengster, P.; Margreiter, R. The cell type specificity of mitochondrial dynamics. *Int. J. Biochem. Cell Biol.* **2009**, *41*, 1928–1939. [CrossRef]
90. Hudder, A.; Nathanson, L.; Deutscher, M.P. Organization of mammalian cytoplasm. *Mol. Cell Biol.* **2003**, *23*, 9318–9326. [CrossRef]
91. Toivola, D.M.; Tao, G.Z.; Habtezion, A.; Liao, J.; Omary, M.B. Cellular integrity plus: Organelle-related and protein-targeting functions of intermediate filaments. *Trends Cell Biol.* **2005**, *15*, 608–617. [CrossRef] [PubMed]
92. Mado, K.; Chekulayev, V.; Shevchuk, I.; Puurand, M.; Tepp, K.; Kaambre, T. On the role of tubulin; plectin; desmin; and vimentin in the regulation of mitochondrial energy fluxes in muscle cells. *Am. J. Physiol. Cell Physiol.* **2019**, *316*, C657–C667. [CrossRef] [PubMed]
93. Hayashi, T.; Martone, M.E.; Yu, Z.; Thor, A.; Doi, M.; Holst, M.J.; Ellisman, M.H.; Hoshijima, M. Three-dimensional electron microscopy reveals new details of membrane systems for Ca^{2+} signaling in the heart. *J. Cell Sci.* **2009**, *122*, 1005–1013. [CrossRef] [PubMed]
94. Lebiedzinska, M.; Szabadkai, G.; Jones, A.W.; Duszynski, J.; Wieckowski, M.R. Interactions between the endoplasmic reticulum; mitochondria; plasma membrane and other subcellular organelles. *Int. J. Biochem. Cell Biol.* **2009**, *41*, 1805–1816. [CrossRef] [PubMed]
95. Viola, H.M.; Hool, L.C. How does calcium regulate mitochondrial energetics in the heart?—New insights. *Heart Lung Circ.* **2014**, *23*, 602–609. [CrossRef]
96. Van Vliet, A.R.; Agostinis, P. Mitochondria-Associated Membranes and ER Stress. *Curr. Top. Microbiol. Immunol.* **2018**, *414*, 73–102.
97. Zhu, L.; Ling, S.; Yu, X.-D.; Venkatesh, L.K.; Subramanian, T.; Chinnadurai, G.; Kuo, T.H. Modulation of Mitochondrial Ca^{2+} Homeostasis by Bcl-2. *J. Biol. Chem.* **1999**, *274*, 33267–33273. [CrossRef]
98. Pinton, P.; Ferrari, D.; Rapizzi, E.; Virgilio, F.D.; Pozzan, T.; Rizzuto, R. The Ca2+ concentration of the endoplasmic reticulum is a key determinant of ceramide-induced apoptosis: Significance for the molecular mechanism of Bcl-2 action. *EMBO J.* **2001**, *20*, 2690–2701. [CrossRef]
99. Szymański, J.; Janikiewicz, J.; Michalska, B.; Patalas-Krawczyk, P.; Perrone, M.; Ziółkowski, W.; Duszyński, J.; Pinton, P.; Dobrzyń, A.; Więckowski, M.R. Interaction of Mitochondria with the Endoplasmic Reticulum and Plasma Membrane in Calcium Homeostasis; Lipid Trafficking and Mitochondrial Structure. *Int. J. Mol. Sci.* **2017**, *18*, 1576. [CrossRef]
100. Simmen, T.; Tagaya, M. Organelle Communication at Membrane Contact Sites (MCS): From Curiosity to Center Stage in Cell Biology and Biomedical Research. *Adv. Exp. Med. Biol.* **2017**, *997*, 1–12.
101. Henderson, C.A.; Gomez, C.G.; Novak, S.M.; Mi-Mi, L.; Gregorio, C.C. Overview of the Muscle Cytoskeleton. *Compr. Physiol.* **2017**, *7*, 891–944. [PubMed]
102. Costa, M.L.; Escaleira, R.; Cataldo, A.; Oliveira, F.; Mermelstein, C.S. Desmin: Molecular interactions and putative functions of the muscle intermediate filament protein. *Braz. J. Med. Biol. Res.* **2004**, *37*, 1819–1830. [CrossRef] [PubMed]
103. Tang, H.L.; Lung, H.L.; Wu, K.C.; Le, A.H.P.; Tang, H.M.; Fung, M.C. Vimentin Supports Mitochondrial Morphology and Organization. *Biochem. J.* **2008**, *410*, 141–146. [CrossRef] [PubMed]

104. Schwarz, N.; Leube, R.E. Intermediate Filaments as Organizers of Cellular Space: How They Affect Mitochondrial Structure and Function. *Cells* **2016**, *5*, 30. [CrossRef] [PubMed]
105. Thornell, L.-E.; Carlsson, L.; Li, Z.; Mericskay, M.; Paulin, D. Null Mutation in the Desmin Gene Gives Rise to a Cardiomyopathy. *J. Mol. Cell. Cardiol.* **1997**, *29*, 2107–2124. [CrossRef] [PubMed]
106. Kay, L.; Nicolay, K.; Wieringa, B.; Saks, V.; Wallimann, T. Direct evidence for the control of mitochondrial respiration by mitochondrial creatine kinase in oxidative muscle cells in situ. *J. Biol. Chem.* **2000**, *275*, 6937–6944. [CrossRef]
107. Dolder, M.; Wendt, S.; Wallimann, T. Mitochondrial creatine kinase in contact sites: Interaction with porin and adenine nucleotide translocase, role in permeability transition and sensitivity to oxidative damage. *Biol. Signals Recept.* **2001**, *10*, 93–111. [CrossRef]
108. Dolder, M.; Walzel, B.; Speer, O.; Schlattner, U.; Wallimann, T. Inhibition of the mitochondrial permeability transition by creatine kinase substrates. Requirement for microcompartmentation. *J. Biol. Chem.* **2003**, *278*, 17760–17766. [CrossRef]
109. Matveeva, E.A.; Venkova, L.S.; Chernoivanenko, I.S.; Minin, A.A. Vimentin is involved in regulation of mitochondrial motility and membrane potential by Rac1. *Biol. Open* **2015**, *4*, 1290–1297. [CrossRef]
110. Chernoivanenko, I.S.; Matveeva, E.A.; Gelfand, V.I.; Goldman, R.D.; Minin, A.A. Mitochondrial membrane potential is regulated by vimentin intermediate filaments. *FASEB J.* **2015**, *29*, 820–827. [CrossRef]
111. Seppet, E.K.; Eimre, M.; Anmann, T.; Seppet, E.; Peet, N.; Käämbre, T.; Paju, K.; Piirsoo, A.; Kuznetsov, A.V.; Vendelin, M.; et al. Intracellular energetic units in healthy and diseased hearts. *Exp. Clin. Cardiol.* **2005**, *10*, 173–183. [PubMed]
112. Saks, V.; Kuznetsov, A.V.; Gonzalez-Granillo, M.; Tepp, K.; Timohhina, N.; Karu-Varikmaa, M.; Kaambre, T.; Dos Santos, P.; Boucher, F.; Guzun, R. Intracellular Energetic Units regulate metabolism in cardiac cells. *J. Mol. Cell. Cardiol.* **2012**, *52*, 419–436. [CrossRef] [PubMed]
113. Summerhayes, I.C.; Wong, D.; Chen, L.B. Effect of microtubules and intermediate filaments on mitochondrial distribution. *J. Cell Sci.* **1983**, *61*, 87–105. [PubMed]
114. Saetersdal, T.; Greve, G.; Dalen, H. Associations between beta-tubulin and mitochondria in adult isolated heart myocytes as shown by immunofluorescence and immunoelectron microscopy. *Histochemistry* **1990**, *95*, 1–10. [CrossRef]
115. Winter, L.; Abrahamsberg, C.; Wiche, G. Plectin isoform 1b mediates mitochondrion-intermediate lament network linkage and controls organelle shape. *J. Cell Biol.* **2008**, *181*, 903–911. [CrossRef]
116. Redeker, V. Mass spectrometry analysis of C-terminal posttranslational modifications of tubulins. *Methods Cell Biol.* **2010**, *95*, 77–103.
117. Hein, S.; Kostin, S.; Heling, A.; Maeno, Y.; Schaper, J. The role of the cytoskeleton in heart failure. *Cardiovasc. Res.* **2000**, *45*, 273–278. [CrossRef]
118. Kostin, S.; Hein, S.; Arnon, E.; Scholz, D.; Schaper, J. The cytoskeleton and related proteins in the human failing heart. *Heart Fail. Rev.* **2000**, *5*, 271–280. [CrossRef]
119. Tagawa, H.; Koide, M.; Sato, H.; Zile, M.R.; Carabello, B.A.; Cooper, G. Cytoskeletal role in the transition from compensated to decompensated hypertrophy during adult canine left ventricular pressure overloading. *Circ. Res* **1998**, *82*, 751–761. [CrossRef]
120. Guerrero, K.; Monge, C.; Bruckner, A.; Puurand, U.; Kadaja, L.; Kaambre, T.; Seppet, E.; Saks, V. Study of possible interactions of tubulin; microtubular network; and STOP protein with mitochondria in muscle cells. *Mol. Cell. Biochem.* **2010**, *337*, 239–249. [CrossRef]
121. Carré, M.; André, N.; Carles, G.; Borghi, H.; Brichese, L.; Briand, C.; Braguer, D. Tubulin is an inherent component of mitochondrial membranes that interacts with the voltage-dependent anion channel. *J. Biol. Chem.* **2002**, *277*, 33664–33669. [CrossRef] [PubMed]
122. Rostovtseva, T.K.; Bezrukov, S.M. VDAC regulation: Role of cytosolic proteins and mitochondrial lipids. *J. Bioenerg. Biomembr.* **2008**, *40*, 163–170. [CrossRef] [PubMed]
123. Gurnev, P.A.; Queralt-Martin, M.; Aguilella, V.M.; Rostovtseva, T.K.; Bezrukov, S.M. Probing tubulin-blocked state of VDAC by varying membrane surface charge. *Biophys. J.* **2012**, *102*, 2070–2076. [CrossRef] [PubMed]
124. Monge, C.; Beraud, N.; Kuznetsov, A.V.; Rostovtseva, T.; Sackett, D.; Schlattner, U.; Vendelin, M.; Saks, V.A. Regulation of respiration in brain mitochondria and synaptosomes: Restrictions of ADP diffusion in situ, roles of tubulin, and mitochondrial creatine kinase. *Mol. Cell. Biochem.* **2008**, *318*, 147–165. [CrossRef]

125. Janke, C.; Kneussel, M. Tubulin post-translational modifications: Encoding functions on the neuronal microtubule cytoskeleton. *Trends Neurosci.* **2010**, *33*, 362–372. [CrossRef]
126. Luduena, R.F. Multiple forms of tubulin: Different gene products and covalent modifications. *Int. Rev. Cytol.* **1998**, *178*, 207–275.
127. Verhey, K.J.; Gaertig, J. The tubulin code. *Cell Cycle* **2007**, *6*, 2152–2160. [CrossRef]
128. Kuznetsov, A.V.; Tiivel, T.; Sikk, P.; Kaambre, T.; Kay, L.; Daneshrad, Z.; Rossi, A.; Kadaja, L.; Peet, N.; Seppet, E.; et al. Striking difference between slow and fast twitch muscles in the kinetics of regulation of respiration by ADP in the cells in vivo. *Eur. J. Biochem.* **1996**, *241*, 909–915. [CrossRef]
129. Warburg, O. On respiratory impairment in cancer cells. *Science* **1956**, *124*, 269–270.
130. Gogvadze, V.; Zhivotovsky, B.; Orrenius, S. The Warburg effect and mitochondrial stability in cancer cells. *Mol. Asp. Med.* **2010**, *31*, 60–74. [CrossRef]
131. Hsu, P.P.; Sabatini, D.M. Cancer cell metabolism: Warburg and beyond. *Cell* **2008**, *134*, 703–707. [CrossRef] [PubMed]
132. Vander Heiden, M.G.; Cantley, L.C.; Thompson, C.B. Understanding the Warburg effect: The metabolic requirements of cell proliferation. *Science* **2009**, *324*, 1029–1033. [CrossRef] [PubMed]
133. Kuznetsov, A.V.; Mayboroda, O.; Kunz, D.; Winkler, K.; Schubert, W.; Kunz, W.S. Functional imaging of mitochondria in saponin-permeabilized mice muscle fibers. *J. Cell Biol.* **1998**, *140*, 1091–1099. [CrossRef] [PubMed]
134. Kuznetsov, A.V.; Usson, Y.; Leverve, X.; Margreiter, R. Subcellular heterogeneity of mitochondrial function and dysfunction: Evidence obtained by confocal imaging. *Mol. Cell. Biochem.* **2004**, *256*, 359–365. [CrossRef]
135. Romashko, D.N.; Marban, E.; O'Rourke, B. Subcellular metabolic transients and mitochondrial redox waves in heart cells. *Proc. Natl. Acad. Sci. USA* **1998**, *95*, 1618–1623. [CrossRef]
136. Anmann, T.; Guzun, R.; Beraud, N.; Pelloux, S.; Kuznetsov, A.V.; Kogerman, L.; Kaambre, T.; Sikk, P.; Paju, K.; Peet, N.; et al. Different kinetics of the regulation of respiration in permeabilized cardiomyocytes and in HL-1 cardiac cells. Importance of cell structure/organization for respiration regulation. *Biochim. Biophys. Acta* **2006**, *1757*, 1597–1606. [CrossRef]
137. Kuznetsov, A.V.; Javadov, S.; Sickinger, S.; Frotschnig, S.; Grimm, M. H9c2 and HL-1 cells demonstrate distinct features of energy metabolism, mitochondrial function and sensitivity to hypoxia-reoxygenation. *Biochim. Biophys. Acta* **2015**, *1853*, 276–284. [CrossRef]
138. Konieczny, P.; Fuchs, P.; Reipert, S.; Kunz, W.S.; Zeöld, A.; Fischer, I.; Paulin, D.; Schröder, R.; Wiche, G. Myofiber integrity depends on desmin network targeting to Z-disks and costameres via distinct plectin isoforms. *J. Cell Biol.* **2008**, *181*, 667–681. [CrossRef]
139. Fuchs, E.; Yang, Y. Crossroads on cytoskeletal highways. *Cell* **1999**, *98*, 547–550. [CrossRef]
140. Rezniczek, G.A.; Abrahamsberg, C.; Fuchs, P.; Spazierer, D.; Wiche, G. Plectin 5′-transcript diversity: Short alternative sequences determine stability of gene products, initiation of translation and subcellular localization of isoforms. *Hum. Mol. Genet.* **2003**, *12*, 3181–3194. [CrossRef]
141. Rezniczek, G.A.; Konieczny, P.; Nikolic, B.; Reipert, S.; Schneller, D.; Abrahamsberg, C.; Davies, K.E.; Winder, S.J.; Wiche, G. Plectin 1f scaffolding at the sarcolemma of dystrophic (mdx) muscle fibers through multiple interactions with beta-dystroglycan. *J. Cell Biol.* **2007**, *176*, 965–977. [CrossRef] [PubMed]
142. Reimann, J.; Kunz, W.S.; Vielhaber, S.; Kappes-Horn, K.; Schröder, R. Mitochondrial dysfunction in myofibrillar myopathy. *Neuropathol. Appl. Neurobiol.* **2003**, *29*, 45–51. [CrossRef] [PubMed]
143. Schröder, R.; Kunz, W.S.; Rouan, F.; Pfendner, E.; Tolksdorf, K.; Kappes-Horn, K.; Altenschmidt-Mehring, M.; Knoblich, R.; Van der Ven, P.F.M.; Reimann, J.; et al. Disorganization of the desmin cytoskeleton and mitochondrial dysfunction in plectin-related epidermolysis bullosa simplex with muscular dystrophy. *J. Neuropathol. Exp. Neurol.* **2002**, *61*, 520–530. [CrossRef] [PubMed]
144. Prosser, B.L.; Ward, C.W.; Lederer, W.J. X-ROS signaling: Rapid mechano-chemo transduction in heart. *Science* **2011**, *333*, 1440–1445. [CrossRef]
145. Miragoli, M.; Cabassi, A. Mitochondrial Mechanosensor Microdomains in Cardiovascular Disorders. *Adv. Exp. Med. Biol.* **2017**, *982*, 247–264.
146. Iribe, G.; Kaihara, K.; Yamaguchi, Y.; Nakaya, M.; Inoue, R.; Naruse, K. Mechano-sensitivity of mitochondrial function in mouse cardiac myocytes. *Prog. Biophys. Mol. Biol.* **2017**, *130 Pt B*, 315–322. [CrossRef]
147. Bartolák-Suki, E.; Imsirovic, J.; Nishibori, Y.; Krishnan, R.; Suki, B. Regulation of Mitochondrial Structure and Dynamics by the Cytoskeleton and Mechanical Factors. *Int. J. Mol. Sci.* **2017**, *18*, 1812. [CrossRef]

148. Kaasik, A.; Kuum, M.; Joubert, F.; Wilding, J.; Ventura-Clapier, R.; Veksler, V. Mitochondria as a source of mechanical signals in cardiomyocytes. *Cardiovasc. Res.* **2010**, *87*, 83–91. [CrossRef]
149. Khurana, T.S.; Davies, K.E. Pharmacological strategies for muscular dystrophy. *Nat. Rev. Drug Discov.* **2003**, *2*, 379–390. [CrossRef]
150. Prins, K.W.; Humston, J.L.; Mehta, A.; Tate, V.; Ralston, E.; Ervasti, J.M. Dystrophin is a microtubule-associated protein. *J. Cell Biol.* **2009**, *186*, 363–369. [CrossRef]
151. Allen, D.G.; Whitehead, N.P.; Froehner, S.C. Absence of Dystrophin Disrupts Skeletal Muscle Signaling: Roles of Ca^{2+}, Reactive Oxygen Species, and Nitric Oxide in the Development of Muscular Dystrophy. *Physiol. Rev.* **2016**, *96*, 253–305. [CrossRef]
152. Kuznetsov, A.V.; Winkler, K.; Wiedemann, F.; Von Bossanyi, P.; Dietzmann, K.; Kunz, W.S. Impaired mitochondrial oxidative phosphorylation in skeletal muscle of the dystrophin-deficient mdx mouse. *Mol. Cell. Biochem.* **1998**, *183*, 87–96. [CrossRef]
153. Randazzo, D.; Khalique, U.; Belanto, J.J.; Kenea, A.; Talsness, D.M.; Olthoff, J.T.; Tran, M.D.; Zaal, K.J.; Pak, K.; Pinal-Fernandez, I.; et al. Persistent upregulation of the β-tubulin tubb6, linked to muscle regeneration, is a source of microtubule disorganization in dystrophic muscle. *Hum. Mol. Genet.* **2019**, *28*, 1117–1135. [CrossRef] [PubMed]
154. Ganote, C.; Armstrong, S. Ischaemia and the myocyte cytoskeleton: Review and speculation. *Cardiovasc. Res.* **1993**, *27*, 1387–1403. [CrossRef] [PubMed]
155. Bagur, R.; Tanguy, S.; Foriel, S.; Grichine, A.; Sanchez, C.; Pernet-Gallay, K.; Kaambre, T.; Kuznetsov, A.V.; Usson, Y.; Boucher, F.; et al. The impact of cardiac ischemia/reperfusion on the mitochondria-cytoskeleton interactions. *Biochim. Biophys. Acta* **2016**, *1862*, 1159–1171. [CrossRef] [PubMed]
156. Perricone, A.J.; Vander Heide, R.S. Novel therapeutic strategies for ischemic heart disease. *Pharm. Res.* **2014**, *89*, 36–45. [CrossRef]
157. Kuznetsov, A.V.; Javadov, S.; Margreiter, R.; Grimm, M.; Hagenbuchner, J.; Ausserlechner, M.J. The Role of Mitochondria in the Mechanisms of Cardiac Ischemia-Reperfusion Injury. *Antioxidants* **2019**, *8*, 454. [CrossRef]
158. Saks, V.A.; Belikova, Y.O.; Kuznetsov, A.V.; Khuchua, Z.A.; Branishte, T.; Semenovsky, M.L.; Naumov, V.G. Phosphocreatine pathway for intracellular energy transport: Facilitation of restricted diffusion of ADP in cardiomyocytes and alterations in cardiomyopathy. *Am. J. Physiol.* **1991**, *261*, 30–38.
159. Khuchua, Z.A.; Kuznetsov, A.V.; Grishin, M.N.; Ventura-Clapier, R.; Saks, V.A. Alterations in the creatine kinase system in the cardiomyopathic hamsters. *Biochem. Biophys. Res. Commun.* **1989**, *165*, 748–757. [CrossRef]
160. Ventura-Clapier, R.; Garnier, A.; Veksler, V.; Joubert, F. Bioenergetics of the failing heart. *Biochim. Biophys. Acta* **2011**, *1813*, 1360–1372. [CrossRef]
161. Cao, F.; Zervou, S.; Lygate, C.A. The creatine kinase system as a therapeutic target for myocardial ischaemia-reperfusion injury. *Biochem. Soc. Trans.* **2018**, *46*, 1119–1127. [CrossRef] [PubMed]
162. Pucar, D.; Dzeja, P.P.; Bast, P.; Juranic, N.; Macura, S.; Terzic, A. Cellular energetics in the preconditioned state: Protective role for phosphotransfer reactions captured by ^{18}O-assisted ^{31}P NMR. *J. Biol. Chem.* **2001**, *276*, 44812–44819. [CrossRef] [PubMed]
163. Devillard, L.; Vandroux, D.; Tissier, C.; Brochot, A.; Voisin, S.; Rochette, L.; Athias, P. Tubulin ligands suggest a microtubule-NADPH oxidase relationship in postischemic cardiomyocytes. *Eur. J. Pharm.* **2006**, *548*, 64–73. [CrossRef]
164. Devillard, L.; Vandroux, D.; Tissier, C.; Dumont, L.; Borgeot, J.; Rochette, L.; Athias, P. Involvement of microtubules in the tolerance of cardiomyocytes to cold ischemia-reperfusion. *Mol. Cell. Biochem.* **2008**, *307*, 149–157. [CrossRef] [PubMed]
165. Decker, R.S.; Decker, M.L.; Nakamura, S.; Zhao, Y.-S.; Hedjbeli, S.; Harris, K.R.; Klocke, F.J. HSC73-tubulin complex formation during low-flow ischemia in the canine myocardium. *Am. J. Physiol. Heart Circ. Physiol.* **2002**, *283*, H1322–H1333. [CrossRef]
166. Kay, L.; Rossi, A.; Saks, V. Detection of early ischemic damage by analysis of mitochondrial function in skinned fibers. *Mol. Cell. Biochem.* **1997**, *174*, 79–85. [CrossRef]
167. Boudina, S.; Laclau, M.N.; Tariosse, L.; Daret, D.; Gouverneur, G.; Bonoron-Adèle, S.; Saks, V.A.; Dos Santos, P. Alteration of mitochondrial function in a model of chronic ischemia in vivo in rat heart. *Am. J. Physiol. Heart Circ. Physiol.* **2002**, *282*, H821–H831. [CrossRef]

168. Ichas, F.; Mazat, J.P. From calcium signaling to cell death: Two conformations for the mitochondrial permeability transition pore. Switching from low- to high-conductance state. *Biochim. Biophys. Acta* **1998**, *1366*, 33–50. [CrossRef]
169. Halestrap, A.P. Regulation of mitochondrial metabolism through changes in matrix volume. *Biochem. Soc. Trans.* **1994**, *22*, 522–529. [CrossRef]
170. Ichas, F.; Jouaville, L.S.; Mazat, J.P. Mitochondria are excitable organelles capable of generating and conveying electrical and calcium signals. *Cell* **1997**, *89*, 1145–1153. [CrossRef]
171. Szabo, I.; Zoratti, M. Mitochondrial channels: Ion fluxes and more. *Physiol. Rev.* **2014**, *94*, 519–608. [CrossRef] [PubMed]
172. Halestrap, A.P.; Kerr, P.M.; Javadov, S.; Woodfield, K.Y. Elucidating the molecular mechanism of the permeability transition pore and its role in reperfusion injury of the heart. *Biochim. Biophys. Acta* **1998**, *1366*, 79–94. [CrossRef]
173. Bernardi, P.; Di Lisa, F. The mitochondrial permeability transition pore: Molecular nature and role as a target in cardioprotection. *J. Mol. Cell. Cardiol.* **2015**, *78*, 100–106. [CrossRef] [PubMed]
174. Javadov, S.; Karmazyn, M.; Escobales, N. Mitochondrial permeability transition pore opening as a promising therapeutic target in cardiac diseases. *J. Pharm. Exp.* **2009**, *330*, 670–678. [CrossRef] [PubMed]
175. Halestrap, A.P.; Clarke, S.J.; Javadov, S.A. Mitochondrial permeability transition pore opening during myocardial reperfusion—A target for cardioprotection. *Cardiovasc. Res.* **2004**, *61*, 372–385. [CrossRef]
176. Javadov, S.; Jang, S.; Parodi-Rullán, R.; Khuchua, Z.; Kuznetsov, A.V. Mitochondrial permeability transition in cardiac ischemia-reperfusion: Whether cyclophilin D is a viable target for cardioprotection? *Cell. Mol. Life Sci.* **2017**, *74*, 2795–2813. [CrossRef]
177. Ramos, S.V.; Hughes, M.C.; Perry, C.G.R. Altered skeletal muscle microtubule-mitochondrial VDAC2 binding is related to bioenergetic impairments after paclitaxel but not vinblastine chemotherapies. *Am. J. Physiol. Cell Physiol.* **2019**, *316*, C449–C455. [CrossRef]
178. Santulli, G.; Xie, W.; Reiken, S.R.; Marks, A.R. Mitochondrial calcium overload is a key determinant in heart failure. *Proc. Natl. Acad. Sci. USA* **2015**, *112*, 11389–11394. [CrossRef]
179. Tahrir, F.G.; Shanmughapriya, S.; Ahooyi, T.M.; Knezevic, T.; Gupta, M.K.; Kontos, C.D.; McClung, J.M.; Madesh, M.; Gordon, J.; Feldman, A.M.; et al. Dysregulation of mitochondrial bioenergetics and quality control by HIV-1 Tat in cardiomyocytes. *J. Cell. Physiol.* **2018**, *233*, 748–758. [CrossRef]
180. Sun, W.; Zhang, J.P.; Zhao, X.Y.; Guo, W.S. A chemical kinetic model for Ca^{2+} induced spontaneous oscillatory contraction of myocardium. *Biophys. Chem.* **2019**, *253*, 106221.
181. Yang, Y.; Tian, Y.; Hu, S.; Bi, S.; Li, S.; Hu, Y.; Kou, J.; Qi, J.; Yu, B. Extract of Sheng-Mai-San Ameliorates Myocardial Ischemia-Induced Heart Failure by Modulating Ca^{2+}-Calcineurin-Mediated Drp1 Signaling Pathways. *Int. J. Mol. Sci.* **2017**, *18*, 1825. [CrossRef] [PubMed]
182. Cerrone, M.; Montnach, J.; Lin, X.; Zhao, Y.-T.; Zhang, M.; Agullo-Pascual, E.; Leo-Macias, A.; Alvarado, F.J.; Dolgalev, I.; Karathanos, T.V.; et al. Plakophilin-2 is required for transcription of genes that control calcium cycling and cardiac rhythm. *Nat. Commun.* **2017**, *8*, 106. [CrossRef] [PubMed]
183. Yuan, F.; Woollard, J.R.; Jordan, K.L.; Lerman, A.; Lerman, L.O.; Eirin, A. Mitochondrial targeted peptides preserve mitochondrial organization and decrease reversible myocardial changes in early swine metabolic syndrome. *Cardiovasc. Res.* **2018**, *114*, 431–442. [CrossRef] [PubMed]
184. Gambardella, J.; Trimarco, B.; Iaccarino, G.; Santulli, G. New Insights in Cardiac Calcium Handling and Excitation-Contraction Coupling. *Adv. Exp. Med. Biol.* **2018**, *1067*, 373–385.
185. Chaanine, A.H.; Kohlbrenner, E.; Gamb, S.I.; Guenzel, A.J.; Klaus, K.; Fayyaz, A.U.; Nair, K.S.; Hajjar, R.J.; Redfield, M.M. FOXO3a regulates BNIP3 and modulates mitochondrial calcium, dynamics, and function in cardiac stress. *Am. J. Physiol. Heart Circ. Physiol.* **2016**, *311*, H1540–H1559. [CrossRef]
186. Kuznetsov, A.V.; Schneeberger, S.; Seiler, R.; Brandacher, G.; Mark, W.; Steurer, W.; Saks, V.; Usson, Y.; Margreiter, R.; Gnaiger, E. Mitochondrial defects and heterogeneous cytochrome c release after cardiac cold ischemia and reperfusion. *Am. J. Physiol.* **2004**, *286*, H1633–H1641. [CrossRef]
187. Beraud, N.; Pelloux, S.; Usson, Y.; Kuznetsov, A.V.; Ronot, X.; Tourneur, Y.; Saks, V. Mitochondrial dynamics in heart cells: Very low amplitude high frequency fluctuations in adult cardiomyocytes and flow motion in non-beating Hl-1 cells. *J. Bioenerg. Biomembr.* **2009**, *41*, 195–214. [CrossRef]

188. Yancey, D.M.; Guichard, J.L.; Ahmed, M.I.; Zhou, L.; Murphy, M.P.; Johnson, M.S.; Benavides, G.A.; Collawn, J.; Darley-Usmar, V.; Dell'Italia, L.J. Cardiomyocyte mitochondrial oxidative stress and cytoskeletal breakdown in the heart with a primary volume overload. *Am. J. Physiol. Heart Circ. Physiol.* **2015**, *308*, H651–H663. [CrossRef]
189. Tsutsui, H.; Tagawa, H.; Kent, R.L.; McCollam, P.L.; Ishihara, K.; Nagatsu, M.; Cooper, G. Role of microtubules in contractile dysfunction of hypertrophied cardiocytes. *Circulation* **1994**, *90*, 533–555. [CrossRef]
190. Koide, M.; Hamawaki, M.; Narishige, T.; Sato, H.; Nemoto, S.; DeFreyte, G.; Zile, M.R.; Cooper, G., IV; Carabello, B.A. Microtubule depolymerization normalizes in vivo myocardial contractile function in dogs with pressure-overload left ventricular hypertrophy. *Circulation.* **2000**, *102*, 1045–1052. [CrossRef]
191. Nederlof, R.; Eerbeek, O.; Hollmann, M.W.; Southworth, R.; Zuurbier, C.J. Targeting hexokinase II to mitochondria to modulate energy metabolism and reduce ischaemia-reperfusion injury in heart. *Br. J. Pharmacol.* **2014**, *171*, 2067–2079. [CrossRef] [PubMed]
192. Belmadani, S.; Poüs, C.; Fischmeister, R.; Méry, P.F. Post-translational modifications of tubulin and microtubule stability in adult rat ventricular myocytes and immortalized HL-1 cardiomyocytes. *Mol. Cell. Biochem.* **2004**, *258*, 35–48. [CrossRef] [PubMed]
193. Schaper, J.; Kostin, S.; Hein, A.; Elsasser, E.; Arnon, D.; Zimmermann, R. Structural remodelling in heart failure. *Exp. Clin. Cardiol.* **2002**, *7*, 64–68. [PubMed]

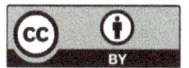

© 2020 by the authors. Licensee MDPI, Basel, Switzerland. This article is an open access article distributed under the terms and conditions of the Creative Commons Attribution (CC BY) license (http://creativecommons.org/licenses/by/4.0/).

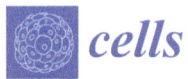

Review

Mitochondrial Gene Expression and Beyond—Novel Aspects of Cellular Physiology

Anna V. Kotrys and Roman J. Szczesny *

Institute of Biochemistry and Biophysics, Polish Academy of Sciences, 02-106 Warsaw, Poland; akotrys@ibb.waw.pl
* Correspondence: rszczesny@ibb.waw.pl; Tel.: +48-22-592-30-23

Received: 28 November 2019; Accepted: 17 December 2019; Published: 19 December 2019

Abstract: Mitochondria are peculiar organelles whose proper function depends on the crosstalk between two genomes, mitochondrial and nuclear. The human mitochondrial genome (mtDNA) encodes only 13 proteins; nevertheless, its proper expression is essential for cellular homeostasis, as mtDNA-encoded proteins are constituents of mitochondrial respiratory complexes. In addition, mtDNA expression results in the production of RNA molecules, which influence cell physiology once released from the mitochondria into the cytoplasm. As a result, dysfunctions of mtDNA expression may lead to pathologies in humans. Here, we review the mechanisms of mitochondrial gene expression with a focus on recent findings in the field. We summarize the complex turnover of mitochondrial transcripts and present an increasing body of evidence indicating new functions of mitochondrial transcripts. We discuss mitochondrial gene regulation in different cellular contexts, focusing on stress conditions. Finally, we highlight the importance of emerging aspects of mitochondrial gene regulation in human health and disease.

Keywords: mitochondria; mitochondrial gene expression; mtDNA; mtDNA transcription; mtRNA; post-transcriptional mtRNA processing; dsRNA; innate immunity; interferon response

1. Introduction: The Role of Mitochondria within the Cell

Mitochondria are present in the majority of eukaryotic cells, where they play a central role in many processes. They are hubs of energy production as sites of oxidative phosphorylation [1]. They are also engaged in maintaining an appropriate redox state and recycling oxidized electron carriers that are important for cell proliferation [2,3]. Moreover, mitochondria play a key role in cellular signaling, buffering calcium ions and regulating apoptosis processes [4,5]. Mitochondria are also the source of most of the cellular reactive oxygen species (ROS), which may impact on various cellular process [6,7]. Mitochondria take part in response to external stimuli, e.g., viral infection [4], and they are also the place where many basic processes related to innate immune intersect [8,9]. Mitochondrial malfunction is related to numerous pathological states in humans, such as cancer and neurodegeneration [10–12]. Furthermore, many human hereditary diseases are caused by mitochondrial dysfunction. Mutations in the mitochondrial genome or nuclear genes that encode mitochondrial proteins lead to primary and secondary mitochondrial diseases connected with improper mitochondrial function [13,14]. In this review, we will focus on the emerging aspects of mitochondrial biology and its implications in human health and we guide interested readers to detailed reviews on mitochondrial disorders [15–17].

Mitochondrial biogenesis is far more complex in comparison to other cellular organelles since they possess their own genome, which requires dedicated gene expression machinery [18–20]. As a consequence, mitochondrial protein production must be coordinated with the nucleocytoplasmic compartment for proper organelle homeostasis. Many nucleus-encoded proteins are needed for mitochondrial transcription, RNA processing, degradation and translation; all to produce just over a dozen proteins that are parts of the oxidative phosphorylation complexes encoded by the mitochondrial genome [18,19]. Recently, new findings deciphering the link between mitochondrial gene expression and cellular homeostasis were reported. Here, we review the basis of mitochondrial gene regulation with a focus on recent findings, highlighting new RNA-driven mechanisms by which mitochondria contribute to the regulation of cell biology in human health and disease.

2. Mitochondrial Genome—A Simple Molecule with Unorthodox Organization

Mitochondria are semiautonomous organelles possessing their own genome. Human mitochondrial DNA (mtDNA) is a ~16 kb circular molecule composed of double-stranded DNA [21]. Human mtDNA contains only a few genes, but all of them are essential for proper cell function, and mutations in mtDNA have dire consequences [13]. Although human mitochondria contain more than 1100 proteins [22], only 13 of them are encoded by mtDNA. The remaining 24 of the 37 genes present in human mtDNA encode RNAs required for the mitochondrial translational apparatus (22 tRNAs and 2 rRNAs) [19] (Figure 1). The rest of the proteins necessary for mitochondrial function are encoded in the nuclear genome and are imported into mitochondria upon synthesis in the cytoplasm [23]. These proteins are key factors in mtDNA replication, transcription and translation processes [23,24]. The presence of a distinct mitochondrial genome is linked to the endosymbiotic origin of this organelle [25,26]. Recent studies of the mitochondrial genome indicated that mitochondria evolved from a proteobacterial lineage [27]. The human mitochondrial genome was first described in the early 1960s and was one of the first genomes to be fully sequenced [28,29]. Since then, the molecular mechanisms of mtDNA expression have been intensively investigated; nevertheless, our knowledge about these processes is still not complete.

The human mitochondrial genome is tightly packed in nucleoprotein complexes called nucleoids [30]. The application of super-resolution microscopy and mass spectrometry-based techniques significantly contributed to the determination of the nucleoid characteristics [31–34]. It was shown that each nucleoid contains one or several copies of mtDNA [33,34] and is spatially organized by DNA-binding proteins [31]. More than 20 proteins were identified to copurify with mitochondrial nucleoids [32], among which the most abundant protein mitochondrial transcription factor A (TFAM) that may serve as a mtDNA copy number regulator [35]. Discrete nucleoid complexes are dispersed among the mitochondrial network in the cell [33]. An estimated number of mtDNA molecules per mitochondrion may vary greatly between tissues and range from less than a hundred to thousands [36–38]. Each mtDNA molecule can be independently segregated in daughter cells, as nucleoids are exchanged within the mitochondrial network upon fusion/fission processes [39,40]. More than one mtDNA sequence can be present within an individual, leading to so-called mitochondrial heteroplasmy. This can be caused by somatic mutations, heteroplasmy of the oocyte or paternal leakage of mtDNA [41,42]. For a long time, mtDNA was considered to be strictly maternally inherited [43]; nevertheless, few reports suggest paternal contribution in the inheritance of the mitochondrial genome [44,45].

There are several models describing the mechanism of mtDNA replication. Notably, the proposed models are not mutually exclusive. Instead, they were proposed to operate in a complementary mode depending on the tissue, cellular state or energy demand [46–48]. For a detailed review of mtDNA replication, please see Holt and Reyes [49] and Gustafsson et al. [50].

Notably, mutations in nuclear-encoded mitochondrial proteins that participate in mtDNA maintenance are implicated in mitochondrial disorders [51]. To date, nearly 300 pathogenic point mutations have been reported in the DNA polymerase gamma (POLG) gene encoding mtDNA replicase, and POLG mutations are one of the main causes of inherited mitochondrial disorders [51,52].

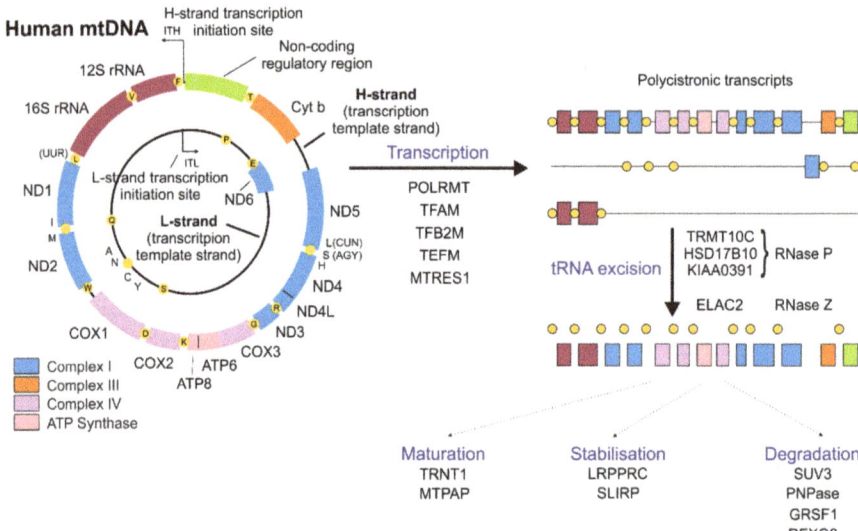

Figure 1. Schematic of human mtDNA and basic steps of mtRNA metabolism. Human mtDNA is a circular double-stranded molecule. Marked are template heavy (H-strand) and light (L-strand) strands of mtDNA. Marked are genes encoding subunits of Complex I (blue), III (orange), IV (violet) and subunits of ATP Synthase (pink). ND4/ND4L and ATP6/ATP8 open reading frames are overlapping and are included in bicistronic mRNAs. Genes encoding rRNAs are colored purple. Genes encoding tRNAs are represented as yellow dots with single letter code depicting their aminoacids. Mitochondrial transcription is initiated from L- and H- strand promoters (ITL and ITH, respectively) located within non-coding regulatory region (NCR). Transcription is driven by DNA-dependent RNA polymerase (POLRMT) with help of its co-factors: TFAM, TFB2M, TEFM and MTRES1. Mitochondrial transcription leads to the formation of three polycistronic transcripts that undergo further processing. Most of mitochondrial mRNAs and rRNAs are punctuated by tRNAs which are excised from the nascent RNA precursors by RNAse P and Z. Arisen transcripts may be subjected to various subsequent processes as maturation, stabilization, degradation, and modification. Selected factors engaged in these processes are presented.

3. Mitochondrial Transcription

MtDNA is composed of heavy (H-strand) and light (L-strand) strands (Figure 1) that can be distinguished by different sedimentation attributes in buoyant density ultracentrifugation due to the uneven distribution of guanines between DNA strands [21]. In humans, the G-rich H-strand serves as a template for the transcription of most mitochondrially encoded genes, while the transcription of the complementary L-strand results in the formation of mostly non-coding RNA (ncRNA) [53]. Only one protein-coding gene and 8 tRNAs are transcribed from the L-strand [53] (Figure 1). The exceptional ~1 kb, non-coding regulatory region (NCR) plays an important role both in mtDNA replication and transcription. The NCR plays an important role as a site of H-strand synthesis initiation [49,54]; moreover, transcription initiation start sites for both mtDNA strands (ITL, light-strand transcription initiation site, ITH, heavy-strand transcription initiation site) are also located within the NCR. The synthesis of RNA starts in both directions within the NCR and leads to the production of long, polycistronic transcripts (Figure 1) [55].

The human transcription apparatus appears to be simple and composed of a monomeric RNA polymerase (POLRMT) that is homologous to bacteriophage polymerases and only a few co-factors [19]. In addition to POLRMT, basic factors participating in the mitochondrial transcription process include TFAM, mitochondrial transcription factor B2 (TFB2M) and mitochondrial transcription elongation factor

(TEFM) (Figure 1) [19,56]. Initial in vitro experiments showed that transcription can proceed with the presence of only two proteins: POLRMT and TFB2M. Nevertheless, the efficiency of this transcription apparatus is rather low [57]. Thanks to recent structural studies, the detailed step-by-step initiation of mitochondrial transcription was revealed [56]. It was shown that mitochondrial transcription is initiated by the binding of TFAM to the promoter region and the following recruitment of POLRMT to TFAM-bound mtDNA near the transcription start site [58,59]. Next, TFB2M is recruited to induce and stabilize the open conformation of mtDNA. After initiation of RNA synthesis, TFAM and TFB2M are subsequently released, and the elongation factor TEFM is recruited to enable the transition into transcription elongation [56]. TEFM was proposed to increase the processivity of POLRMT and to enable nearly whole-genome transcription [60–62]. Additionally, TEFM was shown to participate in the regulation of a replication/transcription switch [62–64]. Recently, TEFM was also proposed to play a role in mitochondrial RNA (mtRNA) processing [65].

Termination of mtDNA transcription is far less understood than its initiation. Mitochondrial transcription termination factor 1 (MTERF1) plays an important role in the termination of mtDNA transcription initiated from the ITL; however, it is not clear which factors take part in the termination of mtDNA transcription initiated from the ITH [56]. MTERF1 binds specific sequences within the tRNA^{Leu} gene, causing DNA unwinding and base flipping (i.e., rotation of the nucleotide base outside the DNA double helix), leading to transcription termination [66,67]. MTERF1 was also suggested to prevent interference of the transcription complexes operating in opposite directions [68] and to prevent collision of transcription and replication machineries [69]. Several other MTERF proteins are conserved in vertebrates and plants [70]. Despite playing a role in mitochondrial gene expression, none of the MTERF2-4 proteins were shown to act as a transcription terminator in mammals [71–73]. This raises the question whether there are other termination factors yet to be discovered in the human mitochondria.

Among mitochondrial transcription machinery constituents, only TFAM mutations are well established to contribute to human disease [17]. TFAM binds DNA in both sequence-specific and nonspecific manners. The former enables the initiation of mitochondrial transcription [58], and the latter enables the compaction of the mitochondrial genome [74,75]. As mtDNA transcription by POLRMT may serve as a source of RNA primers for mtDNA replication [76], it seems that both sequence-specific and nonspecific manners of TFAM DNA-binding contribute to the maintenance of the mtDNA copy number (reviewed in [77]). TFAM knockout in mice causes severe depletion of mtDNA and is embryonically lethal [78]. In humans, mutations in the TFAM gene were shown to cause a decreased mtDNA copy number and impaired cellular respiration underlying progressive liver failure with neonatal onset [79]. Altered TFAM levels and related changes in the mtDNA copy number were also proposed to be associated with neurodegeneration [80].

Recently, some novel factors participating in mitochondrial transcription regulation were reported. Among them, an interesting example pertains to mitochondrial transcription rescue factor 1 (MTRES1), which was shown to interact with POLRMT and TFAM and to prevent stress-induced loss of mtRNAs by acting at the mitochondrial transcription initiation level [81]. Another example refers to mitochondrial ribosomal protein L7/L12 (MRPL12), whose mutations may lead to respiratory chain deficiency that manifest as growth retardation and neurological deterioration [82]. In addition to being a constituent of the mitochondrial ribosome, MRPL12 also exists in a "free", ribosome-unrelated matrix pool [83]. MRPL12 was shown to interact with POLRMT to regulate transcription [84]. It was proposed that MRPL12 may serve to coordinate transcription, ribosome biogenesis and/or protein synthesis processes [83,84]. Different roles of MRPL12 in mitochondrial gene regulation may be connected with the presence of two forms, the short and long forms, generated by proteolytic cleavage upon being imported into mitochondria, which may have distinct properties [85]. Several other factors, such as hormones, nuclear transcription factors and chromatin remodeling enzymes, were proposed to regulate mitochondrial transcription either by direct binding to mtDNA or by indirect regulation (reviewed in [86]).

4. Post-Transcriptional Regulation of mtRNAs

Mitochondrial transcription spans almost the entire mitochondrial genome, leading to the formation of three polycistronic transcripts (Figure 1) [19,55]. Two of them, resulting from transcription of either the H- or L-strand, encompass almost the entire genome and carry sequences corresponding to mRNAs, tRNAs, rRNAs and ncRNAs. The third transcript covers genes for two tRNAs (Phe and Val) and both rRNAs [19]. Further steps of cleavage and processing are required to obtain mature, functional RNAs [87].

In nascent precursor transcripts, most mitochondrial mRNAs and rRNAs are punctuated by tRNAs. The first stage of primary RNA processing is the excision of tRNA molecules from the polycistronic transcript, which leads to the formation of immature mRNAs and rRNAs [19,20]. This is an endonucleolytic cleavage mediated by RNAse P and elaC ribonuclease Z 2 (ELAC2), which act at the 5′ and 3′ ends of tRNAs, respectively, to release individual RNAs from polycistronic precursors [88,89]). Mitochondrial RNAse P, unlike the canonical RNase P present in the nucleus, is a complex of three proteins tRNA methyltransferase 10C (TRMT10C), hydroxysteroid 17-beta dehydrogenase 10 (HSD17B10) and protein-only RNase P catalytic subunit (PRORP) and does not contain an RNA component [88]. Released, immature transcripts undergo further processing steps or, as in the case of the majority of ncRNAs, are rapidly removed [20].

Due to the structural and transcriptional organization of the mitochondrial genome, most genes on the same strand are transcribed with equal efficiency, which leads to the formation of equal amounts of their precursors. Nevertheless, the levels of mature RNAs can differ significantly [90]. Although transcription initiated from the L-strand is more frequent than that of the H-strand [55], emerging non-coding RNAs are barely detectable [91]. These two examples show that post-transcriptional processes, especially mtRNA decay, play an important role in controlling mitochondrial gene expression to regulate steady-state levels of specific transcripts [90,92,93].

4.1. Degradation of mtRNAs

The machinery responsible for RNA decay in human mitochondria has remained unknown for many years. Studies performed within the last several years established that the mitochondrial degradosome, a complex of ATP-dependent RNA helicase SUPV3L1 (SUV3) and polynucleotide phosphorylase (PNPase also known as PNPT1), is a key player in mtRNA degradation [91,94]. The importance of mtRNA decay in maintaining mitochondrial homeostasis is underscored by the fact that the disruption of the SUV3 or PNPase gene is embryonically lethal in mice [95,96].

While SUV3 is a helicase that catalyzes the unwinding of RNA duplexes, an activity dependent on ATP hydrolysis by SUV3 [97], PNPase is a phosphorolytic 3′-5′ exoribonuclease, which catalyzes degradation of phosphodiester bonds in RNA [98]. In vitro experiments showed that PNPase is unable to degrade dsRNA substrates unless it forms a complex with SUV3 that unwinds the substrate for degradation [99]. The interaction between SUV3 and PNPase is a prerequisite for mtRNA degradation in vivo and occurs locally in D-foci [94]. The discovery of these structures shows that the RNA decay process in human mitochondria is spatially organized. Notably, components of the mitochondrial degradosome differ markedly in the submitochondrial localization. While SUV3 localizes only to the mitochondrial matrix [97], most of the PNPase is found in the mitochondrial intermembrane space [94,96]. Thus, only a fraction of the PNPase localizes to the mitochondrial matrix and cooperates with SUV3 in mtRNA degradation [94], whereas the rest of the PNPase functions in an SUV3-independent manner. Crystal structures of both proteins revealed the presence of some peculiarities [98,100]. Human PNPase, such as PNPases from other organisms, forms a trimer but has an untypical arrangement of RNA-binding domains [98]. Human SUV3 also has some distinctive features in terms of substrate binding, and it was even suggested that Suv3-like proteins may constitute a separate subfamily of helicases [100].

The main role of the degradosome appears to be clearing of non-coding mtRNA species, which arise mostly from transcription of the L-strand. Radiolabeling studies showed that under normal conditions, these RNAs are swiftly degraded [101]. Consequently, their steady-state levels are very low, and it is only when the degradosome function is impaired that they become readily detectable [91,94]. The degradosome complex was also found to be important in mt-mRNA turnover [94,102], 16S rRNA decay [103] and the exonucleolytic processing of the ND6 mRNA precursor [104]. The final products of the degradosome-mediated RNA decay are several nucleotides in length. These short RNA degradation intermediates are probably removed by RNA exonuclease 2 (REXO2), which is a postulated mitochondrial oligoribonuclease [105]. The activity of the mitochondrial degradosome is modulated by mtRNA binding proteins. While the complex of leucine rich pentatricopeptide repeat containing and SRA stem-loop interacting RNA binding proteins (LRPPRC-SLIRP complex) was suggested to suppress the degradosome-mediated decay of mitochondrial protein-coding RNAs [102]. G-rich RNA sequence binding factor 1 (GRSF1) was recently found to enhance the degradosome activity towards mtRNAs containing a G-quadruplex (G4), which are mostly non-coding mtRNAs [106].

4.2. Mitochondrial RNA-Binding Proteins (mtRBPs)

LRPPRC and SLIRP are among the best characterized noncatalytic mitochondrial RNA-binding proteins containing known RNA-interacting domains, pentatricopeptide repeats (PPR) and RRM domain, respectively. LRPPRC and SLIRP form a complex involved in the regulation of mtRNA stability, and the levels of both proteins are mutually dependent; silencing of LRPPRC results in the depletion of SLIRP and vice versa [107,108]. A recent study using RNA UV crosslinking and RNase footprinting procedures revealed that the LRPPRC-SLIRP complex modulates the secondary structures of mitochondrial transcripts, suggesting that this complex may serve as a chaperone for mtRNAs [109]. The presence of LRPPRC was shown to be important for the existence of a nontranslated, mitoribosome-unbound pool of mt-mRNAs [110]. In addition, LRPPRC was shown to be required for efficient polyadenylation of mt-mRNAs [108,110]. In mice, LRPPRC knockout is embryonically lethal [110], and in humans, mutations in the LRPPRC gene underlie Leigh syndrome, French Canadian type [111]. Recent studies suggest that LRPPRC may play a role in other various pathological states in humans, such as tumors or neurodegeneration (reviewed in detail by Cui et al. [112], emphasizing the very important role of this protein. SLIRP was shown to regulate the translation process by mediating the association of mtRNAs with mitoribosomes [113]. Surprisingly, although SLIRP knockout in mice results in extensive loss of mtRNAs, it is manifested only as a minor weight loss of the animals without any other observable phenotypes [113].

Another important RNA-binding protein, GRSF1, a member of the quasi-RRM (qRRM) family of RNA-binding proteins, was originally identified as a cytoplasmic poly(A)+ mRNA binding protein interacting with G-rich sequences [114]. Later, it was found that GRSF1 is targeted to mitochondria where it localizes to RNA-containing granules [115,116]. It was postulated that GRSF1 participates in the initial stages of polycistronic mtRNA precursor processing [116] and in the translation of some mt-mRNAs [115]. Recent findings, however, reported that GRSF1 takes part in the RNA surveillance pathway, showing that GRSF1 cooperates with the mitochondrial degradosome to regulate mtRNAs that contain G4s [106]. Vertebrates' mitochondrial genomes have exceptional GC skews, i.e., high guanine content on one strand. As a result, transcripts that are produced by transcription of the G-poor template (i.e., L-strand) are G-rich RNAs; thus, they are prone to form G4s structures. Since G4s are stable, their presence in RNA can hinder its degradation; nevertheless, steady-state levels of mt-ncRNAs that can form G4s are extremely low. GRSF1 was found to positively regulate the degradosome-dependent decay of G4-containing mitochondrial non-coding transcripts by binding and melting G4 structures, which in turn facilitates their degradation [106,117].

Recently, two studies reported novel mtRBP engaged in the regulation of mitochondrial gene expression [81,118]. The level of C6orf203/MTRES1 protein was found to be elevated in cells under stress, and this up-regulation of MTRES1 (mitochondrial transcription rescue factor 1) was shown to prevent mitochondrial transcript loss under perturbed mitochondrial gene expression [81]. MTRES1 associates with the mitochondrial transcription machinery and acts by increasing the mitochondrial transcription without influencing the stability of mitochondrial transcripts [81]. The protective function of MTRES1 depends on its RNA-binding ability since the mutated version incapable of RNA-binding does not prevent a decrease in the mitochondrial RNA [81]. MTRES1 was also shown to associate with a large subunit of the mitochondrial ribosome and to influence mitochondrial translation [118]. Interestingly, silencing of MTRES1 causes the down-regulation of transcripts originating only from NCR without influencing other transcripts [81], which cannot explain the decrease in mitochondrial translation observed in MTRES1 knockout [118]. In contrast, it was reported that the depletion of MTRES1 leads to alterations of the mt-mRNAs' association with the mitoribosome without influencing mitoribosome stability [118]. MTRES1 is an exciting example of mitochondrial RBP that can play a role in the regulation of mitochondrial gene expression at multiple levels. It is tempting to speculate that MTRES1 could serve as a regulatory factor coupling mitochondrial transcription and translation processes. It is possible that MTRES1 could act by interacting with mitochondrial transcription machinery and to facilitate loading of nascent mt-mRNAs on the mitoribosome. It cannot be excluded that MTRES1 could be a key regulator of mitochondrial transcription/translation coupling, especially under stress conditions. Importantly, another mtRBP, MRPL12, was shown to perform double functions in mitochondrial transcription and translation [83,84], highlighting the possible roles of MTRES1.

Another example of important players in the mitochondrial gene expression regulation concerns members of the FASTK family. Fas activated serine/threonine kinase (FASTK) and its homologs FASTKD1-5 are mitochondrially targeted RNA-binding proteins that play various roles in mtRNA metabolism as processing, translation and mitoribosome assembly proteins [104,112,119–121]. The FASTK family was reviewed in detail by Jourdain et al. [122]; therefore, we will not focus on these proteins here.

4.3. mtRNA Modifications

Mitochondrial RNAs undergo diverse modifications. One of the most common is adenylation of the 3' end. Human mt-mRNAs, with the exception of mt-ND6, are adenylated at the 3' ends, and this reaction is catalyzed by a noncanonical mitochondrial poly(A) polymerase (MTPAP) [123]. The role of mt-mRNAs' adenylation is not fully understood. For some mt-mRNAs, the addition of adenine residues at the 3' end is necessary to create a complete termination codon, as it is not encoded in the genome [21]. Initial studies reported some contradictory findings about the role of mt-mRNA polyadenylation, showing that changes in poly(A) tails had diverse effects on mt-mRNAs. Some of the transcripts were up-regulated, some were unaffected, and others were down-regulated [123–126]. This draws a speculation that individual transcripts may be differentially controlled, as it seems that adenylation may stabilize some transcripts while it may also direct other transcripts for degradation [20]. Notably, the polyadenylation pattern may vary within a cell type, and the same mt-mRNA can be adenylated to different extents in various cell types [127]. This individualized regulation is most likely achieved by transcript-specific protein-RNA interactions. In yeast, it was shown that each mt-mRNA has specific translation coactivators; moreover, it was proposed that they can function as a part of feedback control loops regulating translation efficiency according to current cell demands [128]. Similarly, the presence of the specific translation activator of cytochrome c oxidase I (TACO1) [129] was also detected in human cells. In addition to 3'-end adenylation, it was recently shown that human mt-mRNAs may also undergo other modifications, such as methylation [130,131] and pseudouridylation [132,133], unraveling an additional layer of mitochondrial gene expression regulation.

Mitochondrial tRNAs seem to be the most extensively modified among mtRNAs. Precursor tRNAs are modified at the 3' end by tRNA nucleotidyl transferase 1 (TRNT1), which adds the CCA sequence not encoded in the genome [134]. They also undergo several other modifications, which are essential for their stability and proper function [135]. Similarly, mt-rRNAs require several chemical modifications for proper folding, stability and correct mitoribosome assembly, underscoring the important role of RNA modifications in orchestrating various mitochondrial processes [24].

The mitochondrial RNA-binding proteome has been intensely studied, and novel members of this group have been continuously discovered. Among them are mtRNA modifying enzymes, mtRNA processing and mitoribosome assembly factors. Here, we delineated only selected aspects of mtRBP-associated regulation of mitochondrial gene expression, mostly related to mtRNA degradation. For further reading on other aspects of mitochondrial RBP function and detailed insight into mt-tRNA and mt-rRNA editing as well as the mitochondrial epitranscriptome, we guide interested readers to other reviews [136–138].

5. Mitochondrial Non-Coding Transcripts and Their Implications on Human Health

5.1. Mitochondrial Double-Stranded RNA (mt-dsRNA) and the Innate Immune Response

Convergent transcription, synthesis of antisense RNA or expression of hairpin-containing RNAs can result in the formation of double-stranded RNA (dsRNA) [139]. RNA:RNA molecules seem to have important signaling or regulatory roles [140–142], and the function of a particular dsRNA depends on its source and form and the proteins that interacts with it. It is known that the presence of dsRNA can induce the antiviral response and that properly processed dsRNA can regulate gene expression [140–142].

The expression of the human mitochondrial genome is especially prone to produce dsRNA molecules, as this genome is an extraordinary example of convergent transcription. This results in the synthesis of complementary RNAs that can subsequently hybridize and form dsRNA. Under normal conditions, most L-strand transcripts are quickly removed [91,94], which prevents the formation of intermolecular dsRNA. Nevertheless, even in physiological conditions, mt-dsRNAs can be detected [143]. We and others have found that mtDNA transcription is a significant source of dsRNA in humans and have shown that mt-dsRNA can play a signaling role and trigger the interferon response [143,144].

The interferon response pathway is a complex process that is part of the innate immunity response, which together with the adaptive system, provides protection from pathogens. This pathway is far from being fully understood; nevertheless, it can be divided into three major steps: (1) detection of a pathogen, (2) induction of interferon (IFN) expression, and (3) up-regulation of IFN-stimulated genes. Consequently, the cell starts producing anti-pathogen agents and reshapes already active processes to combat a pathogen, or at least hampers its spread [145].

The detection step involves recognition of "pathogen-associated molecular patterns" (PAMPs), which are viral or bacterial nuclei acids, or other molecules specific for microorganisms [146]. The recognition is performed by several families of host sensors collectively called pattern recognition receptors (PRRs), such as interferon induced helicase C domain-containing protein 1 (MDA5) and RNA helicase RIG-I. The binding of immunogenic dsRNA by MDA5 and RIG-I initiates an orchestrated cascade of events that results in the up-regulation of interferon- and interferon-stimulated genes [147]. Normally, this pathway is kept silent due to the mechanisms that help to discriminate between host and foreign nucleic acids, remove potentially immunogenic host-produced nucleic acids or keep them away from PAMP receptors. For example, dsRNA, which can activate MDA5 or RIG-I, is localized in the nucleus and mitochondria, precluding its interaction with MDA5 and RIG-I, which are localized in the cytoplasm.

Recently it was found that mt-dsRNA can be released from mitochondria and, once localized to the cytoplasm, can activate interferon-dependent cellular pathways. Notably degradosome constituents SUV3 and PNPase were established as major actors in the regulation of mt-dsRNA [144]. A crucial role was assigned to PNPase in preventing the induction of the interferon response by mt-dsRNA. PNPase controls mt-dsRNA at two different levels that are spatially separated. First, as a component of the mitochondrial degradosome, it prevents the accumulation of dsRNA by degrading mitochondrial antisense transcripts. The mechanism that determines specificity of PNPase towards antisense transcripts has not been fully uncovered. This may result from targeting of PNPase-SUV3 to G4 mtRNAs by GRSF1. Alternatively, but not mutually exclusive, sense transcripts are protected by mtRBPs, while unprotected antisense mtRNAs are exposed to PNPase-SUV3. This function of PNPase requires cooperation with SUV3 and takes place in the mitochondrial matrix. A second function of PNPase in controlling mt-dsRNAs takes place in the intermembrane space, where a fraction of PNPase prevents the release of mt-dsRNA into the cytosol. This function is SUV3-independent because the helicase is absent from the intermembrane space [97]. The dysfunction of SUV3 thus results in the accumulation of mt-dsRNA exclusively in the matrix but does not lead to the release of mt-dsRNA into the cytosol due to the protective activity of PNPase in the intermembrane space. Therefore, silencing of SUV3 does not stimulate interferon expression, while an increase in interferon levels is observed in PNPase-depleted cells. Since inactivation of the degradosome components causes a vast increase in non-coding L-strand transcripts [91,94,106], it is most likely that the mt-dsRNA that accumulates upon degradosome dysfunction results from intermolecular RNA-RNA interactions. The mechanism by which mt-dsRNA exits mitochondria is unknown, and its identification will be an important step in deciphering a role of mt-dsRNA in cell biology.

The protective role of PNPase is of great importance, as revealed by the fact that mutations in *PNPT1* (PNPase encoding gene) cause pathogenesis associated with the up-regulation of mt-dsRNA and interferon response [144,148]. A comparison of the type I interferon response across species, which involved 10 mammals and one bird, revealed PNPase as one of 62 core vertebrate interferon-stimulated genes [149]. Moreover, the PNPase protein level was observed to be higher in human cells infected by human respiratory syncytial virus (HRSV), a cause of serious infections in infants [150]. Taken together with the results on the protective role of PNPase in mt-dsRNA release, these data suggest that PNPase can be involved in the suppression of the IFN response. In fact, IFN-desensitization is an important process that enables cells to recover from IFN signaling [145]. Otherwise, prolonged activation of IFN-dependent pathways can lead to permanent dysregulation of cellular homeostasis. At the organismal level, this is manifested by the development of pathologies called type I interferonopathies. An example of such a disease is Aicardi–Goutières syndrome [151].

Interestingly, the contribution of mt-dsRNA to innate immunity was also observed in other studies. It was shown that the immune response can be modulated by mt-dsRNA via protein kinase RNA-activated (PKR). The canonical PKR-induced response comprises sensing of viral dsRNA by PKR following phosphorylation of the enzyme and altering cellular signaling pathways to promote an antiviral defense. Recent findings revealed that PKR can also be induced by endogenous RNAs, primarily by mt-dsRNAs [143]. PKR was proposed to associate with mitochondria, and mt-dsRNA sensing was suggested to take part in the mitochondrial matrix [143]. However, the proposed mechanism assumes that PKR needs to be exported to the cytoplasm to induce downstream signaling pathways. How PKR translocation to and from mitochondria is maintained remains unclear. It cannot be excluded that PKR induction may take place during mt-dsRNA escape into the cytoplasm, for example, upon aberrant PNPase function.

Notably, the role of mt-dsRNA in the modulation of innate immunity is not restricted to humans, as similar responses were reported in other species, suggesting that mt-dsRNAs are important regulators of the immune response across species. A study in a fly model demonstrated that disrupted mtRNA turnover leads to mt-dsRNA accumulation and altered immune response once mt-dsRNAs are released into the cytoplasm [152]. A study conducted in a murine model showed that the lack of p53 protein results in the activation of innate immunity by dsRNA of mitochondrial origin [153]. Consistent with previous findings on human cells [144], the immune response was shown to be dependent on MDA5 and RIG-I activation [153]. Altogether, these studies established mt-dsRNAs as important regulators of the immune response and revealed a new RNA-dependent mechanism by which mitochondria regulate cell fate.

5.2. Mitochondrial Long Non-Coding RNAs (mt-lncRNAs)

While most non-coding transcripts are swiftly degraded after synthesis, a pool of antisense mtRNAs exhibits some stability, resulting in their detection under normal conditions. These transcripts, called mirror RNAs, such as mirror ND2 [91,94], or long non-coding RNAs (ncND5, ncND6, and ncCytB) [154], are complementary to sense transcripts. Whether these mt-lncRNAs play any role remains to be elucidated; nevertheless, differential tissue-specific expression of these RNA species [154] suggests their potential regulatory function. One can imagine that by hybridizing to their coding counterparts, mt-lncRNAs could regulate the stability or translation efficiency of corresponding mtRNAs.

Other examples of lncRNAs possibly originating from mitochondrial transcription were proposed [155,156]. An example is a 2374 nt-long transcript containing an antisense 16S mt-rRNA sequence (inverted repeat) linked to the 5' end of the 16S mt-rRNA forming a long double-stranded structure called SncmtRNA (sense non-coding mitochondrial RNA). Interestingly, this transcript was reported to be overexpressed in proliferating but not resting tumor cells [155]. Further studies from the same group reported the presence of 2 other lncRNAs containing inverted repeats linked to the 5' end of the antisense 16S mt-rRNA, called ASncmtRNAs (antisense non-coding mitochondrial RNAs). These transcripts were found in normal proliferating cells and were reported to be down-regulated in tumor cells [156]. Detected transcripts were postulated to be hallmarks of proliferating tumor cells vs nontumor cells, which may play a role in regulating tumor progression [156,157].

A group of lncRNAs mapped to mtDNA was detected in patients with heart disease [158], and these include circulating mitochondria-derived lncRNA LIPCAR (long intergenic non-coding RNA predicting cardiac remodeling) [159]. The 5' end of this 781nt long chimeric lncRNA maps to the antisense of the mt-Cytb gene, while its 3' end maps to the antisense of the mt-COX2 gene. The LIPCAR transcript was shown to be up-regulated in the late stages after myocardial infarction and to be elevated in patients with chronic heart failure, serving as a potential biomarker of cardiac remodeling and cardiovascular mortality [159,160].

As presented here, ncRNAs encompass a group of potentially important molecules that can act in various ways to influence mitochondrial function and cell physiology (Figure 2). Their putative functions involve the regulation of mitochondrial translation and mtRNA stability. They may also function as sponges occupying mtRBPs. Moreover, their ability to form mt-dsRNA together with sense transcripts predisposes them to act as signaling molecules modulating the immune response. Altogether, mitochondrial non-coding RNAs extend the repertoire of potential mechanisms by which mitochondrial gene expression is regulated and influences cell physiology. Thus far, antisense transcripts were mostly studied or linked with non-physiological conditions. It remains to be seen whether this class of RNAs has any roles under normal, nonperturbed conditions.

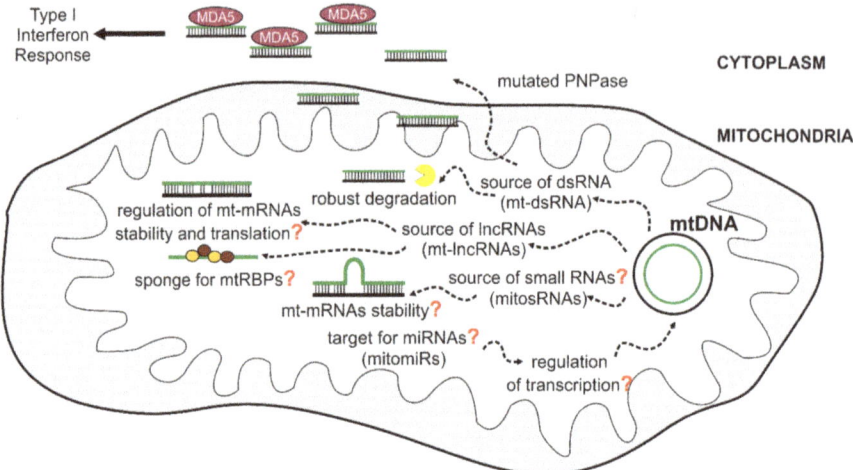

Figure 2. Cellular functions of mitochondria-derived transcripts. MtDNA may be a source and a target for non-coding RNA. Question mark indicates that the process or mechanism is currently undefined. Nucleus-encoded miRNAs (mitomiRs) are suggested to enter mitochondria and regulate mtDNA expression, nevertheless their exact import pathway is currently unexplained. Transcription of mtDNA may result in formation of small non-coding RNAs (mitosRNAs) which may interplay with mt-mRNAs stability. Mechanism of action of mitochondrial small non-coding RNAs is currently undefined. Long non-coding RNAs (mt-lncRNAs) may arise from mtDNA transcription and may regulate stability and transcription of mt-mRNAs or may serve as baits for mitochondrial RNA-binding proteins (mtRBPs). Convergent transcription of mtDNA may result in formation of double-stranded RNA (mt-dsRNA). Under normal conditions, L-strand derived transcripts are swiftly degraded which prevents formation of mt-dsRNAs. Dysfunction of PNPase causes accumulation of mt-dsRNA and its release into cytoplasm. Once released into the cytoplasm, mt-dsRNAs can induce type I interferon response via activation of MDA5 receptors.

6. Emerging Aspects of mtDNA Maintenance and Expression

6.1. mtDNA Polymerases and mtDNA Repair

POLG, responsible for replication of mtDNA, was long believed to be the only DNA polymerase present in mitochondria [161]. In contrast, recent reports suggest that there may be more than one DNA polymerase operating in mammalian mitochondria. Recent studies proposed several additional DNA polymerases to be implicated in mtDNA metabolism; nevertheless, some of those findings require further validation [162]. The most well-documented novel mtDNA polymerase, primase and DNA directed polymerase (PrimPol), takes part both in nuclear and mitochondrial DNA maintenance [163]. PrimPol may act as a primase forming DNA and RNA primers or as a DNA polymerase to extend the DNA primers and it is also able to perform translesion synthesis [164]. It seems that in human mitochondria, the main role of PrimPol is not to prime mtDNA replication but rather to rescue stalled replication forks by bypassing lesions or repriming DNA synthesis at the site of DNA damage. Further polymerases suggested to take part in mtDNA metabolism comprise polymerases Beta (POLB), Zeta (POLZ) and Theta (POLQ) [162]. These polymerases were proposed to participate in mtDNA repair (POLB) [165] (reviewed by Kaufman and Van Houten [166], mtDNA stability (POLZ) [167] and mtDNA maintenance (POLQ) [168].

Importantly, the discovery of novel mtDNA polymerases broadens the horizon for prospective mtDNA repair pathways. Mitochondria are thought to possess a limited DNA repair system comprising mainly base excision repair (BER). In mitochondrial BER, gap filling is driven by POLG assisted by several other proteins engaged in recognition and cleavage of a damaged DNA base, elimination of the abasic site, DNA 5'-end processing to generate substrate for POLG and, finally, ligation [169–174]. Other mtDNA repair pathways are being debated; nucleotide excision repair (NER) is thought to be absent from mitochondria, and only a few studies have reported mismatch repair to be present in mitochondria [52]. It is thus possible that novel enzymes could be engaged in these processes, expanding the repertoire of possible mtDNA repair pathways. This is especially important as mtDNA damage may have significant implications for human health [175].

6.2. mtDNA Editing

As mitochondria are organelles separated with double membranes that harbor strict import machinery, for a long time, it has seemed impossible to stably edit mtDNA in vertebrates. While proteins can efficiently be targeted and delivered into mitochondria, nucleic acid uptake remains controversial. As such, import of the nucleic acid component for mtDNA transformation and editing appeared to be a hurdle [176]. This difficulty can be overcome by the use of protein-only nucleases that can efficiently be engineered to target the mitochondrial matrix and induce sequence-specific double-strand breaks in mtDNA molecules [177]. This strategy takes advantage of mtDNA heteroplasmy and is based on the cleavage of mtDNA molecules harboring certain sequences (for example, pathological mutations). As a double-strand break repair pathway is not present in mitochondria, cleaved mtDNA molecules are rapidly degraded [178–180]. Remaining, noncleaved mtDNA molecules with normal sequences can then be replicated to reconstitute mtDNA content [181–184]. Two DNA editing platforms were introduced into mitochondria: transcription activator-like effector nucleases (TALEN) [185] and zing-finger nucleases (ZFN) [183]; these platforms enabled efficient heteroplasmy shift. In 2018, two breakthrough studies published back-to-back by the Minczuk and Moraes labs showed successful mtDNA editing in vivo [186,187]. In a mouse model of heteroplasmic mitochondrial disease, mitochondrially targeted ZFN [186] and TALENs [187] delivered by the adeno-associated virus led to the successful elimination of mutated mtDNA and subsequent reversion of the pathological phenotype [186,187]. These studies may open a new era for the treatment of heteroplasmic mitochondrial diseases.

6.3. RNA Import into Mitochondria

As mentioned earlier, nucleic acid import into mammalian mitochondria arouses controversy. First, it is not fully clear which RNA molecules can be transported into mitochondria; second, the machinery responsible for this process is debated. PNPase, a component of the mitochondrial degradosome complex, was proposed to play a role in RNA import into mitochondria [96,188]. Indeed, a pool of PNPase is found in the mitochondrial intermembrane space [94,96,189], where it could take part in importing RNA. Nevertheless, the exact mechanism of this process is not known, and it is not certain whether PNPase plays this role alone or cooperates with other proteins. While degradation of mtRNAs is a widely accepted function of PNPase, it is unclear how the enzyme mediates the transport of RNA instead of its destruction. Another suggested pathway of RNA import concerns mitochondrial protein translocase complexes TOM and TIM [190]; however, this has not been confirmed in mammalian cells. Another controversy refers to the RNA species that could potentially be imported into mitochondria. A few studies have indicated the mitochondrial import of recombinant heterologous tRNAs comprising the introduction of motifs derived from yeast tRNA [191–193]. Of note, tRNAs were shown to be imported into mitochondria of trypanosomes and plants [194,195]. Nevertheless, import of endogenous RNAs H1 RNA (as an RNA component of the canonical RNaseP), 7-2 RNA (as an RNA component of the RNase MRP) and 5S rRNA (as a constituent of the mitoribosome) was recently challenged [176], as those RNAs were suggested to be dispensable in human mitochondria. Indeed, it was shown that mitochondrial RNaseP does not possess an RNA moiety [88], RNase MRP localizes predominantly to the nucleolus [196–198] and 5S rRNA is replaced by tRNA in the mitochondrial ribosome [199–201]. Establishing the molecular mechanism of mitochondrial RNA import would be of great value, as it could enable the import of Clustered Regularly Interspaced Short Palindromic Repeats (CRISPR) system constituents for mtDNA manipulation. Although obviously revolutionary and beneficial, introduction of this system in mitochondria seems to be challenging, if not impossible [176].

6.4. Small RNAs in Mitochondrial Biology

Transcription of mtDNA may be a source of distinctive mtRNA species. Recent studies reported that a various range of small ncRNAs may emerge form mitochondrial transcription. A study engaging high-throughput sequencing of small RNA (sRNA) revealed that around 3% of whole-cell sRNAs maps uniquely to the mitochondrial genome in 143B human cells [90]. Interestingly, most of reported unique small RNA sequences were derived from tRNA genes [90]. The functional role of these RNA species is not known and whether they can be a part of RNA interference pathway as it was shown for processed nuclear tRNAs is an open question [90,202,203]. Other reported mitochondrial sRNAs comprise small non-coding transcripts called mitosRNAs (mitochondrial genome-encoded small RNAs) [204] and mitochondrial microRNAs (also called mitomiRs) [205]. Notably, whether the novel sRNA species are just a consequence of mtRNA processing and whether they possess any biological function is currently debated. Small non-coding RNAs appear as a novel class of transcripts that may have regulatory functions in mitochondria, nevertheless their exact mode of action and some aspects of their biogenesis are far from well established and evoke controversies. A canonical function of cytoplasmic microRNA (miRNA) is sequence-specific gene silencing in RNA interference pathway [206]. Several reports suggested presence of microRNAs in mitochondria [207–210] proposed to be either products of mtDNA transcription or an effect of import of cytoplasmic transcripts inside mitochondria [205]. Nevertheless, miRNA biogenesis encompasses multiple steps of processing and require specialized machinery and it is not known which proteins could be engaged in these processes in mitochondria. Moreover, it is not clear how miRNAs could enter mitochondria. These questions need to be answered in order to establish functional potential of mitochondrial small ncRNAs.

Future studies will show whether identified short RNAs have functional importance or they are merely by-products of mtRNA processing and decay. For example, a recently described short RNA called tRNA-like accumulates strongly upon inhibition of mtRNA degradation by the mitochondrial degradosome [106]. This may imply that most, if not all, tRNA-like molecules are just by-products of mtRNA processing which are removed by the degradosome. Or this transcript has functional importance, but its levels need to be strictly controlled.

6.5. 37 or More?

Early studies of the human mitochondrial genome led to the mapping of mtDNA-encoded genes [21]. For a long time, human mtDNA was considered to encode 37 genes; however, a few recent reports suggested that there may be additional coding sequences within human mtDNA. Human mitochondrial genome may harbor nested small open reading frames (sORF) yielding short peptides derived from polycistronic mt-mRNAs. For example, human 16S rRNA gene was suggested to contain sORF encoding 24 amino acid peptide called humanin, which may have cytoprotective properties [211,212]. It is not known, however, whether humanin is translated inside mitochondria or in the cytoplasm and in the latter case, how humanin transcript could be exported from mitochondria and recognized by cytoplasmic translation apparatus [213]. Other mitochondria-derived peptides (MDPs) were proposed to arise from mitochondrial sORFs and were suggested to have regulatory functions within the cell. Among them are mitochondrial open reading frame of the 12S rRNA-c (MOTS-c) and small humanin-like peptides 1–6 (SHLP1-6) located within 12S rRNA and 16S rRNA genes, respectively [214–216]. However, synthesis of MOTS-c would require export of corresponding encoding RNA to the cytoplasm, a process of unknown mechanism. Mitochondrial sORF and sRNAs are intriguing in concept, nonetheless, initial reports of them require further substantiation. It cannot be excluded that mitochondrial sRNAs and MDPs are by-products of mitochondrial gene expression. Therefore, proposed mitochondrial sORF and sRNAs require further studies to be fully embraced by the field.

Author Contributions: Conceptualization, R.J.S. and A.V.K., supervision R.J.S., A.V.K. drafted the manuscript and prepared the figures. R.J.S. reviewed and edited the manuscript. A.V.K. and R.J.S. prepared the final version of the manuscript. All authors have read and agreed to the published version of the manuscript.

Funding: This work was funded by the POIR.04.04.00-00-5E63/18-00 project (to R.J.S.) carried out within the First TEAM programme of the Foundation for Polish Science co-financed by the European Union under the European Regional Development Fund and by the National Science Centre, Poland, grant number UMO-2014/12/W/NZ1/00463 (to R.J.S.).

Conflicts of Interest: The authors declare no conflict of interest.

Abbreviations

ATP	adenosine triphosphate
dsRNA	double-stranded RNA
G4	G-quadruplex
H-strand	heavy-strand
IFN	interferon
ITH	heavy-strand transcription initiation site
ITL	light-strand transcription initiation site
L-strand	light-strand
lncRNA	long non-coding RNA
MDP	mitochondria-derived peptide
miRNA	microRNA
mitomiRs	mitochondrial microRNAs
mitosRNAs	mitochondrial genome-encoded small RNAs
mtDNA	mitochondrial DNA
mtRNA	mitochondrial RNA
NCR	non-coding regulatory region
ncRNA	non-coding RNA
PAMP	pathogen-associated molecular pattern
RBP	RNA-binding protein
sORF	small Open Reading Frame
sRNA	small RNA

References

1. Brown, G.C. Control of respiration and ATP synthesis in mammalian mitochondria and cells. *Biochem. J.* **1992**, *284*, 1–13. [CrossRef] [PubMed]
2. Go, Y.-M.; Jones, D.P. Redox compartmentalization in eukaryotic cells. *Biochim. Biophys. Acta* **2008**, *1780*, 1273–1290. [CrossRef]
3. Titov, D.V.; Cracan, V.; Goodman, R.P.; Peng, J.; Grabarek, Z.; Mootha, V.K. Complementation of mitochondrial electron transport chain by manipulation of the NAD+/NADH ratio. *Science* **2016**, *352*, 231–235. [CrossRef]
4. Galluzzi, L.; Kepp, O.; Trojel-Hansen, C.; Kroemer, G. Mitochondrial control of cellular life, stress, and death. *Circ. Res.* **2012**, *111*, 1198–1207. [CrossRef]
5. Pizzo, P.; Drago, I.; Filadi, R.; Pozzan, T. Mitochondrial Ca^{2+} homeostasis: Mechanism, role, and tissue specificities. *Pflugers Arch.* **2012**, *464*, 3–17. [CrossRef]
6. Brand, M.D.; Orr, A.L.; Perevoshchikova, I.V.; Quinlan, C.L. The role of mitochondrial function and cellular bioenergetics in ageing and disease. *Br. J. Dermatol.* **2013**, *169* (Suppl. 2), 1–8. [CrossRef]
7. Maiese, K. The bright side of reactive oxygen species: Lifespan extension without cellular demise. *J. Transl. Sci.* **2016**, *2*, 185–187. [CrossRef]
8. Arnoult, D.; Soares, F.; Tattoli, I.; Girardin, S.E. Mitochondria in innate immunity. *EMBO Rep.* **2011**, *12*, 901–910. [CrossRef] [PubMed]
9. Sandhir, R.; Halder, A.; Sunkaria, A. Mitochondria as a centrally positioned hub in the innate immune response. *Biochim. Biophys. Acta Mol. Basis Dis.* **2017**, *1863*, 1090–1097. [CrossRef] [PubMed]
10. Czarnecka, A.M.; Golik, P.; Bartnik, E. Mitochondrial DNA mutations in human neoplasia. *J. Appl. Genet.* **2006**, *47*, 67–78. [CrossRef] [PubMed]

11. Lin, M.T.; Beal, M.F. Mitochondrial dysfunction and oxidative stress in neurodegenerative diseases. *Nature* **2006**, *443*, 787–795. [CrossRef] [PubMed]
12. Copeland, W.C.; Wachsman, J.T.; Johnson, F.M.; Penta, J.S. Mitochondrial DNA alterations in cancer. *Cancer Invest.* **2002**, *20*, 557–569. [CrossRef] [PubMed]
13. Schapira, A.H.V. Mitochondrial diseases. *Lancet* **2012**, *379*, 1825–1834. [CrossRef]
14. Nicholls, T.J.; Rorbach, J.; Minczuk, M. Mitochondria: Mitochondrial RNA metabolism and human disease. *Int. J. Biochem. Cell Biol.* **2013**, *45*, 845–849. [CrossRef] [PubMed]
15. Vafai, S.B.; Mootha, V.K. Mitochondrial disorders as windows into an ancient organelle. *Nature* **2012**, *491*, 374–383. [CrossRef] [PubMed]
16. Gorman, G.S.; Chinnery, P.F.; DiMauro, S.; Hirano, M.; Koga, Y.; McFarland, R.; Suomalainen, A.; Thorburn, D.R.; Zeviani, M.; Turnbull, D.M. Mitochondrial diseases. *Nat. Rev. Dis. Primers* **2016**, *2*, 16080. [CrossRef]
17. Rusecka, J.; Kaliszewska, M.; Bartnik, E.; Tońska, K. Nuclear genes involved in mitochondrial diseases caused by instability of mitochondrial DNA. *J. Appl. Genet.* **2018**, *59*, 43–57. [CrossRef]
18. Taanman, J.W. The mitochondrial genome: Structure, transcription, translation and replication. *Biochim. Biophys. Acta* **1999**, *1410*, 103–123. [CrossRef]
19. Fernández-Silva, P.; Enriquez, J.A.; Montoya, J. Replication and transcription of mammalian mitochondrial DNA. *Exp. Physiol.* **2003**, *88*, 41–56. [CrossRef]
20. Rorbach, J.; Minczuk, M. The post-transcriptional life of mammalian mitochondrial RNA. *Biochem. J.* **2012**, *444*, 357–373. [CrossRef]
21. Anderson, S.; Bankier, A.T.; Barrell, B.G.; de Bruijn, M.H.; Coulson, A.R.; Drouin, J.; Eperon, I.C.; Nierlich, D.P.; Roe, B.A.; Sanger, F.; et al. Sequence and organization of the human mitochondrial genome. *Nature* **1981**, *290*, 457–465. [CrossRef] [PubMed]
22. Calvo, S.E.; Clauser, K.R.; Mootha, V.K. MitoCarta2.0: An updated inventory of mammalian mitochondrial proteins. *Nucleic Acids Res.* **2016**, *44*, D1251–D1257. [CrossRef] [PubMed]
23. Schmidt, O.; Pfanner, N.; Meisinger, C. Mitochondrial protein import: From proteomics to functional mechanisms. *Nat. Rev. Mol. Cell Biol.* **2010**, *11*, 655–667. [CrossRef] [PubMed]
24. Van Haute, L.; Pearce, S.F.; Powell, C.A.; D'Souza, A.R.; Nicholls, T.J.; Minczuk, M. Mitochondrial transcript maturation and its disorders. *J. Inherit. Metab. Dis.* **2015**, *38*, 655–680. [CrossRef]
25. Yang, D.; Oyaizu, Y.; Oyaizu, H.; Olsen, G.J.; Woese, C.R. Mitochondrial origins. *Proc. Natl. Acad. Sci. USA* **1985**, *82*, 4443–4447. [CrossRef]
26. Gray, M.W.; Burger, G.; Lang, B.F. Mitochondrial evolution. *Science* **1999**, *283*, 1476–1481. [CrossRef]
27. Martijn, J.; Vosseberg, J.; Guy, L.; Offre, P.; Ettema, T.J.G. Deep mitochondrial origin outside the sampled alphaproteobacteria. *Nature* **2018**, *557*, 101–105. [CrossRef]
28. Nass, M.M.; Nass, S. Intramitochondrial fibers with DNA characteristics. I. fixation and electron staining reactions. *J. Cell Biol.* **1963**, *19*, 593–611. [CrossRef]
29. Anderson, S. Shotgun DNA sequencing using cloned DNase I-generated fragments. *Nucleic Acids Res.* **1981**, *9*, 3015–3027. [CrossRef]
30. Bonekamp, N.A.; Larsson, N.-G. SnapShot: Mitochondrial Nucleoid. *Cell* **2018**, *172*, 388–388.e1. [CrossRef]
31. Garrido, N.; Griparic, L.; Jokitalo, E.; Wartiovaara, J.; van der Bliek, A.M.; Spelbrink, J.N. Composition and dynamics of human mitochondrial nucleoids. *Mol. Biol. Cell* **2003**, *14*, 1583–1596. [CrossRef] [PubMed]
32. Wang, Y.; Bogenhagen, D.F. Human mitochondrial DNA nucleoids are linked to protein folding machinery and metabolic enzymes at the mitochondrial inner membrane. *J. Biol. Chem.* **2006**, *281*, 25791–25802. [CrossRef] [PubMed]
33. Kukat, C.; Wurm, C.A.; Spåhr, H.; Falkenberg, M.; Larsson, N.-G.; Jakobs, S. Super-resolution microscopy reveals that mammalian mitochondrial nucleoids have a uniform size and frequently contain a single copy of mtDNA. *Proc. Natl. Acad. Sci. USA* **2011**, *108*, 13534–13539. [CrossRef] [PubMed]
34. Kukat, C.; Davies, K.M.; Wurm, C.A.; Spåhr, H.; Bonekamp, N.A.; Kühl, I.; Joos, F.; Polosa, P.L.; Park, C.B.; Posse, V.; et al. Cross-strand binding of TFAM to a single mtDNA molecule forms the mitochondrial nucleoid. *Proc. Natl. Acad. Sci. USA* **2015**, *112*, 11288–11293. [CrossRef] [PubMed]
35. Ekstrand, M.I.; Falkenberg, M.; Rantanen, A.; Park, C.B.; Gaspari, M.; Hultenby, K.; Rustin, P.; Gustafsson, C.M.; Larsson, N.-G. Mitochondrial transcription factor A regulates mtDNA copy number in mammals. *Hum. Mol. Genet.* **2004**, *13*, 935–944. [CrossRef] [PubMed]

36. Satoh, M.; Kuroiwa, T. Organization of multiple nucleoids and DNA molecules in mitochondria of a human cell. *Exp. Cell Res.* **1991**, *196*, 137–140. [CrossRef]
37. Legros, F.; Malka, F.; Frachon, P.; Lombès, A.; Rojo, M. Organization and dynamics of human mitochondrial DNA. *J. Cell Sci.* **2004**, *117*, 2653–2662. [CrossRef]
38. Iborra, F.J.; Kimura, H.; Cook, P.R. The functional organization of mitochondrial genomes in human cells. *BMC Biol.* **2004**, *2*, 9. [CrossRef]
39. Jenuth, J.P.; Peterson, A.C.; Fu, K.; Shoubridge, E.A. Random genetic drift in the female germline explains the rapid segregation of mammalian mitochondrial DNA. *Nat. Genet.* **1996**, *14*, 146–151. [CrossRef]
40. Ishihara, T.; Ban-Ishihara, R.; Maeda, M.; Matsunaga, Y.; Ichimura, A.; Kyogoku, S.; Aoki, H.; Katada, S.; Nakada, K.; Nomura, M.; et al. Dynamics of mitochondrial DNA nucleoids regulated by mitochondrial fission is essential for maintenance of homogeneously active mitochondria during neonatal heart development. *Mol. Cell. Biol.* **2015**, *35*, 211–223. [CrossRef]
41. Kvist, L.; Martens, J.; Nazarenko, A.A.; Orell, M. Paternal leakage of mitochondrial DNA in the great tit (Parus major). *Mol. Biol. Evol.* **2003**, *20*, 243–247. [CrossRef] [PubMed]
42. Cree, L.M.; Samuels, D.C.; de Sousa Lopes, S.C.; Rajasimha, H.K.; Wonnapinij, P.; Mann, J.R.; Dahl, H.-H.M.; Chinnery, P.F. A reduction of mitochondrial DNA molecules during embryogenesis explains the rapid segregation of genotypes. *Nat. Genet.* **2008**, *40*, 249–254. [CrossRef] [PubMed]
43. Shoubridge, E.A. Mitochondrial DNA segregation in the developing embryo. *Hum. Reprod.* **2000**, *15* (Suppl. 2), 229–234. [CrossRef] [PubMed]
44. Schwartz, M.; Vissing, J. Paternal inheritance of mitochondrial DNA. *N. Engl. J. Med.* **2002**, *347*, 576–580. [CrossRef] [PubMed]
45. Luo, S.; Valencia, C.A.; Zhang, J.; Lee, N.-C.; Slone, J.; Gui, B.; Wang, X.; Li, Z.; Dell, S.; Brown, J.; et al. Biparental Inheritance of Mitochondrial DNA in Humans. *Proc. Natl. Acad. Sci. USA* **2018**, *115*, 13039–13044. [CrossRef]
46. Pohjoismäki, J.L.O.; Wanrooij, S.; Hyvärinen, A.K.; Goffart, S.; Holt, I.J.; Spelbrink, J.N.; Jacobs, H.T. Alterations to the expression level of mitochondrial transcription factor A, TFAM, modify the mode of mitochondrial DNA replication in cultured human cells. *Nucleic Acids Res.* **2006**, *34*, 5815–5828. [CrossRef]
47. Pohjoismäki, J.L.O.; Goffart, S.; Tyynismaa, H.; Willcox, S.; Ide, T.; Kang, D.; Suomalainen, A.; Karhunen, P.J.; Griffith, J.D.; Holt, I.J.; et al. Human heart mitochondrial DNA is organized in complex catenated networks containing abundant four-way junctions and replication forks. *J. Biol. Chem.* **2009**, *284*, 21446–21457. [CrossRef]
48. Tuppen, H.A.L.; Blakely, E.L.; Turnbull, D.M.; Taylor, R.W. Mitochondrial DNA mutations and human disease. *Biochim. Biophys. Acta* **2010**, *1797*, 113–128. [CrossRef]
49. Holt, I.J.; Reyes, A. Human mitochondrial DNA replication. *Cold Spring Harb. Perspect. Biol.* **2012**, *4*, a012971. [CrossRef]
50. Gustafsson, C.M.; Falkenberg, M.; Larsson, N.-G. Maintenance and Expression of Mammalian Mitochondrial DNA. *Annu. Rev. Biochem.* **2016**, *85*, 133–160. [CrossRef]
51. Young, M.J.; Copeland, W.C. Human mitochondrial DNA replication machinery and disease. *Curr. Opin. Genet. Dev.* **2016**, *38*, 52–62. [CrossRef] [PubMed]
52. Copeland, W.C.; Longley, M.J. Mitochondrial genome maintenance in health and disease. *DNA Repair* **2014**, *19*, 190–198. [CrossRef] [PubMed]
53. Attardi, G.; Chomyn, A.; King, M.P.; Kruse, B.; Polosa, P.L.; Murdter, N.N. Regulation of mitochondrial gene expression in mammalian cells. *Biochem. Soc. Trans.* **1990**, *18*, 509–513. [CrossRef] [PubMed]
54. Fish, J.; Raule, N.; Attardi, G. Discovery of a major D-loop replication origin reveals two modes of human mtDNA synthesis. *Science* **2004**, *306*, 2098–2101. [CrossRef]
55. Aloni, Y.; Attardi, G. Expression of the mitochondrial genome in HeLa cells. II. Evidence for complete transcription of mitochondrial DNA. *J. Mol. Biol.* **1971**, *55*, 251–267. [CrossRef]
56. Hillen, H.S.; Temiakov, D.; Cramer, P. Structural basis of mitochondrial transcription. *Nat. Struct. Mol. Biol.* **2018**, *25*, 754–765. [CrossRef]
57. Fisher, R.P.; Clayton, D.A. A transcription factor required for promoter recognition by human mitochondrial RNA polymerase. Accurate initiation at the heavy- and light-strand promoters dissected and reconstituted in vitro. *J. Biol. Chem.* **1985**, *260*, 11330–11338.

58. Morozov, Y.I.; Parshin, A.V.; Agaronyan, K.; Cheung, A.C.M.; Anikin, M.; Cramer, P.; Temiakov, D. A model for transcription initiation in human mitochondria. *Nucleic Acids Res.* **2015**, *43*, 3726–3735. [CrossRef]
59. Hillen, H.S.; Morozov, Y.I.; Sarfallah, A.; Temiakov, D.; Cramer, P. Structural Basis of Mitochondrial Transcription Initiation. *Cell* **2017**, *171*, 1072.e10–1081.e10. [CrossRef]
60. Minczuk, M.; He, J.; Duch, A.M.; Ettema, T.J.; Chlebowski, A.; Dzionek, K.; Nijtmans, L.G.J.; Huynen, M.A.; Holt, I.J. TEFM (c17orf42) is necessary for transcription of human mtDNA. *Nucleic Acids Res.* **2011**, *39*, 4284–4299. [CrossRef]
61. Posse, V.; Shahzad, S.; Falkenberg, M.; Hällberg, B.M.; Gustafsson, C.M. TEFM is a potent stimulator of mitochondrial transcription elongation in vitro. *Nucleic Acids Res.* **2015**, *43*, 2615–2624. [CrossRef] [PubMed]
62. Yu, H.; Xue, C.; Long, M.; Jia, H.; Xue, G.; Du, S.; Coello, Y.; Ishibashi, T. TEFM Enhances Transcription Elongation by Modifying mtRNAP Pausing Dynamics. *Biophys. J.* **2018**, *115*, 2295–2300. [CrossRef] [PubMed]
63. Agaronyan, K.; Morozov, Y.I.; Anikin, M.; Temiakov, D. Mitochondrial biology. Replication-transcription switch in human mitochondria. *Science* **2015**, *347*, 548–551. [CrossRef] [PubMed]
64. Hillen, H.S.; Parshin, A.V.; Agaronyan, K.; Morozov, Y.I.; Graber, J.J.; Chernev, A.; Schwinghammer, K.; Urlaub, H.; Anikin, M.; Cramer, P.; et al. Mechanism of Transcription Anti-termination in Human Mitochondria. *Cell* **2017**, *171*, 1082–1093.e13. [CrossRef]
65. Jiang, S.; Koolmeister, C.; Misic, J.; Siira, S.; Kühl, I.; Silva Ramos, E.; Miranda, M.; Jiang, M.; Posse, V.; Lytovchenko, O.; et al. TEFM regulates both transcription elongation and RNA processing in mitochondria. *EMBO Rep.* **2019**, *20*, e48101. [CrossRef]
66. Kruse, B.; Narasimhan, N.; Attardi, G. Termination of transcription in human mitochondria: Identification and purification of a DNA binding protein factor that promotes termination. *Cell* **1989**, *58*, 391–397. [CrossRef]
67. Yakubovskaya, E.; Mejia, E.; Byrnes, J.; Hambardjieva, E.; Garcia-Diaz, M. Helix unwinding and base flipping enable human MTERF1 to terminate mitochondrial transcription. *Cell* **2010**, *141*, 982–993. [CrossRef]
68. Terzioglu, M.; Ruzzenente, B.; Harmel, J.; Mourier, A.; Jemt, E.; López, M.D.; Kukat, C.; Stewart, J.B.; Wibom, R.; Meharg, C.; et al. MTERF1 binds mtDNA to prevent transcriptional interference at the light-strand promoter but is dispensable for rRNA gene transcription regulation. *Cell Metab.* **2013**, *17*, 618–626. [CrossRef]
69. Shi, Y.; Posse, V.; Zhu, X.; Hyvärinen, A.K.; Jacobs, H.T.; Falkenberg, M.; Gustafsson, C.M. Mitochondrial transcription termination factor 1 directs polar replication fork pausing. *Nucleic Acids Res.* **2016**, *44*, 5732–5742. [CrossRef]
70. Linder, T.; Park, C.B.; Asin-Cayuela, J.; Pellegrini, M.; Larsson, N.-G.; Falkenberg, M.; Samuelsson, T.; Gustafsson, C.M. A family of putative transcription termination factors shared amongst metazoans and plants. *Curr. Genet.* **2005**, *48*, 265–269. [CrossRef]
71. Pellegrini, M.; Asin-Cayuela, J.; Erdjument-Bromage, H.; Tempst, P.; Larsson, N.-G.; Gustafsson, C.M. MTERF2 is a nucleoid component in mammalian mitochondria. *Biochim. Biophys. Acta* **2009**, *1787*, 296–302. [CrossRef] [PubMed]
72. Cámara, Y.; Asin-Cayuela, J.; Park, C.B.; Metodiev, M.D.; Shi, Y.; Ruzzenente, B.; Kukat, C.; Habermann, B.; Wibom, R.; Hultenby, K.; et al. MTERF4 regulates translation by targeting the methyltransferase NSUN4 to the mammalian mitochondrial ribosome. *Cell Metab.* **2011**, *13*, 527–539. [CrossRef] [PubMed]
73. Wredenberg, A.; Lagouge, M.; Bratic, A.; Metodiev, M.D.; Spåhr, H.; Mourier, A.; Freyer, C.; Ruzzenente, B.; Tain, L.; Grönke, S.; et al. MTERF3 regulates mitochondrial ribosome biogenesis in invertebrates and mammals. *PLoS Genet.* **2013**, *9*, e1003178. [CrossRef] [PubMed]
74. Alam, T.I.; Kanki, T.; Muta, T.; Ukaji, K.; Abe, Y.; Nakayama, H.; Takio, K.; Hamasaki, N.; Kang, D. Human mitochondrial DNA is packaged with TFAM. *Nucleic Acids Res.* **2003**, *31*, 1640–1645. [CrossRef] [PubMed]
75. Kaufman, B.A.; Durisic, N.; Mativetsky, J.M.; Costantino, S.; Hancock, M.A.; Grutter, P.; Shoubridge, E.A. The mitochondrial transcription factor TFAM coordinates the assembly of multiple DNA molecules into nucleoid-like structures. *Mol. Biol. Cell* **2007**, *18*, 3225–3236. [CrossRef] [PubMed]
76. Shadel, G.S.; Clayton, D.A. Mitochondrial DNA maintenance in vertebrates. *Annu. Rev. Biochem.* **1997**, *66*, 409–435. [CrossRef]
77. Campbell, C.T.; Kolesar, J.E.; Kaufman, B.A. Mitochondrial transcription factor A regulates mitochondrial transcription initiation, DNA packaging, and genome copy number. *Biochim. Biophys. Acta* **2012**, *1819*, 921–929. [CrossRef]

78. Larsson, N.G.; Wang, J.; Wilhelmsson, H.; Oldfors, A.; Rustin, P.; Lewandoski, M.; Barsh, G.S.; Clayton, D.A. Mitochondrial transcription factor A is necessary for mtDNA maintenance and embryogenesis in mice. *Nat. Genet.* **1998**, *18*, 231–236. [CrossRef]
79. Stiles, A.R.; Simon, M.T.; Stover, A.; Eftekharian, S.; Khanlou, N.; Wang, H.L.; Magaki, S.; Lee, H.; Partynski, K.; Dorrani, N.; et al. Mutations in TFAM, encoding mitochondrial transcription factor A, cause neonatal liver failure associated with mtDNA depletion. *Mol. Genet. Metab.* **2016**, *119*, 91–99. [CrossRef]
80. Kang, I.; Chu, C.T.; Kaufman, B.A. The mitochondrial transcription factor TFAM in neurodegeneration: Emerging evidence and mechanisms. *FEBS Lett.* **2018**, *592*, 793–811. [CrossRef]
81. Kotrys, A.V.; Cysewski, D.; Czarnomska, S.D.; Pietras, Z.; Borowski, L.S.; Dziembowski, A.; Szczesny, R.J. Quantitative proteomics revealed C6orf203/MTRES1 as a factor preventing stress-induced transcription deficiency in human mitochondria. *Nucleic Acids Res.* **2019**, *47*, 7502–7517. [CrossRef] [PubMed]
82. Serre, V.; Rozanska, A.; Beinat, M.; Chretien, D.; Boddaert, N.; Munnich, A.; Rötig, A.; Chrzanowska-Lightowlers, Z.M. Mutations in mitochondrial ribosomal protein MRPL12 leads to growth retardation, neurological deterioration and mitochondrial translation deficiency. *Biochim. Biophys. Acta* **2013**, *1832*, 1304–1312. [CrossRef] [PubMed]
83. Surovtseva, Y.V.; Shutt, T.E.; Cotney, J.; Cimen, H.; Chen, S.Y.; Koc, E.C.; Shadel, G.S. Mitochondrial ribosomal protein L12 selectively associates with human mitochondrial RNA polymerase to activate transcription. *Proc. Natl. Acad. Sci. USA* **2011**, *108*, 17921–17926. [CrossRef] [PubMed]
84. Wang, Z.; Cotney, J.; Shadel, G.S. Human mitochondrial ribosomal protein MRPL12 interacts directly with mitochondrial RNA polymerase to modulate mitochondrial gene expression. *J. Biol. Chem.* **2007**, *282*, 12610–12618. [CrossRef]
85. Nouws, J.; Goswami, A.V.; Bestwick, M.; McCann, B.J.; Surovtseva, Y.V.; Shadel, G.S. Mitochondrial Ribosomal Protein L12 Is Required for POLRMT Stability and Exists as Two Forms Generated by Alternative Proteolysis during Import. *J. Biol. Chem.* **2016**, *291*, 989–997. [CrossRef]
86. Barchiesi, A.; Vascotto, C. Transcription, Processing, and Decay of Mitochondrial RNA in Health and Disease. *Int. J. Mol. Sci.* **2019**, *20*, 2221. [CrossRef]
87. Ojala, D.; Montoya, J.; Attardi, G. tRNA punctuation model of RNA processing in human mitochondria. *Nature* **1981**, *290*, 470–474. [CrossRef]
88. Holzmann, J.; Frank, P.; Löffler, E.; Bennett, K.L.; Gerner, C.; Rossmanith, W. RNase P without RNA: Identification and functional reconstitution of the human mitochondrial tRNA processing enzyme. *Cell* **2008**, *135*, 462–474. [CrossRef]
89. Brzezniak, L.K.; Bijata, M.; Szczesny, R.J.; Stepien, P.P. Involvement of human ELAC2 gene product in 3′ end processing of mitochondrial tRNAs. *RNA Biol.* **2011**, *8*, 616–626. [CrossRef]
90. Mercer, T.R.; Neph, S.; Dinger, M.E.; Crawford, J.; Smith, M.A.; Shearwood, A.-M.J.; Haugen, E.; Bracken, C.P.; Rackham, O.; Stamatoyannopoulos, J.A.; et al. The human mitochondrial transcriptome. *Cell* **2011**, *146*, 645–658. [CrossRef]
91. Szczesny, R.J.; Borowski, L.S.; Brzezniak, L.K.; Dmochowska, A.; Gewartowski, K.; Bartnik, E.; Stepien, P.P. Human mitochondrial RNA turnover caught in flagranti: Involvement of hSuv3p helicase in RNA surveillance. *Nucleic Acids Res.* **2010**, *38*, 279–298. [CrossRef] [PubMed]
92. Piechota, J.; Tomecki, R.; Gewartowski, K.; Szczesny, R.; Dmochowska, A.; Kudła, M.; Dybczyńska, L.; Stepien, P.P.; Bartnik, E. Differential stability of mitochondrial mRNA in HeLa cells. *Acta Biochim. Pol.* **2006**, *53*, 157–168. [CrossRef] [PubMed]
93. Szczesny, R.J.; Borowski, L.S.; Malecki, M.; Wojcik, M.A.; Stepien, P.P.; Golik, P. RNA degradation in yeast and human mitochondria. *Biochim. Biophys. Acta* **2012**, *1819*, 1027–1034. [CrossRef] [PubMed]
94. Borowski, L.S.; Dziembowski, A.; Hejnowicz, M.S.; Stepien, P.P.; Szczesny, R.J. Human mitochondrial RNA decay mediated by PNPase-hSuv3 complex takes place in distinct foci. *Nucleic Acids Res.* **2013**, *41*, 1223–1240. [CrossRef]
95. Pereira, M.; Mason, P.; Szczesny, R.J.; Maddukuri, L.; Dziwura, S.; Jedrzejczak, R.; Paul, E.; Wojcik, A.; Dybczynska, L.; Tudek, B.; et al. Interaction of human SUV3 RNA/DNA helicase with BLM helicase; loss of the SUV3 gene results in mouse embryonic lethality. *Mech. Ageing Dev.* **2007**, *128*, 609–617. [CrossRef]
96. Wang, G.; Chen, H.-W.; Oktay, Y.; Zhang, J.; Allen, E.L.; Smith, G.M.; Fan, K.C.; Hong, J.S.; French, S.W.; McCaffery, J.M.; et al. PNPASE regulates RNA import into mitochondria. *Cell* **2010**, *142*, 456–467. [CrossRef]

97. Minczuk, M.; Piwowarski, J.; Papworth, M.A.; Awiszus, K.; Schalinski, S.; Dziembowski, A.; Dmochowska, A.; Bartnik, E.; Tokatlidis, K.; Stepien, P.P.; et al. Localisation of the human hSuv3p helicase in the mitochondrial matrix and its preferential unwinding of dsDNA. *Nucleic Acids Res.* **2002**, *30*, 5074–5086. [CrossRef]
98. Lin, C.L.; Wang, Y.-T.; Yang, W.-Z.; Hsiao, Y.-Y.; Yuan, H.S. Crystal structure of human polynucleotide phosphorylase: Insights into its domain function in RNA binding and degradation. *Nucleic Acids Res.* **2012**, *40*, 4146–4157. [CrossRef]
99. Wang, D.D.-H.; Shu, Z.; Lieser, S.A.; Chen, P.-L.; Lee, W.-H. Human mitochondrial SUV3 and polynucleotide phosphorylase form a 330-kDa heteropentamer to cooperatively degrade double-stranded RNA with a 3′-to-5′ directionality. *J. Biol. Chem.* **2009**, *284*, 20812–20821. [CrossRef]
100. Jedrzejczak, R.; Wang, J.; Dauter, M.; Szczesny, R.J.; Stepien, P.P.; Dauter, Z. Human Suv3 protein reveals unique features among SF2 helicases. *Acta Crystallogr. D Biol. Crystallogr.* **2011**, *67*, 988–996. [CrossRef]
101. Aloni, Y.; Attardi, G. Symmetrical in vivo transcription of mitochondrial DNA in HeLa cells. *Proc. Natl. Acad. Sci. USA* **1971**, *68*, 1757–1761. [CrossRef] [PubMed]
102. Chujo, T.; Ohira, T.; Sakaguchi, Y.; Goshima, N.; Nomura, N.; Nagao, A.; Suzuki, T. LRPPRC/SLIRP suppresses PNPase-mediated mRNA decay and promotes polyadenylation in human mitochondria. *Nucleic Acids Res.* **2012**, *40*, 8033–8047. [CrossRef] [PubMed]
103. Tu, Y.-T.; Barrientos, A. The Human Mitochondrial DEAD-Box Protein DDX28 Resides in RNA Granules and Functions in Mitoribosome Assembly. *Cell Rep.* **2015**, *10*, 854–864. [CrossRef] [PubMed]
104. Jourdain, A.A.; Koppen, M.; Rodley, C.D.; Maundrell, K.; Gueguen, N.; Reynier, P.; Guaras, A.M.; Enriquez, J.A.; Anderson, P.; Simarro, M.; et al. A mitochondria-specific isoform of FASTK is present in mitochondrial RNA granules and regulates gene expression and function. *Cell Rep.* **2015**, *10*, 1110–1121. [CrossRef]
105. Bruni, F.; Gramegna, P.; Oliveira, J.M.A.; Lightowlers, R.N.; Chrzanowska-Lightowlers, Z.M.A. REXO2 is an oligoribonuclease active in human mitochondria. *PLoS ONE* **2013**, *8*, e64670. [CrossRef]
106. Pietras, Z.; Wojcik, M.A.; Borowski, L.S.; Szewczyk, M.; Kulinski, T.M.; Cysewski, D.; Stepien, P.P.; Dziembowski, A.; Szczesny, R.J. Dedicated surveillance mechanism controls G-quadruplex forming non-coding RNAs in human mitochondria. *Nat. Commun.* **2018**, *9*, 2558. [CrossRef]
107. Baughman, J.M.; Nilsson, R.; Gohil, V.M.; Arlow, D.H.; Gauhar, Z.; Mootha, V.K. A computational screen for regulators of oxidative phosphorylation implicates SLIRP in mitochondrial RNA homeostasis. *PLoS Genet.* **2009**, *5*, e1000590. [CrossRef]
108. Sasarman, F.; Brunel-Guitton, C.; Antonicka, H.; Wai, T.; Shoubridge, E.A. LSFC Consortium LRPPRC and SLIRP interact in a ribonucleoprotein complex that regulates posttranscriptional gene expression in mitochondria. *Mol. Biol. Cell* **2010**, *21*, 1315–1323. [CrossRef]
109. Siira, S.J.; Spåhr, H.; Shearwood, A.-M.J.; Ruzzenente, B.; Larsson, N.-G.; Rackham, O.; Filipovska, A. LRPPRC-mediated folding of the mitochondrial transcriptome. *Nat. Commun.* **2017**, *8*, 1532. [CrossRef]
110. Ruzzenente, B.; Metodiev, M.D.; Wredenberg, A.; Bratic, A.; Park, C.B.; Cámara, Y.; Milenkovic, D.; Zickermann, V.; Wibom, R.; Hultenby, K.; et al. LRPPRC is necessary for polyadenylation and coordination of translation of mitochondrial mRNAs. *EMBO J.* **2012**, *31*, 443–456. [CrossRef]
111. Mootha, V.K.; Lepage, P.; Miller, K.; Bunkenborg, J.; Reich, M.; Hjerrild, M.; Delmonte, T.; Villeneuve, A.; Sladek, R.; Xu, F.; et al. Identification of a gene causing human cytochrome c oxidase deficiency by integrative genomics. *Proc. Natl. Acad. Sci. USA* **2003**, *100*, 605–610. [CrossRef] [PubMed]
112. Cui, J.; Wang, L.; Ren, X.; Zhang, Y.; Zhang, H. LRPPRC: A Multifunctional Protein Involved in Energy Metabolism and Human Disease. *Front. Physiol.* **2019**, *10*, 595. [CrossRef] [PubMed]
113. Lagouge, M.; Mourier, A.; Lee, H.J.; Spåhr, H.; Wai, T.; Kukat, C.; Silva Ramos, E.; Motori, E.; Busch, J.D.; Siira, S.; et al. SLIRP Regulates the Rate of Mitochondrial Protein Synthesis and Protects LRPPRC from Degradation. *PLoS Genet.* **2015**, *11*, e1005423. [CrossRef] [PubMed]
114. Qian, Z.; Wilusz, J. GRSF-1: A poly(A)+ mRNA binding protein which interacts with a conserved G-rich element. *Nucleic Acids Res.* **1994**, *22*, 2334–2343. [CrossRef] [PubMed]
115. Antonicka, H.; Sasarman, F.; Nishimura, T.; Paupe, V.; Shoubridge, E.A. The mitochondrial RNA-binding protein GRSF1 localizes to RNA granules and is required for posttranscriptional mitochondrial gene expression. *Cell Metab.* **2013**, *17*, 386–398. [CrossRef] [PubMed]

116. Jourdain, A.A.; Koppen, M.; Wydro, M.; Rodley, C.D.; Lightowlers, R.N.; Chrzanowska-Lightowlers, Z.M.; Martinou, J.-C. GRSF1 regulates RNA processing in mitochondrial RNA granules. *Cell Metab.* **2013**, *17*, 399–410. [CrossRef]
117. Pietras, Z.; Wojcik, M.A.; Borowski, L.S.; Szewczyk, M.; Kulinski, T.M.; Cysewski, D.; Stepien, P.P.; Dziembowski, A.; Szczesny, R.J. Controlling the mitochondrial antisense—role of the SUV3-PNPase complex and its co-factor GRSF1 in mitochondrial RNA surveillance. *Mol. Cell. Oncol.* **2018**, *5*, e1516452. [CrossRef]
118. Gopalakrishna, S.; Pearce, S.F.; Dinan, A.M.; Schober, F.A.; Cipullo, M.; Spåhr, H.; Khawaja, A.; Maffezzini, C.; Freyer, C.; Wredenberg, A.; et al. C6orf203 is an RNA-binding protein involved in mitochondrial protein synthesis. *Nucleic Acids Res.* **2019**, *47*, 9386–9399. [CrossRef]
119. Simarro, M.; Gimenez-Cassina, A.; Kedersha, N.; Lazaro, J.-B.; Adelmant, G.O.; Marto, J.A.; Rhee, K.; Tisdale, S.; Danial, N.; Benarafa, C.; et al. Fast kinase domain-containing protein 3 is a mitochondrial protein essential for cellular respiration. *Biochem. Biophys. Res. Commun.* **2010**, *401*, 440–446. [CrossRef]
120. Antonicka, H.; Shoubridge, E.A. Mitochondrial RNA Granules Are Centers for Posttranscriptional RNA Processing and Ribosome Biogenesis. *Cell Rep.* **2015**, *10*, 920–932. [CrossRef]
121. Popow, J.; Alleaume, A.-M.; Curk, T.; Schwarzl, T.; Sauer, S.; Hentze, M.W. FASTKD2 is an RNA-binding protein required for mitochondrial RNA processing and translation. *RNA* **2015**, *21*, 1873–1884. [CrossRef] [PubMed]
122. Jourdain, A.A.; Popow, J.; de la Fuente, M.A.; Martinou, J.-C.; Anderson, P.; Simarro, M. The FASTK family of proteins: Emerging regulators of mitochondrial RNA biology. *Nucleic Acids Res.* **2017**, *45*, 10941–10947. [CrossRef] [PubMed]
123. Tomecki, R.; Dmochowska, A.; Gewartowski, K.; Dziembowski, A.; Stepien, P.P. Identification of a novel human nuclear-encoded mitochondrial poly(A) polymerase. *Nucleic Acids Res.* **2004**, *32*, 6001–6014. [CrossRef] [PubMed]
124. Nagaike, T.; Suzuki, T.; Katoh, T.; Ueda, T. Human mitochondrial mRNAs are stabilized with polyadenylation regulated by mitochondria-specific poly(A) polymerase and polynucleotide phosphorylase. *J. Biol. Chem.* **2005**, *280*, 19721–19727. [CrossRef] [PubMed]
125. Wydro, M.; Bobrowicz, A.; Temperley, R.J.; Lightowlers, R.N.; Chrzanowska-Lightowlers, Z.M. Targeting of the cytosolic poly(A) binding protein PABPC1 to mitochondria causes mitochondrial translation inhibition. *Nucleic Acids Res.* **2010**, *38*, 3732–3742. [CrossRef] [PubMed]
126. Rorbach, J.; Nicholls, T.J.J.; Minczuk, M. PDE12 removes mitochondrial RNA poly(A) tails and controls translation in human mitochondria. *Nucleic Acids Res.* **2011**, *39*, 7750–7763. [CrossRef]
127. Temperley, R.J.; Wydro, M.; Lightowlers, R.N.; Chrzanowska-Lightowlers, Z.M. Human mitochondrial mRNAs–like members of all families, similar but different. *Biochim. Biophys. Acta* **2010**, *1797*, 1081–1085. [CrossRef]
128. Herrmann, J.M.; Woellhaf, M.W.; Bonnefoy, N. Control of protein synthesis in yeast mitochondria: The concept of translational activators. *Biochim. Biophys. Acta* **2013**, *1833*, 286–294. [CrossRef]
129. Weraarpachai, W.; Antonicka, H.; Sasarman, F.; Seeger, J.; Schrank, B.; Kolesar, J.E.; Lochmüller, H.; Chevrette, M.; Kaufman, B.A.; Horvath, R.; et al. Mutation in TACO1, encoding a translational activator of COX I, results in cytochrome c oxidase deficiency and late-onset Leigh syndrome. *Nat. Genet.* **2009**, *41*, 833–837. [CrossRef]
130. Safra, M.; Sas-Chen, A.; Nir, R.; Winkler, R.; Nachshon, A.; Bar-Yaacov, D.; Erlacher, M.; Rossmanith, W.; Stern-Ginossar, N.; Schwartz, S. The m1A landscape on cytosolic and mitochondrial mRNA at single-base resolution. *Nature* **2017**, *551*, 251–255. [CrossRef]
131. Li, X.; Xiong, X.; Zhang, M.; Wang, K.; Chen, Y.; Zhou, J.; Mao, Y.; Lv, J.; Yi, D.; Chen, X.-W.; et al. Base-Resolution Mapping Reveals Distinct m1A Methylome in Nuclear- and Mitochondrial-Encoded Transcripts. *Mol. Cell* **2017**, *68*, 993–1005.e9. [CrossRef] [PubMed]
132. Carlile, T.M.; Rojas-Duran, M.F.; Zinshteyn, B.; Shin, H.; Bartoli, K.M.; Gilbert, W.V. Pseudouridine profiling reveals regulated mRNA pseudouridylation in yeast and human cells. *Nature* **2014**, *515*, 143–146. [CrossRef] [PubMed]
133. Li, X.; Zhu, P.; Ma, S.; Song, J.; Bai, J.; Sun, F.; Yi, C. Chemical pulldown reveals dynamic pseudouridylation of the mammalian transcriptome. *Nat. Chem. Biol.* **2015**, *11*, 592–597. [CrossRef] [PubMed]

134. Nagaike, T.; Suzuki, T.; Tomari, Y.; Takemoto-Hori, C.; Negayama, F.; Watanabe, K.; Ueda, T. Identification and characterization of mammalian mitochondrial tRNA nucleotidyltransferases. *J. Biol. Chem.* **2001**, *276*, 40041–40049. [CrossRef]
135. Suzuki, T.; Nagao, A.; Suzuki, T. Human mitochondrial tRNAs: Biogenesis, function, structural aspects, and diseases. *Annu. Rev. Genet.* **2011**, *45*, 299–329. [CrossRef]
136. Rackham, O.; Mercer, T.R.; Filipovska, A. The human mitochondrial transcriptome and the RNA-binding proteins that regulate its expression. *Wiley Interdiscip. Rev. RNA* **2012**, *3*, 675–695. [CrossRef]
137. Pearce, S.F.; Rebelo-Guiomar, P.; D'Souza, A.R.; Powell, C.A.; Van Haute, L.; Minczuk, M. Regulation of Mammalian Mitochondrial Gene Expression: Recent Advances. *Trends Biochem. Sci.* **2017**, *42*, 625–639. [CrossRef]
138. Lee, R.G.; Rudler, D.L.; Rackham, O.; Filipovska, A. Is mitochondrial gene expression coordinated or stochastic? *Biochem. Soc. Trans.* **2018**, *46*, 1239–1246. [CrossRef]
139. White, E.; Schlackow, M.; Kamieniarz-Gdula, K.; Proudfoot, N.J.; Gullerova, M. Human nuclear Dicer restricts the deleterious accumulation of endogenous double-stranded RNA. *Nat. Struct. Mol. Biol.* **2014**, *21*, 552–559. [CrossRef]
140. Gantier, M.P. Processing of double-stranded RNA in mammalian cells: A direct antiviral role? *J. Interferon Cytokine Res.* **2014**, *34*, 469–477. [CrossRef]
141. Sen, G.C. Biological functions of double-stranded RNA and its binding proteins. *J. Interferon Cytokine Res.* **2014**, *34*, 413–414. [CrossRef] [PubMed]
142. Svoboda, P. Renaissance of mammalian endogenous RNAi. *FEBS Lett.* **2014**, *588*, 2550–2556. [CrossRef] [PubMed]
143. Kim, Y.; Park, J.; Kim, S.; Kim, M.; Kang, M.-G.; Kwak, C.; Kang, M.; Kim, B.; Rhee, H.-W.; Kim, V.N. PKR Senses Nuclear and Mitochondrial Signals by Interacting with Endogenous Double-Stranded RNAs. *Mol. Cell* **2018**, *71*, 1051–1063.e6. [CrossRef] [PubMed]
144. Dhir, A.; Dhir, S.; Borowski, L.S.; Jimenez, L.; Teitell, M.; Rötig, A.; Crow, Y.J.; Rice, G.I.; Duffy, D.; Tamby, C.; et al. Mitochondrial double-stranded RNA triggers antiviral signalling in humans. *Nature* **2018**, *560*, 238–242. [CrossRef]
145. Schneider, W.M.; Chevillotte, M.D.; Rice, C.M. Interferon-stimulated genes: A complex web of host defenses. *Annu. Rev. Immunol.* **2014**, *32*, 513–545. [CrossRef]
146. Medzhitov, R. Recognition of microorganisms and activation of the immune response. *Nature* **2007**, *449*, 819–826. [CrossRef]
147. Belgnaoui, S.M.; Paz, S.; Hiscott, J. Orchestrating the interferon antiviral response through the mitochondrial antiviral signaling (MAVS) adapter. *Curr. Opin. Immunol.* **2011**, *23*, 564–572. [CrossRef]
148. Rius, R.; Van Bergen, N.J.; Compton, A.G.; Riley, L.G.; Kava, M.P.; Balasubramaniam, S.; Amor, D.J.; Fanjul-Fernandez, M.; Cowley, M.J.; Fahey, M.C.; et al. Clinical Spectrum and Functional Consequences Associated with Bi-Allelic Pathogenic PNPT1 Variants. *J. Clin. Med.* **2019**, *8*, 2020. [CrossRef]
149. Shaw, A.E.; Hughes, J.; Gu, Q.; Behdenna, A.; Singer, J.B.; Dennis, T.; Orton, R.J.; Varela, M.; Gifford, R.J.; Wilson, S.J.; et al. Fundamental properties of the mammalian innate immune system revealed by multispecies comparison of type I interferon responses. *PLoS Biol.* **2017**, *15*, e2004086. [CrossRef]
150. Munday, D.C.; Hiscox, J.A.; Barr, J.N. Quantitative proteomic analysis of A549 cells infected with human respiratory syncytial virus subgroup B using SILAC coupled to LC-MS/MS. *Proteomics* **2010**, *10*, 4320–4334. [CrossRef]
151. Crow, Y.J.; Manel, N. Aicardi-Goutières syndrome and the type I interferonopathies. *Nat. Rev. Immunol.* **2015**, *15*, 429–440. [CrossRef] [PubMed]
152. Pajak, A.; Laine, I.; Clemente, P.; El-Fissi, N.; Schober, F.A.; Maffezzini, C.; Calvo-Garrido, J.; Wibom, R.; Filograna, R.; Dhir, A.; et al. Defects of mitochondrial RNA turnover lead to the accumulation of double-stranded RNA in vivo. *PLoS Genet.* **2019**, *15*, e1008240. [CrossRef] [PubMed]
153. Wiatrek, D.M.; Candela, M.E.; Sedmík, J.; Oppelt, J.; Keegan, L.P.; O'Connell, M.A. Activation of innate immunity by mitochondrial dsRNA in mouse cells lacking p53 protein. *RNA* **2019**, *25*, 713–726. [CrossRef] [PubMed]
154. Rackham, O.; Shearwood, A.-M.J.; Mercer, T.R.; Davies, S.M.K.; Mattick, J.S.; Filipovska, A. Long noncoding RNAs are generated from the mitochondrial genome and regulated by nuclear-encoded proteins. *RNA* **2011**, *17*, 2085–2093. [CrossRef] [PubMed]

155. Villegas, J.; Burzio, V.; Villota, C.; Landerer, E.; Martinez, R.; Santander, M.; Martinez, R.; Pinto, R.; Vera, M.I.; Boccardo, E.; et al. Expression of a novel non-coding mitochondrial RNA in human proliferating cells. *Nucleic Acids Res.* **2007**, *35*, 7336–7347. [CrossRef] [PubMed]
156. Burzio, V.A.; Villota, C.; Villegas, J.; Landerer, E.; Boccardo, E.; Villa, L.L.; Martínez, R.; Lopez, C.; Gaete, F.; Toro, V.; et al. Expression of a family of noncoding mitochondrial RNAs distinguishes normal from cancer cells. *Proc. Natl. Acad. Sci. USA* **2009**, *106*, 9430–9434. [CrossRef] [PubMed]
157. Vidaurre, S.; Fitzpatrick, C.; Burzio, V.A.; Briones, M.; Villota, C.; Villegas, J.; Echenique, J.; Oliveira-Cruz, L.; Araya, M.; Borgna, V.; et al. Down-regulation of the antisense mitochondrial non-coding RNAs (ncRNAs) is a unique vulnerability of cancer cells and a potential target for cancer therapy. *J. Biol. Chem.* **2014**, *289*, 27182–27198. [CrossRef]
158. Yang, K.-C.; Yamada, K.A.; Patel, A.Y.; Topkara, V.K.; George, I.; Cheema, F.H.; Ewald, G.A.; Mann, D.L.; Nerbonne, J.M. Deep RNA sequencing reveals dynamic regulation of myocardial noncoding RNAs in failing human heart and remodeling with mechanical circulatory support. *Circulation* **2014**, *129*, 1009–1021. [CrossRef]
159. Kumarswamy, R.; Bauters, C.; Volkmann, I.; Maury, F.; Fetisch, J.; Holzmann, A.; Lemesle, G.; de Groote, P.; Pinet, F.; Thum, T. Circulating long noncoding RNA, LIPCAR, predicts survival in patients with heart failure. *Circ. Res.* **2014**, *114*, 1569–1575. [CrossRef]
160. Dorn, G.W. LIPCAR: A mitochondrial lnc in the noncoding RNA chain? *Circ. Res.* **2014**, *114*, 1548–1550. [CrossRef]
161. Clayton, D.A. Transcription and replication of mitochondrial DNA. *Hum. Reprod.* **2000**, *15* (Suppl. 2), 11–17. [CrossRef] [PubMed]
162. Krasich, R.; Copeland, W.C. DNA polymerases in the mitochondria: A critical review of the evidence. *Front. Biosci.* **2017**, *22*, 692–709.
163. García-Gómez, S.; Reyes, A.; Martínez-Jiménez, M.I.; Chocrón, E.S.; Mourón, S.; Terrados, G.; Powell, C.; Salido, E.; Méndez, J.; Holt, I.J.; et al. PrimPol, an archaic primase/polymerase operating in human cells. *Mol. Cell* **2013**, *52*, 541–553. [CrossRef] [PubMed]
164. Rudd, S.G.; Bianchi, J.; Doherty, A.J. PrimPol-A new polymerase on the block. *Mol. Cell. Oncol.* **2014**, *1*, e960754. [CrossRef] [PubMed]
165. Sykora, P.; Kanno, S.; Akbari, M.; Kulikowicz, T.; Baptiste, B.A.; Leandro, G.S.; Lu, H.; Tian, J.; May, A.; Becker, K.A.; et al. DNA Polymerase Beta Participates in Mitochondrial DNA Repair. *Mol. Cell. Biol.* **2017**, *37*, e00237-17. [CrossRef]
166. Kaufman, B.A.; Van Houten, B. POLB: A new role of DNA polymerase beta in mitochondrial base excision repair. *DNA Repair* **2017**, *60*, A1–A5. [CrossRef]
167. Singh, B.; Li, X.; Owens, K.M.; Vanniarajan, A.; Liang, P.; Singh, K.K. Human REV3 DNA Polymerase Zeta Localizes to Mitochondria and Protects the Mitochondrial Genome. *PLoS ONE* **2015**, *10*, e0140409. [CrossRef]
168. Wisnovsky, S.; Jean, S.R.; Kelley, S.O. Mitochondrial DNA repair and replication proteins revealed by targeted chemical probes. *Nat. Chem. Biol.* **2016**, *12*, 567–573. [CrossRef]
169. Longley, M.J.; Ropp, P.A.; Lim, S.E.; Copeland, W.C. Characterization of the native and recombinant catalytic subunit of human DNA polymerase gamma: Identification of residues critical for exonuclease activity and dideoxynucleotide sensitivity. *Biochemistry* **1998**, *37*, 10529–10539. [CrossRef]
170. Spelbrink, J.N.; Toivonen, J.M.; Hakkaart, G.A.; Kurkela, J.M.; Cooper, H.M.; Lehtinen, S.K.; Lecrenier, N.; Back, J.W.; Speijer, D.; Foury, F.; et al. In vivo functional analysis of the human mitochondrial DNA polymerase POLG expressed in cultured human cells. *J. Biol. Chem.* **2000**, *275*, 24818–24828. [CrossRef]
171. Chattopadhyay, R.; Wiederhold, L.; Szczesny, B.; Boldogh, I.; Hazra, T.K.; Izumi, T.; Mitra, S. Identification and characterization of mitochondrial abasic (AP)-endonuclease in mammalian cells. *Nucleic Acids Res.* **2006**, *34*, 2067–2076. [CrossRef] [PubMed]
172. Akbari, M.; Keijzers, G.; Maynard, S.; Scheibye-Knudsen, M.; Desler, C.; Hickson, I.D.; Bohr, V.A. Overexpression of DNA ligase III in mitochondria protects cells against oxidative stress and improves mitochondrial DNA base excision repair. *DNA Repair* **2014**, *16*, 44–53. [CrossRef] [PubMed]
173. Barchiesi, A.; Wasilewski, M.; Chacinska, A.; Tell, G.; Vascotto, C. Mitochondrial translocation of APE1 relies on the MIA pathway. *Nucleic Acids Res.* **2015**, *43*, 5451–5464. [CrossRef] [PubMed]
174. Szymanski, M.R.; Yu, W.; Gmyrek, A.M.; White, M.A.; Molineux, I.J.; Lee, J.C.; Yin, Y.W. A domain in human EXOG converts apoptotic endonuclease to DNA-repair exonuclease. *Nat. Commun.* **2017**, *8*, 14959. [CrossRef]

175. Sharma, P.; Sampath, H. Mitochondrial DNA Integrity: Role in Health and Disease. *Cells* **2019**, *8*, 100. [CrossRef]
176. Gammage, P.A.; Moraes, C.T.; Minczuk, M. Mitochondrial Genome Engineering: The Revolution May Not Be CRISPR-Ized. *Trends Genet.* **2018**, *34*, 101–110. [CrossRef]
177. Nissanka, N.; Minczuk, M.; Moraes, C.T. Mechanisms of Mitochondrial DNA Deletion Formation. *Trends Genet.* **2019**, *35*, 235–244. [CrossRef]
178. Srivastava, S.; Moraes, C.T. Manipulating mitochondrial DNA heteroplasmy by a mitochondrially targeted restriction endonuclease. *Hum. Mol. Genet.* **2001**, *10*, 3093–3099. [CrossRef]
179. Srivastava, S.; Moraes, C.T. Double-strand breaks of mouse muscle mtDNA promote large deletions similar to multiple mtDNA deletions in humans. *Hum. Mol. Genet.* **2005**, *14*, 893–902. [CrossRef]
180. Bacman, S.R.; Williams, S.L.; Garcia, S.; Moraes, C.T. Organ-specific shifts in mtDNA heteroplasmy following systemic delivery of a mitochondria-targeted restriction endonuclease. *Gene Ther.* **2010**, *17*, 713–720. [CrossRef]
181. Minczuk, M.; Papworth, M.A.; Miller, J.C.; Murphy, M.P.; Klug, A. Development of a single-chain, quasi-dimeric zinc-finger nuclease for the selective degradation of mutated human mitochondrial DNA. *Nucleic Acids Res.* **2008**, *36*, 3926–3938. [CrossRef] [PubMed]
182. Reddy, P.; Ocampo, A.; Suzuki, K.; Luo, J.; Bacman, S.R.; Williams, S.L.; Sugawara, A.; Okamura, D.; Tsunekawa, Y.; Wu, J.; et al. Selective elimination of mitochondrial mutations in the germline by genome editing. *Cell* **2015**, *161*, 459–469. [CrossRef] [PubMed]
183. Gammage, P.A.; Rorbach, J.; Vincent, A.I.; Rebar, E.J.; Minczuk, M. Mitochondrially targeted ZFNs for selective degradation of pathogenic mitochondrial genomes bearing large-scale deletions or point mutations. *EMBO Mol. Med.* **2014**, *6*, 458–466. [CrossRef] [PubMed]
184. Gammage, P.A.; Gaude, E.; Van Haute, L.; Rebelo-Guiomar, P.; Jackson, C.B.; Rorbach, J.; Pekalski, M.L.; Robinson, A.J.; Charpentier, M.; Concordet, J.-P.; et al. Near-complete elimination of mutant mtDNA by iterative or dynamic dose-controlled treatment with mtZFNs. *Nucleic Acids Res.* **2016**, *44*, 7804–7816. [CrossRef]
185. Bacman, S.R.; Williams, S.L.; Pinto, M.; Peralta, S.; Moraes, C.T. Specific elimination of mutant mitochondrial genomes in patient-derived cells by mitoTALENs. *Nat. Med.* **2013**, *19*, 1111–1113. [CrossRef]
186. Gammage, P.A.; Viscomi, C.; Simard, M.-L.; Costa, A.S.H.; Gaude, E.; Powell, C.A.; Van Haute, L.; McCann, B.J.; Rebelo-Guiomar, P.; Cerutti, R.; et al. Genome editing in mitochondria corrects a pathogenic mtDNA mutation in vivo. *Nat. Med.* **2018**, *24*, 1691–1695. [CrossRef]
187. Bacman, S.R.; Kauppila, J.H.K.; Pereira, C.V.; Nissanka, N.; Miranda, M.; Pinto, M.; Williams, S.L.; Larsson, N.-G.; Stewart, J.B.; Moraes, C.T. MitoTALEN reduces mutant mtDNA load and restores tRNAAla levels in a mouse model of heteroplasmic mtDNA mutation. *Nat. Med.* **2018**, *24*, 1696–1700. [CrossRef]
188. Wang, G.; Shimada, E.; Zhang, J.; Hong, J.S.; Smith, G.M.; Teitell, M.A.; Koehler, C.M. Correcting human mitochondrial mutations with targeted RNA import. *Proc. Natl. Acad. Sci. USA* **2012**, *109*, 4840–4845. [CrossRef]
189. Chen, H.-W.; Rainey, R.N.; Balatoni, C.E.; Dawson, D.W.; Troke, J.J.; Wasiak, S.; Hong, J.S.; McBride, H.M.; Koehler, C.M.; Teitell, M.A.; et al. Mammalian polynucleotide phosphorylase is an intermembrane space RNase that maintains mitochondrial homeostasis. *Mol. Cell. Biol.* **2006**, *26*, 8475–8487. [CrossRef]
190. Tarassov, I.; Entelis, N.; Martin, R.P. An intact protein translocating machinery is required for mitochondrial import of a yeast cytoplasmic tRNA. *J. Mol. Biol.* **1995**, *245*, 315–323. [CrossRef]
191. Kolesnikova, O.A.; Entelis, N.S.; Jacquin-Becker, C.; Goltzene, F.; Chrzanowska-Lightowlers, Z.M.; Lightowlers, R.N.; Martin, R.P.; Tarassov, I. Nuclear DNA-encoded tRNAs targeted into mitochondria can rescue a mitochondrial DNA mutation associated with the MERRF syndrome in cultured human cells. *Hum. Mol. Genet.* **2004**, *13*, 2519–2534. [CrossRef] [PubMed]
192. Comte, C.; Tonin, Y.; Heckel-Mager, A.-M.; Boucheham, A.; Smirnov, A.; Auré, K.; Lombès, A.; Martin, R.P.; Entelis, N.; Tarassov, I. Mitochondrial targeting of recombinant RNAs modulates the level of a heteroplasmic mutation in human mitochondrial DNA associated with Kearns Sayre Syndrome. *Nucleic Acids Res.* **2013**, *41*, 418–433. [CrossRef] [PubMed]

193. Tonin, Y.; Heckel, A.-M.; Vysokikh, M.; Dovydenko, I.; Meschaninova, M.; Rötig, A.; Munnich, A.; Venyaminova, A.; Tarassov, I.; Entelis, N. Modeling of antigenomic therapy of mitochondrial diseases by mitochondrially addressed RNA targeting a pathogenic point mutation in mitochondrial DNA. *J. Biol. Chem.* **2014**, *289*, 13323–13334. [CrossRef] [PubMed]
194. Schneider, A.; Martin, J.; Agabian, N. A nuclear encoded tRNA of Trypanosoma brucei is imported into mitochondria. *Mol. Cell. Biol.* **1994**, *14*, 2317–2322. [CrossRef]
195. Kumar, R.; Maréchal-Drouard, L.; Akama, K.; Small, I. Striking differences in mitochondrial tRNA import between different plant species. *Mol. Gen. Genet.* **1996**, *252*, 404–411. [CrossRef]
196. Kiss, T.; Filipowicz, W. Evidence against a mitochondrial location of the 7-2/MRP RNA in mammalian cells. *Cell* **1992**, *70*, 11–16. [CrossRef]
197. Jacobson, M.R.; Cao, L.G.; Wang, Y.L.; Pederson, T. Dynamic localization of RNase MRP RNA in the nucleolus observed by fluorescent RNA cytochemistry in living cells. *J. Cell Biol.* **1995**, *131*, 1649–1658. [CrossRef]
198. Goldfarb, K.C.; Cech, T.R. Targeted CRISPR disruption reveals a role for RNase MRP RNA in human preribosomal RNA processing. *Genes Dev.* **2017**, *31*, 59–71. [CrossRef]
199. Greber, B.J.; Boehringer, D.; Leitner, A.; Bieri, P.; Voigts-Hoffmann, F.; Erzberger, J.P.; Leibundgut, M.; Aebersold, R.; Ban, N. Architecture of the large subunit of the mammalian mitochondrial ribosome. *Nature* **2014**, *505*, 515–519. [CrossRef]
200. Brown, A.; Amunts, A.; Bai, X.-C.; Sugimoto, Y.; Edwards, P.C.; Murshudov, G.; Scheres, S.H.W.; Ramakrishnan, V. Structure of the large ribosomal subunit from human mitochondria. *Science* **2014**, *346*, 718–722. [CrossRef]
201. Greber, B.J.; Bieri, P.; Leibundgut, M.; Leitner, A.; Aebersold, R.; Boehringer, D.; Ban, N. Ribosome. The complete structure of the 55S mammalian mitochondrial ribosome. *Science* **2015**, *348*, 303–308. [CrossRef] [PubMed]
202. Lee, Y.S.; Shibata, Y.; Malhotra, A.; Dutta, A. A novel class of small RNAs: tRNA-derived RNA fragments (tRFs). *Genes Dev.* **2009**, *23*, 2639–2649. [CrossRef] [PubMed]
203. Haussecker, D.; Huang, Y.; Lau, A.; Parameswaran, P.; Fire, A.Z.; Kay, M.A. Human tRNA-derived small RNAs in the global regulation of RNA silencing. *RNA* **2010**, *16*, 673–695. [CrossRef] [PubMed]
204. Ro, S.; Ma, H.-Y.; Park, C.; Ortogero, N.; Song, R.; Hennig, G.W.; Zheng, H.; Lin, Y.-M.; Moro, L.; Hsieh, J.-T.; et al. The mitochondrial genome encodes abundant small noncoding RNAs. *Cell Res.* **2013**, *23*, 759–774. [CrossRef]
205. Geiger, J.; Dalgaard, L.T. Interplay of mitochondrial metabolism and microRNAs. *Cell. Mol. Life Sci.* **2017**, *74*, 631–646. [CrossRef]
206. Bartel, D.P. MicroRNAs: Target recognition and regulatory functions. *Cell* **2009**, *136*, 215–233. [CrossRef]
207. Bandiera, S.; Rüberg, S.; Girard, M.; Cagnard, N.; Hanein, S.; Chrétien, D.; Munnich, A.; Lyonnet, S.; Henrion-Caude, A. Nuclear outsourcing of RNA interference components to human mitochondria. *PLoS ONE* **2011**, *6*, e20746. [CrossRef]
208. Barrey, E.; Saint-Auret, G.; Bonnamy, B.; Damas, D.; Boyer, O.; Gidrol, X. Pre-microRNA and mature microRNA in human mitochondria. *PLoS ONE* **2011**, *6*, e20220. [CrossRef]
209. Sripada, L.; Tomar, D.; Prajapati, P.; Singh, R.; Singh, A.K.; Singh, R. Systematic analysis of small RNAs associated with human mitochondria by deep sequencing: Detailed analysis of mitochondrial associated miRNA. *PLoS ONE* **2012**, *7*, e44873. [CrossRef]
210. Jagannathan, R.; Thapa, D.; Nichols, C.E.; Shepherd, D.L.; Stricker, J.C.; Croston, T.L.; Baseler, W.A.; Lewis, S.E.; Martinez, I.; Hollander, J.M. Translational Regulation of the Mitochondrial Genome Following Redistribution of Mitochondrial MicroRNA in the Diabetic Heart. *Circ. Cardiovasc. Genet.* **2015**, *8*, 785–802. [CrossRef]
211. Hashimoto, Y.; Ito, Y.; Niikura, T.; Shao, Z.; Hata, M.; Oyama, F.; Nishimoto, I. Mechanisms of neuroprotection by a novel rescue factor humanin from Swedish mutant amyloid precursor protein. *Biochem. Biophys. Res. Commun.* **2001**, *283*, 460–468. [CrossRef] [PubMed]
212. Hashimoto, Y.; Niikura, T.; Tajima, H.; Yasukawa, T.; Sudo, H.; Ito, Y.; Kita, Y.; Kawasumi, M.; Kouyama, K.; Doyu, M.; et al. A rescue factor abolishing neuronal cell death by a wide spectrum of familial Alzheimer's disease genes and Abeta. *Proc. Natl. Acad. Sci. USA* **2001**, *98*, 6336–6341. [CrossRef]
213. Lee, C.; Yen, K.; Cohen, P. Humanin: A harbinger of mitochondrial-derived peptides? *Trends Endocrinol. Metab.* **2013**, *24*, 222–228. [CrossRef] [PubMed]

214. Lee, C.; Zeng, J.; Drew, B.G.; Sallam, T.; Martin-Montalvo, A.; Wan, J.; Kim, S.-J.; Mehta, H.; Hevener, A.L.; de Cabo, R.; et al. The mitochondrial-derived peptide MOTS-c promotes metabolic homeostasis and reduces obesity and insulin resistance. *Cell Metab.* **2015**, *21*, 443–454. [CrossRef] [PubMed]
215. Cobb, L.J.; Lee, C.; Xiao, J.; Yen, K.; Wong, R.G.; Nakamura, H.K.; Mehta, H.H.; Gao, Q.; Ashur, C.; Huffman, D.M.; et al. Naturally occurring mitochondrial-derived peptides are age-dependent regulators of apoptosis, insulin sensitivity, and inflammatory markers. *Aging* **2016**, *8*, 796–809. [CrossRef] [PubMed]
216. Kim, S.-J.; Xiao, J.; Wan, J.; Cohen, P.; Yen, K. Mitochondrially derived peptides as novel regulators of metabolism. *J. Physiol.* **2017**, *595*, 6613–6621. [CrossRef] [PubMed]

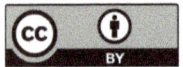

© 2019 by the authors. Licensee MDPI, Basel, Switzerland. This article is an open access article distributed under the terms and conditions of the Creative Commons Attribution (CC BY) license (http://creativecommons.org/licenses/by/4.0/).

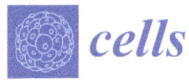

Article

BK$_{Ca}$ (*Slo*) Channel Regulates Mitochondrial Function and Lifespan in *Drosophila melanogaster*

Shubha Gururaja Rao [1,2], Piotr Bednarczyk [3], Atif Towheed [4], Kajol Shah [2], Priyanka Karekar [1,2], Devasena Ponnalagu [1,2], Haley N. Jensen [1], Sankar Addya [5], Beverly A.S. Reyes [2], Elisabeth J. Van Bockstaele [2], Adam Szewczyk [6], Douglas C. Wallace [4,7] and Harpreet Singh [1,2,*]

1. Department of Physiology and Cell Biology, The Ohio State University Wexner Medical Center, Columbus, OH 43210, USA
2. Department of Pharmacology and Physiology, Drexel University College of Medicine, Philadelphia, PA 19102, USA
3. Department of Biophysics, Warsaw University of Life Sciences- SGGW, 02-776 Warsaw, Poland
4. Center for Mitochondrial and Epigenomic Medicine, The Children's Hospital of Philadelphia, Philadelphia, PA 19104, USA
5. Kimmel Cancer Centre, Thomas Jefferson University, Philadelphia, PA 19107, USA
6. Laboratory of Intracellular Ion Channels, Nencki Institute of Experimental Biology, 02-093 Warsaw, Poland
7. Department of Pathology and Laboratory Medicine, University of Pennsylvania, Philadelphia, PA 19104, USA
* Correspondence: harpreet.singh@osumc.edu

Received: 7 June 2019; Accepted: 20 August 2019; Published: 21 August 2019

Abstract: BK$_{Ca}$ channels, originally discovered in *Drosophila melanogaster* as *slowpoke* (*slo*), are recognized for their roles in cellular and organ physiology. Pharmacological approaches implicated BK$_{Ca}$ channels in cellular and organ protection possibly for their ability to modulate mitochondrial function. However, the direct role of BK$_{Ca}$ channels in regulating mitochondrial structure and function is not deciphered. Here, we demonstrate that BK$_{Ca}$ channels are present in fly mitochondria, and *slo* mutants show structural and functional defects in mitochondria. *slo* mutants display an increase in reactive oxygen species and the modulation of ROS affected their survival. We also found that the absence of BK$_{Ca}$ channels reduced the lifespan of *Drosophila*, and overexpression of human BK$_{Ca}$ channels in flies extends life span in males. Our study establishes the presence of BK$_{Ca}$ channels in mitochondria of *Drosophila* and ascertains its novel physiological role in regulating mitochondrial structural and functional integrity, and lifespan.

Keywords: potassium channel; mitochondria; reactive oxygen species; antioxidants; life span; aging; BK$_{Ca}$ channels

---

1. Introduction

The large-conductance potassium channel activated by calcium (Ca^{2+}) and voltage (BK$_{Ca}$/Slo/MaxiK) was originally cloned in *Drosophila* at the *slowpoke* (*slo*) locus [1–3] and addressed as *Kcnma1* in mammals. BK$_{Ca}$ channel is ubiquitously present in the plasma membrane of all eukaryotic cells. In *Drosophila*, extensive work has been performed on *slo* mutants where BK$_{Ca}$ was shown to carry transient Ca^{2+}-dependent K^+ currents (I_{KCa}) in muscles [2,4], and neuronal cells [5]. In addition, *slo* mutant has revealed roles of BK$_{Ca}$ channel in neuronal functions, abnormal circadian activity, and well-characterized locomotor disorder (hence the name *slowpoke*) [3,6].

In mammals, BK$_{Ca}$ is characterized to play similar roles in neuronal and non-neuronal cells [7]. They are the key ion channels with a large conductance, activated by gasses and lipids in addition to sensing changes in Ca^{2+}, and voltage. In the last decade, mutations in *Kcnma1* gene have been associated with a paroxysmal movement disorder, epilepsy, obesity, hypertension, and cancer in humans [8]. BK_{Ca} null mutant mice showed alterations in circadian rhythm, blood pressure, hearing, heart rate, bladder control, locomotion, reproductive function, neurovascular coupling, airway constriction, insulin secretion, and learning and memory [7,9]. In the absence of BK_{Ca}, the survival of mice and weight gain was hampered [10] but in contrast, the absence of Slo-1 in *Caenorhabditis elegans* was associated with slow motor aging and moderate extension of life span [11]. The majority of these functions were shown to be associated with the BK_{Ca} localized to the plasma membrane [9]. One exception to plasma membrane localization of BK_{Ca} channels is their localization to mitochondria of murine and rodent adult cardiomyocytes [8,12]. In the heart, activation of BK_{Ca} is known to play a direct role in cardioprotection from ischemia-reperfusion (IR) injury possibly via regulation of mitochondrial function [8,12–14].

Mitochondria are energy-generating organelles of the cell involved in several metabolic and signaling pathways. The inner mitochondrial membranes support the electron transport chain (ETC) tightly-coupled with membrane potential (ψ_{mito}) that participates in the generation of ATP. Defects in ETC, ψ_{mito}, mitochondrial fusion–fission events, or ionic imbalance can cause mitochondrial permeability transition pore (mPTP) to form, and result in apoptosis [15]. One of the well-established consequences of mitochondrial dysfunction is life span [16]. Several ion channels present in the plasma membrane and intracellular organelle membranes are known to regulate mitochondrial structure as well as functional integrity [8]. Even though BK_{Ca} is shown to regulate mitochondrial function, there is no direct evidence that BK_{Ca} can directly regulate mitochondrial structural and functional integrity. Expression of BK_{Ca} in coronary arteries from old rats, as well as humans, diminishes without showing any changes in biophysical properties [17]. However, whether BK_{Ca} directly affects life span is not well studied. To address this question, we studied the BK_{Ca} channel mutant (*slo*) phenotypes with respect to mitochondrial functional integrity and life span using the *Drosophila* model.

In this study, we found that BK_{Ca}/Slo is present in mitochondria of *Drosophila* as a functional ion channel. The absence of BK_{Ca} results in age-related changes in mitochondrial structural and functional integrity. We also tested whether increased mitochondrial reactive oxygen species (ROS) is responsible for the early death of flies and chelating ROS could partially rescue the aging phenotype. Ablation of BK_{Ca} dramatically reduced the lifespan of *Drosophila*, while overexpression of human BK_{Ca} form surprisingly increased lifespan only in males. In agreement, our microarray data revealed various life span regulated transcripts altered in *slo* mutant flies. Taken together, our results define a novel function for BK_{Ca} channel in regulating mitochondrial structure and function and reduction in life span.

2. Materials and Methods

2.1. Drosophila Stocks, Reagents, Dyes, and Antibodies

All fly stocks were maintained at 25 °C on standard medium (jazz mix, nipagin free) unless otherwise stated. The experiments were carried out at 25 °C or 29 °C (for Gal4 efficiency) as mentioned in the results sections or figures. The Canton S strain served as the wild-type (wt) stock and is indicated as 'wt' through the manuscript. The *slo*^{1} mutants (chemical-induced mutation, originally characterized in Elkins et al. 1986 [3]), RNAi lines, Gal4 lines, and wild type lines (Canton S and W1118) were obtained from the Bloomington Stock Center. UAS Sod2 flies were a gift from Prof. David Walker (UCLA).

2.2. Immuno Cyto/Organelle Chemistry

Flight muscles were dissected and fixed with 4% (*w/v*) paraformaldehyde (PFA), washed and permeabilized with 0.4% (*v/v*) Triton-X100. Mitochondria were isolated from whole flies and loaded with mitotracker as described earlier [18]. Mitochondria and tissues were blocked with normal goat serum (10%) and stained with primary antibodies (anti-ubiquitin 1:100 (FK2), and anti-BK_{Ca} 1:200) and secondary antibodies, followed by DAPI (for tissues) (n = 5 independent experiments).

2.3. Electrophysiology

Patch-clamp experiments using mitoplasts (mitochondria without outer membranes) were performed as described previously [19,20]. Briefly, mitoplasts were prepared from mitochondria isolated from whole *D. melanogaster* placed in a hypotonic solution (5 mM HEPES, 100 µM $CaCl_2$, pH = 7.2) to induce swelling and eventual disruption of the outer membrane. To restore the sample to an isotonic condition (150 mM KCl, 10 mM HEPES, 100 µM $CaCl_2$, pH 7.2) a hypertonic solution (750 mM KCl, 30 mM HEPES, 100 µM $CaCl_2$, pH 7.2) was added. The patch-clamp pipette was filled with an isotonic solution. Mitoplasts are easily recognizable due to their size, round shape, transparency, and the presence of a 'cap', characteristics that distinguish these structures from the cellular debris that is also present in the preparation. The low-calcium solution (1 µM $CaCl_2$) contained the following: 150 mM KCl, 10 mM HEPES, 1 mM EGTA, and 0.752 mM $CaCl_2$ at pH 7.2. An isotonic solution containing 100 µM $CaCl_2$ was used as the control solution for all of the presented data. The experiments to assess the channel activity were carried out in patch-clamp inside-out mode [20]. The electrical circuit was made using Ag/AgCl electrodes and an agar salt bridge (3 M KCl) as the ground electrode. The current was recorded using a patch-clamp amplifier Axopatch 200B. The pipettes had a resistance of about 14 MΩ and were pulled using a vertical puller.

The currents were low-pass filtered at 1 kHz and sampled at a frequency of 100 kHz. The traces of the experiments were recorded in single-channel mode. The conductance of the channel was calculated from the current–voltage relationship (Figure 1I). The probability of channel opening (Po, open probability) was determined using the single-channel search mode of the Clampfit software. Data from the experiments are reported as the mean values $\pm$ standard deviations (S.D.). Student's *t*-test was used for statistical analysis (n = 5 independent experiments comprising of mitochondrial isolation from 100 flies each).

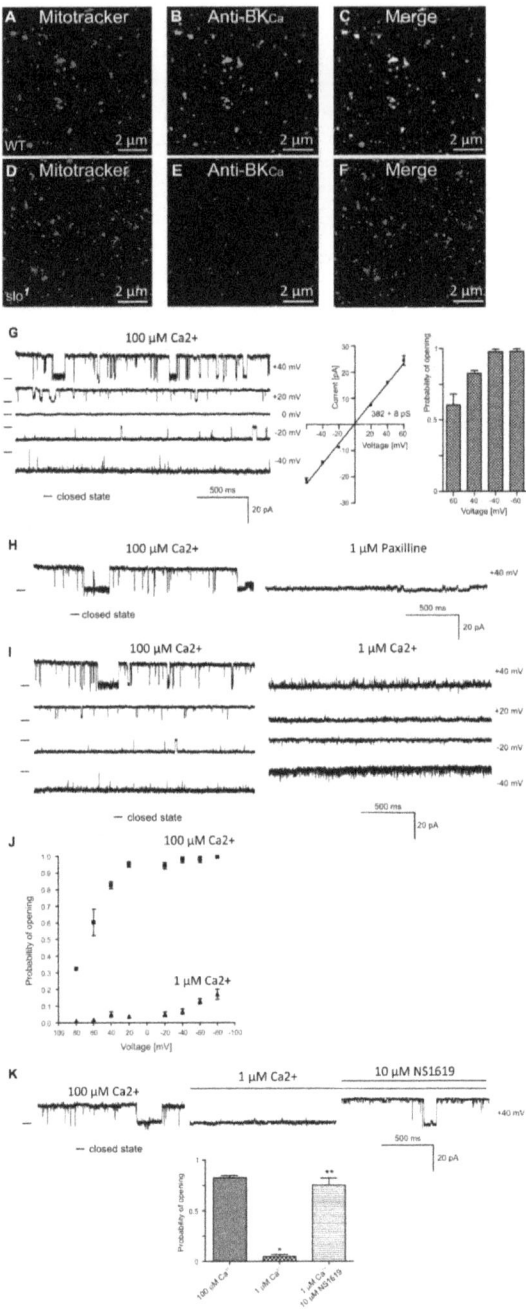

Figure 1. Localization of dSlo in isolated mitochondria. High-resolution confocal images of isolated mitochondria from *Drosophila* (**A–C**, wild type, **D–F** *slo* mutants) loaded with mitotracker (**A,D** red) and labeled with an anti-Slo antibody (**B,E** green). Overlays are shown in (**C,F**). Protein proximity index for dSlo to mitotracker was 0.5 ± 0.1.

(**G**), Single-channel current-time recordings (left panel), current-voltage characteristics (middle panel) and Po analysis of single-channel events in a symmetric 150/150 mM KCl isotonic solution (100 μM Ca^{2+}) at different voltages in mitoplast prepared from whole flies. (**H**), Effects of 1 μM Paxilline on the single-channel activity. (**I**), Single-channel current-time recordings in symmetric 150/150 mM KCl isotonic solution at control (100 μM Ca^{2+}) and after reduction calcium concentration to 1 μM Ca^{2+}. (**J**), Analysis opening probability in the presence of 1 and 100 μM Ca^{2+} at different voltages of the $mitoBK_{Ca}$ channel in mitoplast prepared from whole flies. All data were acquired in a symmetric 150/150 mM KCl isotonic solution (n = 4). (**K**), Current–time recordings of single-channel activity in symmetric 150/150 mM KCl isotonic solution at control (100 μM Ca^{2+}), after reduction calcium concentration to 1 μM Ca^{2+} and after application of 10 μM NS1619. The bar graph shows the distribution of the Po under the conditions above. * $p < 0.001$ vs. the control. ** $p < 0.001$ vs. 1 μM Ca^{2+}. The data in (**G,J,K**) are presented as the means ± S.D. The recordings were low-pass filtered at 1 kHz. "-" indicate a closed state of the channel.

2.4. Reactive Oxygen Species and Quantification

2.4.1. Dihydroethidium (DHE)

Flight muscles were dissected quickly and placed in DHE (molecular probes) in PBS (1:1000 dilution) for 3 min and then washed in PBS three times for 3 min each. The samples were then fixed in 4% (*w/v*) PFA for 3 min and then washed again in PBS twice for 2 min each time. Flight muscles were then mounted in PBS and immediately photographed under a Zeiss confocal microscope (n = 5 independent experiments).

2.4.2. Spectrophotometric Analysis

Flies were homogenized using a pestle, and ROS generation was detected from isolated mitochondria by amplex red using fluorescence spectrophotometer (Hitachi F-2710) described previously [18]. Briefly, 5 μg horseradish peroxidase (Sigma-Aldrich, St. Louis, MO, USA) was added to the ROS buffer (mmol/L, 20 Tris-HCl, 250 sucrose, 1 EGTA-Na_4, 1 EDTA-Na_2, pH 7.4 at 37 °C) and the baseline fluorescence was obtained (excitation at 560 nm and emission at 590 nm) for 30 min (n = 4 independent experiments with 100 flies each to isolate mitochondria). The protein concentration was used to normalize the amount of mitochondria from the same extracts.

2.5. ATP Measurement

ATP was measured from five individual groups of 2-week old females flies (n = 5 independent experiments with 20 flies each), using Roche ATP bioluminescence assay kit CLS II according to manufacturer's instructions. Briefly, flies were homogenized in the lysis buffer and incubated for 5 min at room temperature. The extract was spun down at 10,000 *g* and the supernatant was transferred into a microwell plate. Upon addition of luciferase reagent, the luminescence was measured using a luminometer. The ATP measurements were normalized to protein from the same extract.

2.6. Oxygraph

Mitochondria from 40 flies were harvested and resuspended in 100 μL MiRO5 buffer (mmol/L, 0.5 EGTA, 3 $MgCl_2$, 60 K-lactobionate, 20 taurine, 10 KH_2PO_4, 20 HEPES, 110 sucrose and 1 g/L BSA essentially fatty acid-free adjusted to pH 7.1). The assay was performed using the OROBOROS® Oxygraph-2k (O2k, Oroboros Instruments, Innsbruck, Austria) similar to previously published methods [21]. The oxygen electrodes were calibrated with air-saturated respiration medium (MiRO5) at 25 °C as per manufacturer instructions. SUIT protocol was used to test the activities of Complex I (malate and pyruvate) and Complex II (rotenone and succinate). Following substrates and inhibitors were added sequentially: malate (2 mM) and pyruvate (5 mM), succinate (10 mM), rotenone (0.5 μM), malonic acid (5 mM), and antimycin A (2.5 μM). ADP (1–5 mM) was added at distinct steps after the addition of Complex I and II substrates. FCCP (Carbonyl cyanide 4-(trifluoromethoxy)phenylhydrazone) titrations

(0.05 µM steps) were carefully performed to obtain maximum electron transport capacity. Cytochrome c (10 µM) test was performed in each experiment to make sure that the mitochondrial membrane integrity was not compromised. The rate of oxygen consumption (oxygen flux) as a function of time was normalized to the total protein concentration for each experiment. Background calibration and air calibration were performed as suggested by the manufacturer prior to the experiments. Data were analyzed by DatLab software (v5.0, Oroboros Instruments, Innsbruck, Austria). n = 5 independent experiments from 40 flies each. The protein content was used to normalize the amount of mitochondria from the same extracts.

2.7. Electron Microscopy

Drosophila flight muscles were dissected in PBS and fixed in 2% (*w/v*) glutaraldehyde and 2.5% (*w/v*) formaldehyde in PBS. Embedding, thin sectioning, and staining were carried out according to a standard protocol [22] (n = 5 independent preparations).

2.8. Drosophila Survivorship (Life Span Assays)

Flies were collected upon eclosure and reared in vials (30 flies in each vial, n = 3 independent assays) with food at 25 °C or 29 °C on a standard medium. The media was changed every 3 days and a number of deaths were recorded until all the flies died (for every life span assay, we used at least n ≥ 20 flies per vial and 3 such vials as biological replicates).

2.9. Drosophila Geotaxis

A negative geotaxis assay [23] was performed by counting the number of flies that cross 5 cm mark in 18 s after tapping them to the bottom of the vial (n = 3 independent experiments with 5 flies in each experiment).

2.10. Dye-Feeding Assay

Flies were fed fluorescein (2% (*w/v*) in media) dye for 9 h and imaged under a fluorescent microscope using 10X objective (Zeiss) (n = 5 independent experiments).

2.11. Paraquat/Glutathione Assays

Flies (2–3 days old) were starved for 2 h in 0.5% (*w/v*) agar and transferred into vials containing fiberglass filter papers with 5% (*w/v*) sucrose and 20 mM PQ with or without 220 µM glutathione (reduced). For the glutathione experiments, just eclosed flies were also reared on media containing 220 µM glutathione (reduced) for 1 week prior to PQ survival studies. Numbers of dead flies were counted every 12 h and plotted (n ≥ 20).

2.12. Cloning of Human BK_{Ca}/UAS-Flies

BK_{Ca}-HF full length was cloned in pUASTattb vector between NotI and XhoI restriction enzyme sites. The construct was amplified by PCR using N-terminal c-myc tag pCDNA3BK_{Ca}-HF as a template. Briefly, BK_{Ca}-HF was amplified using sense primer 5′-AAG GAA AAA AGC GGC CGC ATG GGC GCC GAG GAG CAG AAG-3′ and anti-sense primer 5′-CTA GTC TAG ACT CGA GTC AAA GCC GCT CTT CCT G-3′. The PCR conditions were 95 °C for 5 min, 30 cycles of 95 °C for 30 s, 55 °C for 30 s and 72 °C for 7 min followed by extension at 72 °C for 10 min. The clones obtained were confirmed by sequencing (Genewiz). Constructs were injected into *Drosophila* embryos using services from BestGene Inc (Chino Hills, CA, USA).

2.13. Microarray

Total RNA was isolated from 3-week-old female wild type and *slo* mutant flies using Qiagen RNAeasy kit. RNA was treated with RNase-free DNAse I. RNA was quantified on a Nanodrop

ND-100 spectrophotometer (NanoDrop Technologies, Wilmington, DE, USA), followed by RNA quality assessment by analysis on an Agilent 2100 bioanalyzer (Agilent, Palo Alto, CA, USA). Fragmented biotin-labeled cDNA (from 100 ng RNA) were prepared using the GeneChip WT Plus kit.

Each Affymetrix gene chip *Drosophila* array (Affymetrix, Santa Clara, CA, USA) was hybridized with the fragmented and biotin-labeled target (4.5 µg) in 200 µL of hybridization cocktail. Target denaturation was performed at 99 °C for 2 min and then 45 °C for 5 min, followed by hybridization for 18 h. Then the arrays were washed and stained using GeneChip Fluidic Station 450, and hybridization signals were amplified using antibody amplification with goat IgG (Sigma-Aldrich, St. Louis, MO, USA) and anti-streptavidin biotinylated antibody (Vector Laboratories, Burlingame, CA, USA). The chips were scanned on an Affymetrix Gene Chip Scanner 3000, using Command Console Software. Background correction and normalization were done using Robust Multichip Average with Genespring V 14.9 software (Agilent). A 1.5-fold differentially expressed gene ($p \leq 0.05$ values) list was generated. The listing of differentially expressed genes and their fold change were loaded into Ingenuity Pathway Analysis (IPA) 5.0 software (Qiagen Inc., https://www.qiagenbioinformatics.com/products/ingenuity-pathway-analysis) to perform biological network and functional analyses. IPA converts gene sets (with or without expression information) into related molecular networks based on IPA knowledge database. Core analysis was performed for and the genes were categorized based on molecular function, mapped to genetic networks, and ranked by score. The score reflects the probability that a collection of genes equal to or greater than a number in the network could not be achieved by chance alone. A score of more than 10 was used as a cutoff for identifying specific gene networks (n = 3 independent experiments with RNA isolated from 100 flies each).

2.14. Data Analysis

Data were analyzed using Sigma plot. Student's *t*-tests or ANOVA were used for analyzing all the data and reported as mean ± standard error or the mean in text. *p*-values less than 0.05 were considered significant.

3. Results

3.1. Presence of BK_{Ca} Currents in the Drosophila Mitochondria

In addition to the plasma membrane, BK_{Ca} channels are known to be present in the mitochondria of rodent neurons [24] and endothelial cells [19]. In adult cardiomyocytes, they are exclusively present in the mitochondria [12,25] but not in the plasma membrane [12,26]. In *Drosophila*, BK_{Ca} has been well-characterized in the plasma membrane at the biophysical and physiological levels [7,27], however, it is not known whether it is present or active in the mitochondria. In order to test for the presence of BK_{Ca} in mitochondria, we loaded isolated mitochondria with mitotracker [18] and labeled with anti-BK_{Ca} antibodies (Figure 1A,B,D,E). Mitochondria isolated from the whole wild-type but not slo^1 mutant flies [1,3] showed the presence of a BK_{Ca}-specific signal (Figure 1A–F). Protein proximity index (PPI) analysis [12] to estimate colocalization of BK_{Ca} to mitotracker-loaded mitochondria showed a value of ~0.5 ± 0.1 (n = 6), indicating ~50% of BK_{Ca} signal colocalized with mitochondria.

BK_{Ca} has been recorded from cardiac and endothelial mitoplasts [8,19,25], but not in *Drosophila* mitoplast (inner membrane of mitochondria). To examine whether BK_{Ca} is active in *Drosophila* mitoplast (n = 5 independent experiments, mitochondria isolated from 100 flies each), we isolated mitoplast from wild type flies and carried out patch-clamp analysis [19]. Approximately 80% of the currents detected in the mitoplasts were attributed to BK_{Ca}-specific channels. We recorded channel activity (Figure 1G) in the presence of 100 µM Ca^{2+} in the bath pipette at holding potentials ranging from +60 mV to −60 mV in a symmetrical solution (150 mM KCl, 10 mM HEPES, 100 µM Ca^{2+}, pH 7.2). The current (I) vs. voltage (V) curve (Figure 1G) calculated from the single-channel currents showed a conductance of 382 ± 8 pS (n = 5) for mitoBK_{Ca}. Surprisingly, the open probability of single-channel current increases from ~0.6 at +60 mV to ~1.0 at −60 mV holding potentials (Figure 1G). On addition of paxilline (BK$_{Ca}$ antagonist), the large channel conductance was completely blocked (Figure 1H), confirming that the large currents were originated from paxilline-sensitive BK$_{Ca}$.

Since BK$_{Ca}$ is a Ca^{2+}-sensitive channel, we also changed the Ca^{2+} concentration of bath solution from 100 µM to 1 µM. Single-channel recordings showed a decrease in open probability (Po) at holding potentials ranging from −40 mV to 40 mV (Figure 1I). Po vs. V plot shows increase in Po at 100 µM as compared to 1 µM Ca^{2+} (Figure 1J). Large conductance channels were not observed at 1 µM Ca^{2+}. However, on the addition of 1 µM NS1619 (BK$_{Ca}$ agonist), the large-conductance channel reappeared with a high Po (Figure 1K). Our immuno-organelle chemistry data indicate the presence of BK$_{Ca}$ channels in isolated mitochondria. In addition, our electrophysiological approach demonstrates the presence of BK$_{Ca}$ in *Drosophila* mitochondria corroborating the immuno-organelle chemistry data.

3.2. Mitochondrial Functional Aberrations in BK$_{Ca}$ Mutants

Given the presence of BK$_{Ca}$ in the mitochondria, we sought to investigate if BK$_{Ca}$ plays a direct role in its functional integrity using the BK$_{Ca}$ (*slo*^{1}) mutant [1,28].

We tested if ROS, the major byproduct of mitochondria, is altered in *slo*^{1} mutants. The *slo*^{1} mutant showed higher levels of DHE staining (a detector of ROS) in indirect flight muscles indicating significantly ($p < 0.05$, n = 5) increased production and accumulation of ROS (Figure 2A vs. 2B, quantified in 2C). We examined ETC function where ROS is generated and found that *slo*^{1} mutant mitochondria showed a significant increase in ROS production (Figure 2D–G). The increase was significant when pyruvate was used as a substrate (Figure 2D,G, $p < 0.01$). To dissect which complex is generating this ROS, we used specific substrates for complex I and complex II of ETC. With glutamate/malate (substrate for complex I), we did not see any significant difference in ROS generation (Figure 2E,G). However, succinate (substrate for complex II) showed a much higher level of ROS generation (Figure 2F,G) in *slo*^{1} mutants, indicating that increased ROS produced could be due to complex III and or backflow of electrons to complex I [29]. Another mutant for dSlo, *slo[f05915]* [30] also showed the elevated rate as well as the amount of ROS production by complex III (Supplementary Figure S1).

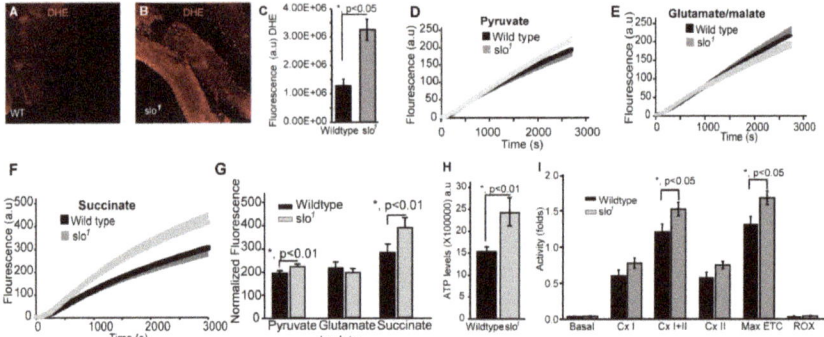

Figure 2. Mitochondrial functional defects in *slo*^{1} mutants. (**A**) (wt) and (**B**) (*slo*^{1}) show indirect flight muscles stained with DHE to detect ROS. (**C**) Quantification of ROS fluorescence in (**A**) and (**B**) (wt-black, *slo*^{1}-grey). The graphs in (**D**–**F**) show ROS generation in isolated wt (black) and *slo*^{1} mutant mitochondria (gray) in the presence of pyruvate (**D**), glutamate/malate (**E**), or succinate (**F**) as substrates. Succinate and pyruvate, but not glutamate/malate show an increase in ROS as detected by the amplex red dye, compared to wt mitochondria. (**G**) Quantification of (**D**,**E**), and (**F**,**H**) shows ATP levels increased in *slo*^{1} mutants (wt-black, *slo*^{1}-grey). (**I**) Quantification of oxygen flux from enriched mitochondria from 40 thoraces of wt (black) and *slo*^{1} mutants (gray) flies. Basal, complex I, complex II, and ROX (non-mitochondrial residual oxygen consumption rate) oxygen consumption rates do not significantly vary between wt and *slo*^{1} mutants but combined complex I and complex II and maximum ETC consumption are significantly higher in *slo*^{1} mutants.

During oxidative phosphorylation, the energy released from oxidation/reduction reactions drives the synthesis of ATP. Mitochondrial disintegration is often associated with a decrease in ATP-generation [31]. We tested ATP-generation by mitochondria from two-week-old wt and slo^1 mutant flies. Surprisingly, slo^1 mutant flies showed a significant increase ($p < 0.001$, n = 5) in ATP-generation compared to wt flies (Figure 2H). We also measured the activity of complexes from both wt and slo^1 mutant flies by measuring substrate driven oxygen consumption rates. In comparison to wt, slo^1 mutant flies had similar basal rates and higher but not significant complex I and complex II oxygen consumption rates (Figure 2I). However, upon substrate saturation of both complex I and II combined, the oxygen consumption rate was highly significant ($p < 0.05$, n = 5, Figure 2I). The maximum electron transport system (ETS) capacity was also increased in slo^1 mutants suggesting a higher index of mitochondrial uncoupling in these mutant mitochondria (Figure 2I). We did not observe a sex-based difference between in slo^1 mutants.

3.3. Absence of BK_{Ca} Renders Flies Susceptible to Oxidative Stress

Our findings indicate abnormally hyper-functional mitochondria, which explain the higher level of ROS production from the mitochondria. To analyze if increased ROS renders slo^1 mutant flies sensitive to oxidative stress, we fed them with paraquat (PQ), a compound known to induce oxidative stress [32]. We found that slo^1 mutants (Figure 3A) are highly sensitive to PQ feeding. Flies (2–3 days old) maintained on starvation media for 2 h followed by exposure to 5% (w/v) sucrose combined with 20 mM PQ showed 50% death of slo^1 flies within 15 h whereas the 50% wt survived up to 25 h (Figure 3A,B). Hypersensitivity of slo^1 mutants to PQ was highly intriguing indicating that ROS plays a detrimental role on the survivability of slo^1 mutants. We tested hypersensitivity to ROS by feeding the flies with reduced glutathione (GSH) to see if glutathione feeding helps them survive in oxidative stress. We observed improved survival of slo^1 mutants similar to wild type in PQ treatment upon feeding of GSH (Figure 3C,D). These results show that increased ROS in slo^1 mutants is responsible for oxidative damage and perhaps influences the survival of flies.

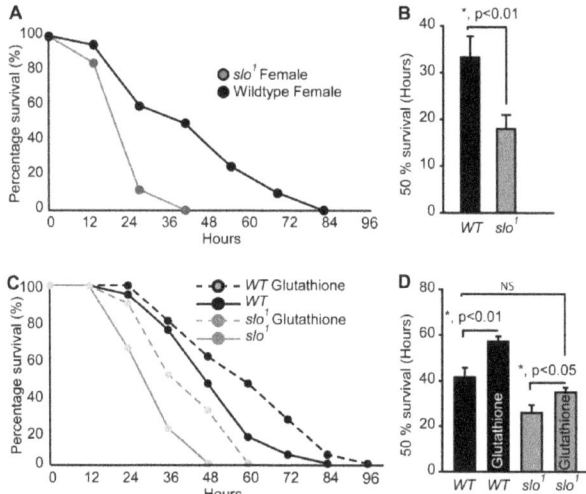

Figure 3. Oxidative stress on fly survival. (**A**) Survival of slo^1 mutants is significantly lower compared to wt flies fed on 20 mM PQ in 5% (w/v) sucrose. (**B**) Histogram shows 50% survival for and slo^1 and wt flies. (**C**) Survival of slo^1 mutants while PQ feeding with or without glutathione. (**D**) Histogram shows 50% survival for and slo^1 mutants with or without reduced glutathione (GSH). GSH increased the survival of wild-type and slo^1 mutants.

3.4. Mitochondrial Structural Abnormalities in BK_{Ca} Mutants

In order to study the structure of mitochondria in slo^1 mutant flies, we analyzed the ultrastructure of mitochondria in wt and slo^1 flies (Figure 4, n = 5). Electron microscopic analysis revealed major differences in the ultrastructure of mitochondria (Figure 4B vs. E). We studied day 1 and day 30 time points based on the differences observed in our initial experiments. The number of mitochondria in slo^1 mutant flies was less compared to wt from older flies (day 30). The mitochondria of older slo^1 mutants showed severe defects in terms of cristae arrangement (Figure 4E). The size of mitochondria in slo^1 mutant older flies was also increased as compared to the young flies, which could be attributed to their swollen appearance and loss of continuous inner mitochondrial membrane (Figure 4D,E,G). No major differences were observed between young (day 1) vs. older wt flies (day 30, Figure 4A,B,G).

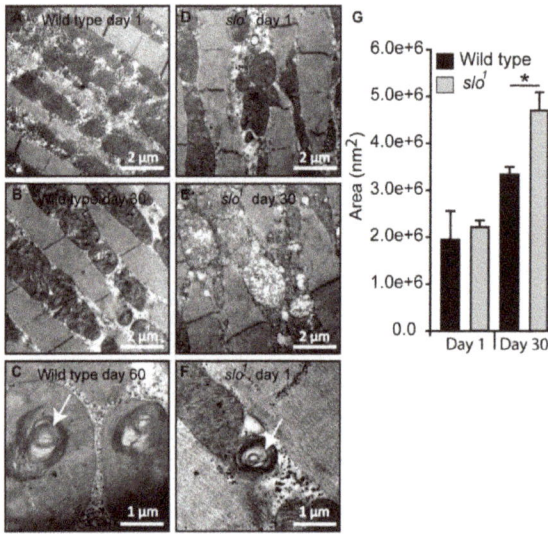

Figure 4. Mitochondrial structural defects in slo^1 mutants. (**A**) Wt mitochondria from indirect flight muscles at age 1 day show normal cristae organization. The slo^1 mutant mitochondria also show normal structure but there are increased numbers of vacuoles in the muscles (**D**). (**B**) Wt mitochondria at the age of day 30 also show a normal cristae organization. However, the slo^1 mutant mitochondria show disorganized cristae and swollen mitochondria (**E**). (**C**) Mitochondria of very old flies (at day 60) in wt show swirling of cristae, a phenotype characteristic of old age but occasionally young (day 1) slo^1 flies also show such swirls (**F**), indicated by white arrows. (**G**) The Average area indicated by histogram showed no difference in day 1 mitochondria in between wt (black) and slo^1 (gray) but significant (* $p < 0.05$) difference at day 30.

Mitochondrial swirls are known to represent early events of deterioration. Unusually close packing of cristae in an onion peel arrangement in the flight muscle mitochondria makes it feasible to detect it by electron micrograph [33]. We observed sporadic mitochondrial swirls in very old wt flies (≥60 days, Figure 4C) but slo^1 mutant showed mitochondrial swirls from day 1 in the flight muscle (Figure 4F, one to two occurrences per field). We have also observed the appearance of vacuoles in young slo^1 mutant flies (Figure 4D) whereas they were not seen in the wt counterparts. Taken together these analyses indicate major disorganization in mitochondrial structure in slo^1 mutant flies, some of them being hallmarks of the early aging phenotype. Mitochondrial structural disintegration, as well as the appearance of swirls, indicated possible oxidative damage to mitochondria consistent with our earlier results. Age-related abnormalities in mitochondria from flight muscles and other tissues of *Drosophila* are well-documented [34,35]. Older flies show severe mitochondrial deterioration; including loss of cristae, increase in size (swelling) and loss of arrangement in muscle fibers [33]. This prompted us to investigate if there are differences in the lifespan of slo^1 mutant flies.

3.5. slo^1 Mutants Show Reduced Lifespan

Mitochondria are energy-generating organelles of the cell involved in several metabolic and signaling pathways [15] such as lifespan. Our results showed mitochondrial structural and functional defects in BK_{Ca} mutants. Hence, we further investigated the consequence of absence of BK_{Ca} in lifespan.

We compared the lifespan of slo^1 mutants with wt flies. Even though flies were cultured in the optimal nutritional conditions and temperature (25 °C), slo^1 mutants surprisingly died within 45 ± 3 days (Figure 5A, B, and Supplementary Figure S2) whereas wt flies survived up to 85 ± 5 days, showing that the slo^1 mutant has only ~50% of lifespan compared to wt flies. There was no significant difference between females (Figure 5A) and males (Figure 5B) slo^1 mutants as they both showed decreased lifespan by ~50%. Reductions in the lifespan of female Drosophila are also associated with mating [36]. To test whether BK_{Ca} has any role in 'cost of mating', we performed a parallel study where males and females were housed together. We did not detect any significant differences in the observed lifespan of flies cultured separately or together (Supplementary Figure S2).

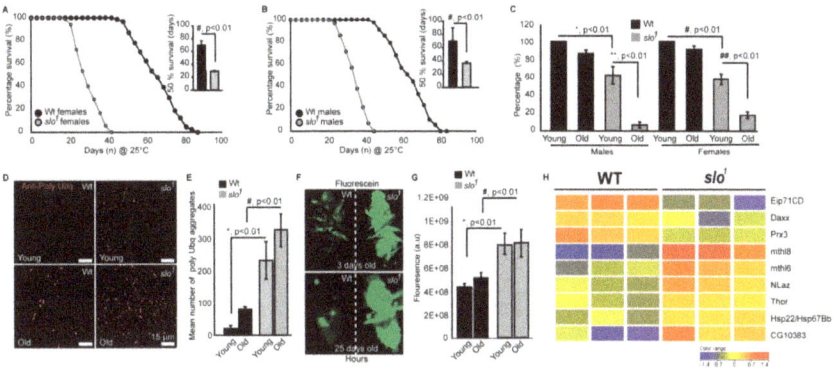

Figure 5. slo^1 mutants reveal accelerated aging. Drosophila BK_{Ca} (slo^1) mutants show significantly reduced lifespan of females (**A**) and males (**B**) by approximately 50% compared to wild-type (wt) flies. The inset shows 50% survival for wt (black) and slo^1 (gray), which was reduced significantly for slo^1 mutants. (**C**) Negative geotaxis assay for wt and slo flies at young (day 3) and older flies (day 30) shows reduced ability of slo^1 mutants to climb the marked distance in a given time in vials compared to their controls. (**D**) Increased polyubiquitination staining is observed in slo^1 mutants (red) as compared to wt in both young and older ages and quantification is provided in (**E**). (**F**) slo^1 mutants show increased intestinal perforations as determined by the leakage of fluorescein dye (green) from the gut unlike control flies, which only show the dye in their gut at both young and older ages. (**G**) Quantification of fluorescein signal from (**F**). (**H**) Microarray data showing differential expression of life span-related genes in wt and slo^1 mutants.

Age-related locomotor impairments including negative geotaxis [23] are well-documented in Drosophila [37]. Drosophila slo^1 mutants are known to have locomotor impairments [38] which were also observed here in both males and females (Figure 5C). No significant changes in negative geotaxis were observed in wt flies in between 3 days and 30 days old in both genders. Wild type flies survive up to ~90 days and our geotaxis assays were performed on comparatively younger wild type flies. However, with age slo^1 mutants showed a dramatic reduction in locomotion (Figure 5C, n = 3, 5 flies each in each trial). Reduction in lifespan is directly associated with increased proteotoxicity [39,40]. We characterized slo^1 mutants at young and old age along with wt flies to study the age-related deposition of protein aggregates in a flight muscle by immunofluorescence (Figure 5D). As shown earlier [39,40] anti-Ubiquitin (Ubq) antibody labels' protein aggregates in indirect flight muscle in old flies, we also observed a significant increase in protein aggregates (Figure 5D,E) in slo^1 mutants. Surprisingly, the slo^1 mutant showed a higher amount of aggregates from a young age which increased with old age (Figure 5D). Integrated fluorescence of protein aggregates showed a significant increase in Poly Ubq fluorescence with age in both wt and slo^1 mutants (Figure 5E) (n = 5). We also observed similar results with western blot studies where poly-Ubq streak was increased in slo^1 mutants. In corroboration, we observed an increase in the levels of refractory to Sigma P, Ref(2)P, a Drosophila orthologue of mammalian p62, which is a major component of protein aggregates in flies [41] (Supplementary Figure S3). Age-dependent intestinal-perforations are utilized as markers of aging and physiological changes associated with aging [42]. We tested age-related intestinal perforation by feeding fluorescein dye to young and old flies from wt as well as slo^1 mutant groups (Figure 5F). Surprisingly, the mutant flies showed fluorescent dye leakage through the intestinal perforations from a young age (3 days) indicating the premature or accelerated aging phenotype (Figure 5F). Taken together, our results suggest that slo^1 mutants not only show shortened lifespan but several accelerated aging phenotypes (n = 5).

We conducted microarray studies using 3-week old wild type and slo mutants (n = 3) to investigate if life span related genes are differentially regulated in the mutants. We found several genes implicated in life span regulation altered in the slo mutants (Figure 5G). Methuselah mutants are well known to expand the life span of Drosophila [43]. We indeed found overexpression of two Methuselah genes explaining the converse phenotype of shortened life span in the slo mutants. Overexpression of methionine sulfoxide reductase A (Epi71CD) is shown to increase life span, whereas in our arrays we found a decrease of this enzyme, along with the mitochondrial antioxidant peroxiredoxin 3 [44]. Several other life span related genes were altered such as Thor, NLaz, Hsp22, and Daxx [45–48] suggesting the absence of BK_{Ca} channel having an important role in regulating life span. In line with the observed mitochondria-related oxidative stress in slo mutants, we also found 63 oxidative stress-related genes altered (Supplementary Figure S4).

We further wanted to investigate if overexpression of BK_{Ca} in flies has a converse effect on life span compared to the slo mutants. We created full-length BK_{Ca} pUAST plasmids and injected into flies. Consistent with our previous results in Figure 5A,B flies overexpressing human BK_{Ca} at 29 °C, at which Gal4 efficiency is maximum, resulted in an increase in a life span of male flies (Figure 6A). The effect was not seen in female flies where they had a similar life span compared to wild type flies (Supplementary Figure S5). This showed that BK_{Ca} has a definitive role in regulating life span and the function is genetically conserved.

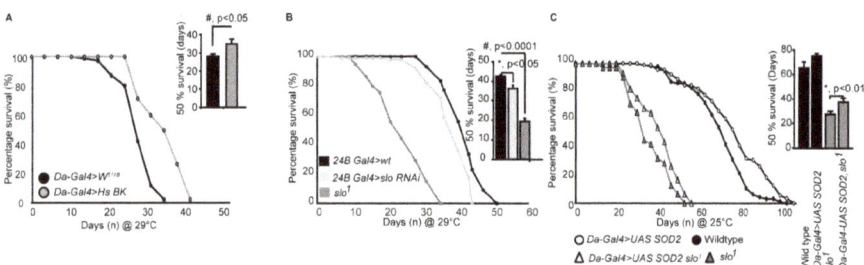

Figure 6. slo^1 expression modulates survival. (**A**) Males overexpressing human (Hs) BK_{Ca} increase life span. Inset shows quantification of 50% survival of control and Hs BK_{Ca} overexpressing flies. (**B**) Lifespan of control, slo RNAi under 24B Gal4 and slo^1 mutants at 29 °C. (**C**) slo^1 mutants are partially rescued by the overexpression of Daughterless Gal4-UAS; Sod2. Inset histograms represent the 50% survivability of the mutants. Histograms represent the 50% survivability of the mutants in both (**B**) and (**C**).

Using RNAis against BK_{Ca} we also narrowed down that the reduction in lifespan is at least partly through its action in the muscles. We tested global (Daughterless Gal4), neuronal (Elav Gal4), and muscle (24B Gal4) knockdown of BK_{Ca} and found that muscle knockdown of BK_{Ca} showed a reduction in lifespan compared to control flies (Figure 6B). We found that *24BGal4>slo* RNAi decreased the lifespan (Figure 6B) from 52 ± 4 days to around 42 ± 3 days at 29 °C, at which Gal4 efficiency is maximum. The 50% survivability bar graphs show a significant decrease in the lifespan of *24BGal4>slo RNAi* (Figure 6B). The reduction in locomotor activity with age could also be associated with loss of BK_{Ca} in the muscles where mitochondria play an important role [49].

As ROS generation was elevated in *slo^1* mutants, we attempted to rescue the reduction in lifespan of BK_{Ca} mutants by chelating ROS. We overexpressed SOD2 using UAS-SOD2 in *slo^1* mutants using a ubiquitous daughterless-Gal4 driver and cultured them to study their lifespan. As shown in Figure 6C, both wt, and *slo^1* mutants showed a modest but significant increase in lifespan on overexpression of SOD2 at 25 °C (we observed similar results at 29 °C as well). We further calculated the time at which 50% of flies survived. Overexpression of SOD2 increased 50% survivability by 10% but for *slo^1* mutants, we observed ~36 ± 8% increase. These results partially implicate ROS in the reduction of the life span of *slo^1* mutants and chelating ROS rescued the lifespan of *slo^1* mutant flies. This suggests, in addition to ROS, other mitochondrial abnormalities observed in *slo^1* mutants could be contributing to the reduction of lifespan.

4. Discussion

The presence of BK_{Ca} in mitochondria has been extensively pursued in the mitochondrial channel field in recent years [8,50]. Hence, we investigated if *Drosophila* mitochondria contain BK_{Ca} currents. Our electrophysiological studies provide clear evidence for the presence of BK_{Ca} channels in the mitochondria of *Drosophila*. The currents measured are of typical BK_{Ca} characteristics and they could be blocked by paxilline, and activated by calcium. Surprisingly, Po decreased at higher voltages which needs further characterization as this phenomenon could result from the presence or absence of additional regulatory subunit. Our immunolabelling of mitochondria also confirmed localization of BK_{Ca} to the mitochondria. These experiments indicate that the large current in *Drosophila* mitoplast is highly sensitive to changes in Ca^{2+} concentrations in the mitochondrial matrix, and could be blocked by highly specific BK_{Ca} inhibitor, paxilline. The large-conductance and sensitivity to NS1619, paxilline as well as Ca^{2+} and voltage in addition to mitochondrial immunocytochemistry indicate that *Drosophila* mitoplast possess functional BK_{Ca} proteins. These experiments for the first time establish BK_{Ca} as a mitochondrial ion channel across the species confirming an evolutionary presence. However, BK_{Ca} is located in several other membranes, for example in plasma membranes in neurons and astrocytes [7,8], along with mitochondrial membranes. It is yet to be deciphered how mitochondrial function is controlled by BK_{Ca} with respect to its various locations.

The absence of BK_{Ca} has several consequences on mitochondria. A dramatic increase in the accumulation of ROS was observed in *slo^1* mutant flies. Increased ROS can be detected in live tissues of mutant flies and also a higher amount of ROS generation was observed in isolated mitochondria. Energized *slo^1* mutant mitochondria produce increased levels of ROS compared to wt mitochondria when provided with specific substrates. This indicates that the increased ROS is a consequence of dysfunctional mitochondria, although it does not rule out the contribution from NOX related enzymes that are capable of producing ROS. However, other mitochondrial readouts such as ATP and oxidative phosphorylation measurements further consolidate the hypothesis that the increased ROS observed in *slo^1* mutant animals is due to mitochondria. The increase in ATP could also be due to sustained membrane potential caused by reduced potassium leak, increasing proton flux from ATP synthase. These results indicate hyper-functional mitochondria, which explain the higher level of ROS production from the mitochondria. We have recently shown that genetic activation of BK_{Ca} channels reduces ROS upon IR injury stress [13], which further supports a role for BK_{Ca} in regulating ROS.

The BK$_{Ca}$ flies also display oxidative stress sensitivity in a ROS-based pathway [51]. When we subjected the flies to oxidative stress using PQ, the BK$_{Ca}$ mutant flies died within 48 h compared to wt flies, which survive for more than 3 days. This indicated that BK$_{Ca}$ flies are under high oxidative stress and any further increase in ROS could be detrimental. The converse experiments by feeding glutathione increased the survivability of *slo*^{1} mutants indicating that ROS is at least a factor that determines the survival of *slo*^{1} mutants.

Consistent with the functional abnormalities of mitochondria, *slo*^{1} mutants also show several structural defects in mitochondria. Although younger flies contain mitochondria of normal appearance, occasional vacuoles and mitochondrial swirls are observed in flies even of day 1 age. As the flies age, mitochondrial structural defects are further enhanced where cristae structure is lost and mitochondrial swelling occurs. This depicts a progressive disintegration of mitochondria in an accelerated manner perhaps one of the causes leading to the early death of flies. Given that mitochondria from *slo*^{1} mutants produced higher amounts of ATP, it is possible that the absence of BK$_{Ca}$ results in changes in cristae as observed here which results in assembly of respiratory chain supercomplexes (RCS). RCS are quaternary supramolecular structures that allow channeling of electrons amongst individual respiratory chain complexes facilitate selective use of RCC subsets for nicotine adenine dinucleotide (NADH)- or flavin adenine dinucleotide (FAD)-derived electrons [52]. These type of supramolecular organization is commonly found in cristae, and the mitochondrial ATP synthase is also assembled as dimers with increased ATPase activity and the dimerization is further augmented during autophagy [53]. Mitochondria are closely associated with lifespan and mitochondrial defects accumulate as the animal ages. Interestingly in *slo*^{1} mutants, mitochondrial abnormalities can be seen on day 1 or birth. Mitochondrial swirls are occasionally seen in *slo*^{1} mutants, a phenotype hallmark of very old/dying flies in wt situations.

Ion channels are reported to alter with age in rats and humans [17,54]. Expression of BK$_{Ca}$ channels was shown to be reduced in aged coronary arteries possibly resulting in decreased vasodilator capacity, increased the risk of coronary spasm and myocardial ischemia in older people [17,54,55]. In mice, the absence of BK$_{Ca}$ causes low body weight and decreased survivability in the first 10 weeks [10,56] but a complete life span analysis has not been reported. In contrast, a recent report indicated a moderate increase in life span and motor neuron activity in *C. elegans* BK$_{Ca}$ mutants [11]. However, broad augmentation of endogenous BK currents in vivo (gain-of-function BK$_{Ca}$ TG mice) resulted in protecting the heart from ischemia-reperfusion injury [13]. In our current study, we have discovered that *Drosophila* lacking BK$_{Ca}$ showed a decrease in lifespan supporting mammalian observations. Flies mutant for BK$_{Ca}$ not only die rapidly but show early and premature accumulation of aging markers. This indicates that the presence of BK$_{Ca}$ is important in the regulation of aging. The key reason for this difference between *C. elegans*, flies, and mammals could be attributed to the role of electron transport chain (ETC) and ROS in aging. In *C. elegans* any perturbation with ETC results in an increase in life span due to their anaerobic energy-producing capacity, which is the exact opposite to what is observed in mammals and *Drosophila* [57]. One of the best examples for this difference is in frataxin homolog gene (frh-1), where knocking down frh-1 significantly increased the life span of *C. elegans* [58], but its ablation in mouse decreased life span [59], and recessive mutations in frataxin cause Friedreich's ataxia [60] in humans.

In agreement with accelerated aging, we observed the accumulation of age-related phenotypes just after the birth of flies such as intestinal perforation and polyubiquitin aggregation accompanied by motor defects in *slo*^{1} mutant flies. This provides evidence that BK$_{Ca}$ channel function is required from an early age, perhaps from developmental stages, for the animal to age in a wild type manner and it regulates life span. Our microarray data intriguing shows increased expression of several methuselah genes whose mutants are known to extend life span [43]. While it is not clearly shown if an increase in methuselah expression reduces the life span, it is consistent with the proposed role of methuselah where lack of it increases life span. We also observed several life span related genes altered in the *slo* mutants along with oxidative stress genes in our microarray [45–48]. These results collectively show that slo is a major regulator of oxidative stress and life span and a detailed study is required in the future to narrow down the direct role of BK_{Ca} in regulating life span. The major limitation is the contribution of mitochondrial vs. non-mitochondrial BKCa in regulation the lifespan of *Drosophila*.

Supporting our observation of ion channels regulating lifespan, it was recently shown that low temperatures activate a cold-sensitive cation channel TRPA-1, which extends a lifespan by triggering cellular signaling pathways [61]. It is also interesting that lack of BK_{Ca} only from the muscles also causes reduced lifespan similar to what is reported in earlier studies [62]. Conversely increasing BK_{Ca} by Gal4-UAS based overexpression increased the life span indicates a true role for BK_{Ca} in regulating life span. Human BK_{Ca} is 70% identical to *Drosophila* BK_{Ca} but is sufficient to rescues as well as augment the life span of *Drosophila* indicating the function could be conserved across species. This result is of relevance given expression of BK_{Ca} goes down with age in humans [63]. However, it is intriguing that only males show this effect while females do not show life span extension upon overexpression. These results are in agreement with increase in a life span of male flies on overexpression of specific DNA repair endonucleases [64]. DNA repair mechanisms are ATP-dependent processes, and dysfunctional mitochondria over a longer period of time could trigger apoptosis and cell death. This indicates gender-based differences in how BK_{Ca} regulates life span or could be involved in DNA repair mechanisms, which needs detailed study.

Taken together, our study establishes BK_{Ca}/Slo as an important player in maintaining the structure and functional integrity of mitochondria in *Drosophila*, and regulating lifespan. These findings also corroborate earlier studies that expression of BK_{Ca} reduces during aging which increases the risk of cardiovascular diseases in older people [17]. Our study also proves the existence of ion channel activity for BK_{Ca} in the *Drosophila* mitochondria. Given the dual cellular localization (intracellular membranes vs. plasma membrane) of BK_{Ca}, it is critical to evaluate its spatial specific role(s) in pathophysiology in future studies. In our findings, we have not ruled out the role of plasma membrane BK_{Ca} but introduced its new physiological role in aging. Presence of BK_{Ca} in the mitochondria and its role in modulation of ROS opens up avenues to explore antioxidant-based therapies in diseases and disorders related to these large conductance potassium channels. In the past decade, studies have indicated that pharmacological and genetic activation of BK_{Ca} results in cellular and organ protection from ischemic injuries. Despite recent successes with animal models, the translational aspect of BK_{Ca} channel openers is still lacking due to poor selectivity of these agonists. With recent advancements in gene delivery and gene therapy, our recent and current work reiterates the importance of expression of BK_{Ca} to protect organs from ischemic insult or increasing life span.

Supplementary Materials: The following are available online at http://www.mdpi.com/2073-4409/8/9/945/s1, Figure S1: *slo^{f05915}* mitochondria produce increased ROS. Figure S2: *slo^1* mutants result in accelerated aging when males and females are grown together. Figure S3: Increased levels of protein aggregates in *slo^1* mutants. Figure S4: Heat map of oxidative stress-related genes altered in *slo^1* mutants in comparison to wt flies. Figure S5: Females overexpressing human (Hs) BK_{Ca} do not show a change in life span as compared to control flies.

Author Contributions: Conceptualization, S.G.R. and H.S.; Methodology, S.G.R., P.B., A.T., K.S., P.K., D.P., H.N.J., S.A., B.A.S.R., and H.S.; Software, H.S.; Validation, S.G.R., E.J.V.B., A.S., D.C.W. and H.S; Formal Analysis, S.G., P.B., A.S., S.A., and H.S.; Investigation, S.G.R., P.B., A.T., and H.S.; Resources, E.J.V.B., A.S., D.C.W., and H.S.; Data Curation, S.G.R. and H.S.; Writing—Original Draft Preparation, S.G.R.; Writing – Review & Editing, S.G.R., A.S., D.C.W., and H.S.; Visualization, S.G.R. and H.S.; Supervision, H.S.; Project Administration, H.S.; Funding Acquisition, S.G.R., D.C.W., and H.S.

Funding: This research was funded by the Commonwealth Universal Research Enhancement (CURE) Program Grants to S.G.R. and H.S., American Heart Association Postdoctoral Fellowship (17POST33670360) to D.P., National Institute of Health (NS021328, CA182384, and MH108592) and Department of Defense (OD10944) to D.C.W., and a grant from the W. W. Smith Charitable Trust, American Heart Association National Scientist Development Grant (11SDG230059), American Heart Association Grant-in-Aid (16GRNT29430000), National Institute of Health (HL133050), and Drexel University College of Medicine startup funds to H.S. Stocks obtained from the Bloomington Drosophila Stock Center (NIH P40OD018537).

Acknowledgments: We thank Nigel Atkinson (University of Texas, Austin) for *slo* mutant flies, David W. Walker (University of California, Los Angeles) for UAS Sod2 flies, and Irwin Levitan (Thomas Jefferson University, Philadelphia) for anti-Slo antibodies.

Conflicts of Interest: The authors declare no conflict of interest.

References

1. Atkinson, N.S.; Robertson, G.A.; Ganetzky, B. A component of calcium-activated potassium channels encoded by the Drosophila slo locus. *Science* **1991**, *253*, 551–555. [CrossRef] [PubMed]
2. Singh, S.; Wu, C.F. Complete separation of four potassium currents in Drosophila. *Neuron* **1989**, *2*, 1325–1329. [CrossRef]
3. Elkins, T.; Ganetzky, B.; Wu, C.F. A Drosophila mutation that eliminates a calcium-dependent potassium current. *Proc. Natl. Acad. Sci. USA* **1986**, *83*, 8415–8419. [CrossRef] [PubMed]
4. Komatsu, A.; Singh, S.; Rathe, P.; Wu, C.F. Mutational and gene dosage analysis of calcium-activated potassium channels in Drosophila: Correlation of micro- and macroscopic currents. *Neuron* **1990**, *4*, 313–321. [CrossRef]
5. Saito, M.; Wu, C.F. Expression of ion channels and mutational effects in giant Drosophila neurons differentiated from cell division-arrested embryonic neuroblasts. *J. Neurosci.* **1991**, *11*, 2135–2150. [CrossRef] [PubMed]
6. Fernandez, M.P.; Chu, J.; Villella, A.; Atkinson, N.; Kay, S.A.; Ceriani, M.F. Impaired clock output by altered connectivity in the circadian network. *Proc. Natl. Acad. Sci. USA* **2007**, *104*, 5650–5655. [CrossRef] [PubMed]
7. Toro, L.; Li, M.; Zhang, Z.; Singh, H.; Wu, Y.; Stefani, E. MaxiK channel and cell signalling. *Eur. J. Physiol.* **2014**, *466*, 875–886. [CrossRef]
8. Singh, H.; Stefani, E.; Toro, L. Intracellular BK(Ca) (iBK(Ca)) channels. *J. Physiol.* **2012**, *590*, 5937–5947. [CrossRef] [PubMed]
9. Latorre, R.; Castillo, K.; Carrasquel-Ursulaez, W.; Sepulveda, R.V.; Gonzalez-Nilo, F.; Gonzalez, C.; Alvarez, O. Molecular Determinants of BK Channel Functional Diversity and Functioning. *Physiol. Rev.* **2017**, *97*, 39–87. [CrossRef] [PubMed]
10. Halm, S.T.; Bottomley, M.A.; Almutairi, M.M.; Di Fulvio, M.; Halm, D.R. Survival and growth of C57BL/6J mice lacking the BK channel, Kcnma1: Lower adult body weight occurs together with higher body fat. *Physiol. Rep.* **2017**, *5*. [CrossRef] [PubMed]
11. Li, G.; Gong, J.; Liu, J.; Liu, J.; Li, H.; Hsu, A.L.; Liu, J.; Xu, X.Z.S. Genetic and pharmacological interventions in the aging motor nervous system slow motor aging and extend life span in C. elegans. *Sci. Adv.* **2019**, *5*, eaau5041. [CrossRef]
12. Singh, H.; Lu, R.; Bopassa, J.C.; Meredith, A.L.; Stefani, E.; Toro, L. mitoBKCa is encoded by the Kcnma1 gene, and a splicing sequence defines its mitochondrial location. *Proc. Natl. Acad. Sci. USA* **2013**, *110*, 10836–10841. [CrossRef]
13. Goswami, S.K.; Ponnalagu, D.; Hussain, A.T.; Shah, K.; Karekar, P.; Gururaja Rao, S.; Meredith, A.L.; Khan, M.; Singh, H. Expression and Activation of BKCa Channels in Mice Protects Against Ischemia-Reperfusion Injury of Isolated Hearts by Modulating Mitochondrial Function. *Front. Cardiovasc. Med.* **2018**, *5*, 194. [CrossRef] [PubMed]
14. Frankenreiter, S.; Bednarczyk, P.; Kniess, A.; Bork, N.I.; Straubinger, J.; Koprowski, P.; Wrzosek, A.; Mohr, E.; Logan, A.; Murphy, M.P.; et al. cGMP-Elevating Compounds and Ischemic Conditioning Provide Cardioprotection Against Ischemia and Reperfusion Injury via Cardiomyocyte-Specific BK Channels. *Circulation* **2017**, *136*, 2337–2355. [CrossRef]
15. Balaban, R.S. Modeling mitochondrial function. *Am. J. Physiology. Cell Physiol.* **2006**, *291*, C1107–C1113. [CrossRef] [PubMed]
16. Balaban, R.S.; Nemoto, S.; Finkel, T. Mitochondria, oxidants, and aging. *Cell* **2005**, *120*, 483–495. [CrossRef]
17. Marijic, J.; Li, Q.; Song, M.; Nishimaru, K.; Stefani, E.; Toro, L. Decreased expression of voltage- and Ca(2+)-activated K(+) channels in coronary smooth muscle during aging. *Circ. Res.* **2001**, *88*, 210–216. [CrossRef]
18. Singh, H.; Lu, R.; Rodriguez, P.F.; Wu, Y.; Bopassa, J.C.; Stefani, E.; Toro, L. Visualization and quantification of cardiac mitochondrial protein clusters with STED microscopy. *Mitochondrion* **2012**, *12*, 230–236. [CrossRef] [PubMed]
19. Bednarczyk, P.; Koziel, A.; Jarmuszkiewicz, W.; Szewczyk, A. Large-conductance Ca(2)(+)-activated potassium channel in mitochondria of endothelial EA.hy926 cells. *Am. J. Physiology. Heart Circ. Physiol.* **2013**, *304*, H1415–H1427. [CrossRef] [PubMed]

20. Bednarczyk, P.; Wieckowski, M.R.; Broszkiewicz, M.; Skowronek, K.; Siemen, D.; Szewczyk, A. Putative Structural and Functional Coupling of the Mitochondrial BK Channel to the Respiratory Chain. *PLoS ONE* **2013**, *8*, e68125. [CrossRef]
21. Pesta, D.; Gnaiger, E. High-resolution respirometry: OXPHOS protocols for human cells and permeabilized fibers from small biopsies of human muscle. *Methods Mol. Biol.* **2012**, *810*, 25–58. [CrossRef] [PubMed]
22. Afzelius, B.A.; Maunsbach, A.B. Biological ultrastructure research; the first 50 years. *Tissue Cell* **2004**, *36*, 83–94. [CrossRef] [PubMed]
23. Nichols, C.D.; Becnel, J.; Pandey, U.B. Methods to assay Drosophila behavior. *J. Vis. Exp.* **2012**. [CrossRef]
24. Singh, H.; Li, M.; Hall, L.; Chen, S.; Sukur, S.; Lu, R.; Caputo, A.; Meredith, A.L.; Stefani, E.; Toro, L. MaxiK channel interactome reveals its interaction with GABA transporter 3 and heat shock protein 60 in the mammalian brain. *Neuroscience* **2016**, *317*, 76–107. [CrossRef] [PubMed]
25. Xu, W.; Liu, Y.; Wang, S.; McDonald, T.; Van Eyk, J.E.; Sidor, A.; O'Rourke, B. Cytoprotective role of Ca2+-activated K+ channels in the cardiac inner mitochondrial membrane. *Science* **2002**, *298*, 1029–1033. [CrossRef]
26. Siemen, D.; Loupatatzis, C.; Borecky, J.; Gulbins, E.; Lang, F. Ca2+-activated K channel of the BK-type in the inner mitochondrial membrane of a human glioma cell line. *Biochem. Biophys. Res. Commun.* **1999**, *257*, 549–554. [CrossRef] [PubMed]
27. Lu, R.; Alioua, A.; Kumar, Y.; Eghbali, M.; Stefani, E.; Toro, L. MaxiK channel partners: Physiological impact. *J. Physiol.* **2006**, *570*, 65–72. [CrossRef] [PubMed]
28. Atkinson, N.S.; Brenner, R.; Chang, W.; Wilbur, J.; Larimer, J.L.; Yu, J. Molecular separation of two behavioral phenotypes by a mutation affecting the promoters of a Ca-activated K channel. *J. Neurosci.* **2000**, *20*, 2988–2993. [CrossRef] [PubMed]
29. Pell, V.R.; Chouchani, E.T.; Murphy, M.P.; Brookes, P.S.; Krieg, T. Moving Forwards by Blocking Back-Flow: The Yin and Yang of MI Therapy. *Circ. Res.* **2016**, *118*, 898–906. [CrossRef] [PubMed]
30. Kwon, Y.; Kim, S.H.; Ronderos, D.S.; Lee, Y.; Akitake, B.; Woodward, O.M.; Guggino, W.B.; Smith, D.P.; Montell, C. Drosophila TRPA1 channel is required to avoid the naturally occurring insect repellent citronellal. *Curr. Biol.* **2010**, *20*, 1672–1678. [CrossRef] [PubMed]
31. Liu, W.; Gnanasambandam, R.; Benjamin, J.; Kaur, G.; Getman, P.B.; Siegel, A.J.; Shortridge, R.D.; Singh, S. Mutations in cytochrome c oxidase subunit VIa cause neurodegeneration and motor dysfunction in Drosophila. *Genetics* **2007**, *176*, 937–946. [CrossRef]
32. Hosamani, R.; Muralidhara. Acute exposure of Drosophila melanogaster to paraquat causes oxidative stress and mitochondrial dysfunction. *Arch. Insect Biochem. Physiol.* **2013**, *83*, 25–40. [CrossRef] [PubMed]
33. Walker, D.W.; Benzer, S. Mitochondrial "swirls" induced by oxygen stress and in the Drosophila mutant hyperswirl. *Proc. Natl. Acad. Sci. USA* **2004**, *101*, 10290–10295. [CrossRef] [PubMed]
34. Guo, M. Drosophila as a model to study mitochondrial dysfunction in Parkinson's disease. *Cold Spring Harb. Perspect. Med.* **2012**, *2*. [CrossRef] [PubMed]
35. Cho, J.; Hur, J.H.; Walker, D.W. The role of mitochondria in Drosophila aging. *Exp. Gerontol.* **2011**, *46*, 331–334. [CrossRef]
36. Fowler, K.; Partidge, L. A cost of mating in female fruitflies. *Nature* **1989**, *338*, 760–761. [CrossRef]
37. Jones, M.A.; Grotewiel, M. Drosophila as a model for age-related impairment in locomotor and other behaviors. *Exp. Gerontol.* **2011**, *46*, 320–325. [CrossRef]
38. Park, H.K. Genetic analysis of the Drosophila slowpoke gene and development of a novel method of targeted downregulation of gene expression by Gal4-repressor. *Dissertation* **2009**, *3363439*, 1–109.
39. Demontis, F.; Perrimon, N. FOXO/4E-BP signaling in Drosophila muscles regulates organism-wide proteostasis during aging. *Cell* **2010**, *143*, 813–825. [CrossRef]
40. Hunt, L.C.; Demontis, F. Whole-mount immunostaining of Drosophila skeletal muscle. *Nat. Protoc.* **2013**, *8*, 2496–2501. [CrossRef]
41. Nezis, I.P.; Simonsen, A.; Sagona, A.P.; Finley, K.; Gaumer, S.; Contamine, D.; Rusten, T.E.; Stenmark, H.; Brech, A. Ref(2)P, the Drosophila melanogaster homologue of mammalian p62, is required for the formation of protein aggregates in adult brain. *J. Cell Biol.* **2008**, *180*, 1065–1071. [CrossRef]
42. Rera, M.; Clark, R.I.; Walker, D.W. Intestinal barrier dysfunction links metabolic and inflammatory markers of aging to death in Drosophila. *Proc. Natl. Acad. Sci. USA* **2012**, *109*, 21528–21533. [CrossRef]
43. Lin, Y.J.; Seroude, L.; Benzer, S. Extended life-span and stress resistance in the Drosophila mutant methuselah. *Science* **1998**, *282*, 943–946. [CrossRef]

44. Odnokoz, O.; Nakatsuka, K.; Klichko, V.I.; Nguyen, J.; Solis, L.C.; Ostling, K.; Badinloo, M.; Orr, W.C.; Radyuk, S.N. Mitochondrial peroxiredoxins are essential in regulating the relationship between Drosophila immunity and aging. *Biochim. Biophys. Acta Mol. Basis Dis.* **2017**, *1863*, 68–80. [CrossRef]
45. Ruiz, M.; Ganfornina, M.D.; Correnti, C.; Strong, R.K.; Sanchez, D. Ligand binding-dependent functions of the lipocalin NLaz: An in vivo study in Drosophila. *FASEB J.* **2014**, *28*, 1555–1567. [CrossRef]
46. Morrow, G.; Samson, M.; Michaud, S.; Tanguay, R.M. Overexpression of the small mitochondrial Hsp22 extends Drosophila life span and increases resistance to oxidative stress. *FASEB J.* **2004**, *18*, 598–599. [CrossRef]
47. Kang, M.J.; Vasudevan, D.; Kang, K.; Kim, K.; Park, J.E.; Zhang, N.; Zeng, X.; Neubert, T.A.; Marr, M.T., 2nd; Ryoo, H.D. 4E-BP is a target of the GCN2-ATF4 pathway during Drosophila development and aging. *J. Cell. Biol.* **2017**, *216*, 115–129. [CrossRef]
48. Bodai, L.; Pardi, N.; Ujfaludi, Z.; Bereczki, O.; Komonyi, O.; Balint, E.; Boros, I.M. Daxx-like protein of Drosophila interacts with Dmp53 and affects longevity and Ark mRNA level. *J. Biol. Chem.* **2007**, *282*, 36386–36393. [CrossRef]
49. Short, K.R.; Bigelow, M.L.; Kahl, J.; Singh, R.; Coenen-Schimke, J.; Raghavakaimal, S.; Nair, K.S. Decline in skeletal muscle mitochondrial function with aging in humans. *Proc. Natl. Acad. Sci. USA* **2005**, *102*, 5618–5623. [CrossRef]
50. Ponnalagu, D.; Singh, H. Anion Channels of Mitochondria. *Handb. Exp. Pharmacol.* **2017**, *240*, 71–101. [CrossRef]
51. Orr, W.C.; Sohal, R.S. Extension of life-span by overexpression of superoxide dismutase and catalase in Drosophila melanogaster. *Science* **1994**, *263*, 1128–1130. [CrossRef]
52. Acin-Perez, R.; Bayona-Bafaluy, M.P.; Fernandez-Silva, P.; Moreno-Loshuertos, R.; Perez-Martos, A.; Bruno, C.; Moraes, C.T.; Enriquez, J.A. Respiratory complex III is required to maintain complex I in mammalian mitochondria. *Mol. Cell* **2004**, *13*, 805–815. [CrossRef]
53. Gomes, L.C.; Di Benedetto, G.; Scorrano, L. During autophagy mitochondria elongate, are spared from degradation and sustain cell viability. *Nat. Cell Biol.* **2011**, *13*, 589–598. [CrossRef]
54. Toro, L.; Marijic, J.; Nishimaru, K.; Tanaka, Y.; Song, M.; Stefani, E. Aging, ion channel expression, and vascular function. *Vasc. Pharmacol.* **2002**, *38*, 73–80. [CrossRef]
55. Nishimaru, K.; Eghbali, M.; Lu, R.; Marijic, J.; Stefani, E.; Toro, L. Functional and molecular evidence of MaxiK channel beta1 subunit decrease with coronary artery ageing in the rat. *J. Physiol.* **2004**, *559*, 849–862. [CrossRef]
56. Meredith, A.L.; Thorneloe, K.S.; Werner, M.E.; Nelson, M.T.; Aldrich, R.W. Overactive bladder and incontinence in the absence of the BK large conductance Ca2+-activated K+ channel. *J. Biol. Chem.* **2004**, *279*, 36746–36752. [CrossRef]
57. Muller, F.L.; Lustgarten, M.S.; Jang, Y.; Richardson, A.; Van Remmen, H. Trends in oxidative aging theories. *Free Radic. Biol. Med.* **2007**, *43*, 477–503. [CrossRef]
58. Ventura, N.; Rea, S.; Henderson, S.T.; Condo, I.; Johnson, T.E.; Testi, R. Reduced expression of frataxin extends the lifespan of Caenorhabditis elegans. *Aging Cell* **2005**, *4*, 109–112. [CrossRef]
59. Puccio, H.; Simon, D.; Cossee, M.; Criqui-Filipe, P.; Tiziano, F.; Melki, J.; Hindelang, C.; Matyas, R.; Rustin, P.; Koenig, M. Mouse models for Friedreich ataxia exhibit cardiomyopathy, sensory nerve defect and Fe-S enzyme deficiency followed by intramitochondrial iron deposits. *Nat. Genet.* **2001**, *27*, 181–186. [CrossRef]
60. Lodi, R.; Tonon, C.; Calabrese, V.; Schapira, A.H. Friedreich's ataxia: From disease mechanisms to therapeutic interventions. *Antioxid. Redox Signal.* **2006**, *8*, 438–443. [CrossRef]
61. Xiao, R.; Zhang, B.; Dong, Y.; Gong, J.; Xu, T.; Liu, J.; Xu, X.Z. A genetic program promotes C. elegans longevity at cold temperatures via a thermosensitive TRP channel. *Cell* **2013**, *152*, 806–817. [CrossRef] [PubMed]
62. Taghli-Lamallem, O.; Akasaka, T.; Hogg, G.; Nudel, U.; Yaffe, D.; Chamberlain, J.S.; Ocorr, K.; Bodmer, R. Dystrophin deficiency in Drosophila reduces lifespan and causes a dilated cardiomyopathy phenotype. *Aging Cell* **2008**, *7*, 237–249. [CrossRef]

63. Farajnia, S.; Meijer, J.H.; Michel, S. Age-related changes in large-conductance calcium-activated potassium channels in mammalian circadian clock neurons. *Neurobiol. Aging* **2015**, *36*, 2176–2183. [CrossRef] [PubMed]
64. Shaposhnikov, M.; Proshkina, E.; Shilova, L.; Zhavoronkov, A.; Moskalev, A. Lifespan and Stress Resistance in Drosophila with Overexpressed DNA Repair Genes. *Sci. Rep.* **2015**, *5*, 15299. [CrossRef]

© 2019 by the authors. Licensee MDPI, Basel, Switzerland. This article is an open access article distributed under the terms and conditions of the Creative Commons Attribution (CC BY) license (http://creativecommons.org/licenses/by/4.0/).

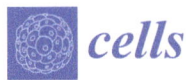

Article

TRPC6-Mediated ERK1/2 Activation Increases Dentate Granule Cell Resistance to Status Epilepticus via Regulating Lon Protease-1 Expression and Mitochondrial Dynamics

Ji-Eun Kim [1,2], Hana Park [1,2], Seo-Hyeon Choi [1,2], Min-Jeong Kong [1,2] and Tae-Cheon Kang [1,2,*]

1. Department of Anatomy and Neurobiology, College of Medicine, Hallym University, Chuncheon 24252, Korea; jieunkim@hallym.ac.kr (J.-E.K.); M19050@hallym.ac.kr (H.P.); 20161239@hallym.ac.kr (S.-H.C.); kmj4180@hallym.ac.kr (M.-J.K.)
2. Institute of Epilepsy Research, College of Medicine, Hallym University, Chuncheon 24252, Korea
* Correspondence: tckang@hallym.ac.kr; Tel.: +82-33-248-2524; Fax: +82-33-248-2525

Received: 7 September 2019; Accepted: 30 October 2019; Published: 1 November 2019

Abstract: Transient receptor potential canonical channel-6 (TRPC6) is one of the Ca^{2+}-permeable non-selective cation channels. TRPC6 is mainly expressed in dentate granule cell (DGC), which is one of the most resistant neuronal populations to various harmful stresses. Although TRPC6 knockdown evokes the massive DGC degeneration induced by status epilepticus (a prolonged seizure activity, SE), the molecular mechanisms underlying the role of TRPC6 in DGC viability in response to SE are still unclear. In the present study, hyperforin (a TRPC6 activator) facilitated mitochondrial fission in DGC concomitant with increases in Lon protease-1 (LONP1, a mitochondrial protease) expression and extracellular-signal-regulated kinase 1/2 (ERK1/2) phosphorylation under physiological conditions, which were abrogated by U0126 (an ERK1/2 inhibitor) co-treatment. TRPC6 knockdown showed the opposite effects on LONP1 expression, ERK1/2 activity, and mitochondrial dynamics. In addition, TRPC6 siRNA and U0126 evoked the massive DGC degeneration accompanied by mitochondrial elongation following SE, independent of seizure severity. However, LONP1 siRNA exacerbated SE-induced DGC death without affecting mitochondrial length. These findings indicate that TRPC6-ERK1/2 activation may increase DGC invulnerability to SE by regulating LONP1 expression as well as mitochondrial dynamics. Therefore, TRPC6-ERK1/2-LONP1 signaling pathway will be an interesting and important therapeutic target for neuroprotection from various neurological diseases.

Keywords: dentate granule cell; epilepsy; hyperforin; LONP1; mitochondrial dynamics; neuroprotection; pilocarpine; seizure; siRNA

---

1. Introduction

Mitochondria are essential organelles for cellular bioenergetics, which are responsible for producing nearly 95% of cellular ATP through oxidative phosphorylation. Under pathological conditions, a progressive decrease in the mitochondrial integrity abrogates respiratory capacities and increases production of free radicals, leading to aberrant structural and/or functional changes in mitochondria. Therefore, the maintenance of mitochondrial redox status is very important for cell viability [1–5].

Lon protease 1 (LONP1) belongs to the ATPases associated with diverse cellular activities (AAA+) protease family in the mitochondrial matrix that has a proteolytic activity of oxidized, dysfunctional, and misfolded proteins in ATP-dependent manner. Thus, LONP1 is rapidly up-regulated to prevent accumulation and aggregation of abnormal mitochondrial proteins under pathophysiological conditions [3–7]. LONP1 over-expression also activates extracellular signal regulated kinase 1/2 (ERK1/2), providing survival advantages and adaptation to cells [8]. Furthermore, ERK1/2 is required for the up-regulation of LONP1 during epidermal growth factor (EGF)-induced tumorigenic transformation [9]. Therefore, it is likely that the reciprocal regulation between ERK1/2 and LONP1 may affect neuron viability against harmful stresses, although the underlying mechanisms have been elusive.

Transient receptor potential canonical channel-6 (TRPC6) is one of Ca^{2+}-permeable non-selective cation channels, which protects neurons from ischemia [10], excitotoxicity [11], and status epilepticus (a prolonged seizure activity, SE) [12]. In the rat hippocampus, TRPC6 is highly expressed in the dentate granule cells (DGC), which are more resistant to various insults than other hippocampal neurons [13,14]. Furthermore, TRPC6 knockdown reduces ERK1/2 activity, and results in the massive DGC degeneration following SE [14–16]. Recently, we have reported that the abrogation of up-regulation of LONP1 expression by its siRNA evokes massive DGC death following SE [17]. Therefore, it is presumable that TRPC6-mediated ERK1/2 activation may be one of the up-stream signaling cascades that protect DGC from SE by regulating LONP1 expression, which is less defined.

Here, we show that TRPC6 knockdown led to mitochondrial elongation in DGC concomitant with decreases in LONP1 expression and ERK1/2 phosphorylation. Hyperforin (a TRPC6 activator) showed the reverse effects on ERK1/2 activity, LONP1 expression, and mitochondrial length. In addition, TRPC6 siRNA and U0126 (an ERK1/2 inhibitor) resulted in massive DGC degeneration following SE. However, LONP1 siRNA evoked SE-induced DGC degeneration without affecting TRPC6 expression, ERK1/2 phosphorylation, or mitochondrial morphologies. These findings for the first time demonstrate TRPC6-ERK1/2 activation may increase DGC invulnerability to SE by regulating LONP1 expression and mitochondrial dynamics.

2. Materials and Methods

2.1. Experimental Animals and Chemicals

Male Sprague–Dawley (SD) rats (7 weeks old) were used in the present study. Animals were kept under controlled environmental conditions (23–25 °C, 12 h light/dark cycle) with free access to water and standard laboratory food. All animal protocols were approved by the Administrative Panel on Laboratory Animal Care of Hallym University (Hallym 2018-2, April, 2018). All possible efforts were taken to avoid animals' suffering and to minimize the number of animals used during the experiment. All reagents were obtained from Sigma-Aldrich (St. Louis, MO, USA), except as noted.

2.2. siRNA and Drug Infusion

Under Isoflurane anesthesia (3% induction, 1.5–2% for surgery, and 1.5% maintenance in a 65:35 mixture of $N_2O:O_2$), animals were stereotaxically implanted with a brain infusion kit 1 (Alzet, Cupertino, CA, USA) into the right lateral ventricle (1 mm posterior; 1.5 mm lateral; −3.5 mm depth to the bregma). The infusion kit was sealed with dental cement and connected to an osmotic pump (1007D, Alzet, Cupertino, CA, USA) containing (1) control siRNA, (2) rat TRPC6 siRNA, (3) rat LONP1 siRNA, (4) vehicle, (5) U0126 (a selective ERK1/2 inhibitor, 25 µM), (6) hyperforin (a TRPC6 activator, 6 µM), or (7) hyperforin + U0126 [12,15,16,18]. Rat TRPC6 siRNA and LONP1 siRNA sequences were 5'-GGAAUAUGCUUGACUUUGGAAUGUUUU-3' [14] and 5'-GAGACAAGUUGCGCAUGAUTT-3' [17], respectively. The non-targeting control siRNA sequence was 5'-GCAACUAACUUCGUUAGAAUCGUUAUU-3'. In a previous study and the present study, 50 µM of U0126 inhibited ERK1/2 phosphorylation in the hippocampus by ~50% after 7 days of over infusion [15]. An osmotic pump was placed in a subcutaneous pocket in the interscapular region. To measure the effect of each siRNA, U0126 or hyperforin on seizure susceptibility in response to pilocarpine, some animals were also implanted with a recording electrode (Plastics One, Roanoke, VA, USA) into the left dorsal hippocampus (−3.8 mm posterior; 2.0 mm lateral; −2.6 mm depth). Before an EEG recording, connecting wire and an electrode socket were inserted in an electrode pedestal (Plastics One, Roanoke, VA, USA).

2.3. SE Induction and EEG Analysis

Three days after surgery, SE was induced by a single dose (30 mg/kg) of pilocarpine in rats pretreated (24 h before pilocarpine injection) with 127 mg/kg LiCl, as previously described [14,15]. Before pilocarpine injection, animals were given atropine methylbromide (5 mg/kg i.p.) to block the peripheral effect of pilocarpine. As controls, rats were treated with saline instead of pilocarpine. After injection, animals were monitored continuously for 2 h to register the extent of behavioral seizure activity. Behavioral seizure severity was also evaluated according to Racine's scale [19]: (1) immobility, eye closure, twitching of vibrissae, sniffing, or facial clonus; (2) head nodding associated with more severe facial clonus; (3) clonus of one forelimb; (4) rearing, often accompanied by bilateral forelimb clonus; and (5) rearing with loss of balance and falling accompanied by generalized clonic seizures. Within 20–45 min of treatment with pilocarpine, animals became catatonic and began staring, followed by myoclonic twitching and often frequent rearing and falling. The behavioral seizure score reached 4–5 in all groups. There was no difference in the behavioral seizure score induced by pilocarpine among all the groups. In some animals, EEG signals were also recorded with a DAM 80 differential amplifier (0.1–3000 Hz bandpass, World Precision Instruments, Sarasota, TL, USA), digitized (sampling rates, 1000 Hz) and analyzed using LabChart Pro v7 (AD Instruments, Bella Vista, NSW, Australia). Total EEG power and spectrograms were automatically calculated in 2-hour recording session using a Hanning sliding window with 50% overlap [14,15]. Two hours after SE, animals received diazepam (Valium; Roche, France; 10 mg/kg, i.p.) to terminate SE.

2.4. Tissue Processing

Seven days after surgery (non-SE induced animals) or three days after SE, rats were perfused transcardially first with phosphate-buffered saline (PBS) followed by a fixative solution (4% paraformaldehyde in 0.1 M phosphate buffer, pH 7.4) during 30 min under urethane anesthesia (1.5 g/kg, i.p.). The brains were removed and submerged in the same fixative solution for 4 h at 4 °C. Following postfixation, brains were cryoprotected overnight in 30% sucrose solution (in 0.1 M PBS), and coronally sectioned with a cryostat at 30 μm, and consecutive sections were contained in six-well plates containing PBS. For western blot, animals were decapitated under urethane anesthesia (1.5 g/kg, i.p.). The hippocampus was rapidly removed and homogenized in lysis buffer. The protein concentration in the supernatant was determined using a Micro BCA Protein Assay Kit (Pierce Chemical, Rockford, IL, USA).

2.5. Western Blot

Western blotting was performed according to standard procedures. Briefly, tissue lysate proteins were blotted onto nitrocellulose transfer membranes (Schleicher and Schuell BioScience Inc., Keene, NH, USA), then incubated with primary antibodies in Table 1. Immunoreactive bands were detected and quantified on ImageQuant LAS4000 system (GE Healthcare, Piscataway, NJ, USA). The values of each sample were normalized with the corresponding amount of β-actin as internal reference.

2.6. Immunohistochemistry and Fluoro-Jade B Staining

As previously described [14–16], free-floating sections were first incubated with 10% normal goat serum (Vector, Burlingame, CA, USA) in PBS for 30 min at room temperature. Sections were then incubated at room temperature for overnight in the mixture of primary antibodies (Table 1) in PBS containing 0.3% triton X-100 (Table 1). After three washes in PBS, sections were incubated for 1 h in fluorescein isothiocyanate (FITC)-, Cy3- or aminomethylcoumarin acetate (AMCA)-conjugated secondary antibodies (Vector, Burlingame, CA, USA). Sections (reacted with TRPC6 antibody only) were reacted with biotinylated secondary antiserum and avidin–biotin complex (Vector, Burlingame, CA, USA). Thereafter, immunoreactivity was developed by standard 3,3'-Diaminobenzidine reaction. The antibody that was preincubated with 1 μg of purified peptide (for TRPC6) or pre-immune serum was used as for negative control. To analyze the neuronal damage, we applied Fluoro-Jade B (FJB) staining (Histo-Chem Inc., Jefferson, AR, USA), according to the manufacturer's instructions. Images were captured using an AxioImage M2 microscope or a confocal laser scanning microscope (LSM 710, Carl Zeiss Inc, Oberkocken, Germany) [14,15].

Table 1. Primary antibodies used in the present study.

Antigen	Host	Manufacturer (Catalog Number)	Dilution Used
ERK1/2	Rabbit	Biorbyt (Orb160960)	1:2000 (WB)
LONP1	Rabbit	Proteintech (15440-1-AP)	1:100 (IF) 1:1000 (WB)
Mitochondrial marker (Mitochondrial complex IV subunit 1, MTCO1)	Mouse	Abcam (#ab14705)	1:500 (IF)
pERK1/2	Rabbit	Bioss (bs-3330R)	1:1000 (WB)
TRPC6	Rabbit	Millipore (AB5574)	1:100 (IHC) 1:1000 (WB)
β-actin	Mouse	Sigma (A5316)	1:5000 (WB)

IF, Immunofluorescence; IHC, immunohistochemistry; WB, Western blot.

2.7. Cell Count and Measurement of Mitochondrial Length

As previously described [14,15], coronal images of the dentate gyrus (3–4 mm posterior to the bregma) were captured (15 sections per each animal) using 20× objectives, and areas of interest (1×10^5 μm^2) were selected from the dentate granule cell layer. Thereafter, FJB-positive neurons were counted on 20× images using AxioVision Rel. 4.8 Software. Individual mitochondrion in DGC ($n = 20$/section) was also captured using 63× or 100× objectives, and each length was measured by using AxioVision Rel. 4.8 Software or ZEN lite (Blue Edition, Carl Zeiss Inc., Oberkocken, Germany) software following 3D-reconstruction. Two different investigators who were blind to the classification of tissues performed cell counts and measurement of mitochondrial length.

2.8. Quantification of Data and Statistical Analysis

All data were analyzed using Student t-test, one-way ANOVA, or one-way repeated measure ANOVA to determine statistical significance. Bonferroni's test was used for post hoc comparisons. A p-value below 0.05 was considered statistically significant.

3. Results

3.1. TRPC6 Knockdown and Hyperforin Reversely Regulate LONP1 Expression, ERK1/2 Phosphorylation, and Mitochondrial Length in DGC under Physiological Conditions

Figure 1A shows that TRPC6 expression was apparently detected in the DGC layer and the molecular layer of the DG rather than other regions. TRPC6 siRNA reduced TRPC6 expression in the hippocampus (Figure 1A). TRPC6 knockdown elongated mitochondrial length (~2.86 μm), as compared to control siRNA (~1.26 μm) ($p < 0.05$ vs. control siRNA, n = 7; Figure 1B,C and Supplementary Figure S1). TRPC6 siRNA decreased LONP1 expressions in mitochondria (Figure 1C). Western blot data demonstrated that TRPC6 knockdown led to ~65% and ~30% reductions of TRPC6 and LONP1 protein levels, respectively ($p < 0.05$ vs. control siRNA, n = 7, respectively; Figure 1D,E). TRPC6 knockdown also declined ERK1/2 phosphorylation ($p < 0.05$ vs. control siRNA, n = 7; Figure 1D E and Supplementary Figure S2). In contrast to TRPC knockdown, hyperforin (a TRPC6 activator) [12,18] decreased mitochondrial length to ~0.54 μm ($p < 0.05$ vs. vehicle, n = 7; Figure 1B,C). Hyperforin increased ERK1/2 phosphorylation and LONP1 expression without altering TRPC6 expression ($p < 0.05$ vs. vehicle, n = 7; Figure 1D,E and Supplementary Figure S2). Since TRPC6 regulates ERK1/2 activity [20], our findings indicate that ERK1/2 may be involved in a potential relationship between TRPC6 and LONP1.

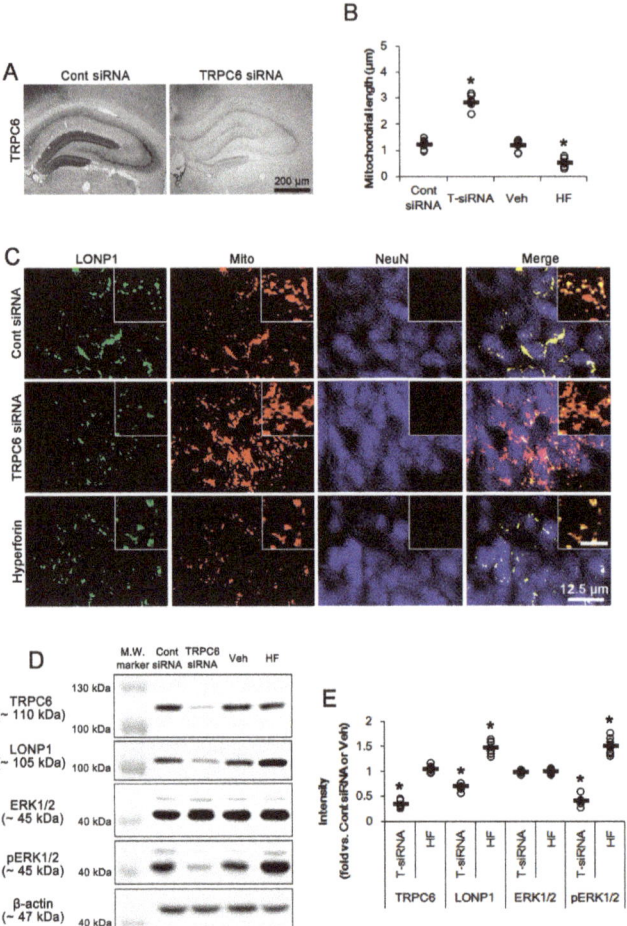

Figure 1. Effects of TRPC6 siRNA and hyperforin on mitochondrial dynamics, LONP1 expression, and ERK1/2 phosphorylation under certain physiological conditions. (**A**) Representative images of control- and TRPC6 siRNA-treated animals. TRPC6 expression is predominantly detected in the molecular layer of the dentate gyrus and DGC. TRPC6 siRNA effectively decreases TRPC6 expression. (**B,C**) Effects of TRPC6 siRNA and hyperforin on mitochondrial length. TRPC6 siRNA (T-siRNA) leads to mitochondrial elongation, while hyperforin (HF) facilitates mitochondrial fragmentation. (**B**) Quantification of mitochondrial length. Open circles indicate each individual value. Horizontal bars indicate mean value (mean ± S.E.M.; * $p < 0.05$ vs. control siRNA and vehicle, respectively; Student *t*-test; n = 7, respectively). (**C**) Representative double immunofluorescent images for LONP1 and mitochondria (Mito). Inserts are high magnification images (insert bar = 1.25 μm). (**D,E**) Effects of TRPC6 siRNA and hyperforin on expressions of TRPC6 and LONP1, and ERK1/2 phosphorylation. TRPC6 siRNA (T-siRNA) decreases protein levels of TRPC6 and LONP1, and ERK1/2 phosphorylation. Hyperforin (HF) increases LONP1 expression and ERK1/2 phosphorylation without changing TRPC6 expression. (**D**) Representative western blots of expressions of TRPC6 and LONP1, and ERK1/2 phosphorylation (M.W. marker, Molecular weight marker). (**E**) Quantification of expressions of TRPC6 and LONP1, and ERK1/2 phosphorylation based on western blot data. Open circles indicate each individual value. Horizontal bars indicate mean value (mean ± S.E.M.; * $p < 0.05$ vs. control siRNA and vehicle, respectively; Student *t*-test; n = 7, respectively).

3.2. LONP1 siRNA Does Not Influence TRPC6 Expression, ERK1/2 Phosphorylation and Mitochondrial Length under Physiological Condition

Next, we applied LONP1 siRNA to confirm whether LONP1 reciprocally influences TRPC6 expression and ERK1/2 phosphorylation. LONP1 knockdown significantly decreased LONP1 expression ($p < 0.05$ vs. control siRNA, n = 7; Figure 2A,B and Supplementary Figure S3). However, LONP1 knockdown did not affect the TRPC6 expression level and mitochondrial length (Figure 2A–D and Supplementary Figure S1). In addition, LONP1 siRNA did not influence ERK1/2 expression and its phosphorylation (Figure 2A,B and Supplementary Figure S3). Thus, these findings suggest that the RPC6-ERK1/2 signaling pathway may be one of the up-steam regulators for LONP1 expression.

3.3. U0126 Abrogates Mitochondrial LONP1 Expression under Physiological Condition and after Hyperforin Treatment

Since hyperforin increases ERK1/2 phosphorylation and LONP1 expression in a previous [16] and the present study, we further investigated whether ERK1/2 activity affects LONP1 expression. U0126 (an ERK1/2 inhibitor) reduced ERK1/2 phosphorylation and LONP1 expression, and led to mitochondrial elongation under physiological condition without affecting TRPC6 expression ($p < 0.05$ vs. vehicle, n = 7; Figure 3A–D and Supplementary Figures S1 and S4). In addition, U0126 co-treatment abolished mitochondrial elongation and up-regulations of LONP1 expression as well as ERK1/2 phosphorylation induced by hyperforin ($p < 0.05$ vs. hyperforin, n = 7; Figure 3A–D and Supplementary Figures S1 and S4). Together with the data obtained from TRPC6 knockdown, these findings indicate that TRPC6 activity may regulate LONP1 expression and mitochondrial dynamics through ERK1/2 activation.

3.4. The TRPC6-ERK1/2-LONP1 Signaling Pathway Inhibits SE-Induced DGC Degeneration, Independent of Seizure Severity

TRPC6 knockdown provokes massive DGC degeneration following pilocarpine-induced SE, although DGC is remarkably resistant to neuronal damage induced by various insults [14,15]. Since seizure severity correlates to neuronal damage [21,22], we explored whether the modulations of the TRPC6-ERK1/2-LONP1 signaling pathway alter seizure susceptibility to pilocarpine. In control siRNA-treated animals, the seizure susceptibility to pilocarpine was similar to that in vehicle-treated animals (Figure 4A,B). TRPC6 siRNA reduced the latency of seizure on-set, and increased total EEG power during SE ($p < 0.05$ vs. control siRNA, n = 7; Figure 4A,B). These findings indicate that TRPC6 knockdown may increase seizure susceptibility. LONP1 siRNA and hyperforin could not affect the seizure susceptibility to pilocarpine (Figure 4A,B). Consistent with our previous study [15], U0126 delayed the seizure on-set, and reduced total EEG power in response to pilocarpine ($p < 0.05$ vs. vehicle, n = 7; Figure 4A,B). Co-treatment of U0126 with hyperforin also reduced seizure activity after pilocarpine injection ($p < 0.05$ vs. vehicle, n = 7; Figure 4A,B). However, TRPC6 siRNA and LONP1 siRNA evoked massive DGC degeneration ($p < 0.05$ vs. control siRNA, n = 7; Figure 5A,B). As compared to vehicle, U0126 aggravated DGC death induced by SE ($p < 0.05$ vs. vehicle, n = 7; Figure 5A,B). Hyperforin attenuated SE-induced DGC degeneration ($p < 0.05$ vs. vehicle, n = 7; Figure 5A,B), which in turn caused deterioration by U0126 co-treatment ($p < 0.05$ vs. hyperforin, n = 7; Figure 5A,B). Therefore, the severity of SE-induced DGC degeneration in each siRNA or compound-treated animals was LONP1 siRNA > U0126 > TRPC6 siRNA > hyperforin + U0126 > control siRNA = vehicle > hyperforin. These findings suggest that the blockade of TRPC6-ERK1/2-LONP1 signaling pathway may increase SE-induced DGC degeneration, independent of seizure susceptibility or its severity.

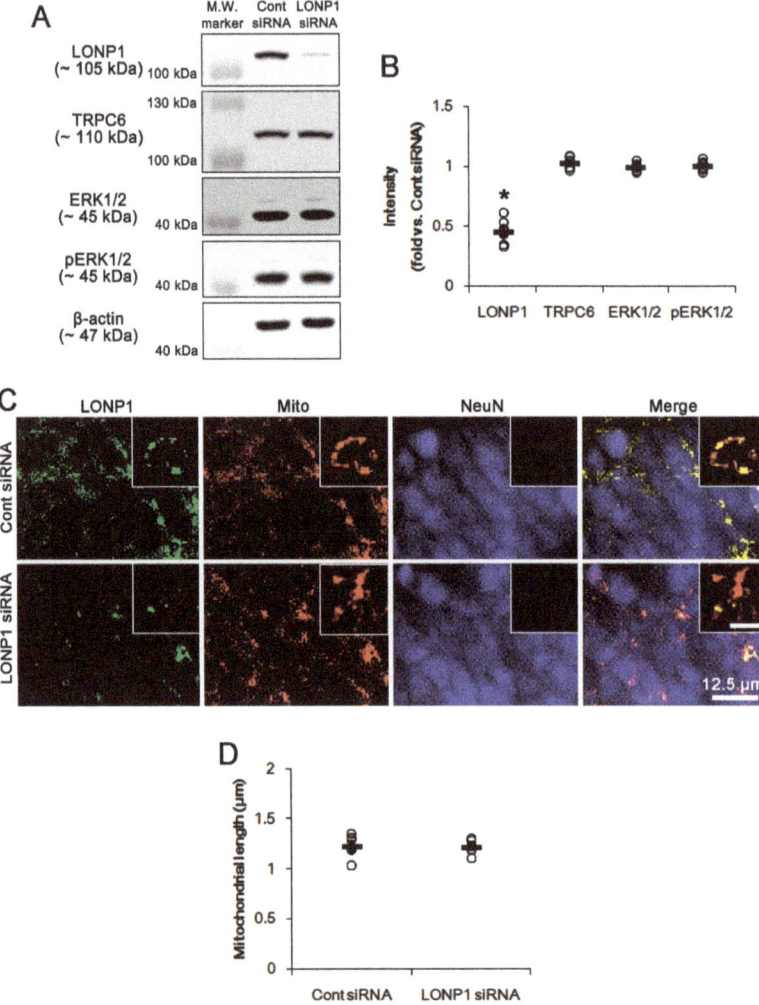

Figure 2. Effects of LONP1 siRNA on expression levels of LONP1 and TRPC6, ERK1/2 phosphorylation and mitochondrial dynamics under physiological condition. (**A,B**) Effects of LONP1 siRNA on expressions of TRPC6 and LONP1, and ERK1/2 phosphorylation. LONP1 siRNA decreases LONP1 expression without affecting TRPC6 expression and ERK1/2 phosphorylation. (**A**) Representative western blots of expressions of LONP1 and TRPC6, and ERK1/2 phosphorylation (M.W. marker, Molecular weight marker). (**B**) Quantification of expressions of LONP1 and TRPC6, and ERK1/2 phosphorylation based on western blot data. Open circles indicate each individual value. Horizontal bars indicate mean value (mean ± S.E.M.; * $p < 0.05$ vs. control siRNA; Student *t*-test; n = 7, respectively). (**C,D**) Effects of LONP1 siRNA on mitochondrial length. LONP1 siRNA does not affect mitochondrial length. (**C**) Representative double immunofluorescent images for LONP1 and mitochondria (Mito). Inserts are high magnification images (insert bar = 1.25 µm). (**D**) Quantification of mitochondrial length. Open circles indicate each individual value. Horizontal bars indicate mean value (mean ± S.E.M.; * $p < 0.05$ vs. control siRNA; Student *t*-test; n = 7, respectively).

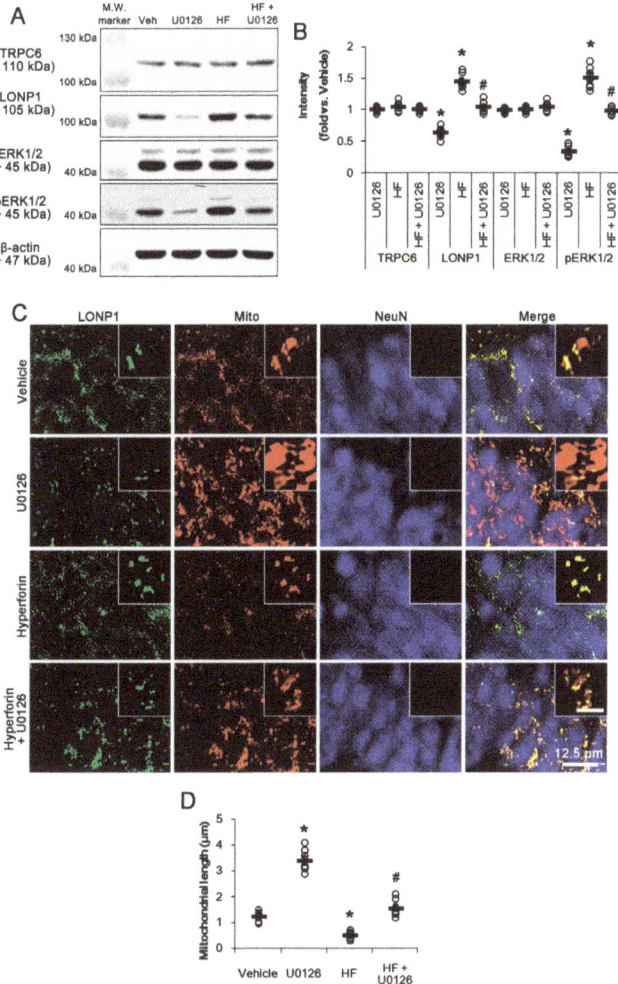

Figure 3. Effects of U0126, hyperforin, and co-treatment of hyperforin and U0126 on expression levels of LONP1 and TRPC6, ERK1/2 phosphorylation and mitochondrial dynamics under physiological condition. (**A**,**B**) Effects of U0126, hyperforin (HF) and co-treatment of hyperforin and U0126 (HF + U0126) on expressions of TRPC6 and LONP1, and ERK1/2 phosphorylation. U0126 decreases LONP1 expression and ERK1/2 phosphorylation without affecting TRPC6 expression. Hyperforin increases LONP1 expression and ERK1/2 phosphorylation, which are abrogated by U0126 co-treatment. (**A**) Representative western blots of expressions of TRPC6 and LONP1, and ERK1/2 phosphorylation (M.W. marker, Molecular weight marker). (**B**) Quantification of expressions of TRPC6 and LONP1, and ERK1/2 phosphorylation based on western blot data. Open circles indicate each individual value. Horizontal bars indicate mean value (mean ± S.E.M.; * $p < 0.05$ vs. control siRNA; one-way ANOVA; n = 7, respectively). (**C**,**D**) Effects of U0126, hyperforin (HF) and co-treatment of hyperforin and U0126 (HF + U0126) on mitochondrial length. U0126 increases mitochondrial length. In contrast, hyperforin diminishes it, which is abrogated by U0126 co-treatment. (**C**) Representative double immunofluorescent images for LONP1 and mitochondria (Mito). Inserts are high magnification images (insert bar = 1.25 μm). (**D**) Quantification of mitochondrial length. Open circles indicate each individual value. Horizontal bars indicate mean value (mean ± S.E.M.; * $p < 0.05$ vs. control siRNA; one-way ANOVA; n = 7, respectively).

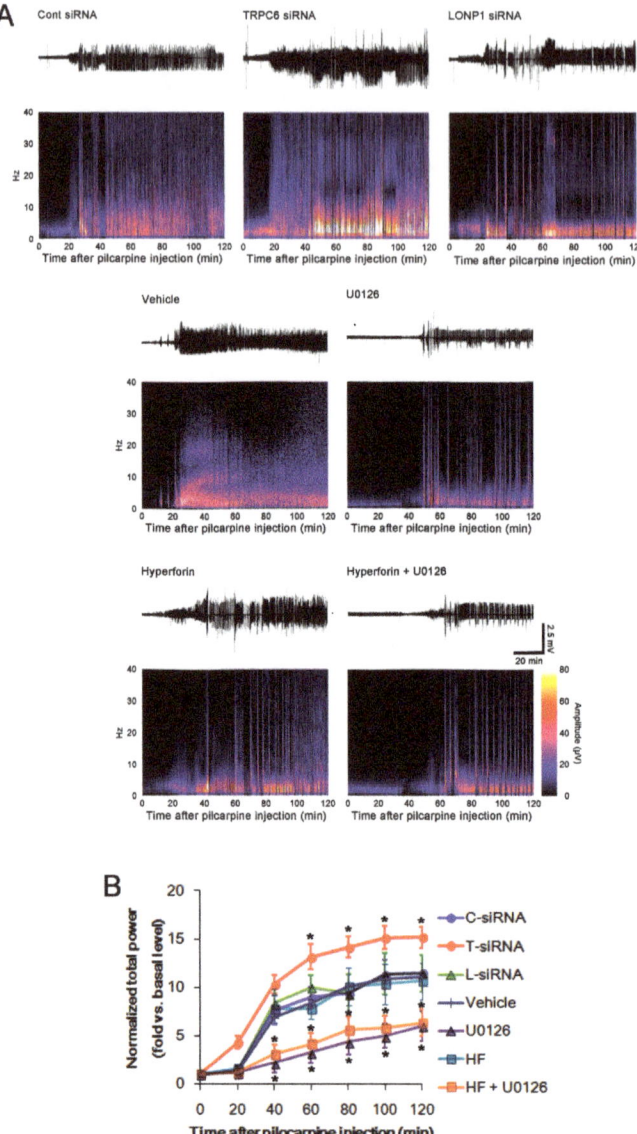

Figure 4. Effects of control siRNA, TRPC6 siRNA, LONP1 siRNA, U0126, hyperforin and co-treatment of hyperforin and U0126 on seizure activity in response to pilocarpine. As compared to control siRNA (C-siRNA), LONP1 siRNA (L-siRNA) does not affect seizure activity induced by pilocarpine. However, TRPC6 siRNA (T-siRNA) reduces seizure latency, and increases seizure severity in response to pilocarpine. No difference in seizure activity is observed between control siRNA and Vehicle (Veh)-treated animals. As compared to vehicle, hyperforin (HF) does not affect seizure activity induced by pilocarpine. However, U0126 and co-treatment of hyperforin and U0126 (HF + U0126) attenuate seizure activity in response to pilocarpine. (**A**) Representative EEG traces and frequency-power spectral temporal maps in response to pilocarpine. (**B**) Quantification of total EEG power (seizure intensity) in response to pilocarpine (mean ± S.E.M.; * $p < 0.05$ vs. control siRNA or vehicle; one-way repeated measure ANOVA; n = 7, respectively).

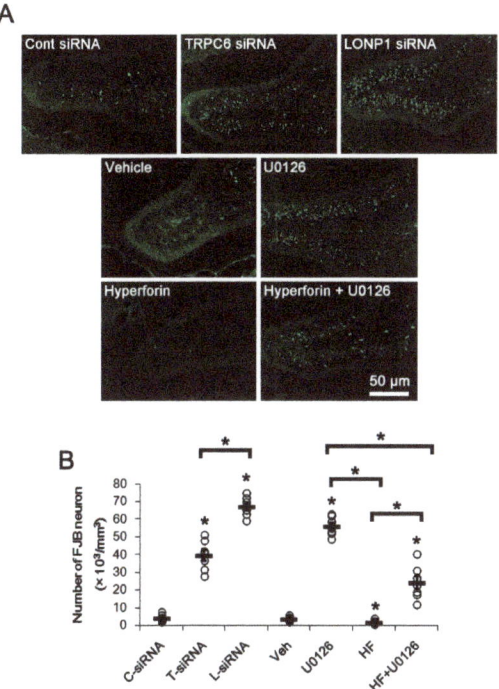

Figure 5. Effects of control siRNA, TRPC6 siRNA, LONP1 siRNA, U0126, hyperforin, and co-treatment of hyperforin and U0126 on SE-induced DGC degeneration. As compared to control siRNA (C-siRNA), TRPC6 siRNA (T-siRNA), LONP1 siRNA (L-siRNA) and U0126 induce massive DGC degeneration induced by SE. Hyperforin (HF) ameliorates SE-induced DGC damage, which is reversed by U0126 co-treatment (HF + U0126). (**A**) Representative images for FJB-positive degenerating DGC. (**B**) Quantification of the number of FJB-positive DGC. Open circles indicate each individual value. Horizontal bars indicate mean value (mean ± S.E.M.; * $p < 0.05$ vs. control siRNA or vehicle; one-way ANOVA; n = 7, respectively).

4. Discussion

The major findings of this study are that TRPC6-mediated ERK1/2 activation regulated LONP1 expression as well as mitochondrial dynamics, which were involved in the invulnerability of DGC to SE (Figure 6).

LONP1 is an inducible ATP-stimulated protease, which plays important roles in cell viability by controlling the maintenance of mitochondrial homeostasis/bioenergetics and DNA integrity [7,23–27]. Therefore, LONP1 expression is up-regulated under some pathological conditions such as hypoxia, oxidative stress, and tumorigenesis [6–9]. However, the underlying mechanisms of regulation of LONP1 expression remain incompletely understood. TRPC6 modulates cell proliferation, differentiation and neuronal vulnerability to various insults [10–12,28,29]. In addition, TRPC6 activates ERK1/2 [15,30], which is involved in mitochondrial dynamics and LONP1 expression [9,31–36]. In the present study, we found that TRPC6 siRNA effectively reduced ERK1/2 activity (phosphorylation) and LONP1 expression under physiological conditions. In contrast, hyperforin, a TRPC6 activator [18,37], increased ERK1/2 activity and LONP1 expression, which were abrogated by U0126 co-treatment. Since LONP1 siRNA did not affect TRPC6 expression and ERK1/2 phosphorylation in the present study, our findings indicate that, at least in DGC, TRPC6-ERK1/2 signaling pathway is one of the up-stream regulators of LONP1 expression.

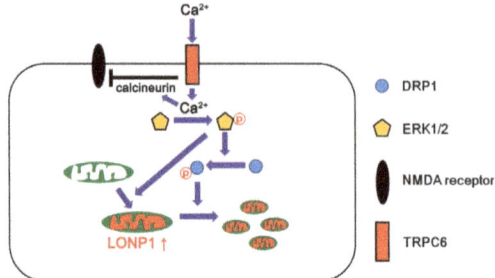

Figure 6. Scheme of roles of TRPC6 in LONP1 expression and mitochondrial dynamics based on the present data and previous reports [11,15,16,20,30]. TRPC6 activation increases Ca^{2+} influx in DGC. Intracellular Ca^{2+} activates calcineurin and ERK1/2. Activated calcineurin inhibits the NMDA receptor. In addition, ERK1/2 activation up-regulates LONP1 expression and DRP1 phosphorylation at the 616 site. Subsequently, phosphorylated DRP1 facilitates mitochondrial fission. Thus, TRPC6 may be involved in the quality controls of mitochondria as well as mitochondrial dynamics, which would enhance DGC invulnerability to SE.

LONP1 is required for the maintenance and expression of the mitochondrial enzymes and genomes [25–27]. In particular, LONP1 plays a direct role in the turnover of cytochrome c oxidase (COX), which is a terminal enzyme of the mitochondrial electron transport chain [38–40]. Under a hypoxic condition, LONP1 degrades isoform 1 of COX subunit 4 (COX4-1) to facilitate the switch from COX4-1 to COX4-2 for enhancing mitochondrial respiration [41]. LONP1 also removes the impaired human mitochondrial transcription factor A (TFAM) that is essential for mitochondrial DNA synthesis and its packaging [42–44]. Thus, deregulation of LONP1 leads to cell death by loss of mitochondrial functions [27,45,46]. In the present study, TRPC6 siRNA, LONP1 siRNA, and U0126 exacerbated SE-induced DGC degeneration. In addition, co-treatment U0126 abrogated the protective effect of hyperforin on DGC damage against SE. Therefore, our findings suggest that the TRPC6-ERK1/2 signaling pathway may play a neuroprotective role against SE by regulating LONP1-mediated mitochondrial homeostasis/bioenergetics. Further studies are needed to elucidate the specific targets controlled by LONP1, which would be involved in SE-induced neuronal death.

On the other hand, ERK1/2 activation accelerates mitochondrial fission via dynamin-related proteins 1 (DRP1)-serine (S) 616 phosphorylation [35,36]. Indeed, the blockade of TRPC6 functionality results in aberrant mitochondrial elongation by abrogating ERK1/2-mediated DRP1 activity in DGC [14,15]. Mitochondria are dynamic organelles responsible for generating ATP. In addition, mitochondrial dynamics participate in the synthesis of reactive oxygen species (ROS). Aberrant mitochondrial elongation inhibits mitochondrial respiratory function that triggers excessive ROS production. Excessive mitochondrial fission also impairs the detoxification of excess ROS and extrusion of intracellular Ca^{2+} [47,48]. Thus, imbalance of mitochondrial fission-fusion induces balance results in neuronal necrosis or apoptosis following SE [15,17,49–53]. Under physiological conditions, furthermore, mitochondrial fission directly enables increases mitochondrial ROS production [1,2]. Considering the relevance between mitochondrial dynamics and ROS syntheses, it is likely that the clearance of oxidized and misfolded proteins generated by ROS may be essential for cell viability. In the present study, TRPC6-mediated ERK1/2 activation facilitated mitochondrial fission, accompanied by LONP1 over-expression. However, LONP1 siRNA resulted in a massive DGC degeneration that was greater than the levels caused by TRPC6 siRNA and U0126, although it did not affect mitochondrial length. Unlike mitochondrial dynamics-related molecules (such as DRP1, optic atrophy 1, and mitofusin 2), LONP1 is up-regulated in response to harmful stresses [54]. Furthermore, LONP1 knockdown does not influence the activities of DRP1 and ERK1/2 under physiological- and post-SE conditions [17]. Since deregulation of LONP1 leads to cell death [17,27,54], the present data indicate that LONP1 may act as one of the important housekeeping antioxidants in mitochondria by limiting oxidative damage to tolerable levels, regardless of aberrant mitochondrial dynamics. Therefore, our findings suggest that TRPC6-ERK1/2-mediated LONP1 regulation may take part in the quality controls of mitochondria via degradation of oxidized/damaged proteins [23–25] and maintenance of mitochondrial DNA levels [27] during mitochondrial fission under physiological- and pathological conditions.

In the present study, TRPC6 siRNA increased seizure susceptibility in response to pilocarpine. TRPC6 inhibits N-methyl-d-aspartate (NMDA) receptor activity mediated by calcineurin [11]. Indeed, TRPC6 knockdown increases the excitability ratio (an index of synaptic efficacy, also referred as excitatory postsynaptic potential-population spike amplitude coupling) [14,16] indicating the lowering intrinsic threshold of neuronal firing in postsynaptic neurons [55]. Therefore, TRPC6 knockdown reduces seizure threshold of DGC via the heightened efficacy of NMDA receptor function in DGC itself [16]. Furthermore, TRPC6 siRNA reduces γ-aminobutyric acid (GABA)-ergic inhibitions onto the DGC during and after high-frequency stimuli due to the impaired repetitive firing of interneurons [16]. However, the present data show that TRPC6 activation by hyperforin did not affect seizure susceptibility in response to pilocarpine. Unlike TRPC6 knockdown, hyperforin shows the distinct effects on evoked potentials in a dose-dependent manner. The higher concentrations of hyperforin (10 and 100 μM) reduce the population spike amplitude (an indicative of synchronous postsynaptic discharges [14,16]), while a lower concentration (1 μM) increases it [56]. Consistent with the present data, the concentration of hyperforin (6 μM) cannot affect GABAergic inhibition and the seizure susceptibility in response to pilocarpine due to the functional saturation of Kv4.3 channels in interneurons, unlike DGC [16,18]. Furthermore, Sell et al. [57] have reported that hyperforin induces TRPC6-independent H^+ currents in HEK-293 cells, cortical microglia, chromaffin cells, and lipid bilayers. This action of hyperforin as a protonophore leads to cytosolic acidification and subsequently increases free intracellular Na^+ concentration via Na^+-H^+ exchanger (NHE). Thus, it is plausible that this unspecific properties of hyperforin as protonophore may be also involved in the ineffectiveness of hyperforin on pilocarpine-induced seizure activity. This is because seizure activity results in biphasic pH shifts, consisting of an initial extracellular alkalinization, followed by a slower acidification. The early extracellular alkalosis increases excitability because of reductions in $GABA_A$ receptor inhibition and enhancement in NMDA receptor currents, and the extracellular acidosis is involved in seizure termination [58]. Thus, it is presumable that hyperforin-induced H^+ efflux from neurons or glia would attenuate seizure activity in response to pilocarpine, independent of TRPC6. However, the simultaneous Na^+ accumulation would offset the inhibitory effect of extracellular acidosis on neuronal excitability by causing a lowering of the threshold for action potential generation in neurons and reducing the driving force for Na^+-dependent re-uptake of glutamate and other excitatory neurotransmitters into glia or neurons [57,59–61]. Thus, it is likely that these discrepancies of hyperforin from TRPC6 siRNA may lead to the ineffectiveness of hyperforin on seizure susceptibility to pilocarpine in the present study.

5. Conclusions

The present data provide novel evidence that TRPC6 regulates LONP1 expression via ERK1/2 activity. In brief, TRPC6-mediated ERK1/2 activation increased LONP1 expression and facilitated mitochondrial fission. Thus, TRPC6 may be involved in the quality controls of mitochondria as well as mitochondrial dynamics, which would enhance DGC invulnerability to SE (Figure 6). To the best of our knowledge, the present study is the first indication of the role of the TRPC6-ERK1/2-LONP1 pathway in neuronal vulnerability to SE. Therefore, this signaling pathway will be an interesting and important therapeutic target for neuroprotection from various neurological diseases.

Supplementary Materials: The following are available online at http://www.mdpi.com/2073-4409/8/11/1376/s1, Figure S1: Representative photos of mitochondria for each siRNA or compound treated-animals. Figure S2: Full-length gel images of Western blot data in Figure 1D. Figure S3: Full-length gel images of Western blot data in Figure 2A. Figure S4: Full-length gel images of Western blot data in Figure 3A.

Author Contributions: T.-C.K. designed and supervised the project. J.-E.K., H.P., S.-H.C. and M.-J.K. performed the experiments described in the manuscript. J.-E.K. and T.-C.K. analyzed the data, and wrote the manuscript.

Funding: This study was supported by a grant of National Research Foundation of Korea (NRF) grant (No. 2018R1C1B6005216 and No. 2018R1A2A2A05018222). The funders had no role in study design, data collection and analysis, decision to publish, or preparation of the manuscript.

Conflicts of Interest: The authors declare that the research was conducted in the absence of any commercial or financial relationships that could be construed as a potential conflict of interest.

References

1. Yu, T.; Robotham, J.L.; Yoon, Y. Increased production of reactive oxygen species in hyperglycemic conditions requires dynamic change of mitochondrial morphology. *Proc. Natl. Acad. Sci. USA* **2006**, *103*, 2653–2658. [CrossRef] [PubMed]
2. Yu, T.; Sheu, S.S.; Robotham, J.L.; Yoon, Y. Mitochondrial fission mediates high glucose-induced cell death through elevated production of reactive oxygen species. *Cardiovasc. Res.* **2008**, *79*, 341–351. [CrossRef] [PubMed]
3. Gibellini, L.; Pinti, M.; Boraldi, F.; Giorgio, V.; Bernardi, P.; Bartolomeo, R.; Nasi, M.; De Biasi, S.; Missiroli, S.; Carnevale, G.; et al. Silencing of mitochondrial Lon protease deeply impairs mitochondrial proteome and function in colon cancer cells. *FASEB J.* **2014**, *28*, 5122–5135. [CrossRef] [PubMed]
4. Marcillat, O.; Zhang, Y.; Lin, S.W.; Davies, K.J. Mitochondria contain a proteolytic system which can recognize and degrade oxidatively-denatured proteins. *Biochem. J.* **1988**, *254*, 677–683. [CrossRef] [PubMed]
5. Gur, E.; Sauer, R.T. Recognition of misfolded proteins by Lon, a AAA(+) protease. *Genes Dev.* **2008**, *22*, 2267–2277. [CrossRef] [PubMed]
6. Bulteau, A.L.; Lundberg, K.C.; Ikeda-Saito, M.; Isaya, G.; Szweda, L.I. Reversible redox-dependent modulation of mitochondrial aconitase and proteolytic activity during in vivo cardiac ischemia/reperfusion. *Proc. Natl. Acad. Sci. USA* **2005**, *102*, 5987–5991. [CrossRef]
7. Hori, O.; Ichinoda, F.; Tamatani, T.; Yamaguchi, A.; Sato, N.; Ozawa, K.; Kitao, Y.; Miyazaki, M.; Harding, H.P.; Ron, D.; et al. Transmission of cell stress from endoplasmic reticulum to mitochondria: Enhanced expression of Lon protease. *J. Cell Biol.* **2002**, *157*, 1151–1160. [CrossRef]
8. Cheng, C.W.; Kuo, C.Y.; Fan, C.C.; Fang, W.C.; Jiang, S.S.; Lo, Y.K.; Wang, T.Y.; Kao, M.C.; Lee, A.Y. Overexpression of Lon contributes to survival and aggressive phenotype of cancer cells through mitochondrial complex I-mediated generation of reactive oxygen species. *Cell Death Dis.* **2013**, *4*, e681. [CrossRef]
9. Zhu, Y.; Wang, M.; Lin, H.; Huang, C.; Shi, X.; Luo, J. Epidermal growth factor up-regulates the transcription of mouse lon homology ATP-dependent protease through extracellular signal-regulated protein kinase- and phosphatidylinositol-3-kinase-dependent pathways. *Exp. Cell Res.* **2002**, *280*, 97–106. [CrossRef]
10. Du, W.; Huang, J.; Yao, H.; Zhou, K.; Duan, B.; Wang, Y. Inhibition of TRPC6 degradation suppresses ischemic brain damage in rats. *J. Clin. Investig.* **2010**, *120*, 3480–3492. [CrossRef]
11. Li, H.; Huang, J.; Du, W.; Jia, C.; Yao, H.; Wang, Y. TRPC6 inhibited NMDA receptor activities and protected neurons from ischemic excitotoxicity. *J. Neurochem.* **2012**, *123*, 1010–1018. [CrossRef] [PubMed]
12. Kim, D.S.; Ryu, H.J.; Kim, J.E.; Kang, T.C. The reverse roles of transient receptor potential canonical channel-3 and -6 in neuronal death following pilocarpine-induced status epilepticus. *Cell Mol. Neurobiol.* **2013**, *33*, 99–109. [CrossRef] [PubMed]
13. Nagy, G.A.; Botond, G.; Borhegyi, Z.; Plummer, N.W.; Freund, T.F.; Hájos, N. DAG-sensitive and Ca^{2+} permeable TRPC6 channels are expressed in dentate granule cells and interneurons in the hippocampal formation. *Hippocampus* **2013**, *23*, 221–232. [CrossRef] [PubMed]
14. Kim, Y.J.; Kang, T.C. The role of TRPC6 in seizure susceptibility and seizure-related neuronal damage in the rat dentate gyrus. *Neuroscience* **2015**, *307*, 215–230. [CrossRef] [PubMed]
15. Ko, A.R.; Kang, T.C. TRPC6-mediated ERK1/2 phosphorylation prevents dentate granule cell degeneration via inhibiting mitochondrial elongation. *Neuropharmacology* **2017**, *121*, 120–129. [CrossRef]
16. Kim, J.E.; Park, J.Y.; Kang, T.C. TRPC6-mediated ERK1/2 activation regulates neuronal excitability via subcellular Kv4.3 localization in the rat hippocampus. *Front. Cell. Neurosci.* **2017**, *11*, 413. [CrossRef]

17. Kim, J.E.; Park, H.; Choi, S.H.; Kong, M.J.; Kang, T.C. CDDO-Me selectively attenuates CA1 neuronal death induced by status epilepticus via facilitating mitochondrial fission independent of LONP1. *Cells* **2019**, *8*, 833. [CrossRef]
18. Lee, S.K.; Kim, J.E.; Kim, Y.J.; Kim, M.J.; Kang, T.C. Hyperforin attenuates microglia activation and inhibits p65-Ser276 NFκB phosphorylation in the rat piriform cortex following status epilepticus. *Neurosci. Res.* **2014**, *85*, 39–50. [CrossRef]
19. Racine, R.J. Modification of seizure activity by electrical stimulation. II. Motor seizure. *Electroencephalogr. Clin. Neurophysiol.* **1972**, *32*, 281–294. [CrossRef]
20. Heiser, J.H.; Schuwald, A.M.; Sillani, G.; Ye, L.; Müller, W.E.; Leuner, K. TRPC6 channel-mediated neurite outgrowth in PC12 cells and hippocampal neurons involves activation of RAS/MEK/ERK, PI3K, and CAMKIV signaling. *J. Neurochem.* **2013**, *127*, 303–313. [CrossRef]
21. Do Val-da Silva, R.A.; Peixoto-Santos, J.E.; Kandratavicius, L.; De Ross, J.B.; Esteves, I.; De Martinis, B.S.; Alves, M.N.; Scandiuzzi, R.C.; Hallak, J.E.; Zuardi, A.W.; et al. Protective effects of cannabidiol against seizures and neuronal death in a rat model of mesial temporal lobe epilepsy. *Front. Pharmacol.* **2017**, *8*, 131. [CrossRef] [PubMed]
22. Min, S.J.; Hyun, H.W.; Kang, T.C. Leptomycin B attenuates neuronal death via PKA- and PP2B-mediated ERK1/2 activation in the rat hippocampus following status epilepticus. *Brain Res.* **2017**, *1670*, 14–23. [CrossRef] [PubMed]
23. Gottesman, S. Proteases and their targets in Escherichia coli. *Ann. Rev. Genet.* **1996**, *30*, 465–506. [CrossRef] [PubMed]
24. Ngo, J.K.; Pomatto, L.C.; Davies, K.J. Upregulation of the mitochondrial Lon Protease allows adaptation to acute oxidative stress but dysregulation is associated with chronic stress, disease, and aging. *Redox Biol.* **2013**, *1*, 258–264. [CrossRef] [PubMed]
25. Bota, D.A.; Davies, K.J.A. Lon protease preferentially degrades oxidized mitochondrial aconitase by an ATP-stimulated mechanism. *Nat. Cell Biol.* **2002**, *4*, 674–680. [CrossRef] [PubMed]
26. Luciakova, K.; Sokolikova, B.; Chloupkova, M.; Nelson, B.D. Enhanced mitochondrial biogenesis is associated with increased expression of the mitochondrial ATP-dependent Lon protease. *FEBS Lett.* **1999**, *444*, 186–188. [CrossRef]
27. Bota, D.A.; Ngo, J.K.; Davies, K.J. Downregulation of the human Lon protease impairs mitochondrial structure and function and causes cell death. *Free Radic. Biol. Med.* **2005**, *38*, 665–677. [CrossRef]
28. Graham, S.; Ding, M.; Sours-Brothers, S.; Yorio, T.; Ma, J.X.; Ma, R. Downregulation of TRPC6 protein expression by high glucose, a possible mechanism for the impaired Ca^{2+} signaling in glomerular mesangial cells in diabetes. *Am. J. Physiol. Renal Physiol.* **2007**, *293*, F1381–F1390. [CrossRef]
29. Zhou, J.; Du, W.; Zhou, K.; Tai, Y.; Yao, H.; Jia, Y.; Ding, Y.; Wang, Y. Critical role of TRPC6 channels in the formation of excitatory synapses. *Nat. Neurosci.* **2008**, *11*, 741–743. [CrossRef]
30. Chiluiza, D.; Krishna, S.; Schumacher, V.A.; Schlöndorff, J. Gain-of-function mutations in transient receptor potential C6 (TRPC6) activate extracellular signal-regulated kinases 1/2 (ERK1/2). *J. Biol. Chem.* **2013**, *288*, 18407–18420. [CrossRef]
31. Agell, N.; Bachs, O.; Rocamora, N.; Villalonga, P. Modulation of the Ras/Raf/MEK/ERK pathway by Ca^{2+}, and calmodulin. *Cell Signal* **2002**, *14*, 649–654. [CrossRef]
32. Cheung, E.C.; Slack, R.S. Emerging role for ERK as a key regulator of neuronal apoptosis. *Sci. STKE.* **2004**, *2004*, PE45. [CrossRef] [PubMed]
33. Hossain, M.S.; Ifuku, M.; Take, S.; Kawamura, J.; Miake, K.; Katafuchi, T. Plasmalogens rescue neuronal cell death through an activation of AKT and ERK survival signaling. *PLoS ONE* **2013**, *8*, e83508. [CrossRef] [PubMed]
34. Ortuño-Sahagún, D.; González, R.M.; Verdaguer, E.; Huerta, V.C.; Torres-Mendoza, B.M.; Lemus, L.; Rivera-Cervantes, M.C.; Camins, A.; Zárate, C.B. Glutamate excitotoxicity activates the MAPK/ERK signaling pathway and induces the survival of rat hippocampal neurons in vivo. *J. Mol. Neurosci.* **2014**, *52*, 366–377. [CrossRef] [PubMed]
35. Prieto, J.; León, M.; Ponsoda, X.; Sendra, R.; Bort, R.; Ferrer-Lorente, R.; Raya, A.; López-García, C.; Torres, J. Early ERK1/2 activation promotes DRP1-dependent mitochondrial fission necessary for cell reprogramming. *Nat. Commun.* **2016**, *7*, 11124. [CrossRef] [PubMed]

36. Serasinghe, M.N.; Wieder, S.Y.; Renault, T.T.; Elkholi, R.; Asciolla, J.J.; Yao, J.L.; Jabado, O.; Hoehn, K.; Kageyama, Y.; Sesaki, H.; et al. Mitochondrial division is requisite to RAS-induced transformation and targeted by oncogenic MAPK pathway inhibitors. *Mol. Cell* **2015**, *57*, 521–536. [CrossRef]
37. Leuner, K.; Li, W.; Amaral, M.D.; Rudolph, S.; Calfa, G.; Schuwald, A.M.; Harteneck, C.; Inoue, T.; Pozzo-Miller, L. Hyperforin modulates dendritic spine morphology in hippocampal pyramidal neurons by activating Ca^{2+}-permeable TRPC6 channels. *Hippocampus* **2013**, *23*, 40–52. [CrossRef]
38. Wong-Riley, M.T. Cytochrome oxidase: An endogenous metabolic marker for neuronal activity. *Trends Neurosci.* **1989**, *12*, 94–101. [CrossRef]
39. Wong-Riley, M.T. Bigenomic regulation of cytochrome c oxidase in neurons and the tight coupling between neuronal activity and energy metabolism. *Adv. Exp. Med. Biol.* **2012**, *748*, 283–304.
40. Sepuri, N.B.V.; Angireddy, R.; Srinivasan, S.; Guha, M.; Spear, J.; Lu, B.; Anandatheerthavarada, H.K.; Suzuki, C.K.; Avadhani, N.G. Mitochondrial LON protease-dependent degradation of cytochrome c oxidase subunits under hypoxia and myocardial ischemia. *Biochim. Biophys. Acta Bioenerg.* **2017**, *1858*, 519–528. [CrossRef]
41. Fukuda, R.; Zhang, H.; Kim, J.W.; Shimoda, L.; Dang, C.V.; Semenza, G.L. HIF-1 regulates cytochrome oxidase subunits to optimize efficiency of respiration in hypoxic cells. *Cell* **2007**, *129*, 111–122. [CrossRef] [PubMed]
42. Kaufman, B.A.; Durisic, N.; Mativetsky, J.M.; Costantino, S.; Hancock, M.A.; Grutter, P.; Shoubridge, E.A. The mitochondrial transcription factor TFAM coordinates the assembly of multiple DNA molecules into nucleoid-like structures. *Mol. Biol. Cell.* **2007**, *18*, 3225–3236. [CrossRef] [PubMed]
43. Kukat, C.; Wurm, C.A.; Spåhr, H.; Falkenberg, M.; Larsson, N.G.; Jakobs, S. Super-resolution microscopy reveals that mammalian mitochondrial nucleoids have a uniform size and frequently contain a single copy of mtDNA. *Proc. Natl. Acad. Sci. USA* **2011**, *108*, 13534–13539. [CrossRef] [PubMed]
44. Lu, B.; Lee, J.; Nie, X.; Li, M.; Morozov, Y.I.; Venkatesh, S.; Bogenhagen, D.F.; Temiakov, D.; Suzuki, C.K. Phosphorylation of human TFAM in mitochondria impairs DNA binding and promotes degradation by the AAA+ Lon protease. *Mol. Cell.* **2013**, *49*, 121–132. [CrossRef] [PubMed]
45. Bernstein, S.H.; Venkatesh, S.; Li, M.; Lee, J.; Lu, B.; Hilchey, S.; Morse, K.M.; Metcalfe, H.M.; Andreeff, M.; Brookes, P.S.; et al. The mitochondrial ATP-dependent Lon protease: A novel target in lymphoma death mediated by the synthetic triterpenoid CDDO and its derivatives. *Blood* **2012**, *119*, 3321–3329. [CrossRef]
46. Wang, H.M.; Cheng, K.C.; Lin, C.J.; Hsu, S.W.; Fang, W.C.; Hsu, T.F.; Chiu, C.C.; Chang, H.W.; Hsu, C.H.; Lee, Y.L. Obtusilactone A and (−)-sesamin induce apoptosis in human lung cancer cells by inhibiting mitochondrial Lon protease and activating DNA damage checkpoints. *Cancer Sci.* **2010**, *101*, 2612–2620. [CrossRef]
47. Flippo, K.H.; Strack, S. Mitochondrial dynamics in neuronal injury, development and plasticity. *J. Cell Sci.* **2017**, *130*, 671–681. [CrossRef]
48. Campello, S.; Scorrano, L. Mitochondrial shape changes: Orchestrating cell pathophysiology. *EMBO Rep.* **2010**, *11*, 678–684. [CrossRef]
49. Kim, J.E.; Kang, T.C. p47Phox/CDK5/DRP1-mediated mitochondrial fission evokes PV cell degeneration in the rat dentate gyrus following status epilepticus. *Front. Cell. Neurosci.* **2017**, *11*, 267. [CrossRef]
50. Kim, J.E.; Kang, T.C. Differential roles of mitochondrial translocation of active caspase-3 and HMGB1 in neuronal death induced by status epilepticus. *Front. Cell. Neurosci.* **2018**, *12*, 301. [CrossRef]
51. DuBoff, B.; Götz, J.; Feany, M.B. Tau promotes neurodegeneration via DRP1 mislocalization in vivo. *Neuron* **2012**, *75*, 618–632. [CrossRef] [PubMed]
52. Kageyama, Y.; Zhang, Z.; Roda, R.; Fukaya, M.; Wakabayashi, J.; Wakabayashi, N.; Kensler, T.W.; Reddy, P.H.; Iijima, M.; Sesaki, H. Mitochondrial division ensures the survival of postmitotic neurons by suppressing oxidative damage. *J. Cell Biol.* **2012**, *197*, 535–551. [CrossRef] [PubMed]
53. Kim, J.E.; Ryu, H.J.; Kim, M.J.; Kang, T.C. LIM kinase-2 induces programmed necrotic neuronal death via dysfunction of DRP1-mediated mitochondrial fission. *Cell Death Differ.* **2014**, *21*, 1036–1049. [CrossRef] [PubMed]
54. Polo, M.; Alegre, F.; Moragrega, A.B.; Gibellini, L.; Marti-Rodrigo, A.; Blas-Garcia, A.; Esplugues, J.V.; Apostolova, N. Lon protease: A novel mitochondrial matrix protein in the interconnection between drug-induced mitochondrial dysfunction and endoplasmic reticulum stress. *Br. J. Pharmacol.* **2017**, *174*, 4409–4429. [CrossRef] [PubMed]

55. Staff, N.P.; Spruston, N. Intracellular correlate of EPSP-spike potentiation in CA1 pyramidal neurons is controlled by GABAergic modulation. *Hippocampus* **2003**, *13*, 801–805. [CrossRef] [PubMed]
56. Langosch, J.M.; Zhou, X.Y.; Heinen, M.; Kupferschmid, S.; Chatterjee, S.S.; Nöldner, M.; Walden, J. St John's wort (*Hypericum perforatum*) modulates evoked potentials in guinea pig hippocampal slices via AMPA and GABA receptors. *Eur. Neuropsychopharmacol.* **2002**, *12*, 209–216. [CrossRef]
57. Sell, T.S.; Belkacemi, T.; Flockerzi, V.; Beck, A. Protonophore properties of hyperforin are essential for its pharmacological activity. *Sci. Rep.* **2014**, *4*, 7500. [CrossRef]
58. Xiong, Z.Q.; Stringer, J.L. Extracellular pH responses in CA1 and the dentate gyrus during electrical stimulation, seizure discharges, and spreading depression. *J. Neurophysiol.* **2000**, *83*, 3519–3524. [CrossRef]
59. Chatterjee, S.S.; Biber, A.; Weibezahn, C. Stimulation of glutamate, aspartate and gamma-aminobutyric acid release from synaptosomes by hyperforin. *Pharmacopsychiatry* **2001**, *34*, S11–S19. [CrossRef]
60. Vance, K.M.; Ribnicky, D.M.; Hermann, G.E.; Rogers, R.C. St. John's Wort enhances the synaptic activity of the nucleus of the solitary tract. *Nutrition* **2014**, *30*, S37–S42. [CrossRef]
61. Singer, A.; Wonnemann, M.; Müller, W.E. Hyperforin, a major antidepressant constituent of St. John's Wort, inhibits serotonin uptake by elevating free intracellular Na^{+1}. *J. Pharmacol. Exp. Ther.* **1999**, *290*, 1363–1368. [PubMed]

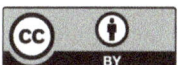

© 2019 by the authors. Licensee MDPI, Basel, Switzerland. This article is an open access article distributed under the terms and conditions of the Creative Commons Attribution (CC BY) license (http://creativecommons.org/licenses/by/4.0/).

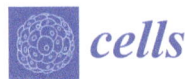

Article

CDDO-Me Selectively Attenuates CA1 Neuronal Death Induced by Status Epilepticus via Facilitating Mitochondrial Fission Independent of LONP1

Ji-Eun Kim [1,2], Hana Park [1,2], Seo-Hyeon Choi [1,2], Min-Jeong Kong [1,2] and Tae-Cheon Kang [1,2,*]

1. Department of Anatomy and Neurobiology, College of Medicine, Hallym University, Chuncheon 24252, Korea
2. Institute of Epilepsy Research, College of Medicine, Hallym University, Chuncheon 24252, Korea
* Correspondence: tckang@hallym.ac.kr; Tel.: +82-33-248-2524; Fax: +82-33-248-2525

Received: 26 June 2019; Accepted: 3 August 2019; Published: 5 August 2019

Abstract: 2-Cyano-3,12-dioxo-oleana-1,9(11)-dien-28-oic acid methyl ester (CDDO-Me) is a triterpenoid analogue of oleanolic acid that exhibits promising anti-cancer, anti-inflammatory, antioxidant and neuroprotective activities. In addition, CDDO-Me affects cellular differentiation and cell cycle arrest, and irreversibly inhibits Lon protease-1 (LONP1). In the present study, we evaluate the effects of CDDO-Me on mitochondrial dynamics and its downstream effectors in order to understand the underlying mechanism of the neuronal death following status epilepticus (SE, a prolonged seizure activity). CDDO-Me increased dynamin-related proteins 1 (DRP1)-serine 616 phosphorylation via activating extracellular-signal-regulated kinase 1/2 (ERK1/2) and c-Jun N-terminal kinase (JNK), but not protein kinase A (PKA) or protein phosphatases (PPs). In addition, CDDO-Me facilitated DRP1-mediated mitochondrial fissions, which selectively attenuated SE-induced CA1 neuronal death. Unlike CDDO-Me, LONP1 knockdown led to SE-induced massive degeneration of dentate granule cells, CA1 neurons and hilus interneurons without altering the expression and phosphorylation of DRP1, ERK1/2, JNK and PP2B. LONP1 knockdown could not inhibit SE-induced mitochondrial elongation in CA1 neurons. Co-treatment of CDDO-Me with LONP1 siRNA ameliorated only CA1 neuronal death, concomitant with abrogation of mitochondrial elongation induced by SE. Thus, our findings suggest that CDDO-Me may selectively attenuate SE-induced CA1 neuronal death by rescuing the abnormal mitochondrial machinery, independent of LONP1 activity.

Keywords: 4-HNE; DRP1; ERK1/2; hippocampus; JNK; mitochondrial dynamics; PKA; protein phosphatases; TUNEL

1. Introduction

Status epilepticus (SE) is a condition which shows prolonged and uncontrolled seizure activity [1]. One of the most remarkable SE-induced consequences is a massive neuronal death, which triggers long-term and profound alterations in the neuronal network that lead to the development of temporal lobe epilepsy (TLE) [2–4]. The neuronal death pattern and susceptibility to SE shows the regional specific heterogeneity: Neurons in the hilus region of the dentate gyrus, such as mossy cells and hilus interneurons (in particular parvalbumin (PV) interneurons), are the most vulnerable to SE insults, while dentate granule cells are less vulnerable. Furthermore, SE induces programmed necrotic CA1 neuronal death, while it evokes apoptosis in the hilus region [5–10]. Therefore, information regarding the molecular events underlying neuron-specific vulnerability may be one of the therapeutic strategies for neuroprotection against SE, which inhibits undesirable output including epileptogenesis.

Mitochondria are dynamic organelles of eukaryotic cells responsible for generating ATP. In addition, mitochondria participate in the synthesis of reactive oxygen species (ROS), cell homeostasis and calcium buffering. In the process of supplying ATP, mitochondria produce ROS through the electron transport chain, which induces oxidative stress. ROS production and oxidative damage induced by neuronal insults rapidly change mitochondrial morphologies, although mitochondria-derived ROS act as homeostatic signaling molecules in various physiological processes [11–15]. To exert their functions properly, mitochondria change their morphologies by two continuous antagonistic processes: fusion and fission (mitochondrial dynamics) [11]. As vital determinants of the fission-fusion balance, various proteins share reciprocal relationships [12]. Briefly, mitochondrial fusion (elongation) is regulated by mitofusin 1/2 (MFN1/2) and optic atrophy 1 (OPA1), while fission (fragmentation) is modulated by dynamin-related proteins 1 (DRP1) [11–13]. Thus, perturbation of mitochondrial dynamics and the altered expressions/activities of regulatory enzymes lead to neurodegeneration. In particular, the post-translational modification of DRP1 is focused on various neurodegenerative disorders. DRP1 activity is reversely regulated by phosphorylation of serine (S) 616 and 637 sites: DRP1-S616 phosphorylation facilitates mitochondrial fission. However, DRP1-S637 phosphorylation leads to DRP1 detaching from mitochondria, which subsequently inhibits mitochondrial fission. S-nitrosylation of cysteine 644 by nitric oxide (NO) also facilitates mitochondrial fragmentation by increasing S616 phosphorylation. Thus, the imbalance of DRP1 phosphorylation and S-nitrosylation evokes dysfunctions of mitochondrial dynamics, which are involved in pathological processes such as cancer and neurological diseases [14,15].

Interestingly, the impaired mitochondrial dynamics distinctly participate in heterogeneous neuronal death patterns in the hippocampus. Briefly, PV interneurons in the hilus regions show apoptotic degeneration following SE, accompanied by extensive mitochondrial fission [10]. In contrast, the abnormal elongation of swollen mitochondria contributes to CA1 neuronal necrosis, which is initiated by aberrant cell cycle entry in post-mitotic neurons [7,8,16–18]. Given these previous reports, the stoichiometric relationship between fission and fusion plays an important role in neuronal viability. Thus, insight into the molecular mechanism responsible for the impaired mitochondrial dynamics provides a deeper understanding of the distinct vulnerability of a neuronal subpopulation to SE.

2-Cyano-3,12-dioxo-oleana-1,9(11)-dien-28-oic acid methyl ester (CDDO-Me) is a triterpenoid analogue of oleanolic acid that exhibits promising anti-cancer, anti-inflammatory, antioxidant and neuroprotective activities. CDDO-Me affects cellular differentiation and cell cycle arrest [19,20]. CDDO-Me also irreversibly inhibits Lon protease-1 (LONP1) activity by forming covalent LONP1-CDDO adducts [21,22]. LONP1 is a highly conserved serine peptidase that contributes to protein quality control processes [23], which play a crucial role in maintaining mitochondrial morphology and function [24]. With respect to these previous studies, exploring the effects of CDDO-Me on mitochondrial dynamics is noteworthy in order to understand the mechanism of the distinct neuronal death that occurs in response to SE, which has been elusive.

Here, we demonstrate previously unsuspected effects of CDDO-Me on DRP1-mediated mitochondrial fissions, which selectively attenuated SE-induced CA1 neuronal death via activating extracellular-signal-regulated kinase 1/2 (ERK1/2) and c-Jun N-terminal kinase (JNK). In contrast to CDDO-Me, LONP1 knockdown aggravated SE-induced neuronal death without changing ERK1/2 and JNK activities. Co-treatment of CDDO-Me with LONP1 siRNA ameliorated only CA1 neuronal death, concomitant with abrogation of mitochondrial elongation induced by SE. Thus, our findings suggest CDDO-Me may abrogate abnormal mitochondrial machinery-mediated neuronal death induced by SE, independent of LONP1 activity.

2. Materials and Methods

2.1. Experimental Animals and Chemicals

Male Sprague–Dawley (SD) rats (7 weeks old, Daehan Biolink, South Korea) were used in the present study. Animals were given a commercial diet and water ad libitum under controlled conditions (22 ± 2 °C, 55 ± 5% and a 12:12 light/dark cycle with lights). Animal protocols were approved by the Institutional Animal Care and Use Committee of Hallym University (Chuncheon, Republic of Korea). The number of animals used and their suffering were minimized in all cases. All reagents were obtained from Sigma-Aldrich (St. Louis, MO, USA), except as noted.

2.2. Surgery, CDDO-Me Infusion and LONP1 Knockdown

Under Isoflurane anesthesia (3% induction, 1.5–2% for surgery and 1.5% maintenance in a 65:35 mixture of $N_2O:O_2$), animals were infused with each chemical or siRNA into the right lateral ventricle (1 mm posterior; 1.5 mm lateral; −3.5 mm depth to the bregma) with a brain infusion kit 1 and an Alzet 1007D osmotic pump (Alzet, Cupertino, CA, USA). The osmotic pump contained (1) vehicle, (2) CDDO-Me (10 μM), (3) a non-targeting control siRNA (5-GCAACUAACUUCGUUAGAAUCGUUAUU-3), (4) LONP1 siRNA (5-GAGACAAGUUGCGCAUGAUTT-3) and (5) CDDO-Me + LONP1 siRNA. The pump was placed in a subcutaneous pocket in the dorsal region. Some animals were also implanted with a monopolar stainless steel electrode (Plastics One, USA) into the left dorsal hippocampus (−3.8 mm posterior; 2.0 mm lateral; −2.6 mm depth). The connecting wire and electrode socket were then inserted in an electrode pedestal (Plastics One, USA) and secured to the exposed skull with dental acrylic [8,16–18]. Three days after surgery, rats were induced with SE by lithium chloride (LiCl)-pilocarpine.

2.3. SE Induction and Electroencephalogram (EEG) Analysis

SE was induced by a single dose (30 mg/kg) of pilocarpine in rats pretreated (24 h before pilocarpine injection) with 127 mg/kg LiCl, as previously described [8,16–18]. Before pilocarpine injection, animals were given atropine methylbromide (5 mg/kg i.p.) to block the peripheral effect of pilocarpine. Two hours after SE, animals received diazepam (10 mg/kg, i.p.) to terminate SE. As controls, rats were treated with saline instead of pilocarpine. For evaluation of the effects of CDDO-Me infusion and LONP1 siRNA knockdown on seizure susceptibility in response to pilocarpine, some animals' EEG signals were recorded with a DAM 80 differential amplifier (0.1–3000 Hz bandpass; World Precision Instruments, Sarasota, FL, USA). EEG activity was measured during the 2 h recording session from each animal. The data were digitized (400 Hz) and analyzed using LabChart Pro v7 (AD Instruments, New South Wales, Australia). Time of seizure onset was defined as the time point showing paroxysmal depolarizing shift, which lasted more than 3 seconds and consisted of a rhythmic discharge between 4 and 10 Hz with an amplitude of at least two times higher than the baseline EEG. EEG activity was measured during the 2 h recording session from each animal. Spectrograms were also automatically calculated using a Hanning sliding window with 50% overlap. Two hours after SE onset, diazepam (Valium; Roche, France; 10 mg/kg, i.p.) was administered and repeated, as needed [18].

2.4. Tissue Processing

Three days after SE induction, animals were perfused transcardially with phosphate-buffered saline (PBS, pH 7.4) followed by 4% paraformaldehyde in 0.1 M phosphate buffer (PB, pH 7.4) under urethane anesthesia (1.5 g/kg i.p.). The brains were removed, postfixed in the same fixative for 4 h and rinsed in PB containing 30% sucrose at 4 °C for 2 days. Thereafter, the tissues were frozen and sectioned with a cryostat at 30 μm, and consecutive sections were collected in six-well plates containing PBS. For western blot, animals were decapitated under urethane anesthesia. The hippocampus was rapidly removed and homogenized in lysis buffer. The protein concentration in the supernatant was determined using a Micro BCA Protein Assay Kit (Pierce Chemical, USA).

2.5. Immunohistochemistry and Measurements of Mitochondrial Length and Neuronal Damage

After incubation with 10% normal goat serum (Vector, Burlingame, CA, USA), sections were incubated in a mixture of primary antibodies shown in Table 1 (in PBS containing 0.3% triton X-100) at room temperature, overnight. After washing, sections were incubated for 1 h in a fluorescein isothiocyanate (FITC, green)-, Cy3 (red)- or aminomethylcoumarin acetate (AMCA, blue)-conjugated secondary antibodies (Vector, Burlingame, CA, USA). For negative control, tissues were incubated in pre-immune serum instead of primary antibody. Negative control tissues did not show any immunoreactivity for the primary antibody (data not shown). Images were captured using an AxioImage M2 microscope or a confocal laser scanning microscope (LSM 710, Carl Zeiss Inc., Oberkocken, Germany). Individual mitochondrion length in PV cells and CA1 neurons ($n = 20$/section) was measured using ZEN lite software (Blue Edition, Carl Zeiss Inc., Oberkocken, Germany) following 3D-reconstruction. Based on our previous study [10,18], twenty-five serial images (z-stack, 1 μm) were obtained from each hippocampal section. Serial images were stacked, aligned, visualized and converted to 3D images using the ZEN lite program. Thereafter, individual mitochondrial length (long axis) was measured. In addition, Fluoro-Jade B (FJB) and terminal deoxynucleotidyl transferase dUTP nick end labeling (TUNEL) staining were performed according to the manufacturer's instructions to analyze the neuronal damage. Two different investigators who were blind to the classification of tissues performed the measurement of mitochondrial length and the cell count of FJB and TUNEL positive neurons based on the lamellar structure of the hippocampus. For quantitative analysis of fluorescent intensity, sections (15 sections per each animal) were viewed through a microscope connected via Axiocam camera (Carl Zeiss Korea, Seoul, South Korea). Thereafter, fluorescent intensity measurements were represented as the number of a 256-gray scale using AxioVision Rel. 4.8 software (Carl Zeiss Korea, Seoul, South Korea). Intensity values were corrected by subtracting the average values of background noise obtained from five image inputs. The optical density was then standardized by setting the threshold levels.

2.6. Western Blot

Western blot was performed by the standard protocol. The primary antibodies used in the present study are listed in Table 1. The bands were detected and quantified on ImageQuant LAS4000 system (GE Healthcare, USA). As an internal reference, rabbit anti-β-actin primary antibody (1:5000) was used. The values of each sample were normalized with the corresponding amount of β-actin. The ratio of phosphoprotein to total protein was described as the phosphorylation level.

Table 1. Primary antibodies used in the present study.

Antigen	Host	Manufacturer (Catalog Number)	Dilution Used
DRP1	Rabbit	Thermo (PA1-16987)	1:1000 (WB)
ERK1/2	Rabbit	Biorbyt (Orb160960)	1:2000 (WB)
JNK	Rabbit	Protein tech (10023-1-AP)	1:1000 (WB)
LONP1	Rabbit	Proteintech (15440-1-AP)	1:100 (IF) 1:1000 (WB)
MFN1	Rabbit	Proteintech (13798-1-AP)	1:1000 (WB)
MFN2	Rabbit	Proteintech (12186-1-AP)	1:1000 (WB)
Mitochondrial marker (Mitochondrial complex IV subunit 1, MTCO1)	Mouse	Abcam (#ab14705)	1:500 (IF)
OPA1	Rabbit	Abcam (ab42364)	1:1000 (WB)
pDRP1 S616	Rabbit	Cell Signaling (4494)	1:500 (WB)
pDRP1 S637	Rabbit	Cell Signaling (4867)	1:500 (WB)
pERK1/2	Rabbit	Bioss (bs-3330R)	1:1000 (WB)

Table 1. Cont.

Antigen	Host	Manufacturer (Catalog Number)	Dilution Used
PKA catalytic subunit	Rabbit	BioVision (3115-100)	1:1000 (WB)
PKA regulatory subunit	Rabbit	Santa Cruz (sc-909)	1:1000 (WB)
PP1	Rabbit	Abcam (ab52619)	1:5000 (WB)
PP2A	Rabbit	Cell Signaling (#2038)	1:5000 (WB)
PP2B	Rabbit	Millipore (07-068-I)	1:1000 (WB)
pPKA catalytic subunit	Rabbit	Assay Biotec (A0548)	1:1000 (WB)
pPKA regulatory subunit	Rabbit	GeneTex (GTX61061)	1:2500 (WB)
pPP1	Rabbit	Abcam (ab62334)	1:5000 (WB)
pPP2A	Rabbit	Sigma (SAB4503975)	1:1000 (WB)
pPP2B	Rabbit	Badrilla (A010-80)	1:1000 (WB)
PV	Goat	Swant (#PVG213)	1:10,000 (IF)
β-actin	Mouse	Sigma (A5316)	1:5000 (WB)
4-HNE	Rabbit	Alpha Diagnostic (# HNE11-S)	1:1000 (IF)

IF, Immunofluorescence; WB, Western blot.

2.7. Quantification of Data and Statistical Analysis

All data were analyzed using the Mann-Whitney test or ANOVA to determine statistical significance. Bonferroni's test was used for post hoc comparisons. A p-value below 0.05 was considered statistically significant.

3. Results

3.1. CDDO-Me Distinctly Affects SE-Induced Neuronal Death in the Hippocampus

Figure 1 shows that SE resulted in up-regulation of LONP1 to ~1.5-fold of the control level in the whole hippocampus, accompanied by massive neuronal death in the CA1 region and the hilus of the dentate gyrus ($p < 0.05$ vs. control animals, respectively; Figure 1A,B,E,F). CDDO-Me did not affect the seizure latency and its severity in response to pilocarpine (Figure 1C,D). Consistent with a previous report [22], CDDO-Me did not affect LONP1 protein levels in the whole hippocampus of control- and post-SE animals, as compared to vehicle (Figure 1A,B). CDDO-Me effectively attenuated SE-induced neuronal loss in the CA1 region, but not in the hilus region ($p < 0.05$ vs. vehicle; Figure 1E–F), although it abolished 4-hydroxy-2-nonenal (4-HNE, the end-product of lipid peroxidation) signals in both regions ($p < 0.05$ vs. vehicle; Figure 1E,G). These findings indicate that CDDO-Me may differently affect the regional specific neuronal death following SE, independent of ROS generation.

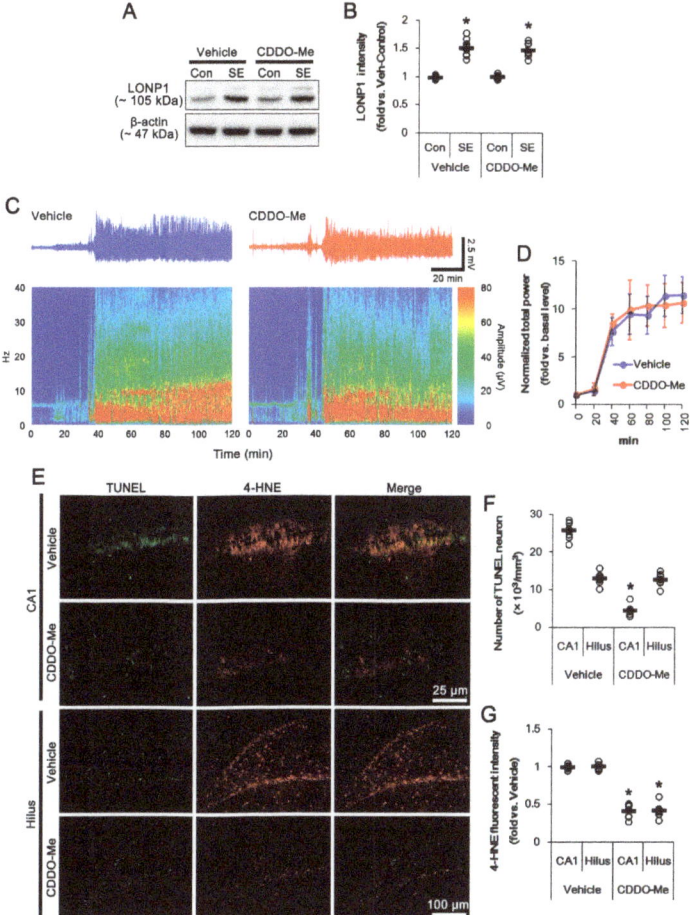

Figure 1. Effects of 2-Cyano-3,12-dioxo-oleana-1,9(11)-dien-28-oic acid methyl ester (CDDO-Me) on Lon protease-1 (LONP1) expression, seizure activity and neuronal damage in response to pilocarpine. (**A–B**) Effect of CDDO-Me on LONP1 expression in response to pilocarpine. Pilocarpine-induced status epilepticus (SE) increases LONP1 expression, which is not affected by CDDO-Me. (**A**) Representative western blots of LONP1 expression. (**B**) Quantification of LONP1 expression based on western blot data. Open circles indicate each individual value. Horizontal bars indicate mean value (mean ± S.E.M.; * $p < 0.05$ vs. control animals, respectively; $n = 7$). (**C–D**) Effect of CDDO-Me on seizure activity in response to pilocarpine. CDDO-Me does not influence seizure activity induced by pilocarpine. (**C**) Representative electroencephalogram (EEG) traces and frequency-power spectral temporal maps in response to pilocarpine. (**D**) Quantification of total EEG power (seizure intensity) in response to pilocarpine. Open circles indicate each individual value. Horizontal bars indicate mean value (mean ± S.E.M.; $n = 7$, respectively). (**E–G**) Effects of CDDO-Me on neuronal death and 4-hydroxy-2-nonenal (4-HNE) signals following SE. CDDO-Me mitigates CA1 neuronal damage, but not hilus interneurons, although it reduces 4-HNE signals in both neurons. (**E**) Representative photos of double immunofluorescent staining for terminal deoxynucleotidyl transferase dUTP nick end labeling (TUNEL) and 4-HNE. (**F**) Quantifications of the number of TUNEL positive neurons and (**G**) and the fluorescent intensity of 4-HNE in response to pilocarpine. Open circles indicate each individual value. Horizontal bars indicate mean value (mean ± S.E.M.; * $p < 0.05$ vs. vehicle; $n = 7$, respectively).

3.2. CDDO-Me Induces Mitochondrial Fission in CA1 Neuron and PV Cells without Altering LONP1 Expression

As mentioned previously, the dysfunctions of mitochondrial dynamics induced by SE lead to apoptosis and programmed necrosis in PV cells and CA1 neurons, respectively [7,8,10,16–18]. Thus, we evaluated the effects of CDDO-Me on mitochondrial dynamics in control- and post-SE animals. In control animals, CDDO-Me reduced mitochondrial length in CA1 neurons without altering mitochondrial LONP1 expression ($p < 0.05$ vs. vehicle; Figure 2A–D). Following SE, CDDO-Me significantly inhibited mitochondrial elongation, but not mitochondrial LONP1 over-expression, in these neurons ($p < 0.05$ vs. control animals; Figure 2A–D). Similarly, CDDO-Me led to mitochondrial fragmentation in PV cells in control animals without changing mitochondrial LONP1 expression ($p < 0.05$ vs. vehicle; Figure 3A–D), while it could not affect SE-induced excessive mitochondrial fission and LONP1 over-expression (Figure 3A–D). These findings indicate that CDDO-Me may facilitate mitochondrial fission in CA1 neurons as well as PV cells, which reversely influences neuronal death in both neuronal subpopulations following SE [10,25].

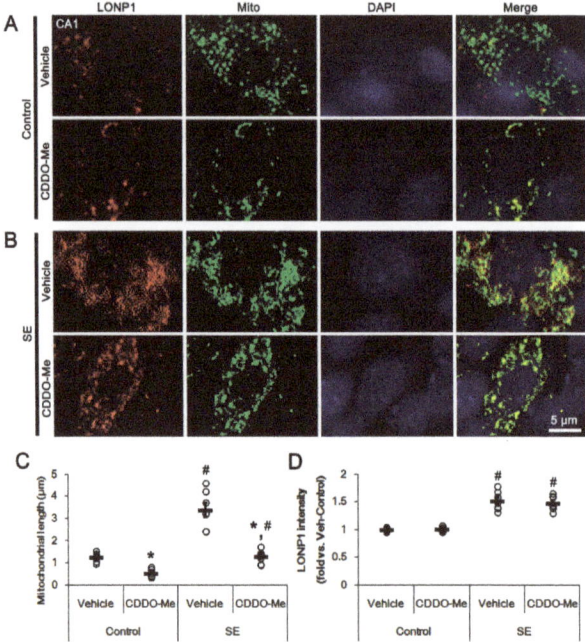

Figure 2. Effects of CDDO-Me on mitochondrial length and LONP1 expression in CA1 neurons. CDDO-Me reduces mitochondrial length in CA1 neurons of (**A**) control- and (**B**) post-SE animals. CDDO-Me does not affect the increased LONP1 expression following SE. (**A**,**B**) Representative photos of LONP1, mitochondria (Mito) and nuclei (DAPI) in CA1 neurons. (**C**,**D**) Quantifications of (**C**) the mitochondrial length and (**D**) LONP1 fluorescent intensity in CA1 neurons. Open circles indicate each individual value. Horizontal bars indicate mean value. Error bars indicate SEM (*,# $p < 0.05$ vs. vehicle and control animals, respectively; $n = 7$, respectively).

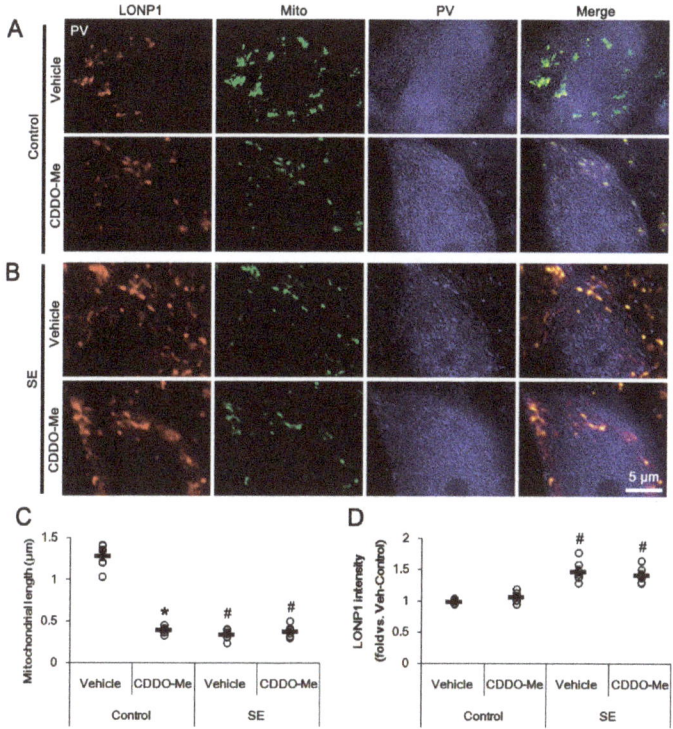

Figure 3. Effects of CDDO-Me on mitochondrial length and LONP1 expression in parvalbumin (PV) cells. CDDO-Me reduces mitochondrial length in CA1 neurons of (**A**) control- and (**B**) post-SE animals. CDDO-Me does not affect the increased LONP1 expression following SE. (**A**,**B**) Representative photos of LONP1, mitochondria (Mito) and PV. (**C**,**D**) Quantifications of (**C**) the mitochondrial length and (**D**) LONP1 fluorescent intensity in PV cells. Open circles indicate each individual value. Horizontal bars indicate mean value. Error bars indicate SEM (*,# $p < 0.05$ vs. vehicle and control animals, respectively; $n = 7$, respectively).

3.3. CDDO-Me Enhances DRP1-S616 Phosphorylation in Control- and Post-SE Animals

Since CDDO-Me exerted mitochondrial fragmentation in control and post-SE animals, we explored whether CDDO-Me influences the machinery molecules of mitochondrial dynamics. SE did not affect OPA1 and MFN1/2 expression levels (Figure 4A–D). Consistent with our previous studies [8,10,16–18,25], DRP1 expression was reduced to 0.68-fold of the control level following SE ($p < 0.05$ vs. control animals; Figure 4A,E). Furthermore, SE decreased the DRP1-S616 phosphorylation level to 0.67-fold of the control level ($p < 0.05$ vs. control animals; Figure 4A,F), while it did not affect the DRP1-S637 phosphorylation level (Figure 4A,G). These findings indicate a reduction in the DRP1-S616/S637 phosphorylation ratio following SE. In control animals, CDDO-Me did not influence OPA1, MFN1/2 and DRP1 expression levels (Figure 4A–E). However, CDDO-Me increased the DRP1-S616, but not S637, phosphorylation level to 1.5-fold of the vehicle level ($p < 0.05$ vs. vehicle; Figure 4A,F,G). In addition, CDDO-Me attenuated the down-regulation of DRP1 expression and its S616 phosphorylation level induced by SE. ($p < 0.05$ vs. control animals and vehicle, respectively; Figure 4A,F,G). Therefore, CDDO-Me increased the DRP1-S616/S637 phosphorylation ratio under physiological- and post-SE conditions. Since S616 site phosphorylation of DRP1 facilitates mitochondrial fission [26], our findings suggest that CDDO-Me may result in mitochondrial fragmentation via the enhancement of DRP1-S616 phosphorylation.

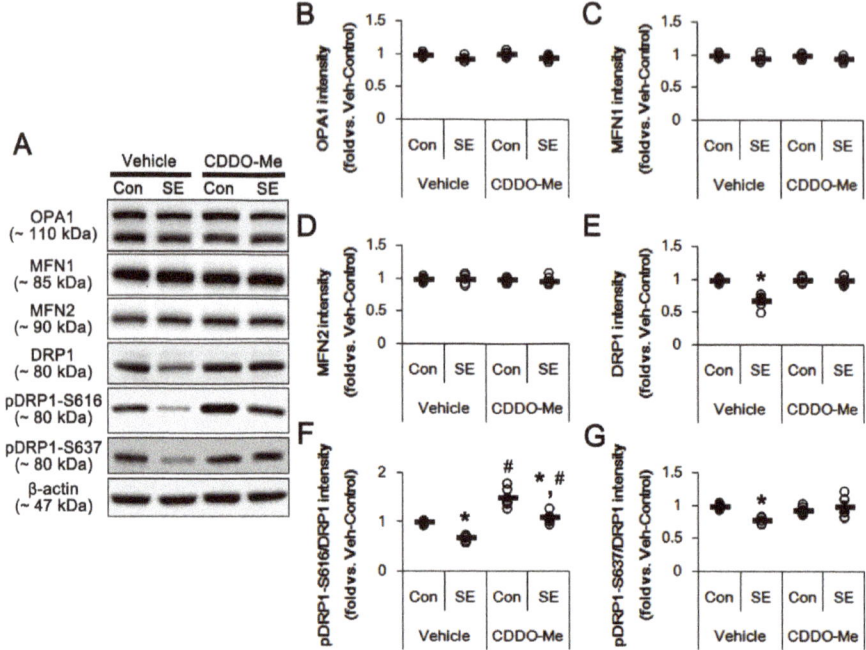

Figure 4. Effects of CDDO-Me on the expression and phosphorylation of mitochondrial dynamics-related molecules. CDDO-Me increases only the dynamin-related proteins 1 (DRP1)-S616 phosphorylation level under physiological- and post-SE conditions. (**A**) Representative images for western blots of optic atrophy 1 (OPA1), mitofusin 1 (MFN1), MFN2, DRP1, phospho (p)-DRP1-S616 and pDRP1-637 in the hippocampal tissues. (**B–G**) Quantifications of OPA1, MFN1 and MFN2, DRP1, pDRP1-S616 and pDRP1-637 levels. Open circles indicate each individual value. Horizontal bars indicate mean value. Error bars indicate SEM (*,# $p < 0.05$ vs. control animals and vehicle, respectively; $n = 7$, respectively).

3.4. CDDO-Me Increases ERK1/2 and JNK Activities in the Hippocampus

DRP1 phosphorylations are modulated by the ERK1/2, PKA and JNK signal pathways [26–30]. Furthermore, CDDO-Me influences ERK1/2 [20,31] and JNK phosphorylations [32,33]. Therefore, we evaluated the effects of CDDO-Me on the activities (phosphorylations) of protein kinases that are involved in DRP1 phosphorylations. In the present study, SE significantly reduced ERK1/2 and JNK phosphorylation levels without changing their expression ($p < 0.05$ vs. control animals, Figure 5A,B,C,F,G), while it did not affect the expression and phosphorylation levels of PKA catalytic and regulatory subunits (Figure 5A,D,E). In control animals, CDDO-Me did not change the protein expression levels of ERK1/2, PKA and JNK (Figure 5A,B,D,F). However, CDDO-Me increased the phosphorylation levels of ERK1/2 and JNK, but not PKA catalytic and regulatory subunits ($p < 0.05$ vs. vehicle; Figure 5A,C,G). Furthermore, CDDO-Me mitigated SE-induced reductions in ERK1/2 and JNK phosphorylations ($p < 0.05$ vs. vehicle; Figure 5A,C,G).

Protein phosphatases also regulate mitochondrial dynamics via DRP1 dephosphorylations. Indeed, protein phosphatase (PP) 2B (calcineurin) facilitates mitochondrial fission by dephosphorylating DRP1-S637 [34]. Thus, we validated whether CDDO-Me affects PP activities in the hippocampus. In control animals, CDDO-Me did not alter the protein expressions of PP1, PP2A and PP2B and their phosphorylation levels (Figure 6A–G). SE significantly reduced PP2B (not PP1 and PP2A) phosphorylation levels in the hippocampus, indicating an increase in its activity ($p < 0.05$ vs. control animals, Figure 6A,C,E,G), which was not affected by CDDO-Me (Figure 6A,C,E,G). Taken together, our findings indicate that CDDO-Me may regulate DRP1 S616 phosphorylation by enhancing ERK1/2 and JNK activities, independent of PP activities.

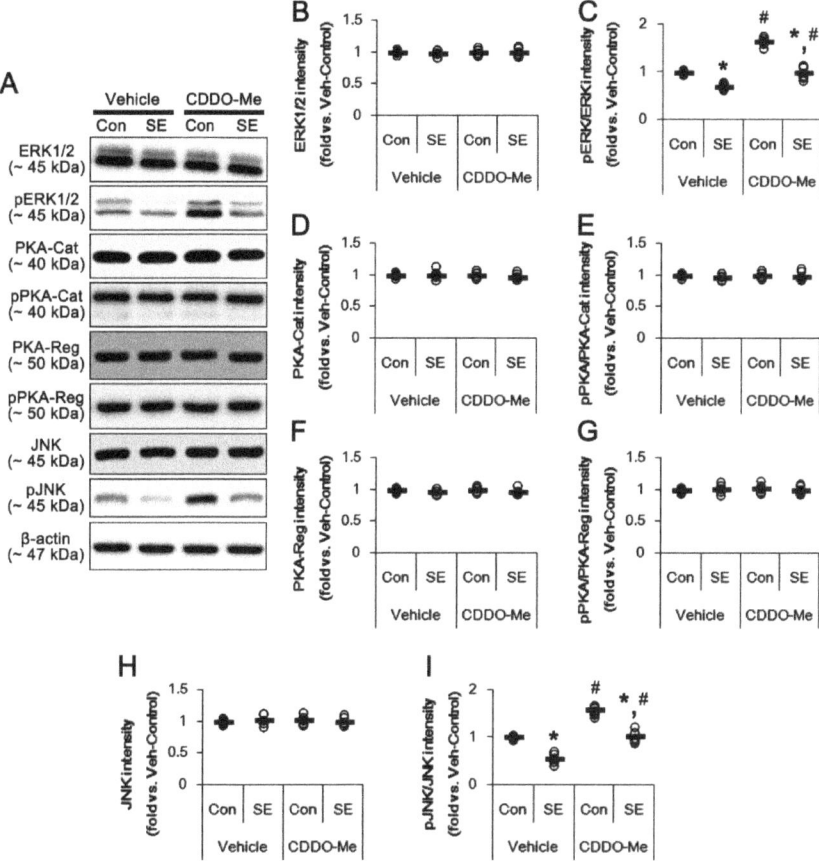

Figure 5. Effects of CDDO-Me on expressions and phosphorylations of extracellular-signal-regulated kinase 1/2 (ERK1/2), protein kinase A (PKA) and c-Jun N-terminal kinase (JNK). CDDO-Me increases ERK1/2 and JNK phosphorylation levels, but not PKA catalytic (PKA-Cat) and regulatory (PKA-Reg) subunits under physiological- and post-SE conditions. (**A**) Representative images for western blot of ERK1/2, phospho (p)-ERK1/2, PKA, pPKA, JNK and pJNK in the hippocampal tissues. (**B–G**) Quantifications of ERK1/2, pERK1/2, PKA, pPKA, JNK and pJNK levels. Open circles indicate each individual value. Horizontal bars indicate mean value. Error bars indicate SEM (*,# $p < 0.05$ vs. control animals and vehicle, respectively; $n = 7$, respectively).

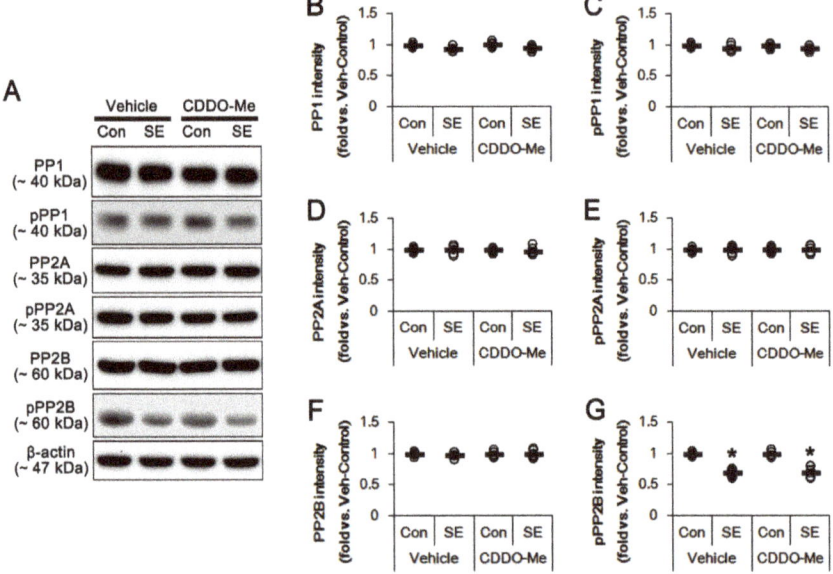

Figure 6. Effects of CDDO-Me on the expression and phosphorylation of protein phosphatase (PP) 1, PP2A and PP2B. CDDO-Me does not affect the expression and phosphorylation levels of protein phosphatase 1 (PP1), PP2A and PP2B under physiological- and post-SE conditions. (**A**) Representative images for western blot of PP1, phospho (p)-PP1, PP2A, pPP2A, PP2B and pPP2B in the hippocampal tissues. (**B–G**) Quantifications of PP1, pPP1, PP2A, pPP2A, PP2B and pPP2B levels. Open circles indicate each individual value. Horizontal bars indicate mean value. Error bars indicate S.E.M. (* $p < 0.05$ vs. control animals; $n = 7$, respectively).

3.5. Effects of CDDO-Me on SE-Induced Neuronal Death and Mitochondrial Dynamics are Independent of LONP1 Activity

In the present study, we found that CDDO-Me facilitated mitochondrial fission by increasing ERK1/2- and JNK-mediated DRP1-S616 phosphorylation. However, it was unclear whether these effects are relevant to the reduced LONP1 activity or the additional CDDO-Me actions. To directly elucidate the role of LONP1 in mitochondrial dynamics, we applied LONP1 siRNA prior to SE induction. In control animals, LONP1 knockdown effectively reduced LONP1 expression in the hippocampus ($p < 0.05$ vs. control siRNA; Figure 7A,B). Although LONP1 knockdown did not affect seizure susceptibility in response to pilocarpine (Figure 7C,D), it attenuated up-regulation of LONP1 expression induced by SE ($p < 0.05$ vs. control siRNA; Figure 7A,B). However, LONP1 siRNA exacerbated SE-induced neuronal damage in the CA1 neurons, hilus neurons and dentate granule cells, unlike CDDO-Me ($p < 0.05$ vs. control siRNA; Figure 7E,F). Co-treatment of CDDO-Me with LONP1 siRNA ameliorated only CA1 neuronal death, but not hilus neurons and dentate granule cells, following SE ($p < 0.05$ vs. LONP1 siRNA; Figure 7E,F). Furthermore, LONP1 siRNA did not influence the expression and phosphorylation of DRP1, ERK1/2, JNK and PP2B under physiological- and post-SE conditions (Figure 8A–J). LONP1 knockdown could not inhibit SE-induced mitochondrial elongation in CA1 neurons (Figure 8K,L). However, co-treatment of CDDO-Me with LONP1 siRNA abrogated mitochondrial elongation induced by SE ($p < 0.05$ vs. LONP1 siRNA; Figure 8K,L). These findings indicate that CDDO-Me-mediated mitochondrial fission may be independent of LONP1 activity, and that up-regulation of LONP1 may be an adaptive response to protect neurons from SE.

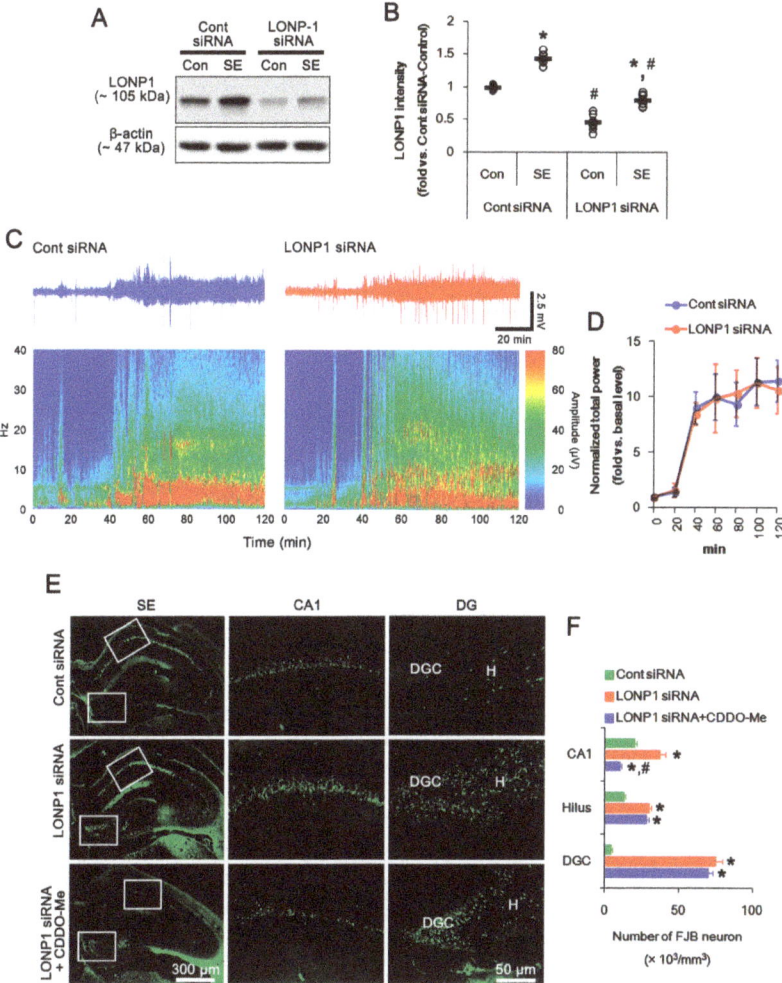

Figure 7. Effects of LONP1 siRNA on LONP1 expression, seizure activity and neuronal damage in response to pilocarpine. (**A,B**) Effect of LONP1 knockdown on LONP1 expression in response to pilocarpine. LONP1 siRNA effectively reduced LONP1 expression under physiological- and post-SE conditions. (**A**) Representative western blots of LONP1 expression. (**B**) Quantification of LONP1 expression based on western blot data. Open circles indicate each individual value. Horizontal bars indicate mean value (mean ± S.E.M.; * $p < 0.05$ vs. control animals, respectively; $n = 7$). (**C,D**) Effect of LONP1 knockdown on seizure activity in response to pilocarpine. LONP1 siRNA does not influence seizure activity induced by pilocarpine. (**C**) Representative EEG traces and frequency-power spectral temporal maps in response to pilocarpine. (**D**) Quantification of total EEG power (seizure intensity) in response to pilocarpine. Open circles indicate each individual value. Horizontal bars indicate mean value (mean ± S.E.M.; $n = 7$, respectively). (**E,F**) Effects of LONP1 siRNA and co-treatment of CDDO-Me on neuronal death induced by pilocarpine. LONP1 knockdown deteriorates degenerations of CA1 neurons, hilus interneurons (**H**) and dentate granule cells (DGC). Co-treatment of CDDO-Me attenuated CA1 neuronal death induced by SE. (**E**) Representative photos of FJB positive degenerating neurons. (**F**) Quantification of the number of FJB positive neurons in response to pilocarpine (mean ± S.E.M.; *,# $p < 0.05$ vs. control siRNA and LONP1 siRNA, respectively; $n = 7$, respectively).

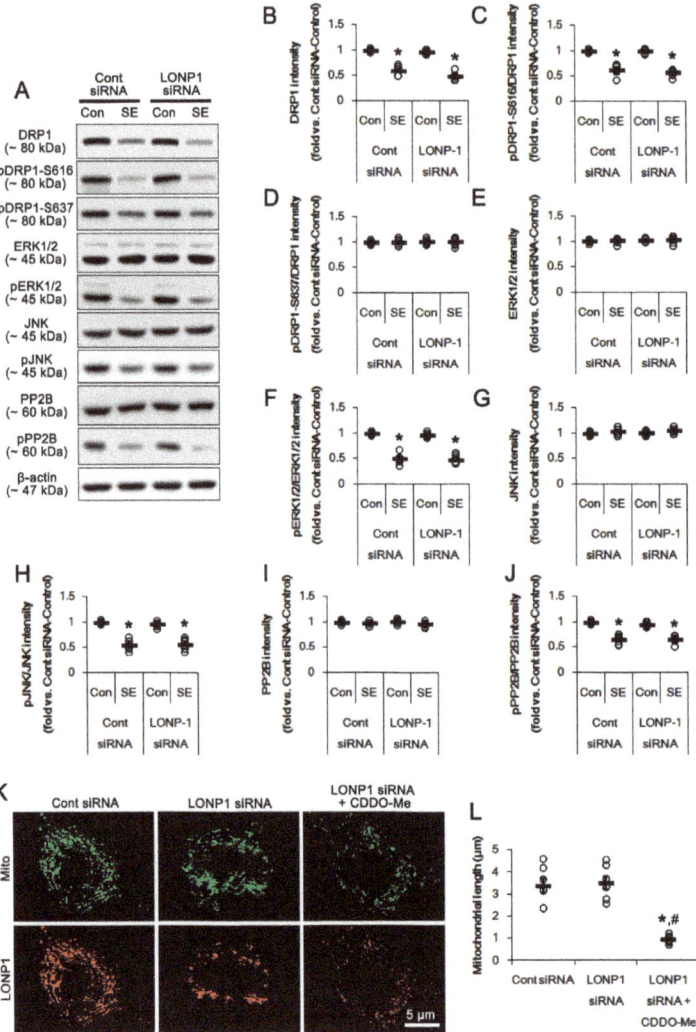

Figure 8. Effects of LONP1 knockdown on expression/phosphorylation of DRP1, ERK1/2, JNK and PP2B, and mitochondrial length in CA1 neurons. LONP1 siRNA does not affect the expression and phosphorylation levels of DRP1, ERK1/2, JNK and PP2B under physiological- and post-SE conditions. In addition, LONP1 knockdown does not influence SE-induced mitochondrial elongation in CA1 neurons, although it reduces LONP1 expression. However, co-treatment of CDDO-Me ameliorates mitochondrial elongation. (**A**) Representative images for western blots of DRP1, phospho (p)-DRP1-S616, pDRP1-637, ERK1/2, pERK1/2, JNK, pJNK, PP2B and pPP2B in the hippocampal tissues. (**B–J**) Quantifications of DRP1, pDRP1-S616, pDRP1-637, ERK1/2, pERK1/2, JNK, pJNK, PP2B and pPP2B levels. Open circles indicate each individual value. Horizontal bars indicate mean value. Error bars indicate S.E.M. (* $p < 0.05$ vs. control animals; $n = 7$, respectively). (**K**) Representative photos of mitochondria (Mito) and LONP1 in CA1 neurons following SE. (**L**) Quantification of the mitochondrial length in CA1 neurons. Open circles indicate each individual value. Horizontal bars indicate mean value. Error bars indicate S.E.M. (*,# $p < 0.05$ vs. control siRNA and LONP1 siRNA, respectively; $n = 7$, respectively).

4. Discussion

Aberrant cell cycle entry in post-mitotic neurons leads to neuronal death in various neurological diseases [35,36]. Similarly, SE increases the expression of cell cycle regulatory molecules such as cyclin D1 and CDK4, and evokes programmed necrosis in CA1 neurons through dysfunction of mitochondrial fission [8,10,16–18]. Imbalance of mitochondrial fusion/fission rate evokes cell degeneration: Dysfunction of mitochondrial fission (aberrant mitochondrial elongation) results in improper segregation of mitochondria and a decrease in ATP levels, which abrogates mitochondrial transports in dendrites or axons, and subsequently induces ATP deficiency in peripheral sites. Impaired mitochondrial fission also inhibits respiratory function in mitochondria that triggers excessive ROS production. Therefore, dysregulation of mitochondrial fission leads to cell degeneration [37–39]. Excessive mitochondrial fission (impaired mitochondrial fusion) also results in cell death. This is because fragmented mitochondria are not able to produce ATP, which impairs the detoxification of excess ROS and extrusion of intracellular Ca^{2+}, and in turn increases mitochondrial ROS and susceptibility to apoptosis [15,34,40,41]. Indeed, abnormal mitochondrial fission induces PV cell apoptosis following SE [10,25]. Since CDDO-Me inhibits cyclin D1 and induces cell cycle arrest [19,20], it is likely that CDDO-Me would affect aberrant mitochondrial dynamics induced by SE. In the present study, we found that CDDO-Me reduced mitochondrial length in CA1 neurons and PV cells without altering mitochondrial LONP1 expression in control animals. Furthermore, CDDO-Me effectively ameliorated SE-induced CA1 neuronal death, but not PV cell loss, accompanied by abrogating abnormal mitochondrial elongation. Since CDDO-Me induces mitochondrial fission in cancer cells [22,31,32] and WY14643 (an enhancer of mitochondrial fission) attenuates SE-induced CA1 neuronal death by rescuing aberrant mitochondrial elongation [8,25], our findings indicate that CDDO-Me-induced mitochondrial fission may have a selective neuroprotective effect against SE-induced CA1 necrosis, but not PV cell apoptosis.

In the present study, CDDO-Me increased DRP1-S616, but not S637, phosphorylation without changing the expression of other molecular components of mitochondrial dynamics, such as OPA1 and MFN1/2. Thus, CDDO-Me increased the DRP1-S616/S637 phosphorylation ratio. In our previous studies [8,16,17], SE decreased DRP1 expression and the DRP1-S616/S637 phosphorylation ratio, accompanied by increased mitochondrial length and sphere formation in CA1 neurons. Furthermore, WY 14643 increases DRP1-S616 phosphorylation and the DRP1-S616/S637 phosphorylation ratio [8]. Therefore, it is likely that the decreased DRP1-S616/S637 phosphorylation ratio may lead to aberrant mitochondrial elongation following SE. Consistent with these previous reports, the present study reveals that SE diminished the DRP1-S616/S637 phosphorylation ratio, concomitant with abnormal mitochondrial elongation, which were abolished by CDDO-Me. These findings indicate that CDDO-Me may facilitate mitochondrial DRP1 localization via the increased DRP1-S616/S637 phosphorylation ratio, although we could not confirm the subcellular localization of DRP1.

DRP1-S616 phosphorylation is regulated by the ERK1/2 and JNK signal pathways, which facilitate mitochondrial fission [27,29,30]. However, DRP1-S637 phosphorylation by PKA leads to detached DRP1 from mitochondria, thus inhibiting mitochondrial fission [26,28]. Indeed, DRP1-S637 dephosphorylation by PP2B accelerates mitochondrial fission [34]. Consistent with previous studies demonstrating that CDDO-Me regulates ERK1/2 [20,31] and JNK phosphorylation [32,33], the present data also reveal that CDDO-Me activated ERK1/2 and JNK under physiological conditions, and mitigated SE-induced reductions in ERK1/2 and JNK phosphorylation. However, CDDO-Me did not influence PKA and PP phosphorylation under physiological- and post-SE conditions. Since ERK1/2 inhibitor deteriorated SE-induced CA1 neuronal damage concomitant with mitochondrial elongation [18], our findings indicate that CDDO-Me may facilitate DRP1-mediated mitochondrial fission by activating ERK1/2 and JNK, which may attenuate CA1 neuronal degenerations following SE.

The present study also reveals that SE increased LONP1 expression in CA1 neurons as well as PV cells. LONP1 is one of the quality control proteins in the mitochondria supporting cell viability via the degradation of misfolded and damaged proteins under oxidative, hypoxic and endoplasmic reticulum-stress conditions [42,43]. Indeed, LONP1 expression is up-regulated under these stressful conditions [44,45]. Thus, LONP1 knockdown results in the disruption of mitochondrial function, reduced proliferation and the fragmented shape of the mitochondrial network [22,24,46]. With respect to these reports, it is likely that the up-regulation of LONP1 in PV cells and CA1 neurons may be an adaptive response to protect these neurons from SE. Considering this hypothesis and CDDO-Me as a LONP1 inhibitor [21,22], it is plausible that CDDO-Me would exacerbate degenerations of hilus interneurons and CA1 neurons by inhibiting LONP1 activity following SE. In the present study, however, CDDO-Me selectively alleviated CA1 neuronal damage without affecting the up-regulation of LONP1 expression induced by SE. In contrast, LONP1 knockdown aggravated neuronal loss of CA1 neurons. What makes these discrepancies in the effects of CDDO-Me and LONP1 siRNA on neuronal viability? In previous studies [21,22,24,46], CDDO-Me and LONP1 siRNA induced apoptosis of various cancer cells that have potent proliferative and differentiating abilities by inhibiting mitochondrial functionality. However, we applied CDDO-Me and LONP1 knockdown to post-mitotic neurons in the present study. Therefore, it is presumable that the differential proliferating ability of cancer cells and neurons would lead to the distinct effects of CDDO-Me and LONP1 siRNA on neuronal damage. Conversely, it is also considerable that LONP1 would not be a specific target of CDDO-Me. Indeed, the present data show that CDDO-Me affected ERK1/2 and JNK phosphorylation, while LONP1 siRNA did not influence the expression and phosphorylation of DRP1, ERK1/2, JNK, PKA and PPs under physiological- and post-SE conditions. In addition, co-treatment of CDDO-Me with LONP1 siRNA ameliorated only CA1 neuronal death, but not hilus neurons and dentate granule cells, following SE. Although LONP1 knockdown did not affect mitochondrial length in CA1 neurons, co-treatment of COOD-Me abrogated mitochondrial elongation induced by SE. Therefore, the present findings indicate that the neuroprotective effects of CDDO-Me may not be relevant to LONP1 inhibition. Since SE leads to programmed necrosis in CA1 neurons [8,16,17] and apoptosis in hilus interneurons, respectively [10], it cannot be excluded that CDDO-Me may selectively attenuate programmed necrosis rather than apoptosis. Taken together, the data from previous reports [8,25] and the present study identically suggest that the repair of dysfunction of mitochondrial fission may selectively rescue SE-induced CA1 neuronal death.

The heterogeneous vulnerability of hippocampal neurons in response to various insults has been reported. Briefly, dentate granule cells are remarkably resistant to various insults when compared to CA1 neurons or hilus interneurons [8,10,16,17,47–49]. Consistent with these previous studies, the present data show that SE induced a massive neuronal loss of hilus interneurons and CA1 neurons, although the degeneration of dentate granule cells was negligible. However, LONP1 knockdown provoked the massive degeneration of dentate granule cells, and aggravated loss of CA1 neurons and hilus interneurons. These findings indicate that LONP1 may be one of the important housekeeping molecules for neuronal viability, regardless of the heterogeneous vulnerability in response to harmful stimuli. Thus, it is likely that the regulation of LONP1 may be a useful therapeutic strategy for prevention of neurodegeneration. Future studies are needed to elucidate the role of LONP1 in other neurological diseases and the underlying regulatory mechanisms for its expression and activity.

5. Conclusions

To the best of our knowledge, the present data demonstrate, for the first time, the selective neuroprotective effects of CDDO-Me against SE. Briefly, CDDO-Me attenuated SE-induced CA1 neuronal death, but not hilus interneurons, by facilitating DRP1-mediated mitochondrial fission via ERK1/2 and JNK activation. Unlike CDDO-Me, LONP1 siRNA did not influence the expression and phosphorylation of DRP1, ERK1/2, JNK and PP2B under physiological- and post-SE conditions. In addition, LONP1 knockdown induced massive degeneration of dentate granule cells, and aggravated loss of CA1 neurons and hilus interneurons following SE. Co-treatment of CDDO-Me with LONP1 siRNA ameliorated CA1 neuronal death concomitant with abrogation of mitochondrial elongation induced by SE. Therefore, we provide an underlying mechanism of CDDO-Me for mitochondrial fission independent of LONP1 activity, and propose the availability of CDDO-Me for various neurological diseases relating to aberrant mitochondrial dynamics.

Author Contributions: T.-C.K. designed and supervised the project. J.-E.K., H.P., S.-H.C. and M.-J.K. performed the experiments described in the manuscript. J.-E.K. and T.-C.K. analyzed the data, and wrote the manuscript.

Funding: This study was supported by a grant of National Research Foundation of Korea (NRF) grant (No. 2018R1A2A2A05018222). The funders had no role in study design, data collection and analysis, decision to publish or preparation of the manuscript.

Conflicts of Interest: The authors declare that the research was conducted in the absence of any commercial or financial relationships that could be construed as a potential conflict of interest.

References

1. Trinka, E.; Cock, H.; Hesdorffer, D.; Rossetti, A.O.; Scheffer, I.E.; Shinnar, S.; Shorvon, S.; Lowenstein, D.H. A definition and classification of status epilepticus—Report of the ILAE Task Force on Classification of Status Epilepticus. *Epilepsia* **2015**, *56*, 1515–1523. [CrossRef] [PubMed]
2. Scharfman, H.E. Epileptogenesis in the parahippocampal region. Parallels with the dentate gyrus. *Ann. N. Y. Acad. Sci. USA* **2000**, *911*, 305–327. [CrossRef] [PubMed]
3. Cossart, R.; Bernard, C.; Ben-Ari, Y. Multiple facets of GABAergic neurons and synapses: Multiple fates of GABA signalling in epilepsies. *Trends. Neurosci.* **2005**, *28*, 108–115. [CrossRef] [PubMed]
4. Ribak, C.E.; Dashtipour, K. Neuroplasticity in the damaged dentate gyrus of the epileptic brain. *Prog. Brain Res.* **2005**, *136*, 319–328.
5. Tan, Z.; Sankar, R.; Shin, D.; Sun, N.; Liu, H.; Wasterlain, C.G.; Schreiber, S.S. Differential induction of p53 in immature and adult rat brain following lithium-pilocarpine status epilepticus. *Brain Res.* **2002**, *928*, 187–193. [CrossRef]
6. Kang, T.C.; Kim, D.S.; Kwak, S.E.; Kim, J.E.; Won, M.H.; Kim, D.W.; Choi, S.Y.; Kwon, O.S. Epileptogenic roles of astroglial death and regeneration in the dentate gyrus of experimental temporal lobe epilepsy. *Glia* **2006**, *54*, 258–271. [CrossRef] [PubMed]
7. Seo, D.W.; Lopez-Meraz, M.L.; Allen, S.; Wasterlain, C.G.; Niquet, J. Contribution of a mitochondrial pathway to excitotoxic neuronal necrosis. *J. Neurosci. Res.* **2009**, *87*, 2087–2094. [CrossRef] [PubMed]
8. Kim, J.E.; Ryu, H.J.; Kim, M.J.; Kang, T.C. LIM kinase-2 induces programmed necrotic neuronal death via dysfunction of DRP1-mediated mitochondrial fission. *Cell Death Differ.* **2014**, *21*, 1036–1049. [CrossRef] [PubMed]
9. Niquet, J.; Auvin, S.; Archie, M.; Seo, D.W.; Allen, S.; Sankar, R.; Wasterlain, C.G. Status epilepticus triggers caspase-3 activation and necrosis in the immature rat brain. *Epilepsia* **2007**, *48*, 1203–1206. [CrossRef]
10. Kim, J.E.; Kang, T.C. p47Phox/CDK5/DRP1-mediated mitochondrial fission evokes PV cell degeneration in the rat dentate gyrus following status epilepticus. *Front. Cell. Neurosci.* **2017**, *11*, 267. [CrossRef]
11. Chan, D.C. Mitochondrial fusion and fission in mammals. *Annu. Rev. Cell. Dev. Biol.* **2006**, *22*, 79–99. [CrossRef] [PubMed]
12. Karbowski, M.; Lee, Y.J.; Gaume, B.; Jeong, S.Y.; Frank, S.; Nechushtan, A.; Santel, A.; Fuller, M.; Smith, C.L.; Youle, R.J. Spatial and temporal association of Bax with mitochondrial fission sites, Drp1, and Mfn2 during apoptosis. *J. Cell Biol.* **2002**, *159*, 931–938. [CrossRef] [PubMed]
13. Song, Z.; Ghochani, M.; McCaffery, J.M.; Frey, T.G.; Chan, D.C. Mitofusins and OPA1 mediate sequential steps in mitochondrial membrane fusion. *Mol. Biol. Cell.* **2009**, *20*, 3525–3532. [CrossRef] [PubMed]
14. Lee, D.S.; Kim, J.E. PDI-mediated S-nitrosylation of DRP1 facilitates DRP1-S616 phosphorylation and mitochondrial fission in CA1 neurons. *Cell Death Dis.* **2018**, *9*, 869. [CrossRef] [PubMed]
15. Flippo, K.H.; Strack, S. Mitochondrial dynamics in neuronal injury, development and plasticity. *J. Cell Sci.* **2017**, *130*, 671–681. [CrossRef] [PubMed]
16. Ko, A.R.; Hyun, H.W.; Min, S.J.; Kim, J.E.; Kang, T.C. Endothelin-1 induces LIMK2-mediated programmed necrotic neuronal death independent of NOS activity. *Mol. Brain* **2015**, *8*, 58. [CrossRef]
17. Hyun, H.W.; Ko, A.R.; Kang, T.C. Mitochondrial translocation of high mobility group box 1 facilitates LIM Kinase 2-mediated programmed necrotic neuronal death. *Front. Cell. Neurosci.* **2016**, *10*, 99. [CrossRef]
18. Ko, A.R.; Kang, T.C. TRPC6-mediated ERK1/2 phosphorylation prevents dentate granule cell degeneration via inhibiting mitochondrial elongation. *Neuropharmacology* **2017**, *121*, 120–129. [CrossRef]

19. Tran, T.A.; McCoy, M.K.; Sporn, M.B.; Tansey, M.G. The synthetic triterpenoid CDDO-methyl ester modulates microglial activities, inhibits TNF production, and provides dopaminergic neuroprotection. *J. Neuroinflammation* **2008**, *5*, 14. [CrossRef]
20. Wang, X.Y.; Zhang, X.H.; Peng, L.; Liu, Z.; Yang, Y.X.; He, Z.X.; Dang, H.W.; Zhou, S.F. Bardoxolone methyl (CDDO-Me or RTA402) induces cell cycle arrest, apoptosis and autophagy via PI3K/Akt/mTOR and p38 MAPK/Erk1/2 signaling pathways in K562 cells. *Am. J. Transl. Res.* **2017**, *9*, 4652–4672.
21. Bernstein, S.H.; Venkatesh, S.; Li, M.; Lee, J.; Lu, B.; Hilchey, S.P.; Morse, K.M.; Metcalfe, H.M.; Skalska, J.; Andreeff, M.; et al. The mitochondrial ATP-dependent Lon protease: A novel target in lymphoma death mediated by the synthetic triterpenoid CDDO and its derivatives. *Blood* **2012**, *119*, 3321–3329. [CrossRef] [PubMed]
22. Gibellini, L.; Pinti, M.; Bartolomeo, R.; De Biasi, S.; Cormio, A.; Musicco, C.; Carnevale, G.; Pecorini, S.; Nasi, M.; De Pol, A.; et al. Inhibition of Lon protease by triterpenoids alters mitochondria and is associated to cell death in human cancer cells. *Oncotarget* **2015**, *6*, 25466–25483. [CrossRef] [PubMed]
23. Lu, B.; Liu, T.; Crosby, J.A.; Thomas-Wohlever, J.; Lee, I.; Suzuki, C.K. The ATP-dependent Lon protease of Mus musculus is a DNA-binding protein that is functionally conserved between yeast and mammals. *Gene* **2003**, *306*, 45–55. [CrossRef]
24. Gibellini, L.; Pinti, M.; Boraldi, F.; Giorgio, V.; Bernardi, P.; Bartolomeo, R.; Nasi, M.; De Biasi, S.; Missiroli, S.; Carnevale, G.; et al. Silencing of mitochondrial Lon protease deeply impairs mitochondrial proteome and function in colon cancer cells. *FASEB J.* **2014**, *28*, 5122–5135. [CrossRef] [PubMed]
25. Kim, J.E.; Kang, T.C. Differential roles of mitochondrial translocation of active caspase-3 and HMGB1 in neuronal death induced by status epilepticus. *Front. Cell. Neurosci.* **2018**, *12*, 301. [CrossRef] [PubMed]
26. Kashatus, D.F.; Lim, K.H.; Brady, D.C.; Pershing, N.L.; Cox, A.D.; Counter, C.M. RALA and RALBP1 regulate mitochondrial fission at mitosis. *Nat. Cell Biol.* **2011**, *13*, 1108–1115. [CrossRef] [PubMed]
27. Prieto, J.; León, M.; Ponsoda, X.; Sendra, R.; Bort, R.; Ferrer-Lorente, R.; Raya, A.; López-García, C.; Torres, J. Early ERK1/2 activation promotes DRP1-dependent mitochondrial fission necessary for cell reprogramming. *Nat. Commun.* **2016**, *7*, 11124. [CrossRef]
28. Wang, Z.; Jiang, H.; Chen, S.; Du, F.; Wang, X. The mitochondrial phosphatase PGAM5 functions at the convergence point of multiple necrotic death pathways. *Cell* **2012**, *148*, 228–243. [CrossRef]
29. Wang, H.; Zhao, X.; Ni, C.; Dai, Y.; Guo, Y. Zearalenone regulates endometrial stromal cell apoptosis and migration via the promotion of mitochondrial fission by activation of the JNK/Drp1 pathway. *Mol. Med. Rep.* **2018**, *17*, 7797–7806. [CrossRef]
30. Feng, M.; Wang, L.; Chang, S.; Yuan, P. Penehyclidine hydrochloride regulates mitochondrial dynamics and apoptosis through p38MAPK and JNK signal pathways and provides cardioprotection in rats with myocardial ischemia-reperfusion injury. *Eur. J. Pharm. Sci.* **2018**, *121*, 243–250. [CrossRef]
31. Konopleva, M.; Contractor, R.; Kurinna, S.M.; Chen, W.; Andreeff, M.; Ruvolo, P.P. The novel triterpenoid CDDO-Me suppresses MAPK pathways and promotes p38 activation in acute myeloid leukemia cells. *Leukemia* **2005**, *19*, 1350–1354. [CrossRef] [PubMed]
32. Ikeda, T.; Sporn, M.; Honda, T.; Gribble, G.W.; Kufe, D. The novel triterpenoid CDDO and its derivatives induce apoptosis by disruption of intracellular redox balance. *Cancer Res.* **2003**, *63*, 5551–5558. [PubMed]
33. Zou, W.; Yue, P.; Khuri, F.R.; Sun, S.Y. Coupling of endoplasmic reticulum stress to CDDO-Me-induced up-regulation of death receptor 5 via a CHOP-dependent mechanism involving JNK activation. *Cancer Res.* **2008**, *68*, 7484–7492. [CrossRef] [PubMed]
34. Campello, S.; Scorrano, L. Mitochondrial shape changes: Orchestrating cell pathophysiology. *EMBO Rep.* **2010**, *11*, 678–684. [CrossRef] [PubMed]
35. Greene, L.; Biswas, S.; Liu, D. Cell cycle molecules and vertebrate neuron death: E2F at the hub. *Cell Death Differ.* **2004**, *11*, 49–60. [CrossRef] [PubMed]
36. Nguyen, M.; Boudreau, M.; Kriz, J.; Couillard-Despres, S.; Kaplan, D.; Julien, J. Cell cycle regulators in the neuron death pathway of amyotrophic lateral sclerosis caused by mutant superoxide dismutase. *J. Neurosci.* **2003**, *23*, 2131–2140. [CrossRef] [PubMed]
37. DuBoff, B.; Götz, J.; Feany, M.B. Tau promotes neurodegeneration via DRP1 mislocalization *in vivo*. *Neuron* **2012**, *75*, 618–632. [CrossRef]

38. Kageyama, Y.; Zhang, Z.; Roda, R.; Fukaya, M.; Wakabayashi, J.; Wakabayashi, N.; Kensler, T.W.; Reddy, P.H.; Iijima, M.; Sesaki, H. Mitochondrial division ensures the survival of postmitotic neurons by suppressing oxidative damage. *J. Cell Biol.* **2012**, *197*, 535–551. [CrossRef]
39. Parone, P.A.; Da Cruz, S.; Tondera, D.; Mattenberger, Y.; James, D.I.; Maechler, P.; Barja, F.; Martinou, J.C. Preventing mitochondrial fission impairs mitochondrial function and leads to loss of mitochondrial DNA. *PLoS ONE* **2008**. [CrossRef]
40. Yu, T.; Robotham, J.L.; Yoon, Y. Increased production of reactive oxygen species in hyperglycemic conditions requires dynamic change of mitochondrial morphology. *Proc. Natl. Acad. Sci. USA* **2006**, *103*, 2653–2658. [CrossRef]
41. Yu, T.; Sheu, S.S.; Robotham, J.L.; Yoon, Y. Mitochondrial fission mediates high glucose-induced cell death through elevated production of reactive oxygen species. *Cardiovasc. Res.* **2008**, *79*, 341–351. [CrossRef] [PubMed]
42. Rugarli, E.I.; Langer, T. Mitochondrial quality control: A matter of life and death for neurons. *EMBO J.* **2012**, *31*, 1336–1349. [CrossRef] [PubMed]
43. Venkatesh, S.; Lee, J.; Singh, K.; Lee, I.; Suzuki, C.K. Multitasking in the mitochondrion by the ATP-dependent Lon protease. *Biochim. Biophys. Acta* **2012**, *1823*, 56–66. [CrossRef] [PubMed]
44. Fukuda, R.; Zhang, H.; Kim, J.W.; Shimoda, L.; Dang, C.V.; Semenza, G.L. HIF-1 regulates cytochrome oxidase subunits to optimize efficiency of respiration in hypoxic cells. *Cell* **2007**, *129*, 111–122. [CrossRef] [PubMed]
45. Ngo, J.K.; Pomatto, L.C.; Davies, K.J. Upregulation of the mitochondrial Lon Protease allows adaptation to acute oxidative stress but dysregulation is associated with chronic stress, disease, and aging. *Redox Biol.* **2013**, *1*, 258–264. [CrossRef]
46. Quirós, P.M.; Español, Y.; Acín-Pérez, R.; Rodríguez, F.; Bárcena, C.; Watanabe, K.; Calvo, E.; Loureiro, M.; Fernández-García, M.S.; Fueyo, A.; et al. ATP-dependent Lon protease controls tumor bioenergetics by reprogramming mitochondrial activity. *Cell Rep.* **2014**, *8*, 542–556. [CrossRef] [PubMed]
47. Ordy, J.M.; Wengenack, T.M.; Bialobok, P.; Coleman, P.D.; Rodier, P.; Baggs, R.B.; Dunlap, W.P.; Kates, B. Selective vulnerability and early progression of hippocampal CA1 pyramidal cell degeneration and GFAP-positive astrocyte reactivity in the rat four-vessel occlusion model of transient global ischemia. *Exp. Neurol.* **1993**, *119*, 128–139. [CrossRef]
48. Soukupová, M.; Binaschi, A.; Falcicchia, C.; Zucchini, S.; Roncon, P.; Palma, E.; Magri, E.; Grandi, E.; Simonato, M. Impairment of GABA release in the hippocampus at the time of the first spontaneous seizure in the pilocarpine model of temporal lobe epilepsy. *Exp. Neurol.* **2014**, *257*, 39–49. [CrossRef]
49. Wittner, L.; Maglóczky, Z.; Borhegyi, Z.; Halász, P.; Tóth, S.; Eross, L.; Szabó, Z.; Freund, T.F. Preservation of perisomatic inhibitory input of granule cells in the epileptic human dentate gyrus. *Neuroscience* **2001**, *108*, 587–600. [CrossRef]

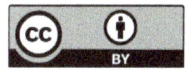

© 2019 by the authors. Licensee MDPI, Basel, Switzerland. This article is an open access article distributed under the terms and conditions of the Creative Commons Attribution (CC BY) license (http://creativecommons.org/licenses/by/4.0/).

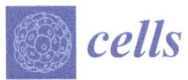

Article

The Effects of Sodium Dichloroacetate on Mitochondrial Dysfunction and Neuronal Death Following Hypoglycemia-Induced Injury

A Ra Kho [1], Bo Young Choi [1], Song Hee Lee [1], Dae Ki Hong [1], Jeong Hyun Jeong [1], Beom Seok Kang [1], Dong Hyeon Kang [2], Kyoung-Ha Park [3], Jae Bong Park [4] and Sang Won Suh [1,*]

1. Department of Physiology, College of Medicine, Hallym University, Chuncheon 24252, Kangwon-Do, Korea; rnlduadkfk136@hallym.ac.kr (A.R.K.); bychoi@hallym.ac.kr (B.Y.C.); sshlee@hallym.ac.kr (S.H.L.); zxnm01220@gmail.com (D.K.H.); jd1422@hanmail.net (J.H.J.); ttiger1993@gmail.com (B.S.K.)
2. Department of Medical science, College of Medicine, Hallym University, Chuncheon 24252, Kangwon-Do, Korea; ehdgus6312@gmail.com
3. Division of Cardiovascular Disease, Hallym University Medical Center, Anyang 14068, Korea; pkhmd@naver.com
4. Department of Biochemistry, College of Medicine, Hallym University, Chuncheon 24252, Kangwon-Do, Korea; jbpark@hallym.ac.kr
* Correspondence: swsuh@hallym.ac.kr; Tel.: +82-10-8573-6364

Received: 15 March 2019; Accepted: 1 May 2019; Published: 1 May 2019

Abstract: Our previous studies demonstrated that some degree of neuronal death is caused by hypoglycemia, but a subsequent and more severe wave of neuronal cell death occurs due to glucose reperfusion, which results from the rapid restoration of low blood glucose levels. Mitochondrial dysfunction caused by hypoglycemia leads to increased levels of pyruvate dehydrogenase kinase (PDK) and suppresses the formation of ATP by inhibiting pyruvate dehydrogenase (PDH) activation, which can convert pyruvate into acetyl-coenzyme A (acetyl-CoA). Sodium dichloroacetate (DCA) is a PDK inhibitor and activates PDH, the gatekeeper of glucose oxidation. However, no studies about the effect of DCA on hypoglycemia have been published. In the present study, we hypothesized that DCA treatment could reduce neuronal death through improvement of glycolysis and prevention of reactive oxygen species production after hypoglycemia. To test this, we used an animal model of insulin-induced hypoglycemia and injected DCA (100 mg/kg, i.v., two days) following hypoglycemic insult. Histological evaluation was performed one week after hypoglycemia. DCA treatment reduced hypoglycemia-induced oxidative stress, microglial activation, blood–brain barrier disruption, and neuronal death compared to the vehicle-treated hypoglycemia group. Therefore, our findings suggest that DCA may have the therapeutic potential to reduce hippocampal neuronal death after hypoglycemia.

Keywords: hypoglycemia; sodium dichloroacetate; pyruvate dehydrogenase kinase; pyruvate dehydrogenase; oxidative stress; neuron death

1. Introduction

Hypoglycemia is a potentially serious condition that occurs when blood glucose levels quickly fall below a specific threshold concentration. The most common cause of hypoglycemia is misuse of medications such as insulin and sulfonylureas to control blood glucose levels [1,2]. Medications that cause blood glucose levels to fall sharply or repeatedly can lead to hypoglycemic shock. In these cases, the first treatment for patients who present at the hospital in a hypoglycemic state of shock is to rapidly raise blood glucose levels, which is essential for resuscitating the patient and impossible to avoid. Clinically, patients display decreased cognitive abilities over time following such episodes [3], and our previous paper revealed that this condition causes an increase in neuronal cell death [4]. Therefore, this study is important to identify means to minimize neuronal cell death caused by hypoglycemia and glucose reperfusion, which is performed as an essential step in treating hypoglycemia.

Therefore, type 1 and type 2 diabetic patients are at an increased risk of experiencing hypoglycemia. Hypoglycemia is classified into three categories depending on the level of blood glucose: mild, moderate, and severe. Mild hypoglycemia occurs when the concentration of blood glucose falls below 70 mg/dL, leading to symptoms such as headache, sweating, and irritation. Moderate hypoglycemia (below 55 mg/dL) is more severe; thus, people need to regulate this condition carefully. The most serious form of hypoglycemia occurs when blood glucose levels fall below 35 mg/dL. Severe hypoglycemia can lead to seizure, loss of consciousness, and death in the most extreme cases. Previous studies demonstrated that some degree of the observed neuronal death is caused by hypoglycemia itself, but glucose reperfusion to recover the patient from critically low glucose levels acts to drive secondary injury, thereby inducing a second, more severe wave of neuronal death [5,6]. This process is called "glucose-reperfusion injury" after hypoglycemia by our laboratory [4,7]. This injury promotes an imbalance in several cellular programs that can cause neuronal cell death, including the production of reactive oxygen species (ROS), destruction of the blood–brain barrier (BBB), microglial activation associated with inflammation [8], and excessive zinc release [9].

The enzyme pyruvate dehydrogenase (PDH) has three main components: E1, decarboxylates pyruvate and acetylates lipoic acid; E2, dihydrolipoamide acetyltransferase, which uses covalently bound lipoic acid; and lipoic acid is reoxidized by E3, dihydrolipoyl dehydrogenase. In addition, there are other subunits, the E3 binding protein and two complex-controlling enzymes: PDH kinases (PDKs), which inactivate PDH, and PDH phosphatase, which reactivates the PDH. PDH is a key enzyme that catalyzes the oxidative decarboxylation of pyruvate to form acetyl-coenzyme A (acetyl-CoA) under normal conditions. PDH controls the influx of pyruvate into the mitochondria to initiate oxidative metabolism and is an important regulator of the citric acid cycle [10,11]. PDH dysfunction or deficiency most often arise due to mutations or inactivation by PDKs via E1, which causes malfunction of the citric acid cycle due to PDH inactivation and leads to cell death [12]. Previous studies reported that starvation and diabetes lead to enhanced PDK activity, leading to decreased activity of PDH [13–18]. This decreased PDH activity results from increased PDK expression. Starvation increases the level of PDK2 expression in liver and kidney [19].

PDKs have four isoforms: PDK1, PDK2, PDK3, and PDK4. PDK1 is expressed in the heart, pancreatic islet cells, and in muscles [20–22]. PDK3 is only been found in the testis and kidneys in small quantities [23]. PDK4 expression was observed in the heart, skeletal muscles, liver, and brain [19,22,24]. PDK2 is the most abundant isoenzyme in the rat brain [23], with PDK4 hardly being expressed under basal physiological conditions. PDKs phosphorylate the E1 subunit, thus inactivating PDH [25].

In general, previous studies showed that PDK inhibits PDH via phosphorylating PDH after brain injuries, such as ischemia or epilepsy, thereby restricting the pyruvate oxidation (PO) pathway available to brain cells. As a result, under this pathological condition, the citric acid cycle cannot proceed and the production of ATP decreases, leading to cell death [26,27].

Sodium dichloroacetate (DCA) has been studied for a long time, especially in cancer research. DCA, a known activator of PDH and inhibitor of PDK, is a mitochondria-targeting small molecule that can penetrate most tissues even after oral administration [28]. It is responsible for maintaining PDH in the dephosphorylated active form and improving the oxidation of pyruvate via inhibition of PDK [29]. DCA has been shown to instigate inhibition of fatty acid oxidation, which eventually can lead to an increase in acetyl-CoA concentration [30]. DCA stimulates glucose and lactate oxidation, thereby improving recovery of injury after ischemia [31–33]. Although DCA has toxic side effects in high doses, it has highly beneficial effects on outcomes for many diseases such as ischemia and cardiac arrest [34,35].

In our laboratory, we have suggested a number of possible methods for aiding in the prevention of hippocampal neuron death after hypoglycemia [4,8,9,36–39]. In our previous studies, we revealed that administration of pyruvate reduced severe hypoglycemia-induced neuronal cell death and cognitive impairment [37]. Therefore, we questioned whether supplementation of DCA (100 mg/kg, i.v., two days) could improve the oxidation of pyruvate and reduce severe hypoglycemia-induced neuronal cell death.

We found that DCA treatment inhibited PDK and significantly reduced oxidative stress, microglial activation, BBB disruption, and thus hippocampal neuronal death after severe hypoglycemia via enhancing PDH activation.

2. Materials and Methods

2.1. Ethics Statement

This study was conducted in strict accordance with the recommendation of the Institutional Animal Studies Care and Use Committee of the Hallym University in Chuncheon, Korea (Protocol # Hallym-2017-3). Animal sacrifice was conducted using isoflurane anesthesia and all attempts were made to minimize pain or distress.

2.2. Experimental Animals

We used adult male Sprague-Dawley rats (8 weeks old, 250–350 g, DBL Co., Eumseong, Korea). We accommodated the animals in a continuous temperature- and humidity-controlled environment (22 ± 2 °C, 55 ± 5% humidity, and a 12-h light:12-h dark cycle), and fed them with Purina diet (Purina, Gyeonggi, Korea) and water, both provided ad libitum. This study was written in accordance with the Animal Research: Reporting in Vivo Experiments (ARRIVE) guidelines.

2.3. Animal Surgery and Severe Hypoglycemia Induction

We induced hypoglycemia (HG) using human insulin [5,36]. Before inducing hypoglycemia, rats were fasted for 15–16 h. The next day, we performed intraperitoneal injection of 10 U/kg regular insulin (Novolin-R, Novo Nordisk, Bagsværd, Denmark). We conducted hypoglycemia surgeries under controlled ventilation with a small rodent respirator (Harvard Apparatus, South Natick, MA, USA). We inserted a catheter into the femoral artery to continuously monitor the arterial blood pressure and into the femoral vein for glucose infusion after hypoglycemia. To monitor electroencephalogram (EEG) signals, we pierced a small hole in the skull bilaterally and then inserted a reference needle in the neck muscle. We measured the blood pressure and EEG using the BIOPAC System (BIOPAC System Inc., Santa Barbara, CA, USA) in succession. We maintained the core temperature of animals at 36.5–37.5 °C and measured blood glucose levels at 30-min intervals to monitor induction of hypoglycemia.

When insulin reduces blood glucose levels to a level low enough to induce hypoglycemia, an isoelectric state is observed. Arterial blood pressure was sustained between 160 and 200 mmHg during the entire EEG isoelectric period. The severity of hypoglycemia-induced neuronal cell death is strongly related to the duration of the isoelectric (iso-EEG) period. We abruptly ended the hypoglycemic state at 30 min from initiation of iso-EEG [5,36] by suppling 25% glucose solution intravenously for 2 h (2.5 mL/h, i.v.) to recover normal blood glucose levels.

2.4. Injection of DCA

To ascertain the effect of DCA on hypoglycemia-induced neuronal death, the experimental group was divided into 4 groups: Sham (Vehicle, DCA) and Hypoglycemia (Vehicle, DCA). The control group was injected with 0.9% normal saline. Following hypoglycemia, animals were treated with DCA (100 mg/kg, i.v.) once a day for 2 days.

2.5. Brain Sample Preparation

To estimate the neuroprotective effects of DCA, we sacrificed animals 1 week after injury. Animals were deeply anesthetized with urethane injection (1.5 g/kg, i.p.). Brains were transcardially perfused with 500–600 mL of 0.9% saline and this was followed by 600 mL of 4% formaldehyde (FA). After perfusion, we removed the brain and then proceeded to post-fixation in the same fixative solution for roughly 1 h. After that, brains were immersed for cryoprotection in 30% sucrose for 2–3 days until the samples sank to the bottom. After cryoprotection, brain samples were frozen using freezing medium and were cut on a cryostat into 30-µm thicknesses and then kept in storage solution.

2.6. Detection of PDH and PDK2

To confirm PDH and PDK2 levels, we performed PDH and PDK2 staining with primary antibodies for each. Immunohistochemistry with PDH and PDK2 antibodies (Abcam, Cambridge, UK) was performed. Brain tissues were incubated in monoclonal rabbit antibody to rat PDH (diluted 1:100, ab168379) and a monoclonal rabbit antibody to rat PDK2 (diluted 1:100, ab68164) overnight in a 4 °C incubator. After washing, the sections were immersed in secondary antibody (PDH: Alexa Fluor 594-conjugated donkey anti-rabbit IgG secondary antibody, PDK2: Alexa Fluor 488-conjugated donkey anti-rabbit IgG secondary antibody, respectively, both diluted 1:250; Molecular Probes, Invitrogen, Carlsbad, CA, USA) for 2 h at room temperature (RT). The brain tissues were placed on gelatin-coated slides for observation under a microscope. To check the intensity of fluorescence of PDH and PDK2, we used ImageJ (version 1.47c; NIH, Bethesda, MD, USA) and the following steps were executed: select 100 cells in one brain tissue and then click the menu option Analyze → Measurement. (magnification = 80×).

2.7. Detection of Neuronal Death

To investigate neuronal death, brain samples were cut into 30 µm thicknesses on gelatin-coated slides for staining (Fisher Scientific, Pittsburgh, PA, USA). Fluoro-Jade B (FJB) staining was performed as descried by Hopkins and Schmued [40]. First, the slides were immersed in a basic alcohol solution (100→70%) and then washed with distilled water. After that, the slides were submerged in 0.06% potassium permanganate for 15 min. Secondly, the slides were dipped in 0.001% Fluoro-Jade B (Histo-Chem Inc., Jefferson AR, USA) for 30 min and washed 3 times for 10 min each in distilled water. After drying, we mounted a cover glass on each slide with a mixture of distyrene, a plasticizer, and xylene (DPX) solution and then observed the signals with a fluorescence microscope using blue (450–490 nm) excitation light. To quantify the result, we selected five coronal brain sections that were gathered from each animal starting 4.0 mm posterior to Bregma and collecting 5 sections at 75 µm intervals. A blind researcher counted the number of degenerating neurons in the same scope (magnification = 10×) of the hippocampal subiculum (900 × 1200 µm), CA1 (900 × 400 µm), and dentate gyrus (900 × 1200 µm) from both hemispheres. The total average number of degenerating neurons from each region was used for statistical analysis.

2.8. Detection of Live Neurons

To determine the number of live neurons present, we performed NeuN staining with a monoclonal anti-NeuN, clone A60 antibody (diluted 1:500, EMD Millipore, Billerica, MA, USA). We used it as the primary antibody in PBS with 30% Triton X-100 overnight in a 4 °C incubator. After washing three times for 10 min with PBS, and then incubating in anti-mouse IgG secondary antibody (diluted 1:250, Vector Laboraorise, Burlingame, CA, USA) for 2 h at RT, then, the samples were washed again. Next, the brain samples were put into the ABC solution (Burlingame, vector, CA, USA) for 2 h at RT on the shaker. After that, the samples were washed repeatedly three time for 10 min. To activate immune responses, we put samples in 0.01 M PBS buffer (100 mL) with 3,30-diaminobenzidine (0.06% DAB agar, Sigma-Aldrich Co., St. Louis, MO, USA) and 30% H_2O_2 (50 µL) for 1 min. After mounting the sample on the slides, we then used an Axioscope microscope to analyze the immunoreaction. A blinded experimenter counted the number of live neurons in a constant area (magnification = 10×) of the hippocampal subiculum (900 × 1200 µm), CA1 (900 × 400 µm), and dentate gyrus (900 × 1200 µm) from both hemispheres. The total average number of live neurons from each region was used for statistical analysis.

2.9. Detection of Oxidative Injury

To estimate oxidative injury after hypoglycemia, we conducted immunofluorescence staining with 4-hydroxy-2-nonenal (4HNE) antibodies (diluted 1:500, Alpha Diagnostic Intl. Inc., San Antonio, TX, USA) as described previously [4]. Brain sections were incubated in a mixture of polyclonal rabbit anti-HNE anti-serum and phosphate buffered saline (PBS) containing 0.3% TritonX-100 overnight in a 4 °C incubator. After washing three times for 10 min each with PBS, samples were also immersed in a mixture of Alexa Fluor 594-conjugated goat-anti rabbit IgG secondary antibody (diluted 1:250, Invitrogen, Grand Island, NY, USA) for two hours at room temperature. Finally, the sections were placed on gelatin-coated slides. To measure the oxidative stress signals, we used ImageJ using the following order of commands: click the menu option Image → Adjust → Color threshold and dark background. Then, we modulated brightness according to the intensity of oxidative stress. The image was converted to 8-bit images (magnification = 10×). The fluorescence intensity was expressed as mean gray value.

2.10. Detection of Microglia and Astrocyte Activation

To semi-quantitatively measure inflammation after injury, we performed CD11b and GFAP staining, a well-described indicator of the inflammatory response. Immunohistochemical staining was conducted with a mouse antibody to rat CD11b (diluted 1:500; AbD Serotec, Raleigh, NC, USA) and of goat antibody to rat GFAP (diluted 1:1000; Abcam, Cambridge, UK) in PBS containing 0.3% TritonX-100 overnight in a 4 °C incubator. After rinsing, the sections were immersed in Alexa Fluor 488-conjugated donkey anti-mouse IgG secondary antibody and Alexa Fluor 594-conjugated donkey anti-goat IgG secondary antibody (both diluted 1:250; Molecular Probes, Invitrogen) for two hours at RT. A randomly blinded experimenter then measured the intensity of astrocytes in the CA1 region. In the case of microglia, we used five sections from each animal to estimate scoring within the same CA1 region (magnification = 20×). To quantify microglial activation, a randomly blinded observer performed the measurements. Microglial activation criteria based on the number and intensity of CD11b positive cells and on their morphology are as follows [41,42]. The scores for each criterion are as follows: for *CD11b-positive cells number*, a score of 0 denotes no cells with continuously stained processes are present, score 1 denotes 1–9 cells with continuous processes per 100 μm^2, score of 2 denotes 10–20 cells with continuous processes per 100 μm^2, and score of 3 denotes >20 cells with continuous processes per 100 μm^2; for *Intensity*, a score of 0 denotes no expression, 1 denotes weak expression, 2 denotes average expression, and a score of 3 denotes intense expression. When ImageJ is used, based on the max value 225, a score of 1 has intensity to mean value 1–50, a score of 2 has intensity to 51–100 and the last score of 3 has intensity to 100–max value 225.; and for *Morphology*, a score of 0 denotes 0% have activated morphology (amoeboid morphology with enlarged soma and thickened processes), 1 denotes 1–45% of microglia have the activated morphology, 2 denotes 45–90% of microglia, and a score of 3 denotes >90% of microglia have the activated morphology. Therefore, the total score includes the combination of three individual scores (CD11b-immunoreactive cell number, morphology and intensity), ranging from 0 to 9 (magnification = 20×).

2.11. Detection of BBB Disruption and Neutrophils

To check the degree of BBB disruption, we evaluated leakage of endogenous serum IgG after hypoglycemia [43]. We conducted IgG staining with anti-rat IgG, which detects serum IgG released when the BBB is disrupted. Brain sections were incubated in a mixture of anti-rat IgG serum (diluted 1:250, Burlingame, Vector, CA, USA) in PBS containing 0.3% TritonX-100 on a shaking shelf for 2 h at RT. After rinsing three times for 10 min each with PBS, we treated ABC solution for two hours at RT on a shaker. The ABC immunoperoxidase was used to reveal IgG-like immunoreactivity [44]. After that, the sections were exposed to 3,3′-diaminobenzidine (DAB ager, Sigma-Aldrich Co., St. Louis, MO, USA) in 0.1 M PBS buffer to trigger immune responses. After mounting, we observed the immune responses using an Axioscope microscope (Carl Zeiss, Munich, Germany) and quantified extravasation of endogenous serum IgG in the whole brain using the Image J program. The procedure for measuring IgG is as follows: Click the menu option Image→Type→8 bits and then, edit→invert. To measure the area, the menu option Analyze→Measure was selected. Mean gray values (magnification = 4×) were used. In addition, to measure the degree of BBB disruption, we evaluated any influx of neutrophils after hypoglycemia. We conducted myeloperoxidase (MPO) staining with rabbit anti-MPO (diluted 1:100, Invitrogen, Grand Island, NY, USA). The brain sections were soaked in the primary antibody solution with PBS containing 0.3% TritonX-100 overnight in a 4 °C incubator. After washing, samples were immersed in a mixture of Alexa Fluor 594-conjugated goat-anti rabbit IgG secondary antibody (diluted 1:250, Invitrogen, Grand Island, NY, USA) for two hours at room temperature. We put the sample on the slides and then, the blinded tester counted the number of neutrophils in the hippocampus from both hemispheres under fluorescent microscope. The total average number of neutrophils from the hippocampus region was used for statistical analysis.

2.12. Data Analysis

Data are displayed as the mean ± S.E.M. Statistical significance between experimental groups was measured by analysis of variance (ANOVA) in accordance with the Bonferroni post-hoc test. Differences were considered statistically significant at $p < 0.05$.

3. Results

3.1. DCA Inhibits PDK2 after Hypoglycemia

In previous studies, PDKs were shown to be key regulators in glucose metabolism and to inhibit PDH by phosphorylating the enzyme during brain injury [26,45]. In the present study, we hypothesized that PDKs activation blocks entry of pyruvate into the citrate acid cycle in mitochondria, leading to reduction of ATP formation, and thus, causes neuronal cell death in hypoglycemia. As a result of PDK2 immunostaining, we found that the level of PDK2 significantly increased in the hypoglycemia-induced group compared to the sham group. However, DCA, the inhibitor of PDK2, reduced the level of PDK2, and consequently reduced neuronal cell death (Figure 1A,C).

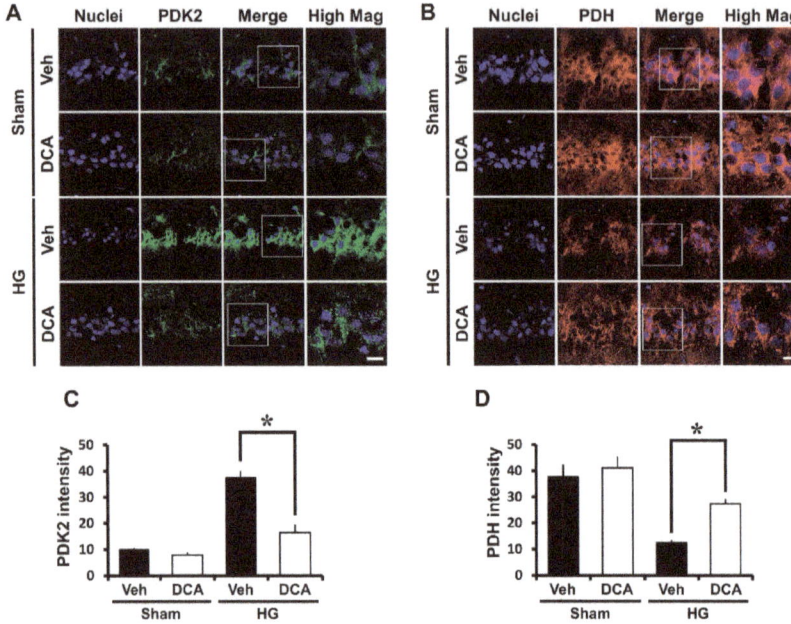

Figure 1. Effects of sodium dichloroacetate (DCA) on hypoglycemia-induced pyruvate dehydrogenase kinase 2 (PDK2) activation and pyruvate dehydrogenase (PDH) reduction. Fluorescent images show the effect of DCA treatment on PDK2 level after hypoglycemia. (**A**) Difference in PDK2 intensity between vehicle- and DCA-treated groups in the vulnerable CA1 after hypoglycemia. Scale bar = 10 μm. (**B**) Difference in PDH intensity between vehicle- and DCA-treated groups in the vulnerable CA1 after hypoglycemia. In normal state, neuronal cells maintain an adequate amount of active PDH, while hypoglycemia causes a significant reduction of active PDH. However, DCA administration recovers PDH activity. Scale bar = 10 μm. Bar graph shows quantification of (**C**) PDK2 or (**D**) PDH intensity in CA1 region. Data are mean ± S.E.M., n = 3 from each group. * Significantly different from vehicle treated group, $p < 0.05$.

3.2. DCA Increases PDH after Hypoglycemia

To continually maintain life, cells must use glucose as a fuel. This process is mainly controlled by the enzyme PDH, which regulates the entry of glycolytic products into the citric acid cycle by converting pyruvate into acetyl-CoA in the mitochondria [46]. PDH is usually suppressed by PDH-induced phosphorylation [47]. According to previous studies, pyruvate dehydrogenase activity is reduced in neurodegenerative brain diseases such as Huntington and Alzheimer's [48,49]. Based on these previous results, we conducted PDH staining to investigate if active PDH is similarly inhibited after hypoglycemia and to determine if this results in the loss of neuronal cells. We discovered that the level of PDH significantly decreased in the hippocampal CA1 region in the hypoglycemia-induced group compared with the sham group. In the present study we found that the administration of DCA increased the level of PDH and reduced hypoglycemia-induced neuronal death (Figure 1B,D).

3.3. DCA Decreases Neuronal Death after Hypoglycemia

Severe neuronal death is caused by hypoglycemia and subsequent glucose reperfusion when estimated at seven days after injury [4]. After hypoglycemia, we performed NeuN staining in order to confirm the number of surviving neurons, and also Fluoro-Jade B (FJB) staining in order to detect degenerating neurons in the hippocampal subiculum (sub), CA1 and dentate gyrus (DG). First, Fluoro-Jade B staining, a selective marker of degenerating neurons, exposed broad hippocampal neuronal cell death in the subiculum (sub), CA1, and dentate gyrus (DG) after insult. Rats treated with DCA (100 mg/kg, i.v., two days) displayed a significant reduction in hippocampal neuronal death after hypoglycemia (Figure 2A). As demonstrated in Figure 2B, rats given DCA showed reduced FJB (+) neurons in the subiculum, CA1, and DG by 53%, 76%, and 76%, respectively, compared with rats given only saline plus glucose. Moreover, sham-operated groups showed live neurons in the hippocampal subiculum, CA1 and dentate gyrus via NeuN staining. There were no significant differences in the NeuN (+) cell numbers between vehicle- and DCA- treated group. Compared to the sham group, the number of surviving neurons was significantly decreased at 1 week after hypoglycemia. However, the number of surviving neurons in the DCA-treated group was significantly higher than in the vehicle-treated group (Figure 2C). As shown in Figure 2D, rats given DCA showed increased NeuN (+) neurons in the subiculum, CA1, and DG by 35%, 51%, and 35%, respectively, compared with rats given only saline plus glucose.

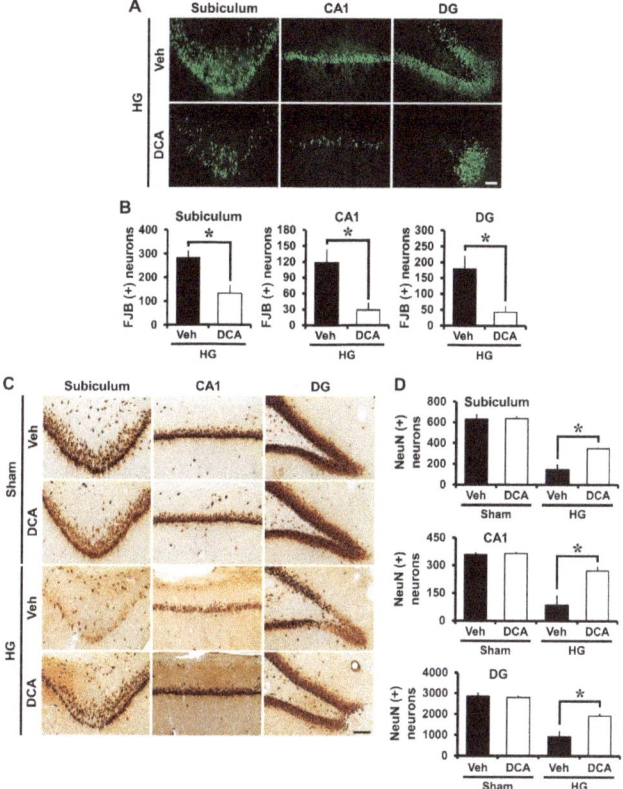

Figure 2. Effects of DCA on hypoglycemia-induced neuronal death. Hypoglycemia resulted in neuronal death in the subiculum (sub), CA1, and dentate gyrus (DG) of hippocampus one week after hypoglycemia. (**A**) Fluoro-Jade B (FJB) positive neuronal cells are observed in the CA1, subiculum, and DG one week after hypoglycemia. Scale bar = 50 μm. (**B**) The number of FJB (+) cells were significantly lower in the DCA-treated group than that in the control group after insult. Data are mean ± S.E.M., n = 8 from each hypoglycemia group. (**C**) NeuN (+) cells show live neurons in the hippocampal subiculum, CA1 and DG. Scale bar = 100 μm. (**D**) The number of NeuN (+) cells were considerably more increased in the DCA-treated group than in the control group after insult. Data are mean ± S.E.M., n = 3 for each sham group and hypoglycemia group. * Significantly different from vehicle treated group, $p < 0.05$.

3.4. DCA Reduces Hypoglycemia-Induced Oxidative Injury

Mitochondria are the main sources of ROS production in many disorders such as ischemia, traumatic brain injury, or seizure [50]. Mitochondria taken from brain during hypoglycemia exhibit increased capacity to produce ROS [51]. Our previous study suggested that ROS can be produced by NADPH oxidase activation after hypoglycemia, so the production of ROS causes oxidative stress-induced neuronal cell death in the hippocampus [4]. We conducted 4-hydroxynonenal (4HNE) staining to estimate the degree of oxidative damage after hypoglycemia. Rat brains were immunohistochemically stained with a 4HNE antibody one week after injury to reveal whether oxidative stress had occurred in the hippocampal neurons and whether DCA can reduce this negative effect on neurons. In the sham-operated group, both saline controls and DCA-treated rats demonstrated no difference in the fluorescence intensity of the 4HNE staining in the subiculum, CA1, and DG. In the hypoglycemia-operated group, 4HNE fluorescence intensity increased in the hippocampus region of the saline only group and but decreased in the DCA-treated group after hypoglycemia (Figure 3A). As demonstrated in Figure 3B, group treated with DCA and then 25% glucose showed an approximately 53% reduction in the intensity of 4HNE in the subiculum, 60% in the CA1, and 56% in the DG compared with the group provided only glucose (Figure 3B). Therefore, this result indicates that DCA can reduce oxidative injury, and thus spare hippocampal neurons from hypoglycemic insult.

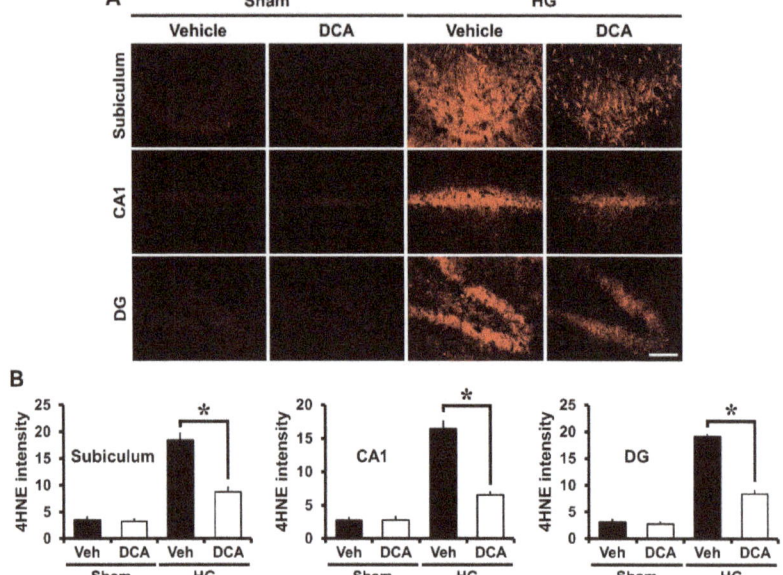

Figure 3. Administration of DCA decreases oxidative injury after hypoglycemia. Neuronal oxidative injury was determined by 4-hydroxy-2-nonenal (4HNE) (red color) staining in the hippocampal regions seven days after hypoglycemia. (**A**) Sham-operated groups rarely displayed the 4HNE signal in the hippocampus. DCA decreased the intensity of 4HNE fluorescence in the hippocampus compared with the saline-treated group after hypoglycemia. Scale bar = 100 μm. (**B**) 4HNE fluorescence intensity in the hippocampus. The fluorescence intensity indicates a significant gap between saline- and DCA-treated groups. Data are mean ± S.E.M., n = 5 for each sham group. n = 8 for each hypoglycemia group. * Significantly different from vehicle treated group, $p < 0.05$.

3.5. DCA Reduces Hypoglycemia-Induced Microglia and Astrocyte Activation

Another study showed that hypoglycemia induces microglia and astrocyte activation in the cerebral cortex and the hippocampus [52]. Severe hypoglycemia was induced in rats and then brains were harvested one week after insult. We therefore evaluated the degree of microglia and astrocyte activation between four groups: Sham (Vehicle, DCA) and Hypoglycemia (Vehicle, DCA). As a result of the staining, sham-operated groups showed resting microglia and small astrocytes. Also, activated astrocytes have the potential to be harmful because they can express NOS and produce neurotoxic NO [53,54]. Compared with the sham-operated groups, microglia and astrocyte activation in the CA1 increased by approximately 66% and 60%, respectively, in the hypoglycemia-operated group. However, after insult, microglia and astrocyte activation decreased around 56% and 46% in the DCA-treated group compared to the saline-treated group. Therefore, administration of DCA can decrease microglia and astrocyte activation associated with inflammation (Figure 4A–D).

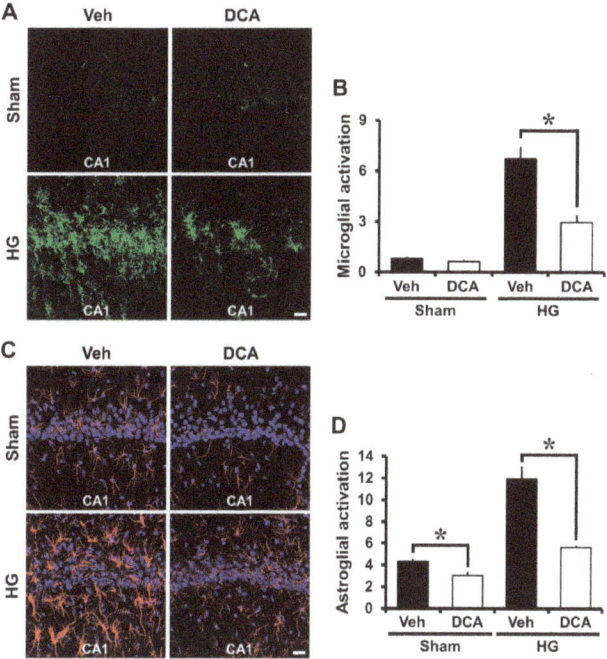

Figure 4. Administration of DCA decreases microglia and astrocyte activation after hypoglycemia. To detect microglia activation, we conducted CD11b staining. Hypoglycemia-induced microglia activation triggers an immune response. CA1 is vulnerable to damage by activated microglia. (**A**) The green fluorescence (CD11b staining) shows activated microglia in the hippocampal CA1 area. Sham-operated group shows almost no microglial activation. However, after hypoglycemia, microglia cell number, intensity, and morphology were greatly enhanced in the vehicle-treated group compared to the DCA-treated group. Scale bar = 20 µm. Data are mean ± S.E.M., n = 5 for each sham group, n = 8 for each hypoglycemia group. (**B**) The grade of microglia activation in the CA1. (**C**) The red fluorescence (GFAP staining) shows activated astrocyte in the hippocampal CA1 area. The sham-operated group shows almost no astrocyte activation. However, after insult, DCA administration prevented astrocyte activation in the CA1. Scale bar = 20 µm. (**D**) The graph represents the intensity of activated astrocytes in the CA1 region. Data are mean ± S.E.M., n = 3 for each sham group and hypoglycemia group. * Significantly different from vehicle treated group, $p < 0.05$.

3.6. DCA Prevents Hypoglycemia-Induced Blood-Brain Barrier (BBB) Disruption

Many other studies reported that blood-brain barrier (BBB) disruption occurs under brain injury conditions such as ischemia, traumatic brain injury, and seizure [55–57]. In severe hypoglycemia, BBB is destroyed as early critical events, because glucose deprivation destroys endothelial cells that make up BBB [58–60]. To determine disruption of the BBB, we conducted IgG staining by detecting the degree of extravasation of serum immunoglobulin G (IgG) with a previously described method [43] and myeloperoxidase (MPO) staining to look for an influx of neutrophils after hypoglycemia. Firstly, IgG produced coronas with a concentration gradient around the blood vessels in the hippocampus area, and IgG staining was observed in broad areas in the brain due to hypoglycemia. Generally, in the sham-operated group, little leakage of IgG occurred, but the group experiencing hypoglycemic status experienced IgG leakage from damaged vessels. Figure 5 shows that a significant difference was found in the concentration gradient of IgG leakage between the sham and hypoglycemia-induced groups. IgG leakage via BBB disruption was apparent in the vehicle-treated group following hypoglycemia. However, administration of DCA significantly decreased hypoglycemia-induced IgG leakage through BBB disruption in the hippocampus (Figure 5A,B). In additionally, we conducted MPO staining to check BBB permeability increased by the destruction of BBB after hypoglycemia. The increase of BBB permeability causes an influx of neutrophils, and neutrophils are identified through MPO staining. As a result of the MPO staining, sham-operated groups did not show MPO (+) cells. After hypoglycemia, compared with the sham-operated groups, MPO (+) cells were found to be significantly increased, but DCA administration reduced the infiltration of neutrophils in the hippocampus (Figure 5C,D).

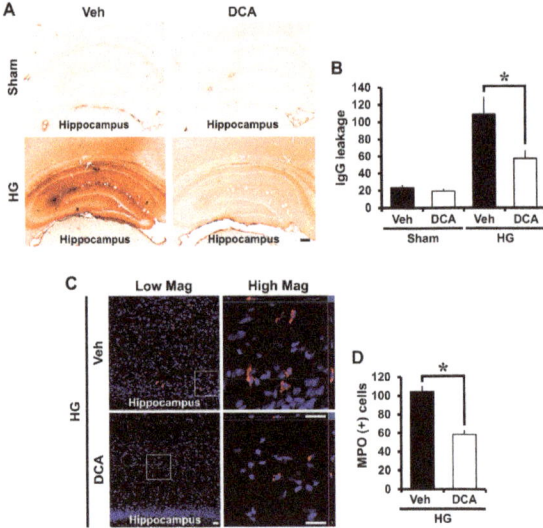

Figure 5. Administration of DCA decreases blood-brain barrier (BBB) breakdown and an influx of neutrophils after hypoglycemia. (**A**) Whereas sham-operated group had little leakage of IgG, the hypoglycemia group had a large quantity of IgG leakage when the BBB broke down. However, the DCA–treated group had significantly reduced IgG leakage. Scale bar = 200 μm (4×). (**B**) The quantification of IgG leakage in the whole hippocampus. Data are mean ± S.E.M., n = 5 for each sham group, n = 8 for each hypoglycemia group. Data are mean ± S.E.M., n = 5 for each sham group, n = 8 for each hypoglycemia group. (**C**) Representative immunofluorescence images show expression of the neutrophil marker MPO in the cortex and hippocampus. DCA prevent Scale bar = 20 μm. (**D**) The bar graph indicates the number of MPO (+) cells in the cortex and hippocampus. Data are mean ± S.E.M., n = 3 for each sham group and hypoglycemia group. * Significantly different from vehicle treated group, $p < 0.05$.

4. Discussion

Previous studies showed that severe hypoglycemia can cause seizure, unconsciousness, and neuronal death as extreme end-points [8,38,39]. The mechanisms of hypoglycemia-induced neuronal cell death are still unclear. Our previous study demonstrated that neuronal cell death induced by hypoglycemia is caused not only by the low glucose level itself but also by glucose reperfusion [37]. Hypoglycemia causes excessive vesicular zinc release, which leads to NADPH oxidase activation and causes neurotoxicity [4,9]. Zinc influx into neurons after hypoglycemia can lead to mitochondrial dysfunction, resulting in reduced ATP levels in the brain [61]. Therefore, we investigated whether treatment with DCA, an activator of ATP formation, has neuroprotective effects in the hippocampus after severe hypoglycemia.

The ATP required for neurological function in the brain is predominantly generated by glucose oxidation (GO) and pyruvate oxidation (PO) in mitochondria [62] and it is closely related to hypoglycemic state. Under physiological conditions, formation of pyruvate increase rates of glycolysis and enhances glucose oxidation by way of activation of PDH, which converts pyruvate into Acetyl-CoA. However, under pathophysiological conditions such as hypoglycemia (HG) and ischemia-reperfusion (IR), it decreases the rates of glucose oxidation due to mitochondrial dysfunction [62,63]. Depressed glucose oxidation can lead to neuronal cell death [49,64].

Dysfunction of mitochondrial metabolism is central to the pathological results following brain injury, such as traumatic brain injury or ischemia [65,66]. Previous studies reported that PDH is important in altered brain energy metabolism in diverse brain injuries [67–69]. Traumatic brain injury is reported to enhance the expression of PDK and phosphorylate PDH, leading to inhibition of PDH-regulated glucose metabolism [45]. Bowker-Kinley et al. mentioned that when they looked at levels of PDK mRNA, PDK1 (heart), PDK3 (testis), PDK4 (skeletal muscle and heart) was found in certain tissues, whereas PDK2 was found in all tissues. Also, they indicated that in the brain, for example, PDK activity corresponds primarily to the isoenzyme PDK2. In addition, they showed that DCA, a structural analog of pyruvate, attaches to the pyruvate-binding site, resulting in inhibition of PDKs with the order of inhibition being PDK2 > PDK1~PDK4 >> PDK3 [23]. In the present study, we confirmed that hypoglycemic insult increased the level of PDK2 in the hippocampus and thus reduced PDH, causing inhibition of glucose metabolism. However, administration of DCA decreased PDK2 levels in the hippocampus.

After several brain insults, mitochondrial damage induces excessive PDK activation, which restricts ATP formation and results in more severe neuronal death [26,45]. In the case of severe hypoglycemic animal models, neuronal death occurs, and given the result, mitochondrial dysfunction occurs in both the hypoglycemic state itself and also during the hyperglycemic state when glucose is reperfused [51,70–72]. DCA is known to be neurotoxic when high doses, above 500 mg/kg, are used, or if 300 mg/kg is administered for more than 10 weeks [73,74]. However, many previous animal studies have confirmed the beneficial effects of administering DCA at dose of 50 to 200 mg/kg [75–79], and our previous study also confirmed that treatment with a dose of 100 mg/kg after ischemia reduced neuronal death [26]. According to the paper by Stacpoole, it was noted that DCA was rapidly absorbed following treatment, crosses the blood-brain barrier and activates PDH within a few minutes [80].

In the present study, we found that DCA, a PDK inhibitor, significantly reduces the number of degenerating neurons after hypoglycemia. FJB staining demonstrated a decline in the number of degenerating neurons in the hippocampus in the DCA-treated group compared to the vehicle-treated group after hypoglycemia. This trend correlated with the NeuN staining, which indicated an increase of surviving neurons in the DCA group. This result suggests that DCA increases PDH levels by inhibiting PDK2, which may result in increased ATP synthesis, reducing neuronal cell death in the subiculum, CA1 and dentate gyrus of hippocampus compared with the vehicle-treated group, after hypoglycemia (Figure 6).

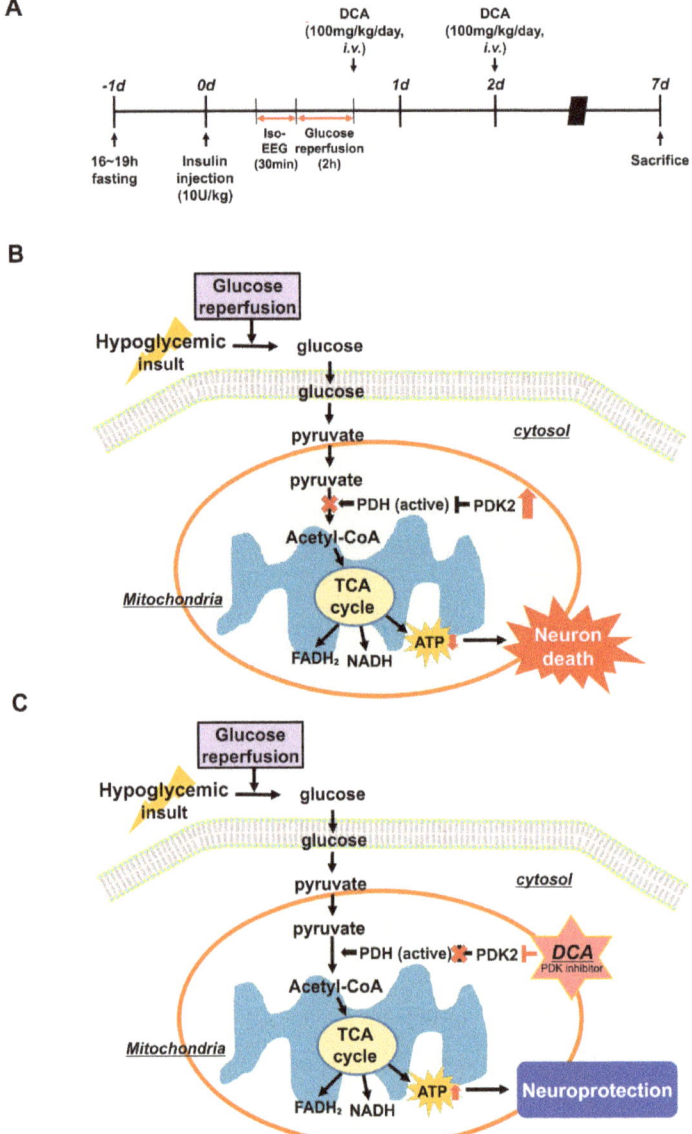

Figure 6. Possible association of PDK2, PDH, DCA, and neuronal death under hypoglycemic conditions. This schematic illustration shows the effects of DCA on the process of hypoglycemia-induced hippocampal neuronal death. (**A**) Experimental timeline. (**B**) Neuronal cell death mechanism caused by hypoglycemia: (1) After hypoglycemia, mitochondria disruption occurs and then PDK2 increase abnormally (2) An abnormally increased PDK2 inhibits the activity of PDH by phosphating PDH (3) The conversion from pyruvate to acetyl-CoA is unsuccessful due to the inhibition of PDH (4) The rate of synthesis of ATP through the TCA cycle significantly reduces. When these conditions dominate, neuronal death is more likely to occur. (**C**) Effects of DCA on hypoglycemia-induced neuronal cell death: administration of DCA can inhibit PDK2 and thus prevent hippocampal neuronal death after hypoglycemia.

D'Alessandro et al. stated that mitochondrial impairment induced by the reduction of the glucose-derived pyruvate results in decreased glutathione synthesis [39,81]. Glutathione plays an important role in the cells, which reduces the oxidative stress by acting as an antioxidant. This synthesis of glutathione requires glycine, glutamate and cysteine, and consumes ATP [82]. Mitochondrial dysfunction after hypoglycemic insult contributes to oxidative stress by activating NADPH oxidase, leading to ROS formation, which is heavily associated with neurodegenerative diseases [4,9,83]. Therefore, we conducted 4HNE staining to confirm whether DCA decreases oxidative stress in the hippocampus. We found that DCA administration successfully reduced oxidative injury in the hippocampus compared to the vehicle-treated group after hypoglycemia. Therefore, we assumed that the administration of DCA increases the level of ATP, and this has resulted in the reduction of the oxidative stress due to the efficient supply of ATP for glutathione formation.

Neural or immune cells participating in neuroinflammation experience metabolic changes including a glycolytic metabolic shift. The altered glycolytic metabolism leads to promotion or inhibition of neuroinflammation [84,85]. PDKs have been reported to control functional polarization of macrophages [86]. Macrophage polarization toward the pro-inflammatory M1 phenotype is usually followed by a cellular metabolic change from oxidative phosphorylation to aerobic glycolysis, as well as nitric oxide (NO) production [86]. Likewise, NO produced by brain diseases suppresses enzyme activity in PDH [87]. Jha et al. suggested that PDK2/4 play vital roles in the inflammatory infiltration of immune cells, in the induction of the pro-inflammatory macrophages, and in inhibition of the anti-inflammatory phenotype of peripheral macrophages [88]. Microglia and astrocyte can be activated immediately during brain injury and induce pro-inflammatory molecules such as tumor necrosis factor-α (TNF-α) or NO [89,90]. Therefore, brain inflammation has been considered to be a potential target in treating brain diseases for several years, and various approaches have been implemented to suppress disease-induced brain inflammation [91–93]. The selective vulnerability of CA1 hippocampus is very well studied in rodents and CA1 is known to have the highest susceptibility to damaging conditions [94–96]. We performed CD11b and GFAP staining, which is an inflammatory marker, to confirm the neuroprotective effects of DCA on inflammation induced by microglia and astrocyte activation after hypoglycemia. Thus, we found that DCA reduced microglia and astrocyte activation by inhibiting PDK2 in the hippocampal CA1 region after hypoglycemia.

BBB disruption was assessed on the basis of IgG extravasation [43] and is related to an influx of neutrophils after brain insult [97]. Generally, IgG concentration and an infiltration of neutrophils in the brain is rare because it exists in the blood vessels when undamaged. However, under pathological conditions, IgG leakage and neutrophils influx occur as the BBB is disrupted by brain injuries such as seizure, ischemia, or traumatic brain injury [55,98–100]. Doll et al. reported that mitochondria play an important role in the opening of the BBB [101]. If mitochondria are destroyed by lack of oxygen or glucose, ATP production decreases in the endothelial cells surrounding the blood vessels in the brain, resulting in the disruption of the BBB, which exacerbates brain injury [102]. Mitochondrial dysfunction also causes the collapse of the BBB because it further reduces the rate of ATP synthesis [101,103]. Therefore, we conducted IgG and MPO staining to confirm whether DCA prevents the BBB breakdown by increasing the formation of ATP. Here, we found that DCA decreased IgG leakage in the whole brain and the number of MPO (+) cells in the hippocampus after hypoglycemia. This result demonstrates that DCA has the capability to prevent BBB disruption by enhancing ATP production in brain endothelial cells after hypoglycemia.

In conclusion, we found that DCA treatment can alleviate hippocampal neuronal death by inhibiting PDK activity following hypoglycemia. It is unclear exactly how PDK2 is increased by hypoglycemia/glucose reperfusion. We speculate that a complex signaling pathway may be generated by the hypoglycemic insult inside mitochondria. Therefore, our findings suggest that DCA may be a vital therapeutic tool for preventing neuronal death induced by hypoglycemia.

Author Contributions: A.R.K. researched data and reviewed and edited the manuscript. B.Y.C., K.-H.P. and J.B.P. reviewed and edited the manuscript. S.H.L., D.K.H., J.H.J., B.S.K. and D.H.K. researched the data. S.W.S.

contributed to the discussion and wrote/reviewed and edited the manuscript. S.W.S. is the person who takes full responsibility for the manuscript and its originality. All authors read and approved the final manuscript.

Funding: This research was supported by the Brain Research Program through the National Research Foundation of Korea (NRF), funded by the Ministry of Science, Information and Communication Technology and Future Planning (NRF-2017M3C7A1028937 and 2018R1A4A1020922) to Sang Won Suh.

Conflicts of Interest: The authors declare no conflict of interest.

References

1. Seltzer, H.S. Drug-induced hypoglycemia. A review of 1418 cases. *Endocrinol. Metab. Clin. North. Am.* **1989**, *18*, 163–183. [CrossRef]
2. Tallroth, G.; Lindgren, M.; Stenberg, G.; Rosen, I.; Agardh, C.D. Neurophysiological changes during insulin-induced hypoglycaemia and in the recovery period following glucose infusion in type 1 (insulin-dependent) diabetes mellitus and in normal man. *Diabetologia* **1990**, *33*, 319–323. [CrossRef] [PubMed]
3. Graveling, A.J.; Deary, I.J.; Frier, B.M. Acute hypoglycemia impairs executive cognitive function in adults with and without type 1 diabetes. *Diabetes Care* **2013**, *36*, 3240–3246. [CrossRef]
4. Suh, S.W.; Gum, E.T.; Hamby, A.M.; Chan, P.H.; Swanson, R.A. Hypoglycemic neuronal death is triggered by glucose reperfusion and activation of neuronal NADPH oxidase. *J. Clin. Invest.* **2007**, *117*, 910–918. [CrossRef] [PubMed]
5. Auer, R.N.; Olsson, Y.; Siesjo, B.K. Hypoglycemic brain injury in the rat. Correlation of density of brain damage with the EEG isoelectric time: A quantitative study. *Diabetes* **1984**, *33*, 1090–1098. [CrossRef]
6. Auer, R.N.; Hall, P.; Ingvar, M.; Siesjo, B.K. Hypotension as a complication of hypoglycemia leads to enhanced energy failure but no increase in neuronal necrosis. *Stroke* **1986**, *17*, 442–449. [CrossRef] [PubMed]
7. Suh, S.W.; Shin, B.S.; Ma, H.; Van Hoecke, M.; Brennan, A.M.; Yenari, M.A.; Swanson, R.A. Glucose and NADPH oxidase drive neuronal superoxide formation in stroke. *Ann. Neurol.* **2008**, *64*, 654–663. [CrossRef] [PubMed]
8. Kim, J.H.; Yoo, B.H.; Won, S.J.; Choi, B.Y.; Lee, B.E.; Kim, I.Y.; Kho, A.; Lee, S.H.; Sohn, M.; Suh, S.W. Melatonin Reduces Hypoglycemia-Induced Neuronal Death in Rats. *Neuroendocrinology* **2015**, *102*, 300–310. [CrossRef] [PubMed]
9. Suh, S.W.; Garnier, P.; Aoyama, K.; Chen, Y.; Swanson, R.A. Zinc release contributes to hypoglycemia-induced neuronal death. *Neurobiol. Dis.* **2004**, *16*, 538–545. [CrossRef] [PubMed]
10. Martin, E.; Rosenthal, R.E.; Fiskum, G. Pyruvate dehydrogenase complex: Metabolic link to ischemic brain injury and target of oxidative stress. *J. Neurosci. Res.* **2005**, *79*, 240–247. [CrossRef]
11. Sun, W.; Liu, Q.; Leng, J.; Zheng, Y.; Li, J. The role of Pyruvate Dehydrogenase Complex in cardiovascular diseases. *Life Sci.* **2015**, *121*, 97–103. [CrossRef] [PubMed]
12. Sidhu, S.; Gangasani, A.; Korotchkina, L.G.; Suzuki, G.; Fallavollita, J.A.; Canty, J.M., Jr.; Patel, M.S. Tissue-specific pyruvate dehydrogenase complex deficiency causes cardiac hypertrophy and sudden death of weaned male mice. *Am. J. Physiol. Heart Circ. Physiol.* **2008**, *295*, H946–H952. [CrossRef]
13. Holness, M.J.; Sugden, M.C. Regulation of pyruvate dehydrogenase complex activity by reversible phosphorylation. *Biochem. Soc. Trans.* **2003**, *31*, 1143–1151. [CrossRef]
14. Hutson, N.J.; Randle, P.J. Enhanced activity of pyruvate dehydrogenase kinase in rat heart mitochondria in alloxan-diabetes or starvation. *FEBS Lett.* **1978**, *92*, 73–76. [CrossRef]
15. Jha, M.K.; Lee, I.K.; Suk, K. Metabolic reprogramming by the pyruvate dehydrogenase kinase-lactic acid axis: Linking metabolism and diverse neuropathophysiologies. *Neurosci. Biobehav. Rev.* **2016**, *68*, 1–19. [CrossRef]
16. Holness, M.J.; Kraus, A.; Harris, R.A.; Sugden, M.C. Targeted upregulation of pyruvate dehydrogenase kinase (PDK)-4 in slow-twitch skeletal muscle underlies the stable modification of the regulatory characteristics of PDK induced by high-fat feeding. *Diabetes* **2000**, *49*, 775–781. [CrossRef]
17. Sugden, M.C.; Kraus, A.; Harris, R.A.; Holness, M.J. Fibre-type specific modification of the activity and regulation of skeletal muscle pyruvate dehydrogenase kinase (PDK) by prolonged starvation and refeeding is associated with targeted regulation of PDK isoenzyme 4 expression. *Biochem. J.* **2000**, *346*, 651–657. [CrossRef] [PubMed]

18. Peters, S.J.; Harris, R.A.; Heigenhauser, G.J.; Spriet, L.L. Muscle fiber type comparison of PDH kinase activity and isoform expression in fed and fasted rats. *Am. J. Physiol. Regul. Integr. Comp. Physiol.* **2001**, *280*, R661–R668. [CrossRef]
19. Wu, P.; Blair, P.V.; Sato, J.; Jaskiewicz, J.; Popov, K.M.; Harris, R.A. Starvation increases the amount of pyruvate dehydrogenase kinase in several mammalian tissues. *Arch. Biochem. Biophys.* **2000**, *381*, 1–7. [CrossRef]
20. Di, R.M.; Feng, Q.T.; Chang, Z.; Luan, Q.; Zhang, Y.Y.; Huang, J.; Li, X.L.; Yang, Z.Z. PDK1 plays a critical role in regulating cardiac function in mice and human. *Chin. Med. J.* **2010**, *123*, 2358–2363.
21. Sugden, M.C.; Bulmer, K.; Augustine, D.; Holness, M.J. Selective modification of pyruvate dehydrogenase kinase isoform expression in rat pancreatic islets elicited by starvation and activation of peroxisome proliferator-activated receptor-alpha: Implications for glucose-stimulated insulin secretion. *Diabetes* **2001**, *50*, 2729–2736. [CrossRef] [PubMed]
22. Spriet, L.L.; Tunstall, R.J.; Watt, M.J.; Mehan, K.A.; Hargreaves, M.; Cameron-Smith, D. Pyruvate dehydrogenase activation and kinase expression in human skeletal muscle during fasting. *J. Appl. Physiol. (1985)* **2004**, *96*, 2082–2087. [CrossRef] [PubMed]
23. Bowker-Kinley, M.M.; Davis, W.I.; Wu, P.; Harris, R.A.; Popov, K.M. Evidence for existence of tissue-specific regulation of the mammalian pyruvate dehydrogenase complex. *Biochem. J.* **1998**, *329*, 191–196. [CrossRef] [PubMed]
24. Wu, P.; Sato, J.; Zhao, Y.; Jaskiewicz, J.; Popov, K.M.; Harris, R.A. Starvation and diabetes increase the amount of pyruvate dehydrogenase kinase isoenzyme 4 in rat heart. *Biochem. J.* **1998**, *329*, 197–201. [CrossRef] [PubMed]
25. Jha, M.K.; Jeon, S.; Suk, K. Pyruvate Dehydrogenase Kinases in the Nervous System: Their Principal Functions in Neuronal-glial Metabolic Interaction and Neuro-metabolic Disorders. *Curr. Neuropharmacol.* **2012**, *10*, 393–403. [CrossRef] [PubMed]
26. Hong, D.K.; Kho, A.R.; Choi, B.Y.; Lee, S.H.; Jeong, J.H.; Lee, S.H.; Park, K.H.; Park, J.B.; Suh, S.W. Combined Treatment With Dichloroacetic Acid and Pyruvate Reduces Hippocampal Neuronal Death After Transient Cerebral Ischemia. *Front. Neurol.* **2018**, *9*, 137. [CrossRef] [PubMed]
27. McDonald, T.S.; Borges, K. Impaired hippocampal glucose metabolism during and after flurothyl-induced seizures in mice: Reduced phosphorylation coincides with reduced activity of pyruvate dehydrogenase. *Epilepsia* **2017**, *58*, 1172–1180. [CrossRef]
28. Bonnet, S.; Archer, S.L.; Allalunis-Turner, J.; Haromy, A.; Beaulieu, C.; Thompson, R.; Lee, C.T.; Lopaschuk, G.D.; Puttagunta, L.; Bonnet, S.; et al. A mitochondria-K+ channel axis is suppressed in cancer and its normalization promotes apoptosis and inhibits cancer growth. *Cancer Cell* **2007**, *11*, 37–51. [CrossRef]
29. Lewandowski, E.D.; Johnston, D.L. Reduced substrate oxidation in postischemic myocardium: 13C and 31P NMR analyses. *Am. J. Physiol.* **1990**, *258*, H1357–H1365. [CrossRef]
30. Saddik, M.; Gamble, J.; Witters, L.A.; Lopaschuk, G.D. Acetyl-CoA carboxylase regulation of fatty acid oxidation in the heart. *J. Biol. Chem.* **1993**, *268*, 25836–25845.
31. Wahr, J.A.; Childs, K.F.; Bolling, S.F. Dichloroacetate enhances myocardial functional and metabolic recovery following global ischemia. *J. Cardiothorac. Vasc. Anesth.* **1994**, *8*, 192–197. [CrossRef]
32. Lewandowski, E.D.; White, L.T. Pyruvate dehydrogenase influences postischemic heart function. *Circulation* **1995**, *91*, 2071–2079. [CrossRef] [PubMed]
33. McVeigh, J.J.; Lopaschuk, G.D. Dichloroacetate stimulation of glucose oxidation improves recovery of ischemic rat hearts. *Am. J. Physiol.* **1990**, *259*, H1079–H1085. [CrossRef] [PubMed]
34. Stacpoole, P.W.; Henderson, G.N.; Yan, Z.; James, M.O. Clinical pharmacology and toxicology of dichloroacetate. *Environ. Health Perspect.* **1998**, *106* (Suppl. 4), 989–994.
35. Yang, H.M.; Davis, M.E. Dichloroacetic acid pretreatment of male and female rats increases chloroform metabolism in vitro. *Toxicology* **1997**, *124*, 53–62. [CrossRef]
36. Suh, S.W.; Aoyama, K.; Chen, Y.; Garnier, P.; Matsumori, Y.; Gum, E.; Liu, J.; Swanson, R.A. Hypoglycemic neuronal death and cognitive impairment are prevented by poly(ADP-ribose) polymerase inhibitors administered after hypoglycemia. *J. Neurosci.* **2003**, *23*, 10681–10690. [CrossRef] [PubMed]
37. Suh, S.W.; Aoyama, K.; Matsumori, Y.; Liu, J.; Swanson, R.A. Pyruvate administered after severe hypoglycemia reduces neuronal death and cognitive impairment. *Diabetes* **2005**, *54*, 1452–1458. [CrossRef] [PubMed]

38. Suh, S.W.; Hamby, A.M.; Gum, E.T.; Shin, B.S.; Won, S.J.; Sheline, C.T.; Chan, P.H.; Swanson, R.A. Sequential release of nitric oxide, zinc, and superoxide in hypoglycemic neuronal death. *J. Cereb. Blood Flow Metab.* **2008**, *28*, 1697–1706. [CrossRef]
39. Kho, A.R.; Choi, B.Y.; Kim, J.H.; Lee, S.H.; Hong, D.K.; Lee, S.H.; Jeong, J.H.; Sohn, M.; Suh, S.W. Prevention of hypoglycemia-induced hippocampal neuronal death by N-acetyl-L-cysteine (NAC). *Amino Acids* **2017**, *49*, 367–378. [CrossRef]
40. Schmued, L.C.; Hopkins, K.J. Fluoro-Jade B: A high affinity fluorescent marker for the localization of neuronal degeneration. *Brain Res.* **2000**, *874*, 123–130. [CrossRef]
41. Kauppinen, T.M.; Swanson, R.A. Poly(ADP-ribose) polymerase-1 promotes microglial activation, proliferation, and matrix metalloproteinase-9-mediated neuron death. *J. Immunol.* **2005**, *174*, 2288–2296. [CrossRef] [PubMed]
42. Kauppinen, T.M.; Higashi, Y.; Suh, S.W.; Escartin, C.; Nagasawa, K.; Swanson, R.A. Zinc triggers microglial activation. *J. Neurosci.* **2008**, *28*, 5827–5835. [CrossRef] [PubMed]
43. Ruth, R.E.; Feinerman, G.S. Foreign and endogenous serum protein extravasation during harmaline tremors or kainic acid seizures in the rat: A comparison. *Acta Neuropathol.* **1988**, *76*, 380–387. [CrossRef]
44. Hsu, S.M.; Raine, L.; Fanger, H. Use of avidin-biotin-peroxidase complex (ABC) in immunoperoxidase techniques: A comparison between ABC and unlabeled antibody (PAP) procedures. *J. Histochem. Cytochem.* **1981**, *29*, 577–580. [CrossRef]
45. Xing, G.; Ren, M.; O'Neill, J.T.; Verma, A.; Watson, W.D. Controlled cortical impact injury and craniotomy result in divergent alterations of pyruvate metabolizing enzymes in rat brain. *Exp. Neurol.* **2012**, *234*, 31–38. [CrossRef]
46. Jeong, J.Y.; Jeoung, N.H.; Park, K.G.; Lee, I.K. Transcriptional regulation of pyruvate dehydrogenase kinase. *Diabetes Metab. J.* **2012**, *36*, 328–335. [CrossRef] [PubMed]
47. Zhang, S.; Hulver, M.W.; McMillan, R.P.; Cline, M.A.; Gilbert, E.R. The pivotal role of pyruvate dehydrogenase kinases in metabolic flexibility. *Nutr. Metab.* **2014**, *11*, 10. [CrossRef] [PubMed]
48. Sorbi, S.; Bird, E.D.; Blass, J.P. Decreased pyruvate dehydrogenase complex activity in Huntington and Alzheimer brain. *Ann. Neurol.* **1983**, *13*, 72–78. [CrossRef] [PubMed]
49. Sheu, K.F.; Kim, Y.T.; Blass, J.P.; Weksler, M.E. An immunochemical study of the pyruvate dehydrogenase deficit in Alzheimer's disease brain. *Ann. Neurol.* **1985**, *17*, 444–449. [CrossRef]
50. Chinopoulos, C.; Adam-Vizi, V. Calcium, mitochondria and oxidative stress in neuronal pathology. Novel aspects of an enduring theme. *FEBS J.* **2006**, *273*, 433–450. [CrossRef] [PubMed]
51. McGowan, J.E.; Chen, L.; Gao, D.; Trush, M.; Wei, C. Increased mitochondrial reactive oxygen species production in newborn brain during hypoglycemia. *Neurosci. Lett.* **2006**, *399*, 111–114. [CrossRef] [PubMed]
52. Won, S.J.; Yoo, B.H.; Kauppinen, T.M.; Choi, B.Y.; Kim, J.H.; Jang, B.G.; Lee, M.W.; Sohn, M.; Liu, J.; Swanson, R.A.; et al. Recurrent/moderate hypoglycemia induces hippocampal dendritic injury, microglial activation, and cognitive impairment in diabetic rats. *J. Neuroinflammation* **2012**, *9*, 182. [CrossRef] [PubMed]
53. Ali, S.M.; Dunn, E.; Oostveen, J.A.; Hall, E.D.; Carter, D.B. Induction of apolipoprotein E mRNA in the hippocampus of the gerbil after transient global ischemia. *Brain Res. Mol. Brain Res.* **1996**, *38*, 37–44. [CrossRef]
54. Hirsch, E.C.; Hunot, S. Neuroinflammation in Parkinson's disease: A target for neuroprotection? *Lancet Neurol.* **2009**, *8*, 382–397. [CrossRef]
55. Kho, A.R.; Choi, B.Y.; Lee, S.H.; Hong, D.K.; Lee, S.H.; Jeong, J.H.; Park, K.H.; Song, H.K.; Choi, H.C.; Suh, S.W. Effects of Protocatechuic Acid (PCA) on Global Cerebral Ischemia-Induced Hippocampal Neuronal Death. *Int. J. Mol. Sci.* **2018**, *19*. [CrossRef] [PubMed]
56. Choi, B.Y.; Jang, B.G.; Kim, J.H.; Lee, B.E.; Sohn, M.; Song, H.K.; Suh, S.W. Prevention of traumatic brain injury-induced neuronal death by inhibition of NADPH oxidase activation. *Brain Res.* **2012**, *1481*, 49–58. [CrossRef]
57. Kim, J.H.; Jang, B.G.; Choi, B.Y.; Kim, H.S.; Sohn, M.; Chung, T.N.; Choi, H.C.; Song, H.K.; Suh, S.W. Post-treatment of an NADPH oxidase inhibitor prevents seizure-induced neuronal death. *Brain Res.* **2013**, *1499*, 163–172. [CrossRef]
58. Deng, J.; Zhao, F.; Yu, X.; Zhao, Y.; Li, D.; Shi, H.; Sun, Y. Expression of aquaporin 4 and breakdown of the blood-brain barrier after hypoglycemia-induced brain edema in rats. *PLoS ONE* **2014**, *9*, e107022. [CrossRef]

59. Zhao, F.; Deng, J.; Yu, X.; Li, D.; Shi, H.; Zhao, Y. Protective effects of vascular endothelial growth factor in cultured brain endothelial cells against hypoglycemia. *Metab. Brain Dis.* **2015**, *30*, 999–1007. [CrossRef]
60. Luo, S.; Li, S.; Zhu, L.; Fang, S.H.; Chen, J.L.; Xu, Q.Q.; Li, H.Y.; Luo, N.C.; Yang, C.; Luo, D.; et al. Effect of baicalin on oxygen-glucose deprivation-induced endothelial cell damage. *Neuroreport* **2017**, *28*, 299–306. [CrossRef]
61. Murakami, K.; Yoshino, M. Zinc inhibition of pyruvate kinase of M-type isozyme. *Biometals* **2017**, *30*, 335–340. [CrossRef]
62. Stanley, W.C.; Lopaschuk, G.D.; Hall, J.L.; McCormack, J.G. Regulation of myocardial carbohydrate metabolism under normal and ischaemic conditions. Potential for pharmacological interventions. *Cardiovasc. Res.* **1997**, *33*, 243–257. [CrossRef]
63. Ussher, J.R.; Wang, W.; Gandhi, M.; Keung, W.; Samokhvalov, V.; Oka, T.; Wagg, C.S.; Jaswal, J.S.; Harris, R.A.; Clanachan, A.S.; et al. Stimulation of glucose oxidation protects against acute myocardial infarction and reperfusion injury. *Cardiovasc. Res.* **2012**, *94*, 359–369. [CrossRef]
64. Pulsinelli, W.A.; Levy, D.E.; Duffy, T.E. Regional cerebral blood flow and glucose metabolism following transient forebrain ischemia. *Ann. Neurol.* **1982**, *11*, 499–502. [CrossRef] [PubMed]
65. Yokobori, S.; Mazzeo, A.T.; Gajavelli, S.; Bullock, M.R. Mitochondrial neuroprotection in traumatic brain injury: Rationale and therapeutic strategies. *CNS Neurol. Disord. Drug Targets* **2014**, *13*, 606–619. [CrossRef]
66. Fiskum, G.; Rosenthal, R.E.; Vereczki, V.; Martin, E.; Hoffman, G.E.; Chinopoulos, C.; Kowaltowski, A. Protection against ischemic brain injury by inhibition of mitochondrial oxidative stress. *J. Bioenerg. Biomembr.* **2004**, *36*, 347–352. [CrossRef] [PubMed]
67. Opii, W.O.; Nukala, V.N.; Sultana, R.; Pandya, J.D.; Day, K.M.; Merchant, M.L.; Klein, J.B.; Sullivan, P.G.; Butterfield, D.A. Proteomic identification of oxidized mitochondrial proteins following experimental traumatic brain injury. *J. Neurotrauma* **2007**, *24*, 772–789. [CrossRef] [PubMed]
68. Roche, T.E.; Hiromasa, Y. Pyruvate dehydrogenase kinase regulatory mechanisms and inhibition in treating diabetes, heart ischemia, and cancer. *Cell. Mol. Life Sci.* **2007**, *64*, 830–849. [CrossRef]
69. Xing, G.; Ren, M.; Watson, W.D.; O'Neill, J.T.; Verma, A. Traumatic brain injury-induced expression and phosphorylation of pyruvate dehydrogenase: A mechanism of dysregulated glucose metabolism. *Neurosci. Lett.* **2009**, *454*, 38–42. [CrossRef]
70. Leinninger, G.M.; Backus, C.; Sastry, A.M.; Yi, Y.B.; Wang, C.W.; Feldman, E.L. Mitochondria in DRG neurons undergo hyperglycemic mediated injury through Bim, Bax and the fission protein Drp1. *Neurobiol. Dis.* **2006**, *23*, 11–22. [CrossRef] [PubMed]
71. Katyare, S.S.; Patel, S.P. Insulin status differentially affects energy transduction in cerebral mitochondria from male and female rats. *Brain Res. Bull.* **2006**, *69*, 458–464. [CrossRef]
72. Otera, H.; Ishihara, N.; Mihara, K. New insights into the function and regulation of mitochondrial fission. *Biochim. Biophys. Acta* **2013**, *1833*, 1256–1268. [CrossRef]
73. Calcutt, N.A.; Lopez, V.L.; Bautista, A.D.; Mizisin, L.M.; Torres, B.R.; Shroads, A.L.; Mizisin, A.P.; Stacpoole, P.W. Peripheral neuropathy in rats exposed to dichloroacetate. *J. Neuropathol. Exp. Neurol.* **2009**, *68*, 985–993. [CrossRef]
74. Moser, V.C.; Phillips, P.M.; McDaniel, K.L.; MacPhail, R.C. Behavioral evaluation of the neurotoxicity produced by dichloroacetic acid in rats. *Neurotoxicol. Teratol.* **1999**, *21*, 719–731. [CrossRef]
75. Sun, X.Q.; Zhang, R.; Zhang, H.D.; Yuan, P.; Wang, X.J.; Zhao, Q.H.; Wang, L.; Jiang, R.; Jan Bogaard, H.; Jing, Z.C. Reversal of right ventricular remodeling by dichloroacetate is related to inhibition of mitochondria-dependent apoptosis. *Hypertens Res.* **2016**, *39*, 302–311. [CrossRef]
76. Durie, D.; McDonald, T.S.; Borges, K. The effect of dichloroacetate in mouse models of epilepsy. *Epilepsy Res.* **2018**, *145*, 77–81. [CrossRef] [PubMed]
77. Staneviciute, J.; Jukneviciene, M.; Palubinskiene, J.; Balnyte, I.; Valanciute, A.; Vosyliute, R.; Suziedelis, K.; Lesauskaite, V.; Stakisaitis, D. Sodium Dichloroacetate Pharmacological Effect as Related to Na-K-2Cl Cotransporter Inhibition in Rats. *Dose Response* **2018**, *16*, 1559325818811522. [CrossRef] [PubMed]
78. Li, X.; Liu, J.; Hu, H.; Lu, S.; Lu, Q.; Quan, N.; Rousselle, T.; Patel, M.S.; Li, J. Dichloroacetate Ameliorates Cardiac Dysfunction Caused by Ischemic Insults Through AMPK Signal Pathway-Not Only Shifts Metabolism. *Toxicol. Sci.* **2019**, *167*, 604–617. [CrossRef] [PubMed]

79. Martinez-Palma, L.; Miquel, E.; Lagos-Rodriguez, V.; Barbeito, L.; Cassina, A.; Cassina, P. Mitochondrial Modulation by Dichloroacetate Reduces Toxicity of Aberrant Glial Cells and Gliosis in the SOD1G93A Rat Model of Amyotrophic Lateral Sclerosis. *Neurotherapeutics* **2019**, *16*, 203–215. [CrossRef] [PubMed]
80. Stacpoole, P.W. The pharmacology of dichloroacetate. *Metabolism* **1989**, *38*, 1124–1144. [CrossRef]
81. D'Alessandro, G.; Calcagno, E.; Tartari, S.; Rizzardini, M.; Invernizzi, R.W.; Cantoni, L. Glutamate and glutathione interplay in a motor neuronal model of amyotrophic lateral sclerosis reveals altered energy metabolism. *Neurobiol. Dis.* **2011**, *43*, 346–355. [CrossRef]
82. Jozefczak, M.; Remans, T.; Vangronsveld, J.; Cuypers, A. Glutathione is a key player in metal-induced oxidative stress defenses. *Int. J. Mol. Sci.* **2012**, *13*, 3145–3175. [CrossRef]
83. Choi, B.Y.; Kim, I.Y.; Kim, J.H.; Lee, B.E.; Lee, S.H.; Kho, A.R.; Jung, H.J.; Sohn, M.; Song, H.K.; Suh, S.W. Decreased cysteine uptake by EAAC1 gene deletion exacerbates neuronal oxidative stress and neuronal death after traumatic brain injury. *Amino Acids* **2016**, *48*, 1619–1629. [CrossRef] [PubMed]
84. Jha, M.K.; Park, D.H.; Kook, H.; Lee, I.K.; Lee, W.H.; Suk, K. Metabolic Control of Glia-Mediated Neuroinflammation. *Curr. Alzheimer Res.* **2016**, *13*, 387–402.
85. O'Neill, L.A.; Hardie, D.G. Metabolism of inflammation limited by AMPK and pseudo-starvation. *Nature* **2013**, *493*, 346–355. [CrossRef]
86. Orihuela, R.; McPherson, C.A.; Harry, G.J. Microglial M1/M2 polarization and metabolic states. *Br. J. Pharmacol.* **2016**, *173*, 649–665. [CrossRef] [PubMed]
87. Klimaszewska-Lata, J.; Gul-Hinc, S.; Bielarczyk, H.; Ronowska, A.; Zysk, M.; Gruzewska, K.; Pawelczyk, T.; Szutowicz, A. Differential effects of lipopolysaccharide on energy metabolism in murine microglial N9 and cholinergic SN56 neuronal cells. *J. Neurochem.* **2015**, *133*, 284–297. [CrossRef]
88. Jha, M.K.; Song, G.J.; Lee, M.G.; Jeoung, N.H.; Go, Y.; Harris, R.A.; Park, D.H.; Kook, H.; Lee, I.K.; Suk, K. Metabolic Connection of Inflammatory Pain: Pivotal Role of a Pyruvate Dehydrogenase Kinase-Pyruvate Dehydrogenase-Lactic Acid Axis. *J. Neurosci.* **2015**, *35*, 14353–14369. [CrossRef]
89. Liu, W.; Wang, X.; Yang, S.; Huang, J.; Xue, X.; Zheng, Y.; Shang, G.; Tao, J.; Chen, L. Electroacupunctre improves motor impairment via inhibition of microglia-mediated neuroinflammation in the sensorimotor cortex after ischemic stroke. *Life Sci.* **2016**, *151*, 313–322. [CrossRef]
90. Ghaemi, A.; Alizadeh, L.; Babaei, S.; Jafarian, M.; Khaleghi Ghadiri, M.; Meuth, S.G.; Kovac, S.; Gorji, A. Astrocyte-mediated inflammation in cortical spreading depression. *Cephalalgia* **2018**, *38*, 626–638. [CrossRef]
91. Dvoriantchikova, G.; Barakat, D.; Brambilla, R.; Agudelo, C.; Hernandez, E.; Bethea, J.R.; Shestopalov, V.I.; Ivanov, D. Inactivation of astroglial NF-kappa B promotes survival of retinal neurons following ischemic injury. *Eur. J. Neurosci.* **2009**, *30*, 175–185. [CrossRef]
92. Kirkley, K.S.; Popichak, K.A.; Afzali, M.F.; Legare, M.E.; Tjalkens, R.B. Microglia amplify inflammatory activation of astrocytes in manganese neurotoxicity. *J. Neuroinflammation* **2017**, *14*, 99. [CrossRef]
93. Liddelow, S.A.; Guttenplan, K.A.; Clarke, L.E.; Bennett, F.C.; Bohlen, C.J.; Schirmer, L.; Bennett, M.L.; Munch, A.E.; Chung, W.S.; Peterson, T.C.; et al. Neurotoxic reactive astrocytes are induced by activated microglia. *Nature* **2017**, *541*, 481–487. [CrossRef] [PubMed]
94. Blumcke, I.; Pauli, E.; Clusmann, H.; Schramm, J.; Becker, A.; Elger, C.; Merschhemke, M.; Meencke, H.J.; Lehmann, T.; von Deimling, A.; et al. A new clinico-pathological classification system for mesial temporal sclerosis. *Acta Neuropathol.* **2007**, *113*, 235–244. [CrossRef]
95. Mueller, S.G.; Stables, L.; Du, A.T.; Schuff, N.; Truran, D.; Cashdollar, N.; Weiner, M.W. Measurement of hippocampal subfields and age-related changes with high resolution MRI at 4T. *Neurobiol. Aging* **2007**, *28*, 719–726. [CrossRef]
96. West, M.J.; Kawas, C.H.; Stewart, W.F.; Rudow, G.L.; Troncoso, J.C. Hippocampal neurons in pre-clinical Alzheimer's disease. *Neurobiol. Aging* **2004**, *25*, 1205–1212. [CrossRef]
97. Chodobski, A.; Zink, B.J.; Szmydynger-Chodobska, J. Blood-brain barrier pathophysiology in traumatic brain injury. *Transl. Stroke Res.* **2011**, *2*, 492–516. [CrossRef]
98. Tomkins, O.; Shelef, I.; Kaizerman, I.; Eliushin, A.; Afawi, Z.; Misk, A.; Gidon, M.; Cohen, A.; Zumsteg, D.; Friedman, A. Blood-brain barrier disruption in post-traumatic epilepsy. *J. Neurol. Neurosurg. Psychiatry* **2008**, *79*, 774–777. [CrossRef]
99. Scholz, M.; Cinatl, J.; Schadel-Hopfner, M.; Windolf, J. Neutrophils and the blood-brain barrier dysfunction after trauma. *Med. Res. Rev.* **2007**, *27*, 401–416. [CrossRef]
100. Alves, J.L. Blood-brain barrier and traumatic brain injury. *J. Neurosci. Res.* **2014**, *92*, 141–147. [CrossRef]

101. Doll, D.N.; Hu, H.; Sun, J.; Lewis, S.E.; Simpkins, J.W.; Ren, X. Mitochondrial crisis in cerebrovascular endothelial cells opens the blood-brain barrier. *Stroke* **2015**, *46*, 1681–1689. [CrossRef]
102. Hu, H.; Doll, D.N.; Sun, J.; Lewis, S.E.; Wimsatt, J.H.; Kessler, M.J.; Simpkins, J.W.; Ren, X. Mitochondrial Impairment in Cerebrovascular Endothelial Cells is Involved in the Correlation between Body Temperature and Stroke Severity. *Aging Dis.* **2016**, *7*, 14–27. [CrossRef]
103. Salmina, A.B.; Kuvacheva, N.V.; Morgun, A.V.; Komleva, Y.K.; Pozhilenkova, E.A.; Lopatina, O.L.; Gorina, Y.V.; Taranushenko, T.E.; Petrova, L.L. Glycolysis-mediated control of blood-brain barrier development and function. *Int. J. Biochem. Cell Biol.* **2015**, *64*, 174–184. [CrossRef] [PubMed]

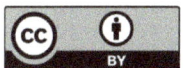

© 2019 by the authors. Licensee MDPI, Basel, Switzerland. This article is an open access article distributed under the terms and conditions of the Creative Commons Attribution (CC BY) license (http://creativecommons.org/licenses/by/4.0/).

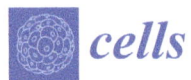

Article

Perilipin 5 Protects against Cellular Oxidative Stress by Enhancing Mitochondrial Function in HepG2 Cells

Yanjie Tan [1,†], Yi Jin [1,†], Qian Wang [1], Jin Huang [1], Xiang Wu [1] and Zhuqing Ren [1,2,*]

1. Key Laboratory of Agriculture Animal Genetics, Breeding and Reproduction of the Ministry of Education, College of Animal Science, Huazhong Agricultural University, Wuhan 430070, China; tanyanjie@webmail.hzau.edu.cn (Y.T.); hyj_1900@webmail.hzau.edu.cn (Y.J.); wangqian58@webmail.hzau.edu.cn (Q.W.); 13164367031@163.com (J.H.); wx1078724218@163.com (X.W.)
2. The Cooperative Innovation Center for Sustainable Pig Production, Huazhong Agricultural University, Wuhan 430070, China
* Correspondence: renzq@mail.hzau.edu.cn; Tel.: +86-132-9798-0341; Fax: +86-027-8728-2091
† These two authors contributed equally to this work.

Received: 12 July 2019; Accepted: 8 October 2019; Published: 11 October 2019

Abstract: Non-alcoholic fatty liver disease (NAFLD) is one of the most common liver diseases worldwide. Reactive oxygen species (ROS), as potent oxidants in cells, have been shown to promote the development of NAFLD. Previous studies reported that for ROS-induced cellular oxidative stress, promoting lipid droplet (LD) accumulation is associated with the cellular antioxidation process. However, the regulatory role of LDs in relieving cellular oxidative stress is poorly understood. Here, we showed that *Perilipin 5* (*PLIN5*), a key LD protein related to mitochondria–LD contact, reduced ROS levels and improved mitochondrial function in HepG2 cells. Both mRNA and protein levels of *PLIN5* were significantly increased in cells with hydrogen peroxide or lipopolysaccharide (LPS) treatment ($p < 0.05$). Additionally, the overexpression of *PLIN5* promoted LD formation and mitochondria–LD contact, reduced cellular ROS levels and up-regulated mitochondrial function-related genes such as *COX* and *CS*. Knockdown *PLIN5*, meanwhile, showed opposite effects. Furthermore, we identified that cellular oxidative stress up-regulated *PLIN5* expression via the JNK-p38-ATF pathway. This study shows that the up-regulation of *PLIN5* is a kind of survival strategy for cells in response to stress. *PLIN5* can be a potential therapeutic target in NAFLD.

Keywords: perilipin 5; lipid droplet; mitochondria; ROS

---

1. Introduction

There are a large number of patients suffering from non-alcoholic fatty liver disease (NAFLD) all over the world. This disease increases the risk of non-alcoholic hepatitis (NASH), chronic interstitial hepatitis, hepatic failure, and even hepatocellular carcinoma [1–3]. One of the characterizations of NAFLD is increased levels of reactive oxygen species (ROS) [4]. Some studies have shown that high levels of ROS promote the development of NAFLD/NASH and hepatocellular carcinoma by inducing ER stress [5] or regulating the AMPK signaling pathway [6]. There are several antioxidant enzymes such as superoxide dismutase (*SOD*), catalase (*CAT*), and glutathione peroxidase (*GPX*) responsible for scavenging cellular ROS. Meanwhile, the expression levels of *SOD* and other antioxidant enzymes are decreased in NAFLD/NASH [4]. Interestingly, lipid droplets (LDs) have been shown to be involved in the cellular stress response process. Bailey et al. demonstrated that lipid droplets can act as antioxidant organelles that protect *Drosophila* neural stem cells from hypoxia-triggered ROS [7], by allowing neuronal stem cells to keep proliferating under hypoxic conditions, and protection likely involves sequestering vulnerable membrane lipids away from ROS [8]. Furthermore, LDs also respond to starvation-induced stress by increasing their contact with mitochondria and lysosomes, which could consist in the role of these contacts in transferring fatty acids from LDs to mitochondria or lysosomes for energy supply [9]. Moreover, the formation of nuclear LDs is related to the stress induced by phospholipid shortages [10,11]. Our previous study has shown that hydrogen peroxide promoted the formation of cellular LDs [12]. However, whether the increased cellular LDs play a role as anti-oxidants is largely unknown.

Perilipin 5 (*PLIN5*) is one of the conserved LD proteins, which belongs to the PAT (*perilipin, adipophilin,* and *TIP47*) protein family [13]. Oxidative tissues such as skeletal muscle, liver, and brown fat have high expression levels of *PLIN5*, indicating that *PLIN5* plays an important role in lipid storage and LD function [14–16]. Previous studies identified that *PLIN5* regulated triglyceride contents in hepatocytes [17] and skeletal muscle [18]. Overexpression of *PLIN5* in skeletal muscle promotes oxidative gene expression and lipid content [19]. Recently, *PLIN5* was reported to be the key factor that regulated LD contacting mitochondria [20,21]. The N-terminal (1-188aa) of *PLIN5* is the conserved PAT domain, and 189-391aa is the domain contacting with patatin like phospholipase domain containing 2 (*PNPLA2, ATGL*). The C-terminal of *PLIN5* (443-463aa) is the key sequence related to mitochondrial recruiting [22]. LD–mitochondria contact is important for the energy supply during starvation stress, which promotes lipid β-oxidation [9,23], and the transfer process of fatty acids from LDs to mitochondria was also observed by probe imaging [24,25]. Recently, a study also found that LD–mitochondria contact contributed to lipid synthesis and LD expansion [22]. Furthermore, LDs are able to protect against cellular apoptosis by clearing harmful proteins from outer mitochondrial membranes [26]. Moreover, *PLIN5* has been shown to limit fatty acid toxicity [27]. These studies suggested that *PLIN5* was involved in the process of cellular anti-oxidation.

In the present study, we found that hydrogen peroxide- or lipopolysaccharide (LPS)-induced oxidative stress up-regulated both mRNA and protein levels of *PLIN5*. The overexpression of *PLIN5* increased the cellular LD content, promoted LD–mitochondria contact, reduced cellular ROS level, and enhanced mitochondrial function-related gene expression, whereas knockdown *PLIN5* indicated opposite phenotypes. Moreover, we identified that the promoter region of *PLIN5* contained the binding sites of *JUN, ATF1, ATF3,* and *ATF4*, and therefore *PLIN5* expression was activated by the JNK-p38-ATF pathway. By bioinformatic analysis, it has been found that *PLIN5* has a high expression in liver hepatocellular carcinoma (LIHC), and additionally, low expression of *PLIN5* is correlated with poor prognosis in LIHC. Therefore, *PLIN5* can be a potential therapeutic target in NAFLD and NAFLD-induced LIHC.

2. Results

2.1. PLIN5 Was Up-Regulated in Liver Tissues of NAFLD Mice

NAFLD is characterized by the accumulation of LDs and a raised ROS level. We induced NAFLD in mice by two classical methods, which were the methionine-choline-deficient diet (MCDD) treatment and high-fat diet (HFD) treatment, respectively. The liver tissues of mice fed with MCDD for 0 week, 1 week, 2 weeks, 3 weeks, 4 weeks, 6 weeks, and 8 weeks, and mice fed with HFD for 0 week and 10 weeks were collected. Then, the changes in hepatic *PLIN5* expression were investigated in these collected samples. The results showed that the mRNA level of *PLIN5* was up-regulated significantly in hepatic tissues of mice fed with MCDD for 4 weeks, 6 weeks, and 8 weeks, and mice fed with HFD for 10 weeks, compared to the corresponding control samples (fed with chow diet, CD; $p < 0.05$; Figure 1A–D). To validate this phenotype and further investigate the localization of *PLIN5*, immunohistochemistry was performed. The hepatic tissues of mice fed with MCDD for 0 week, 1 week, 2 weeks, 3 weeks, 4 weeks, 6 weeks, and 8 weeks were detected. The results showed that *PLIN5* protein was mainly localized surrounding the LDs, and additionally, in mice fed with MCDD, the expression of *PLIN5* was activated (Figure 1E). These results indicate that the expression levels of *PLIN5* were enhanced and *PLIN5* was mainly recruited on the surface of LDs during NAFLD development.

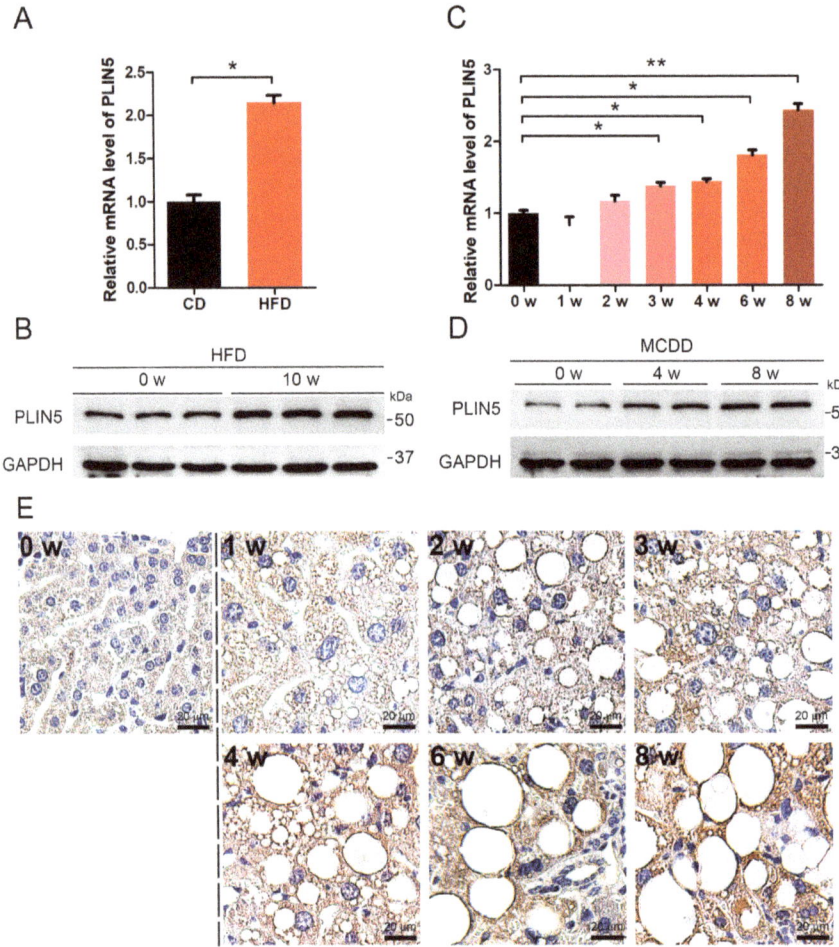

Figure 1. *Perilipin 5 (PLIN5)* was up-regulated in liver tissues of non-alcoholic fatty liver disease (NAFLD) mice. (**A**) Six-week-old C57/bl male mice were fed with a high-fat diet (HFD) or chow diet (CD) for 10 weeks. The mRNA levels of *PLIN5* in liver tissues of mice fed with chow diet (CD) and HFD were detected by qRT-PCR. (**B**) The protein levels of *PLIN5* in liver tissues of mice fed with chow diet (CD) and HFD were detected by Western Blot. (**C**) Six-week-old C57/bl male mice were fed with methionine-choline-deficient diet (MCDD) for 1 week, 2 weeks, 3 weeks, 4 weeks, 6 weeks, and 8 weeks, respectively. The mRNA levels of *PLIN5* were detected by qRT-PCR. (**D**) The protein levels of *PLIN5* were detected by Western Blot. (**E**) Immunohistochemistry analysis of liver tissues of mice fed with MCDD (1–8 weeks) and control mice (0 week). Scale bar, 20 μm. These experiments were performed in triplicate. * $p < 0.05$; and ** $p < 0.01$.

2.2. Hydrogen Peroxide or LPS Treatment Enhanced Expression of PLIN5

It was already well known that ROS levels were increased in hepatic tissues with NAFLD. Moreover, we did not observe any significant up-regulation of hepatic *PLIN5* in mice fed with MCDD for 1 week, 2 weeks, and 3 weeks, although many hepatic LDs had accumulated. Therefore, we assumed that the raised ROS levels activated *PLIN5* expression. ROS represents a variety of molecules and free radicals (chemical species with one unpaired electron) derived from molecular oxygen. Superoxide anion ($O_2^-\bullet$), the product of a one-electron reduction of oxygen, is the precursor of most ROS and a mediator in oxidative chain reactions [28], and then hydrogen peroxide arises from $O_2^-\bullet$ [29,30]. Hydrogen peroxide and LPS are classical regents that induce cellular oxidation. Therefore, we investigated whether inducing cellular oxidative stress affected the expression level of PLIN5. The HepG2 cells were treated with 200 μM hydrogen peroxide for 12 h. qRT-PCR showed that PLIN5 mRNA was up-regulated significantly by hydrogen peroxide treatment ($p < 0.05$; Figure 2A), and, additionally, the Western Blot indicated that PLIN5 protein was also significantly up-regulated ($p < 0.05$; Figure 2B). Furthermore, we also investigated the changes in PLIN5 expression levels with the lipopolysaccharide (LPS) treatment. The results showed that both mRNA and protein levels of PLIN5 were up-regulated significantly ($p < 0.05$; Figure 2C,D). The oleic acid (OA) treatment can induce cells to form more and larger LDs, which is well applicable to observe the subcellular localization of PLIN5. Therefore, we subsequently detected the subcellular localization of PLIN5 in OA treated cells by the PLIN5-EGFP expression vector. The results indicated that PLIN5 was located on the surface of LDs (Figure 2E). To investigate whether hydrogen peroxide treatment changes the localization of PLIN5, we detected subcellular localization of PLIN5 in cells with the 200 μM hydrogen peroxide treatment. We found that hydrogen peroxide treatment did not change the localization of PLIN5 (Figure 2E). These results indicated that increased cellular ROS levels promoted the expression of PLIN5.

2.3. PLIN5 Regulated Cellular ROS Levels

To investigate whether PLIN5 was involved in the anti-oxidant process, we validated the efficiency of PLIN5 overexpression and knockdown by the Western Blot method first. The result showed that PLIN5 was overexpressed and interfered successfully (Figure 3A,B). Subsequently, we knocked down and overexpressed PLIN5 to detect ROS levels by the DCFH-DA (2,7-dichlorodihydrofluorescein diacetate) method, respectively. The results showed that PLIN5 knockdown increased ROS levels, whereas PLIN5 overexpression decreased ROS levels significantly ($p < 0.05$; Figure 3C). Subsequently, we used 200 μM hydrogen peroxide to treat cells with PLIN5 knockdown and overexpression in order to investigate whether PLIN5 expression affected ROS levels of cells in oxidative stress. The results indicated that PLIN5 knockdown increased ROS levels, whereas PLIN5 overexpression decreased ROS levels significantly in cells treated with 200 μM hydrogen peroxide ($p < 0.05$; Figure 3D). To validate the phenotype, we further used the DHE (dihydroethidium) method to detect the $O_2^-\bullet$ levels in PLIN5 knockdown, overexpression, and corresponding control cells, respectively. The microplate reader indicated that PLIN5 knockdown increased ROS levels, whereas PLIN5 overexpression decreased ROS levels (Figure 3E,F). The release level of cytochrome c from mitochondria to cell plasma is the gold standard to reflect the level of cellular oxidative stress. Therefore, we investigated whether PLIN5 knockdown aggravated or whether PLIN5 overexpression reduced hydrogen peroxide-induced cytochrome c release. Firstly, we treated the cells with 200 μM hydrogen peroxide and then isolated the cytosolic and mitochondrial fractions respectively to detect the levels of cytochrome c (Figure 3G). The result showed that hydrogen peroxide treatment increased cytosolic cytochrome c levels and decreased mitochondrial cytochrome c levels, which indicated that hydrogen peroxide treatment increased cytochrome c releasing from mitochondria to cytoplasm. Then we detected the effect of PLIN5 overexpression on the hydrogen peroxide treatment-induced cytochrome c release. The cells were transfected with PLIN5 expression vector or pcDNA3.1 (control) vector, and then treated with 200 μM hydrogen peroxide. The cytoplasm and mitochondria were isolated, and then cytosolic and mitochondrial cytochrome c levels were detected through Western Blot, respectively. The result showed that PLIN5 overexpression decreased cytosolic cytochrome c levels but increased mitochondrial cytochrome c levels compared to the control in the presence of hydrogen peroxide (Figure 3H). Mitochondrial membrane potential is an important indicator for mitochondrial oxidative damage. Therefore, we detected the mitochondrial membrane potential in cells with PLIN5 overexpression or control by the JC-1 (5,5',6,6'-tetrachloro-1,1',3,3'-tetraethyl-imidacarbocyanine) method. As expected, the mitochondrial membrane potential was significantly higher in cells with PLIN5 overexpression than in the corresponding control cells (Figure 3I). Furthermore, we detected the mitochondrial membrane potential in cells with *PLIN5* overexpression or control in the presence of hydrogen peroxide. The result showed that mitochondrial membrane potential of *PLIN5* overexpression group was higher than the control group (Figure 3I).

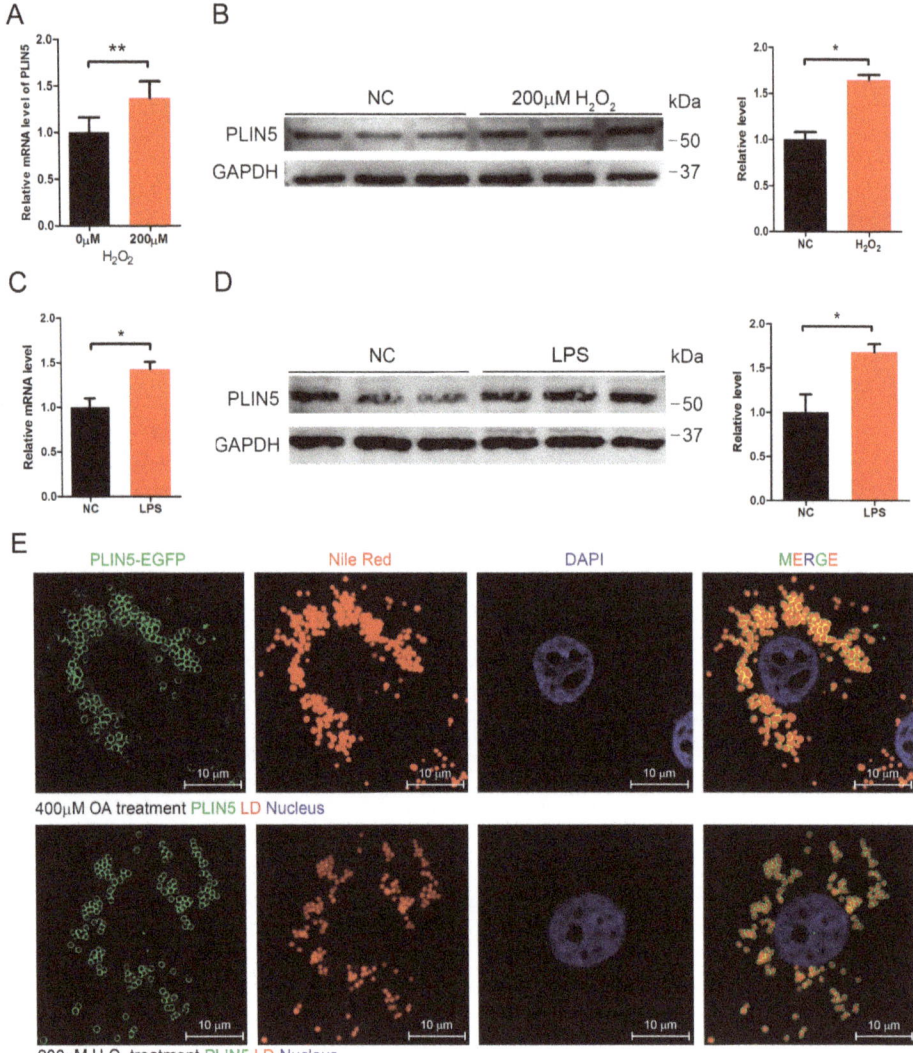

Figure 2. Hydrogen peroxide or lipopolysaccharide (LPS) treatment enhanced the expression of *PLIN5*. Hydrogen peroxide and LPS were used to induce cellular oxidative stress. (**A**) mRNA level of *PLIN5* in cells with H_2O_2 treatment or control (phosphate buffer saline, PBS). (**B**) Western Blot analysis of *PLIN5* protein levels in cells with H_2O_2 treatment or control (PBS). (**C**) mRNA level of *PLIN5* in cells with LPS treatment or control (PBS). (**D**) Western Blot analysis of *PLIN5* protein levels in cells with LPS treatment or control (PBS). (**E**) H_2O_2 treatment did not change the localization of *PLIN5*. *PLIN5* localization analysis of cells with 400 μM oleic acid medium or H_2O_2 treatment. Green, PLIN5-EGFP; red, lipid droplets; blue, nucleus. Bar, 10 μm. These experiments were performed in triplicate. * $p < 0.05$; and ** $p < 0.01$.

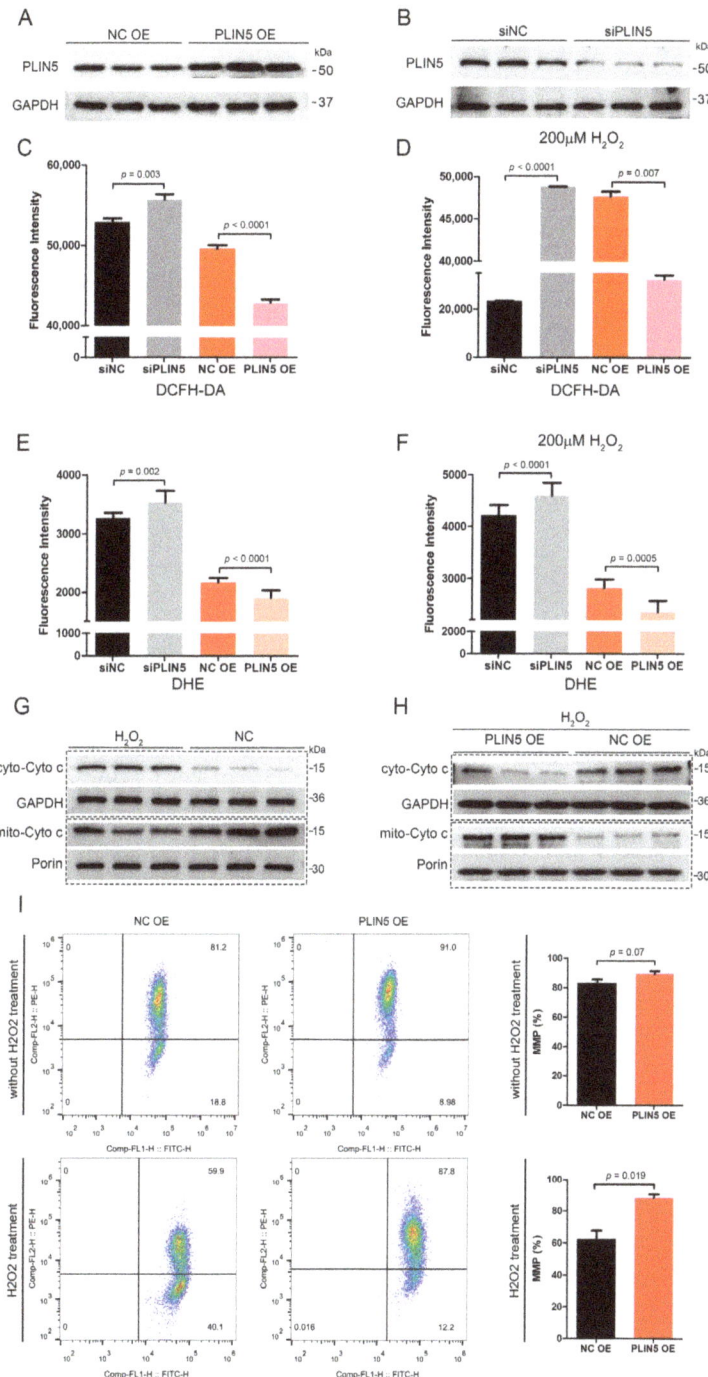

Figure 3. *PLIN5* regulated cellular reactive oxygen species (ROS) levels. (**A**,**B**) Western blot validation of *PLIN5* overexpression (**A**) and RNAi (**B**) efficiency. (**C**) HepG2 cells were transfected with *PLIN5* siRNAs or negative control siRNAs or *PLIN5* expression vector or pcDNA3.1 (control) vector, respectively. Then,

the cellular ROS levels were detected by DCFH-DA probes through a microplate reader (Ex = 488 nm, Em = 525 nm). (**D**) The cells were transfected with *PLIN5* siRNAs or negative control siRNAs or *PLIN5* expression vector or pcDNA3.1 (control) vector, respectively, and then treated with 200 μM H_2O_2. Then, the cellular ROS levels were detected by DCFH-DA probes through a microplate reader (Ex = 488 nm, Em = 525 nm). (**E**) HepG2 cells were transfected with *PLIN5* siRNAs or negative control siRNAs or *PLIN5* expression vector or pcDNA3.1 (control) vector, respectively. Then, the cellular ROS levels were detected by DHE through a microplate reader (Ex = 535 nm, Em = 610 nm). (**F**) The cells were transfected with *PLIN5* siRNAs or negative control siRNAs or *PLIN5* expression vector or pcDNA3.1 (control) vector, respectively, and then treated with 200 μM H_2O_2. Then, the cellular ROS levels were detected by DCFH-DA probes through a microplate reader (Ex = 488 nm, Em = 525 nm). (**G**) The cells were treated with 200 μM H_2O_2. The cytoplasm and mitochondria were isolated respectively, and then cytosolic and mitochondrial cytochrome c levels were detected respectively through Western Blot. (**H**) The cells were transfected with *PLIN5* expression vector or pcDNA3.1 (control) vector, and then treated with 200 μM H_2O_2. The cytoplasm and mitochondria were isolated, and then cytosolic and mitochondrial cytochrome c levels were detected respectively through Western Blot. *GAPDH* was the reference protein of cytosolic component and the *Porin/VDAC1* was the reference protein of mitochondrial component. (**I**) The mitochondrial membrane potential (MMP) was detected by JC-1 probes using the flow cytometry method. These experiments were performed in triplicate. * $p < 0.05$. Ex, excitation wavelength; Em, emission wavelength.

2.4. PLIN5 Promoted LD Formation and Contact with Mitochondria

We have shown that up-regulated *PLIN5* decreased cellular ROS levels, so we then investigated the regulatory mechanism. Our previous study has shown that the up-regulation of *PLIN2* promoted the formation of cellular LDs [12]. Therefore, *PLIN5* was overexpressed in HepG2 cells, and then the cellular LDs were labeled by BODIPY493/503 (4,4-difluoro-1,3,5,7,8-pentamethyl-4-bora-3a,4a-diaza-s-indacene) to reflect the effect of *PLIN5* up-regulation on LD content. As expected, the number of cellular LDs in cells with *PLIN5* overexpression was higher than the LDs in control cells ($p < 0.05$; Figure 4A,B). To validate the phenotype, the LD content was detected in cells transfected with siRNA oligos targeting *PLIN5* and control cells. The result indicated that *PLIN5* knockdown decreased the number of cellular LDs ($p < 0.05$; Figure 4C,D). A previous study showed that *PLIN5* promoted LD contact with mitochondria, and subsequently, we validated this phenotype in HepG2 cells. There was no doubt that the result indicated that the overexpression of *PLIN5* highly enhanced this contact in HepG2 cells ($p < 0.05$; Figure 4E,F). Moreover, we also investigated whether hydrogen peroxide treatment induced LD contact with mitochondria, since the high levels of ROS up-regulated *PLIN5*. The mitochondria were labeled by a mito-tracker, and LDs were marked by BODIPY. After the treatment with hydrogen peroxide, the contact events were increased significantly compared to corresponding cells ($p < 0.05$; Figure 4G,H). The results indicated that high ROS levels enhanced LD formation and promoted LD contact with mitochondria by up-regulating *PLIN5*.

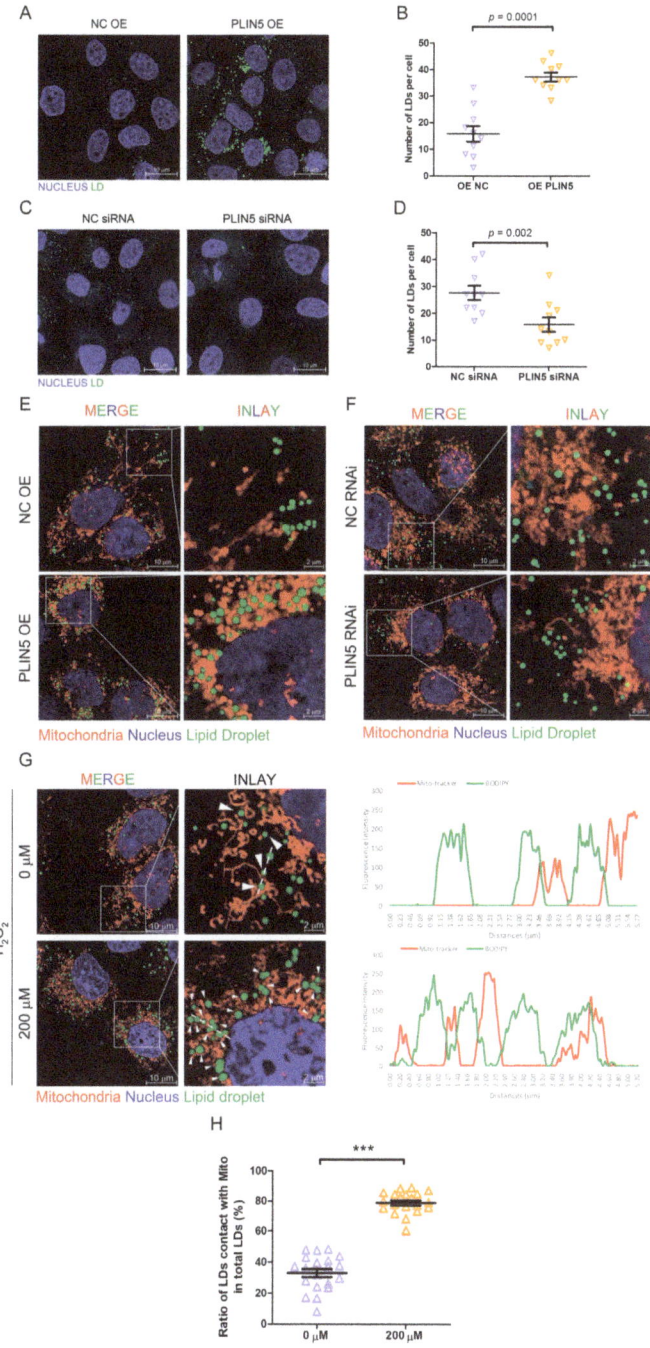

Figure 4. *PLIN5* promoted LD formation and contact with mitochondria. (**A**) HepG2 cells were transfected with *PLIN5* expression vector or pcDNA3.1 (control) vector. Then, the cellular lipid droplets

were stained with BODIPY493/503 and observed by a confocal microscope. (**B**) The counts of cellular LDs in A. (**C**) HepG2 cells were transfected with *PLIN5* siRNAs or negative control siRNAs. Then, the cellular lipid droplets were stained with BODIPY493/503 and observed by a confocal microscope. (**D**) The counts of cellular LDs in C. (**E**) HepG2 cells were transfected with the mito-Dsred vector and *PLIN5* expression vector or pcDNA3.1 (control) vector. Then, the cellular lipid droplets were stained with BODIPY493/503 and observed by a confocal microscope. (**F**) HepG2 cells were transfected with mito-Dsred vector and *PLIN5* siRNAs or negative control siRNAs. Then, the cellular lipid droplets were stained with BODIPY493/503 and observed by a confocal microscope. (**G**) HepG2 cells were transfected with mito-Dsred vector and then treated with 200 μM H_2O_2. Then, the cellular lipid droplets were stained with BODIPY493/503 and observed by a confocal microscope. The fluorescence intensity along with the dotted line was performed to illustrate the contacts between LDs and mitochondria. (**H**) The ratio of contacts between LDs and mitochondria was analyzed. These experiments were performed in triplicate. *** $p < 0.0001$.

2.5. PLIN5 Regulated the Expression Levels of Mitochondrial Function-Related Genes

One of the functions of mitochondria is oxidative metabolism, which requires several mitochondrial respiratory chain oxidases, such as *COX* and *CS*. The expression levels of *COX* and *CS* are related to the mitochondria activity. Therefore, we further investigated whether PLIN5 expression affected the expression of *COX* and *CS*. The qPCR results showed that *COX2*, *COX4*, and *CS* were up-regulated in the cells with *PLIN5* overexpression (Figure 5A), whereas they were down-regulated significantly in cells with *PLIN5* knockdown ($p < 0.05$; Figure 5B). Subsequently, we investigated the effect of *PLIN5* expression on the expression levels of several cellular anti-oxidant genes including *GPX1*, *GPX2*, *SOD1*, *SOD2*, *TXNRD1*, *CAT*, and *PRDX3* through qPCR. The result showed that *GPX2* and *CAT* mRNA levels were increased significantly after *PLIN5* overexpression ($p < 0.05$), but *SOD2* mRNA level was decreased (Figure 5C). After *PLIN5* knockdown, the mRNA levels of *GPX1*, *SOD1*, and *TXNRD1* were decreased significantly ($p < 0.05$; Figure 5D).

2.6. PLIN5 Reduced Apoptotic Rates of HepG2 Cells

The mitochondrial activity is important for the cellular apoptosis process; therefore, we further investigated the effect of *PLIN5* on the regulation of cellular apoptosis. The rates of apoptosis of HepG2 cells were detected by the flow cytometry method. The results showed that *PLIN5* overexpression decreased the apoptotic rates significantly ($p < 0.05$; Figure 5E). Subsequently, a rescue experiment was carried out. *PLIN5* was overexpressed in the cells treated with hydrogen peroxide for 12 h, and then the apoptotic rates were detected. The result indicated that *PLIN5* overexpression rescued the enhancement of cellular apoptosis induced by hydrogen peroxide treatment ($p < 0.05$; Figure 5F).

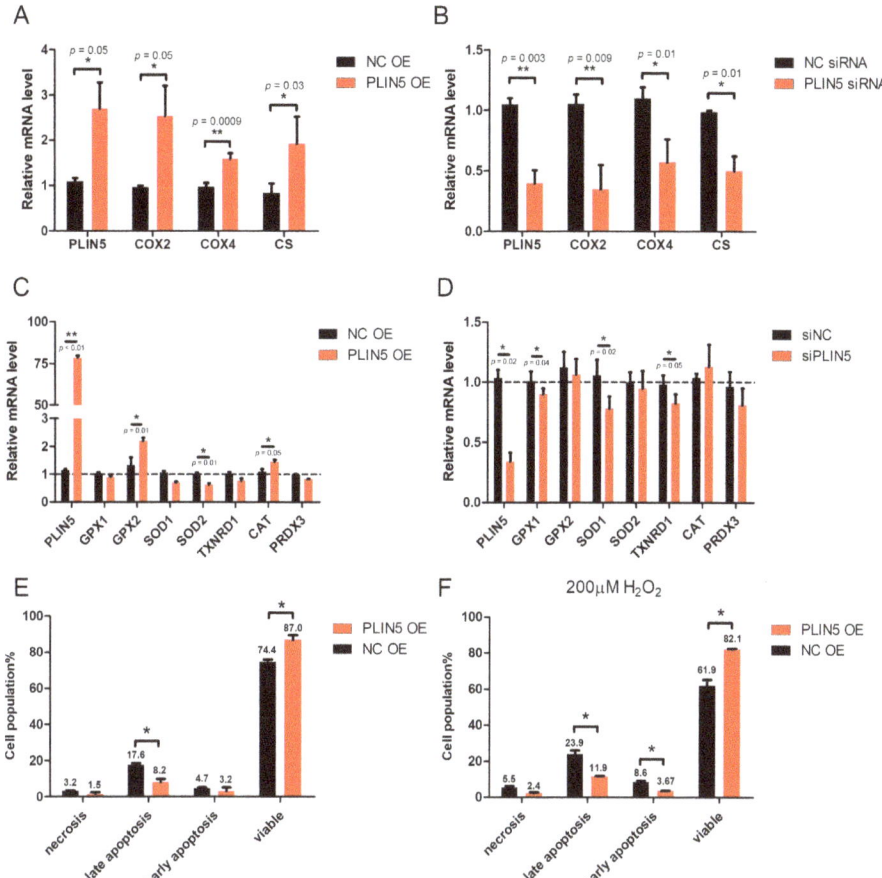

Figure 5. *PLIN5* regulated the expression levels of mitochondrial function-related genes and apoptosis rate. (**A**) mRNA levels of *COX2*, *COX4*, and *CS* in cells transfected with *PLIN5* expression vector or control vector. (**B**) mRNA levels of *COX2*, *COX4*, and *CS* in cells transfected with *PLIN5* siRNAs or control siRNAs. (**C**) mRNA levels of *GPX1*, *GPX2*, *SOD1*, *SOD2*, *TXNRD1*, *CAT*, and *PRDX3* in cells transfected with *PLIN5* expression vector or control vector. (**D**) mRNA levels of *GPX1*, *GPX2*, *SOD1*, *SOD2*, *TXNRD1*, *CAT*, and *PRDX3* in cells transfected with *PLIN5* siRNAs or control siRNAs. (**E**) Apoptosis rate of cells transfected with *PLIN5* expression vector or control vector. (**F**) Cells transfected with *PLIN5* expression vector or control vector were treated with 200 μM H_2O_2 for 12 h. Then, the apoptosis rate was analyzed. These experiments were performed in triplicate. *GAPDH* was used as the reference gene. * $p < 0.05$; and ** $p < 0.01$.

2.7. The Expression of PLIN5 Was Regulated by the JNK-p38-ATF Pathway

We analyzed the promoter region to investigate the transcriptional regulation mechanism of *PLIN5* expression. The GeneHancer dataset showed two potential promoter/enhancer regions (GH19J004539 and GH19J004534) whose distances from TSS (transcription start site) were −5.3 kb and +0.1 kb. Then, the transcription factor binding sites in these two regions were analyzed. We found that these two regions contained *JNK*, *ATF1*, and *ATF4* binding sites. It is well known that JNK-p38 is an important signaling involved in stress response, which is activated by oxidative stress, DNA damage, and UV, and subsequently regulates the downstream targets' expression, such as ATFs and STATs [31–34]. We have shown that *PLIN5* was up-regulated by hydrogen peroxide treatment; therefore, we assumed that

PLIN5 expression was regulated by the JNK-p38-ATF pathway. The phosphorylation levels of *p38* and *JNK* were detected. The Western Blot results indicated that *p-p38* and *p-JNK* levels were significantly increased in cells with hydrogen peroxide treatment ($p < 0.05$; Figure 6A,B). Moreover, the downstream targets of JNK-p38, *ATF1*, and *ATF4* were also up-regulated (Figure 6A,B). To further investigate whether ATFs regulate *PLIN5* expression, we overexpressed ATF1 and ATF4 and detected the *PLIN5* expression levels of both mRNA and protein. The qPCR and WB results showed that both mRNA and protein levels of *PLIN5* were increased significantly by either *ATF1* or *ATF4* overexpression ($p < 0.05$; Figure 6C–E). Subsequently, we cloned the promoter/enhancer regions of *PLIN5* (−2 kb) into pGL3-basic reporter vector to confirm the regulatory role of ATFs in *PLIN5* expression. The dual luciferase reporter gene assay showed that the fluorescence intensity of cells with *ATF1* or *ATF4* overexpression was much higher than that of the control cells (Figure 6F). The results indicated that both *ATF1* and *ATF4* did promote the transcriptional activity of *PLIN5*. To further validate the effect of JNK-p38 pathway on the expression of *PLIN5*, we utilized the p38-JNK pathway inhibitor, GS-4997 (Selonsertib). GS-4997 could inhibit the activity of *ASK1* so that to suppress the phosphorylation of downstream targets, *JNK* and *p38*. We found that hydrogen peroxide treatment activated the JNK-p38 pathway, but the GS-4997 treatment suppressed the JNK-p38 pathway (Figure 6G,H). Furthermore, we also found that hydrogen peroxide treatment increased the expression levels of *PLIN5*, and whereas GS-4997 treatment blocked the upregulation of *PLIN5* induced by hydrogen peroxide treatment (Figure 6G,H).

2.8. Low Expression of PLIN5 Is Associated with Poor Prognosis

We have shown that *PLIN5* expression was enhanced by oxidative stress and *PLIN5* could alleviate cellular ROS levels. We then analyzed the expression level of *PLIN5* in different kinds of tumors via the GEPIA (gene expression profiling interactive analysis) database (http://gepia.cancer-pku.cn/). Interestingly, many kinds of tumor samples showed lower *PLIN5* expression compared to normal samples (Figure 7A). Furthermore, among these kinds of tumor samples, liver hepatocellular carcinoma (LIHC), ovarian serous cystadenocarcinoma (OA), pancreatic adenocarcinoma (PAAD), and stomach adenocarcinoma (STAD) showed the largest differences (Figure 7B). Subsequently, survival analysis showed that the prognosis of LIHC was poor with a low expression level of *PLIN5* (Figure 7C). Then, survival analysis was performed to predicate the prognosis of 31 kinds of tumors with lower expressions of *PLIN5* (including ACC, BLCA, BRCA, CESC, CHOL, COAD, DLBC, ESCA, GBM, HNSC, KICH, KIRC, KIRP, LAML, LGG, LICH, LUAD, LUSC, OV, PPAD, READ, SARC, SKCM, STAD, TGCT, THCA, THYM, UCEC, and UCS; the extension of tumor abbreviations can be referred to in GEPIA). The result indicated that a low expression level of *PLIN5* was associated with poor prognosis (Figure 7D). These results indicated that low expression levels of *PLIN5* were bad for the prognosis of tumors.

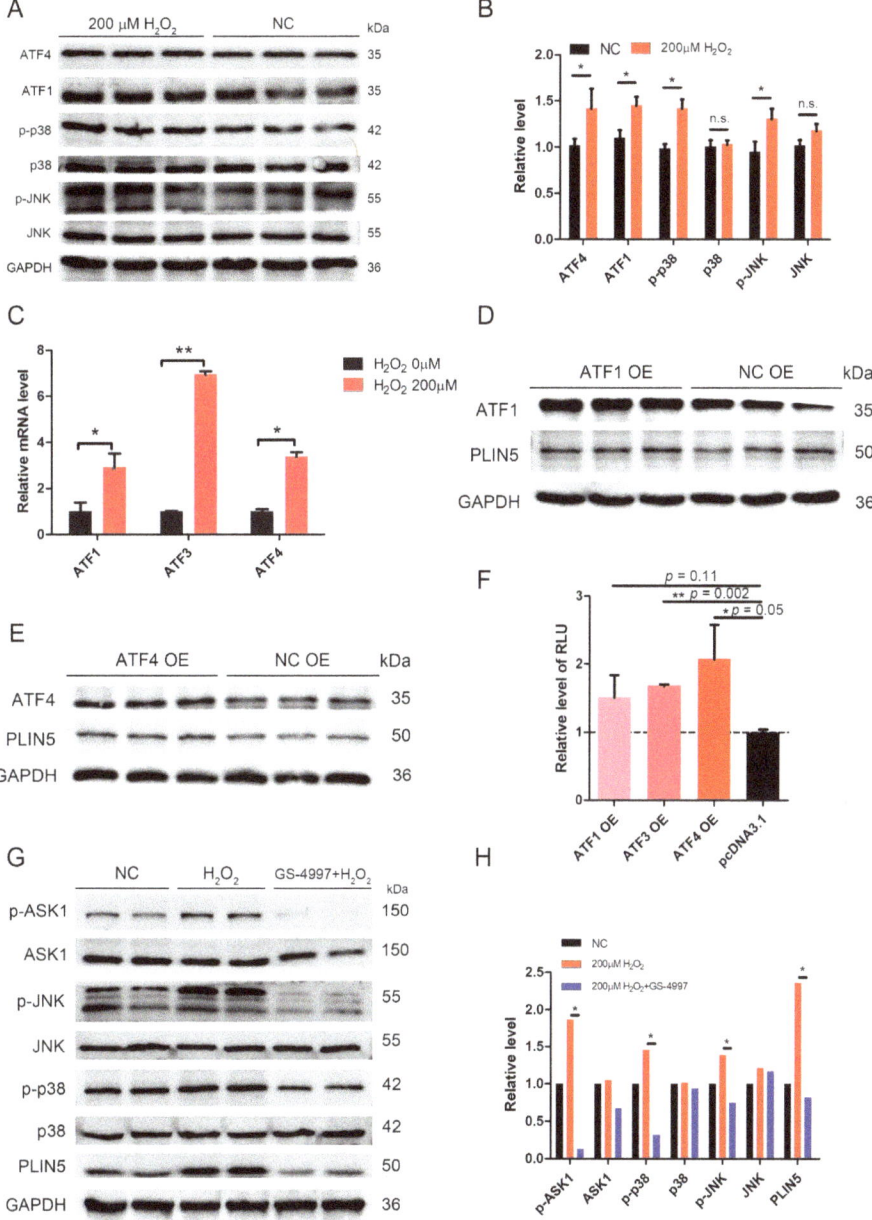

Figure 6. The expression of *PLIN5* was regulated by the JNK-p38-ATF pathway. (**A**) Protein levels of *ATF1, ATF4, p-p38, p38, p-JNK,* and *JNK* were detected by Western Blot. (**B**) The gray value analysis of A. (**C**) mRNA levels of *ATF1, ATF3,* and *ATF4* in cells with 200 μM H_2O_2 treatment were detected by qPCR. (**D**) The cells were transfected with *ATF1* expression vector or pcDNA3.1 vector. The protein levels of *ATF1* and *PLIN5* were detected through Western Blot. (**E**) The cells were transfected with *ATF4* expression vector or pcDNA3.1 vector. The protein levels of *ATF4* and *PLIN5* were detected through Western Blot. (**F**) The effects of ATFs' expression on *PLIN5* transcriptional activity were detected by dual-luciferase reporter assay. (**G**) Protein levels of *p-ASK1, Ask1, p-p38, p38, p-JNK, JNK,* and *PLIN5* were detected by Western Blot. (**H**) The gray value analysis of G. *GAPDH* was used as the reference protein. These experiments were performed in triplicate. * $p < 0.05$; ** $p < 0.01$; and n. s., not significant.

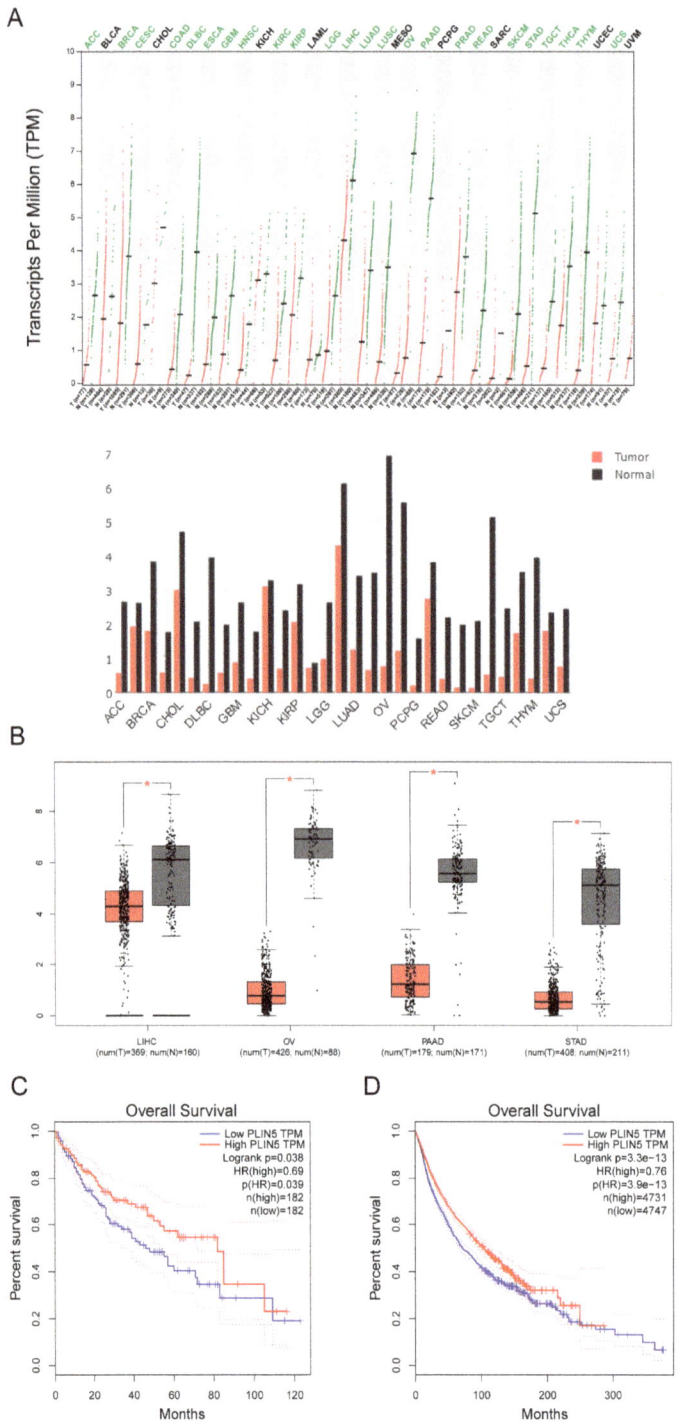

Figure 7. Low expression of *PLIN5* is associated with poor prognosis. Gene expression analysis and survival analysis were performed using the GEPIA database (http://gepia.cancer-pku.cn/). (**A**) Gene

expression analysis of *PLIN5* by cancer type. The lower pattern is the histogram illustration of the upper pattern. (**B**) The expression levels of *PLIN5* in samples with LIHC, OV, PAAD, STAD, and corresponding controls, respectively. (**C**) Survival analysis of *PLIN5* in LIHCtumor samples. (**D**) Survival analysis of PLIN5 in different kinds of tumor samples including ACC, BLCA, BRCA, CESC, CHOL, COAD, DLBC, ESCA, GBM, HNSC, KICH, KIRC, KIRP, LAML, LGG, LICH, LUAD, LUSC, OV, PPAD, READ, SARC, SKCM, STAD, TGCT, THCA, THYM, UCEC and UCS; E, CESC, DLBC, HNSC, LIHC, LUSC, PPAD and THYM; F, ACC, BLCA, BRCA, CESC, CHOL, COAD, DLBC, ESCA, GBM, HNSC, KICH, KIRC, KIRP, LAML, LGG, LICH, LUAD, LUSC, OV, PPAD, READ, SARC, SKCM, STAD, TGCT, THCA, THYM, UCEC, and UCS. The extension of tumor abbreviations can be referred to in the GEPIA database. * $p < 0.05$.

3. Discussion and Conclusions

NAFLD has become one of the most common liver metabolic diseases worldwide. One obvious characterization of NALFD is an accumulation of LDs. A high level of hepatic fat accumulation increased cellular free fatty acids in hepatocytes, which was induced by lipolysis. However, the overaccumulation of free acids is dangerous because of toxic metabolites generated by fatty acid breakdown. Moreover, high lipid content showed higher levels of ROS [35]. Indeed, in liver tissues with NAFLD, a high level of oxidative damage was observed [4]. The enhanced oxidative stress resulted in changes in mitochondrial permeability transition, which was able to decrease the mitochondrial membrane potential and subsequently induce cell apoptosis. It is well known that decreasing the number of hepatocytes impairs the hepatic function and promotes NAFLD/NASH development [36]. Therefore, reducing cellular ROS levels contributed to the alleviation of oxidative damage, which was good for NAFLD/NASH treatment. However, the expression levels of SOD and other antioxidant enzymes, the main scavengers of cellular ROS, were decreased in NAFLD/NASH tissues [4]. Therefore, we considered that a compensation mechanism could exist to respond to this case.

PLIN5 is a conserved LD protein that belongs to the PAT family [13]. *PLIN5* is expressed mainly in tissues with high oxidative metabolism such as liver, skeletal muscle, cardiac muscle, and brown adipose tissues. It is interesting that *PLIN5* was reported to be the key factor regulating LDs contacting mitochondria [37]. 443-463aa is the key region that promotes LDs' recruitment to mitochondria [22]. The deletion of 443-463aa of *PLIN5* deprived the ability of *PLIN5* promoting LDs contacting mitochondria [22]. Additionally, 443-463aa region of *PLIN5* is highly conserved between different species [22]. A previous study has showed that the overexpression of *PLIN5* promoted cellular LD accumulation, whereas knockdown *PLIN5* enhanced fatty acid oxidation metabolism in liver cells [38]. Moreover, an SNP (single nucleotide polymorphism; rs327694326, NC_010444.4:g.74314701T>C) in Italy big white, Italy Duroc, and Peter ran pigs, which induced high expression levels of *PLIN5*, promoted lipid accumulation and decreased the levels of *HSL*, an important lipolysis. Ilan et al. overexpressed *PLIN5* in mouse brown adipocytes and found that more mitochondria surrounded LDs and lipid synthesis was enhanced to promote the expansion of LDs [22]. In our study, we found that the overexpression of *PLIN5* increased the number of cellular LDs, whereas *PLIN5* knockdown decreased the number of cellular LDs (Figure 4C,D). Moreover, we also found that *PLIN5* overexpression promoted LD contact with mitochondria.

It is well known that organelle contacts usually induce the exchange of proteins in the outer membrane. LD is a highly dynamic organelle, which contacts other organelles frequently, such as endoplasmic reticulum (ER), mitochondria, peroxisome, and autolysosome. Many studies have reported that LD–ER contacts resulted in ER proteins, such as lipid synthetases (*DGAT2*, *GPAT4*) transferring to LDs [39–42]. LD contact with ER is important to LDs' expansion and cellular lipid homeostasis. A previous study showed an interesting phenotype involving LDs contacting mitochondria and clearing harmful proteins from the outer mitochondrial membrane [26]. A high level of cellular ROS induced the damage, and when accumulated damage exceeded a certain threshold, the cells would undergo the apoptosis process. During this process, some specific proteins were translocated to mitochondria such as pro- and anti-apoptotic proteins, for example, *BAX*, *BCL-XS*, *BIK*, *BAK*, *BCL-2*,

BCL-XL, and CED [43,44]. Among these proteins, BAX played an important role in leading to a permeabilization of the outer mitochondrial membrane, which was able to subsequently induce the release of cytochrome c and apoptosis [45,46]. Interestingly, BAX and BCL-XL contained a protein domain consisting of two α-helices, which allowed them to localize to LDs. When LDs were in contact with mitochondria, BAX and BCL-XL were translocated to LDs from mitochondria [26]. Therefore, we considered that enhancing LD contact with mitochondria promoted the translocation process, which would subsequently modulate the stress response. In the present study, PLIN5 overexpression enhanced the contacts between LDs and mitochondria, and the cellular ROS levels were significantly decreased ($p < 0.05$; Figures 3 and 4). Moreover, we also detected the influence of PLIN5 expression on the expression of several anti-oxidant genes. The results showed that PLIN5 did affect several anti-oxidant enzymes. We considered that there was a little effect, because not so many anti-oxidant enzymes such as some isoforms of SOD, CAT, and GPX can be influenced by the change of PLIN5 expression. Therefore, the PLIN5-mediated LD contact with mitochondria could be an important mechanism for cells to respond to oxidative stress. For further study, the proteins of mitochondria and LDs in cells with PLIN5 overexpression and control could be isolated, respectively, to investigate whether PLIN5 overexpression promotes the proteins' translocation between these two organelles and to analyze the terms of proteins translocated through the mass spectrum method.

We investigated the regulatory pathway of PLIN5 during the oxidative stress process. It is well known that the JNK-p38 signaling pathway plays an important role in the stress response. When the ROS levels (such as cellular hydrogen peroxide) were elevated, apoptosis signal-regulating kinase 1 (ASK1) was activated and subsequently sustained the activation of JNK and p38 MAPK signaling [47]. The activated JNK and p38 MAPK signaling would further activate ATFs' expression [31–34]. In our study, JNK-p38 MAPK signaling was activated by hydrogen peroxide treatment, and then ATF1 and ATF4 expression levels were significantly increased ($p < 0.05$; Figure 6A), which corresponds to the previous studies. Through bioinformatic analysis, we found that the promoter region of PLIN5 contained the binding sites of ATFs. Therefore, we considered that the expression of ATFs could affect the expression levels of PLIN5. Overexpression of ATF1 or ATF4 indeed up-regulated PLIN5 (Figure 6B,C). Furthermore, we also validated the regulatory role of ATFs on PLIN5 expression experimentally, through dual luciferase reporter gene assay. The results confirmed that ATFs did indeed enhance the transcriptional activity of PLIN5. Therefore, we demonstrated that the ROS-JNK-p38-ATFs regulatory axis modulated the expression of PLIN5 so that it regulated the cellular stress response process. Moreover, many studies have reported that ASK1 signaling played an important role in NAFLD/NASH processes by promoting the inhibition of lipid and glucose metabolism [48–50] and by driving a strong inflammatory response [51]. Currently, ASK1 has become a key therapeutic target for NAFLD/NASH. For example, Selonsertib (GS-4997) is a highly selective and potent ASK1 inhibitor with potential anti-inflammatory, anti-tumor, and anti-fibrotic activities [52]. ASK1-JNK-p38 signaling was activated in NAFLD/NASH; therefore, PLIN5 expression levels were supported to increase also. Our results showed that PLIN5 expression was indeed up-regulated in liver tissues of mice fed with MCDD, which supported our hypothesis. We considered that PLIN5 up-regulation could be a rescue mechanism during NAFLD/NASH processes. Increased PLIN5 expression promoted LDs contacting mitochondria, enhanced the expression of mitochondrial functional genes and subsequently alleviated the cellular oxidative stress. We found that many kinds of tumors cells showed low expression levels of PLIN5 (Figure 7A). Previous studies showed that NAFLD and NASH were well-known risk factors of hepatocellular carcinoma (HCC) [53,54], whereas and HCC was a lipid-rich tumor. Patients with obesity and NAFLD/NASH show an increased intake of dietary fatty acids (FAs). Meanwhile, insulin resistance enhances lipolysis of adipose tissue, which causes an increased exogenous FA supply and results in the development of a "lipid-rich" environment for hepatocytes. As we all know, more FAs would promote cells to generate more ROS through β-oxidation process. High level of cellular ROS often induced cellular stress and promoted cell apoptosis. However, we found that PLIN5 could reduce cellular ROS levels and reduce cell apoptosis in the present study. Moreover, we also found that expression of *PLIN5* could increase cellular lipid content. Previous studies reported that the lipid-rich environment is considered to promote the proliferation and metastasis of tumor cells [55–57]. Therefore, we considered that both functions of *PLIN5*, regulating cellular ROS levels and regulating cellular lipid content and lipolysis, could influence the tumor development process. Consequently, the down-regulation of *PLIN5* could be a predisposition for tumors' occurrence. *PLIN5* can be a good therapeutic target for NAFLD due to its ability to protect against oxidative stress and enhance mitochondrial function.

In the present study, we found that increase of cellular ROS induced by hydrogen peroxide or LPS treatment could up-regulate *PLIN5* expression. We then identified that ROS regulates the expression levels of *PLIN5* through JNK-p38-ATF signaling. Furthermore, we found that *PLIN5* could regulate the expression levels of mitochondrial cytochrome c oxidases (COXs) such as *COX2*, *COX4* and *CS*. Therefore, *PLIN5* could decrease cellular ROS levels through reducing the generation of ROS products by mitochondria, because up-regulation of COXs could reduce ROS products. Above is the novelty of this study. However, there are also several limitations in this study. The regulatory mechanism of *PLIN5* modulating the expression of COXs need further study. For example, studying the mechanism of protein exchange between LD and mitochondria during these two organelles contact. The LDs in cells with *PLIN5* overexpression could be isolated and the LD-related proteins on LD surface could be analyzed by mass spectrometry. Subsequently, whether *PLIN5* could promote protein exchange between LD and mitochondria can be investigated, by detecting the levels of mitochondrial-derived proteins on LD surface. Moreover, we noted that *PLIN5* could influence the expression levels of cellular anti-oxidative enzymes, such as *SOD1*, *SOD2*, *GPX1*, *GPX2*, and *CAT*. Although the effect of *PLIN5* on the expression of these enzymes was very mild, the mechanism is worth further study.

In conclusion, ROS-mediated activation of JNK-p38-ATF signaling up-regulated expression levels of *PLIN5*, and, then, increased *PLIN5* levels enhanced lipid synthesis and promoted LD contact with mitochondria, which helped cells to modulate stress response (Figure 8). Moreover, our study suggests that *PLIN5* could be a therapeutic target for NAFLD.

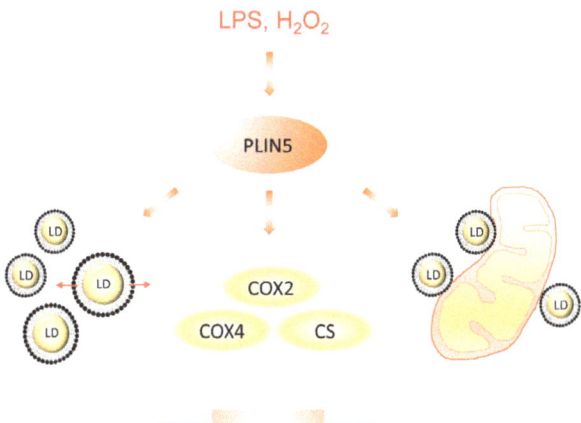

Figure 8. Diagrammatic sketch of this study. *PLIN5* was up-regulated by cellular stress induced by H_2O_2 or LPS treatment. Then, the increased *PLIN5* levels promoted cellular LD formation and expansion, expression levels of COXs and LDs contacting with mitochondria. Subsequently, LD formation and expansion reduced the levels of cellular fatty acids, which promoted the alleviation of stress. COXs' up-regulation reduced the release of cytochrome c from mitochondria to cytoplasm and reduced the mitochondrial damage. The contacts between LDs and mitochondria helped the transfer of potential harmful proteins from mitochondria to LDs. Therefore, cellular stress was alleviated.

4. Materials and Methods

4.1. Animals

Six-week-old c57/bl6 male mice were purchased from Hubei Center for Disease Control and Prevention. All mice were housed in a normal environment and were provided with food and water. The methods were carried out in accordance with approved guidelines from Huazhong Agricultural University and the scientific, ethical, and legal principles of the Hubei Regulations for the Administration of Affairs Concerning Experimental Animals. All of the experimental protocols were subject to approval by the Ethics Committee of Huazhong Agricultural University (HZAUMU2013-0005). The mice were fed with either a methionine-choline-deficient diet (MCDD) or a high-fat diet (HFD) to make a NAFLD phenotype in liver tissue. The mice were divided into nine groups, which were fed with MCDD for 0 week (control groups), 1 week, 2 weeks, 3 weeks, 4 weeks, 6 weeks, 8 weeks, and HFD for 10 weeks. The control groups of mice were fed with chow diet.

4.2. Cell Culture

The HepG2 cell line was gifted by the lab of Prof. Xianghua Yan, Huazhong Agricultural University (Wuhan, China), which was purchased from the Type Culture Collection of the Chinese Academy of Sciences (Wuhan, China). HepG2 cells were cultured in Dulbecco's Modified Eagle Medium (DMEM; HyClone, Logan, UT, USA) with 10% fetal bovine serum (FBS; #SH30396.03, Hyclone, Canada), 100 unit/mL penicillin, and 100 μg/mL streptomycin in dishes at 37 °C, in a humidified atmosphere, with 5% CO_2. For oleic acid treatment, a 20 mM oleic acid-phosphate buffer saline (PBS) mixture and 20% FA-free bovine serum albumin (BSA) medium were prepared, and both media were heated in a 70 °C water bath for 30 min. Finally, the media were mixed. The 10 mM oleic acid-BSA mixture was added to the cell cultural medium at 1:49 (v:v). The cells were then either seeded on slides, or on plates that had been washed three times using PBS. Then, 1 mL oleic acid medium was added to the well, and the cells were cultured for 12 h.

4.3. Antibodies

Rabbit polyclonal antibodies that were used included anti-PLIN5 (#26951-1-AP, Proteintech, Wuhan, China), anti-ATF1 (#11946-1-AP, Proteintech, Wuhan, China), anti-ATF4 (#10835-1-AP, Proteintech, Wuhan, China), anti-MAPK14 (p38; #A10832, Abclonal, Wuhan, China), anti-Phospho-MAPK14-T180/Y182 (#AP0526, Abclonal, Wuhan, China), anti-Phospho-JNK1/2/3-T183/T183/T221 (#AP0631, Abclonal, Wuhan, China), anti-ASK1 (#A6274; rabbit polyclonal antibody; ABclonal; 1:2000 dilution), anti- p-ASK1 (#AP0394; rabbit polyclonal antibody; ABclonal; 1:2000 dilution), anti-VDAC1/Porin (#55259-1-AP, Proteintech, Wuhan, China), and anti-GAPDH (#AC027, Abclonal, Wuhan, China). The mouse monoclonal antibody that was used included anti-JNK1/2/3 (#A11119, Abclonal, Wuhan, China). The following secondary antibodies were used: HRP (horseradish peroxidase)-labeled Goat Anti-Rabbit IgG (H+L; #AS014, Abclonal, Wuhan, China), and HRP-labeled Goat Anti-Mouse IgG (H+L; #AS003, Abclonal, Wuhan, China).

4.4. Transfection Assay

Cells were seeded on a 6-well plate or on slides in a 24-well plate. Then, the cells were transfected with Lipo8000™ Transfection Reagent (#C0533, Beyotime, Nanjing, China). For the preparation of RNAi working solution, 10 μL siRNA oligo (20 μM, Ribobio, Guangzhou, China) was mixed with 10 μL Lipo8000 regent in 100 μL DMEM. For the preparation of the overexpression working solution, 2.5 μg plasmid was mixed with 4 μL Lipo8000 regent in 50 μL DMEM. The working solution was added in the plate well and incubated for 6 h. Then, the plate well was changed with fresh cultural medium (DMEM with 10% FBS) for another 48 h of culture.

4.5. Plasmid DNA Construction

For the overexpression assay and the localization assay, expression vector and fluorescence-labeled vector were constructed. In brief, the *PLIN5/ATF1/ATF4* CDS region was amplified by the cDNA library of HepG2 cells using KOD-Plus-Neo DNA polymerase (#KOD-401, TOYOBO, Shanghai, China). After gel extraction, the *PLIN5* CDS fragment was cloned into the digested pcDNA3.1 vector (digestion sites, HindIII and BamHI) using a seamless cloning kit (#C112-01, ClonExpress II One Step Cloning Kit, Vazyme, Nanjing, China). For the localization assay, the gene CDS region was cloned into the digested pCMV-C-Dsred (#D2624, Beyotime Biotechnology, Nanjing, China) or pCMV-C-EGFP (#D2626, Beyotime Biotechnology, Nanjing, China). For the luciferase reporter assay, the promoter region of *PLIN5* (about 2000 bp upstream of the transcription initiation site of *PLIN5*) was cloned into the digested pGL3-basic vector (digestion sites, KpnI and XhoI).

4.6. Hydrogen Peroxide and LPS Treatment

The treatment process was the same as in our previous study [12]. Briefly, 30% hydrogen peroxide (i.e., 10 M) was diluted 10,000× by DMEM medium to 1 mM concentration, after the medium had been sterilized using a 0.22 µm filter. The hydrogen peroxide was then diluted to 200 µM and the medium was used to treat cells. The cells were then washed three times using PBS and were treated with different concentrations of hydrogen peroxide media; this operation is important for the treatment of hydrogen peroxide, especially if in low concentrations. Due to the significant impacts of small amounts of metals, such as iron and copper, on the outcomes of in vitro experiments, the medium contained ferric nitrate·9H_2O (0.1 mg/L). No other iron or copper was present. The water that was used in this experiment was double distilled and deionized.

4.7. Lipid Droplets Marking and Observation

The cell slides were fixed with 4% paraformaldehyde for 15 min at room temperature. The slides were stained with BODIPY 493/503 (#D3922, Invitrogen, Carlsbad, CA, USA) for 10 min at 37 °C and were then stained with DAPI (#G-1012, Servicebio) for 10 min at 37 °C. After washing three times with PBS for 10 min each, the slides were sealed with an anti-fluorescent quenching solution (#P36961, ProLong™ Diamond Antifade Mountant, Invitrogen, Thermo Fisher, USA) for confocal microscopic observation (63× oil lens, BODIPY FL and DAPI channels, Zeiss LSM 800, Germany).

4.8. Western Blot

Western blotting was performed as reported previously [58]. Briefly, cells were collected and homogenized in lysis buffer (#P0013, Beyotime Biotechnology, Nanjing, China). Then, the homogenates were incubated with an SDS-PAGE sample loading buffer (#P0015A, Beyotime Biotechnology, Nanjing, China) at 98 °C for 10 min. Subsequently, the samples were separated by 10% sodium dodecyl sulfate-polyacrylamide gel electrophoresis (SDS-PAGE) and were transferred to a polyvinylidene fluoride (PVDF) membrane (Biorad, USA) using a semidry electrophoretic apparatus. The blocked membranes (#P0252-100mL, QuickBlock™ Blocking Buffer for Western Blot, Beyotime Biotechnology, Nanjing, China) were incubated with antibodies overnight at 4 °C. The blots were extensively washed three times with tris-buffered saline with tween20 (TBST) buffer for 10 min and were incubated under gentle agitation with the primary antibodies for immunodetection at 37 °C for 1.5 h (diluted in QuickBlock™ Primary Antibody Dilution Buffer for Western Blot, #P0256, Beyotime Biotechnology, Nanjing, China). Then, the blots were extensively washed three times with TBST. Subsequently, blots were incubated under gentle agitation with the secondary antibodies for immunodetection at 37 °C for 1 h (diluted in QuickBlock™ Secondary Antibody Dilution Buffer for Western Blot, #P0258, Beyotime Biotechnology, Nanjing, China). For detection, M5 eECL Western Blot Kit (#MF-078-01, Mei5bio, Beijing, China) and the chemiluminescence imaging system (LAS4000, ImageQuant, Germany) were used.

4.9. Real-Time PCR

Real-time PCR was performed using the QuantStudio 6 Flex Real-Time PCR System (ABI, Thermo Fisher, Shanghai, China) and Roche LightCycler® 480 (Roche, Switzerland), and the following PCR program: Denaturation at 95 °C for 10 min; amplification for 45 cycles at 95 °C for 15 s; annealing and extension at 60 °C for 1 min. 2× SYBR Green qPCR Master Mix (#B21203, Bimake, Shanghai, China) were used for the detection of RT-qPCR. Primer sequences are shown in Table 1. Specific amplifications for certain PCR reactions were assessed using a melting curve. One negative control reaction, in which the cDNA template was replaced by water, was performed to avoid potential contamination. The sample from each well was repeated three times, and the comparative Ct ($2^{-\Delta\Delta Ct}$) value method was used for relative quantification. GAPDH (NM_002046.6) was used as the reference gene.

Table 1. Primer used for SYBR Green I qRT-PCR validation.

Gene Symbol	Primer Sequence 5'-3'
PLIN5 (Perilipin 5)	Forward: AAGGCCCTGAAGTGGGTTC Reverse: GCATGTGGTCTATCAGCTCCA
CS	Forward: GCTCCTGTTTCCATGGGTCA Reverse: TGCCAAAGCATGTCCAGCTA
COX2	Forward: GCTGTCCCCACATTAGGCTT Reverse: ACCGTAGTATACCCCCGGTC
COX4	Forward: CCCGGCATTTTACGACGTTC Reverse: AAAAATGTACACCTGCCGCC
ATF1	Forward: TTCGGATCTACCTGGGAGGG Reverse: CTGATAAAGATGATACCTGTTGAGC
ATF3	Forward: GACCAACCATGCCTTGAGGA Reverse: GGATGGCAAACCTCAGCTCT
ATF4	Forward: TAAGCCATGGCGTGAGTACC Reverse: GCGCTCGTTAAATCGCTTCC
GAPDH	Forward: CTGGGCTACACTGAGCACC Reverse: AAGTGGTCGTTGAGGGCAATG
CAT	Forward: TGGGATCTCGTTGGAAATAACAC Reverse: TCAGGACGTAGGCTCCAGAAG
GPX1	Forward: CAGTCGGTGTATGCCTTCTCG Reverse: GAGGGACGCCACATTCTCG
GPX2	Forward: GAATGGGCAGAACGAGCATC Reverse: CCGGCCCTATGAGGAACTTC
SOD1	Forward: GGTGGGCCAAAGGATGAAGAG Reverse: CCACAAGCCAAACGACTTCC
SOD2	Forward: TTTCAATAAGGAACGGGGACAC Reverse: GTGCTCCCACACATCAATCC
TXNRD1	Forward: ATGGGCAATTTATTGGTCCTCAC Reverse: CCCAAGTAACGTGGTCTTTCAC
PRDX3	Forward: ACTGTGAAGTTGTCGCAGTCT Reverse: CACACCGTAGTCTCGGGAAA

4.10. Apoptosis and Mitochondrial Membrane Potential Analysis

The analysis was performed by Servicebio Co., Ltd. (Wuhan, China). Briefly, the cells with transfections were collected through trypsin digestion. Then, the cells were incubated by annexin V-FITC and propidium iodide (PI). Then, the apoptosis rates were detected through flow cytometry (Ex = 488 nm, FL1 (Em = 525 ± 20 nm) and FL2 (Em = 585 ± 21 nm)). Flow Jo software was used to analysis the rates of cells in different conditions. For mitochondrial membrane potential (MMP) analysis, JC-1 probe was used. Briefly, the cells were collected and counted. The cells were then incubated with 10 μg/mL JC-1 probe at 37 °C for 20 min. Cells were detected through flow cytometry (Ex = 488 nm, FL1 (Em = 525 ± 20 nm) and FL2 (Em = 585 ± 20 nm)). Flow Jo software was used for the analysis.

4.11. Bioinformatics and Data Analysis

The survival predication was performed using the GEPIA database (http://gepia.cancerpku.cn/). The prognosis analysis and gene expression analysis were performed according to the construction of the creator of this database [59].

4.12. Dual-Luciferase Reporter Assay

The promoter region of *PLIN5* was amplified by PCR with total DNA of HepG2 cells. The primers were used as following, F: 5′-GAAAACTGGATCGGATGAATTGG-3′ and R: 5′-CACCCCCGCCGGTCCCGC-3′. Then, the promoter region was cloned into the pGL3-basic vector. Then, the reconstructed vector was co-transfected with the ATFs expression or pcDNA3.1 (control) vectors and TK vector into HepG2 cells seeded into the 12-well plate. Moreover, pGL3-basic vector was used as the negative control and pGL3-CMV vector was used as the positive vector. Luciferase enzymatic activity was measured by a microplate reader from a multi-wavelength measurement system (PE Enspire, PerkinElmer, Germany) using a dual-luciferase reporter assay system (#RG027, Beyotime Biotechnology, Nanjing, China). The relative light unit (RLU) was normalized by a control group. The result was showed by the relative RLU. All transfections were performed in triplicate, and the data are expressed as the means ± SD.

4.13. Immunohistochemistry Assay

Liver tissue samples of MCDD- and HFD-fed mice and control mice were collected. Then, the samples were fixed in 4% paraformaldehyde for 24 h. The immunohistochemistry assay was entrusted by Servicebio (Wuhan, China). The detailed processes of this experiment can be referred to in our previous study [12].

4.14. Isolation of Cytosolic and Mitochondrial Fractions

The cell mitochondria isolation kit (#C3601, Beyotime Biotechnology, Nanjing, China) was utilized to isolate the cytosolic and mitochondrial fractions. Briefly, wash the cells with cold PBS and harvest the cells by trypsin-EDTA solution. Re-wash the cells two times and collect the cells by centrifuge, and then remove the supernatant. Add 1 mL mitochondrial isolation regent (with 1 mM PMSF) and resuspend the cells, and then incubate the suspension in an ice bath. Then the cell suspension was transferred to a glass homogenizer of appropriate size, and the homogenate was about 10–30 times. Centrifuge the cell homogenate at 600× g, 4 °C for 10 min. Then carefully transfer the supernatant to another centrifugal tube and centrifuge for 10 min at 11,000× g, 4 °C. The precipitation was the isolated mitochondria. The supernatant collected was then centrifuged for 10 min at 12,000× g, 4 °C. The supernatant was the cytoplasmic protein without mitochondria.

4.15. Fluorescence Image Analysis

The ImageJ software was utilized to analyze the number of mitochondria interacting LDs. Briefly, the fluorescence intensity was analyzed along with the dotted line (Figure 4G). If the LD is contacting mitochondria, the signal of Dsred (mitochondria) can be detected between or overlap the signal of BODIPY493/503 (lipid droplet). If the LD does not contact mitochondria, the signal of Dsred (mitochondria) is supposed to be losing between the signal of BODIPY493/503 (lipid droplet).

4.16. Survival Analysis and Normal/Cancer Gene Expression Comparison Analysis

The survival predication was performed by the GEPIA database (http://gepia.cancer-pku.cn/). The prognosis analysis and gene expression analysis were performed according to the construction of the creator of this database [59].

4.17. Statistical Analyses

All quantitative experiments were evaluated for statistical significance using the software GraphPad Prism v.5.0 (GraphPad Software, Inc. 7825 Fay Avenue, Suite 230 La Jolla, CA, USA), after verifying the normality of values and equivalence of variances. For lipid droplet counts, pixel quantification, LD-mitochondria contact site counts, fluorescence intensity, and qPCR analyses, means ± s.d. are displayed, and the statistical differences between overexpression or RNAi-treated or peroxide hydrogen-treated samples and controls were addressed using Student's two-tailed *t*-tests. The Student's *t*-test was utilized because the sample size in the experiment was small, and a sample mean and standard deviation can be obtained, and additionally samples came from normal or approximate normal population. A p-value < 0.05 was considered statistically significant.

Author Contributions: Y.J. conceived and designed the experiments. Y.T. and Q.W. performed the experiments (Y.T. performed the main part). Y.T. and Q.W. analyzed data. J.H. and X.W. contributed to the preparation of reagents/materials/analysis tools. Y.T. wrote the manuscript. Z.R. supervised this study.

Funding: This work was supported by the Fundamental Research Funds for the Central Universities (No. 2662018PY043), Hubei Agricultural Sciences and Technology Innovation Center Team of Livestock and Poultry Genetic Improvement and Healthy Breeding (2019-620-000-001-30) and the National Project for Breeding of Transgenic Pig (No. 2016ZX08006-002).

Conflicts of Interest: The authors declare that they have no competing interests.

Abbreviations

AMPK	protein kinase AMP-activated catalytic subunit
ASK	apoptosis signal-regulating kinase
ATF	activating transcription factor
BODIPY	4,4-difluoro-1,3,5,7,8-pentamethyl-4-bora-3a,4a-diaza-s-indacene
CAT	catalase
COX	cytochrome c oxidase subunit IV
CS	citrate synthase
Cyto c	cytochrome c
DCFH-DA	2,7-Dichlorodihydrofluorescein diacetate
GEPIA	gene expression profiling interactive analysis
GPX	glutathione peroxidase
HFD	high-fat diet
JC-1	5,5',6,6'-Tetrachloro-1,1',3,3'-tetraethyl-imidacarbocyanine
JNK	jnk c-Jun N-terminal kinase
LD	lipid droplet
LIHC	liver hepatocellular carcinoma
LPS	lipopolysaccharide
MAPK	mitogen-activated protein kinase
MCDD	methionine-choline-deficient diet
NAFLD	non-alcoholic fatty liver disease
NASH	non-alcoholic hepatitis
P38	mitogen-activated protein kinase 14
PAT	perilipin, adipophilin, and TIP47
PLIN5	perilipin 5
PNPLA2/ATGL	patatin like phospholipase domain containing 2
ROS	reactive oxygen species
SOD	superoxide dismutase

References

1. Anderson, N.; Borlak, J. Molecular Mechanisms and Therapeutic Targets in Steatosis and Steatohepatitis. *Pharmacol. Rev.* **2008**, *60*, 311–357. [CrossRef] [PubMed]

2. Malaguarnera, M.; Di, R.M.; Nicoletti, F.; Malaguarnera, L. Molecular mechanisms involved in NAFLD progression. *J. Mol. Med.* **2009**, *87*, 679. [CrossRef] [PubMed]
3. Wierzbicki, A.S.; Oben, J. Nonalcoholic fatty liver disease and lipids. *Curr. Opin. Lipidol.* **2012**, *23*, 345. [CrossRef] [PubMed]
4. Videla, L.A.; Rodrigo, R.; Orellana, M.; Fernandez, V.; Tapia, G.; Quiñones, L.; Varela, N.; Contreras, J.; Lazarte, R.; Csendes, A. Oxidative stress-related parameters in the liver of non-alcoholic fatty liver disease patients. *Clin. Sci.* **2004**, *106*, 261. [CrossRef] [PubMed]
5. Ashraf, N.U.; Sheikh, T.A. Endoplasmic reticulum stress and Oxidative stress in the pathogenesis of Non-alcoholic fatty liver disease. *Free Radic. Res.* **2015**, *49*, 1405–1418. [CrossRef] [PubMed]
6. Ceni, E.; Mello, T.; Galli, A. Pathogenesis of alcoholic liver disease: Role of oxidative metabolism. *World J. Gastroenterol.* **2014**, *20*, 17756–17772. [CrossRef] [PubMed]
7. Bailey, A.P.; Koster, G.; Guillermier, C.; Hirst, E.M.A.; MacRae, J.I.; Lechene, C.P.; Postle, A.D.; Gould, A.P. Antioxidant Role for Lipid Droplets in a Stem Cell Niche of Drosophila. *Cell* **2015**, *163*, 340–353. [CrossRef]
8. Welte, M.A. How Brain Fat Conquers Stress. *Cell* **2015**, *163*, 269–270. [CrossRef]
9. Valm, A.M.; Cohen, S.; Legant, W.R.; Melunis, J.; Hershberg, U.; Wait, E.; Cohen, A.R.; Davidson, M.W.; Betzig, E.; Lippincott-Schwartz, J. Applying systems-level spectral imaging and analysis to reveal the organelle interactome. *Nature* **2017**, *546*, 162–167. [CrossRef]
10. Romanauska, A.; Kohler, A. The Inner Nuclear Membrane is a Metabolically Active Territory that Generates Nuclear Lipid Droplets. *Cell* **2018**, *174*, 700–715. [CrossRef]
11. Soltysik, K.; Ohsaki, Y.; Tatematsu, T.; Cheng, J.L.; Fujimoto, T. Nuclear lipid droplets derive from a lipoprotein precursor and regulate phosphatidylcholine synthesis. *Nat. Commun.* **2019**, *10*, 473. [CrossRef] [PubMed]
12. Jin, Y.; Tan, Y.; Chen, L.; Liu, Y.; Ren, Z. Reactive Oxygen Species Induces Lipid Droplet Accumulation in HepG2 Cells by Increasing Perilipin 2 Expression. *Int. J. Mol. Sci.* **2018**, *19*, 3445. [CrossRef] [PubMed]
13. Dalen, K.T.; Dahl, T.; Holter, E.; Arntsen, B.; Londos, C.; Sztalryd, C.; Nebb, H.I. LSDP5 is a PAT protein specifically expressed in fatty acid oxidizing tissues. *BBA-Mol. Cell Biol. Lipids* **2007**, *1771*, 210–227. [CrossRef] [PubMed]
14. Mason, R.R.; Watt, M.J. Unraveling the roles of PLIN5: Linking cell biology to physiology. *Trends Endocrinol. Metab.* **2015**, *26*, 144–152. [CrossRef] [PubMed]
15. Wang, H.; Sztalryd, C. Oxidative tissue: Perilipin 5 links storage with the furnace. *Trends Endocrinol. Metab.* **2011**, *22*, 197–203. [CrossRef] [PubMed]
16. Whytock, K.L.; Shepherd, S.O.; Wagenmakers, A.J.M.; Strauss, J.A. Hormone-sensitive lipase preferentially redistributes to lipid droplets associated with perilipin-5 in human skeletal muscle during moderate-intensity exercise. *J. Physiol.* **2018**, *596*, 2077–2090. [CrossRef] [PubMed]
17. Langhi, C.; Marquart, T.J.; Allen, R.M.; Baldan, A. Perilipin-5 is regulated by statins and controls triglyceride contents in the hepatocyte. *J. Hepatol.* **2014**, *61*, 358–365. [CrossRef]
18. Harris, L.A.; Skinner, J.R.; Shew, T.M.; Pietka, T.A.; Abumrad, N.A.; Wolins, N.E. Perilipin 5-Driven Lipid Droplet Accumulation in Skeletal Muscle Stimulates the Expression of Fibroblast Growth Factor 21. *Diabetes* **2015**, *64*, 2757–2768. [CrossRef]
19. Bosma, M.; Sparks, L.M.; Hooiveld, G.J.; Jorgensen, J.A.; Houten, S.M.; Schrauwen, P.; Kersten, S.; Hesselink, M.K.C. Overexpression of PLIN5 in skeletal muscle promotes oxidative gene expression and intramyocellular lipid content without compromising insulin sensitivity. *BBA-Mol. Cell Biol. Lipids* **2013**, *1831*, 844–852. [CrossRef]
20. Bosma, M.; Minnaard, R.; Sparks, L.M.; Schaart, G.; Losen, M.; de Baets, M.H.; Duimel, H.; Kersten, S.; Bickel, P.E.; Schrauwen, P.; et al. The lipid droplet coat protein perilipin 5 also localizes to muscle mitochondria. *Histochem. Cell Biol.* **2012**, *137*, 205–216. [CrossRef]
21. Wang, H.; Sreenevasan, U.; Hu, H.; Saladino, A.; Polster, B.M.; Lund, L.M.; Gong, D.W.; Stanley, W.C.; Sztalryd, C. Perilipin 5, a lipid droplet-associated protein, provides physical and metabolic linkage to mitochondria. *J. Lipid Res.* **2011**, *52*, 2159–2168. [CrossRef] [PubMed]
22. Benador, I.Y.; Veliova, M.; Mahdaviani, K.; Petcherski, A.; Wikstrom, J.D.; Assali, E.A.; Acin-Perez, R.; Shum, M.; Oliveira, M.F.; Cinti, S.; et al. Mitochondria Bound to Lipid Droplets Have Unique Bioenergetics, Composition, and Dynamics that Support Lipid Droplet Expansion. *Cell Metab.* **2018**, *27*, 869–885. [CrossRef]

23. Nguyen, T.B.; Louie, S.M.; Daniele, J.R.; Tran, Q.; Dillin, A.; Zoncu, R.; Nomura, D.K.; Olzmann, J.A. DGAT1-Dependent Lipid Droplet Biogenesis Protects Mitochondrial Function during Starvation-Induced Autophagy. *Dev. Cell* **2017**, *42*, 9–21.e5. [CrossRef] [PubMed]
24. Rambold, A.S.; Cohen, S.; Lippincott-Schwartz, J. Fatty acid trafficking in starved cells: Regulation by lipid droplet lipolysis, autophagy, and mitochondrial fusion dynamics. *Dev. Cell* **2015**, *32*, 678–692. [CrossRef] [PubMed]
25. Herms, A.; Bosch, M.; Ariotti, N.; Reddy, B.J.N.; Fajardo, A.; Fernandez-Vidal, A.; Alvarez-Guaita, A.; Fernandez-Rojo, M.A.; Rentero, C.; Tebar, F.; et al. Cell-to-Cell Heterogeneity in Lipid Droplets Suggests a Mechanism to Reduce Lipotoxicity. *Curr. Biol.* **2013**, *23*, 1489–1496. [CrossRef] [PubMed]
26. Bischof, J.; Salzmann, M.; Streubel, M.K.; Hasek, J.; Geltinger, F.; Duschl, J.; Bresgen, N.; Briza, P.; Haskova, D.; Lejskovas, R.; et al. Clearing the outer mitochondrial membrane from harmful proteins via lipid droplets. *Cell Death Discov.* **2017**, *3*, 17016. [CrossRef] [PubMed]
27. Kimmel, A.R.; Sztalryd, C. Perilipin 5, a lipid droplet protein adapted to mitochondrial energy utilization. *Curr. Opin. Lipidol.* **2014**, *25*, 110–117. [CrossRef] [PubMed]
28. Turrens, J.F. Mitochondrial formation of reactive oxygen species. *J. Physiol.* **2003**, *552*, 335–344. [CrossRef] [PubMed]
29. Forman, H.J.; Kennedy, J.A. Role of Superoxide Radical in Mitochondrial Dehydrogenase Reactions. *Biochem. Biophys. Res. Commun.* **1974**, *60*, 1044–1050. [CrossRef]
30. Loschen, G.; Azzi, A.; Richter, C.; Flohe, L. Superoxide Radicals as Precursors of Mitochondrial Hydrogen-Peroxide. *FEBS Lett.* **1974**, *42*, 68–72. [CrossRef]
31. Bogoyevitch, M.A.; Ngoei, K.R.; Zhao, T.T.; Yeap, Y.Y.; Ng, D.C. c-Jun N-terminal kinase (JNK) signaling: Recent advances and challenges. *Biochim. Biophys. Acta* **2010**, *1804*, 463–475. [CrossRef] [PubMed]
32. Chen, F. JNK-induced apoptosis, compensatory growth, and cancer stem cells. *Cancer Res.* **2012**, *72*, 379–386. [CrossRef] [PubMed]
33. Coulthard, L.R.; White, D.E.; Jones, D.L.; McDermott, M.F.; Burchill, S.A. p38(MAPK): Stress responses from molecular mechanisms to therapeutics. *Trends Mol. Med.* **2009**, *15*, 369–379. [CrossRef] [PubMed]
34. Cuadrado, A.; Nebreda, A.R. Mechanisms and functions of p38 MAPK signalling. *Biochem. J.* **2010**, *429*, 403–417. [CrossRef] [PubMed]
35. Welte, M.A. Expanding Roles for Lipid Droplets. *Curr. Biol.* **2015**, *25*, R470–R481. [CrossRef] [PubMed]
36. Cao, S.S.; Kaufman, R.J. Targeting endoplasmic reticulum stress in metabolic disease. *Expert Opin. Ther. Targets* **2013**, *17*, 437–448. [CrossRef]
37. Olzmann, J.A.; Carvalho, P. Dynamics and functions of lipid droplets. *Nat. Rev. Mol. Cell Biol.* **2018**. [CrossRef] [PubMed]
38. Li, H.; Song, Y.; Zhang, L.J.; Gu, Y.; Li, F.F.; Pan, S.Y.; Jiang, L.N.; Liu, F.; Ye, J.; Li, Q. LSDP5 enhances triglyceride storage in hepatocytes by influencing lipolysis and fatty acid beta-oxidation of lipid droplets. *PLoS ONE* **2012**, *7*, e36712. [CrossRef]
39. Yuki, O.; Jinglei, C.; Michitaka, S.; Akikazu, F.; Toyoshi, F. Lipid droplets are arrested in the ER membrane by tight binding of lipidated apolipoprotein B-100. *J. Cell Sci.* **2008**, *121*, 2415–2422.
40. Jacquier, N.; Choudhary, V.; Mari, M.; Toulmay, A.; Reggiori, F.; Schneiter, R. Lipid droplets are functionally connected to the endoplasmic reticulum in Saccharomyces cerevisiae. *J. Cell Sci.* **2011**, *124*, 2424–2437. [CrossRef]
41. Alexandra, G.; Laura, B.; Gabriel, M.; Charlotta, F.; Fatima-Zahra, I.; Francesco, M.; Raul, G.; Júlia, M.; Eduard, S.; Pedro, C. The seipin complex Fld1/Ldb16 stabilizes ER-lipid droplet contact sites. *J. Cell Biol.* **2015**, *211*, 829–844.
42. Wang, H.; Becuwe, M.; Housden, B.E.; Chitraju, C.; Porras, A.J.; Graham, M.M.; Liu, X.N.; Thiam, A.R.; Savage, D.B.; Agarwal, A.K. Seipin is required for converting nascent to mature lipid droplets. *eLife* **2016**, *5*, e16582. [CrossRef] [PubMed]
43. Lindsay, J.; Esposti, M.D.; Gilmore, A.P. Bcl-2 proteins and mitochondria-Specificity in membrane targeting for death. *BBA-Mol. Cell Res.* **2011**, *1813*, 532–539. [CrossRef] [PubMed]
44. Happo, L.; Strasser, A.; Cory, S. BH3-only proteins in apoptosis at a glance. *J. Cell Sci.* **2012**, *125*, 1081–1087. [CrossRef] [PubMed]
45. Oltvai, Z.N.; Milliman, C.L.; Korsmeyer, S.J. Bcl-2 Heterodimerizes in-Vivo with a Conserved Homolog, Bax, That Accelerates Programmed Cell-Death. *Cell* **1993**, *74*, 609–619. [CrossRef]

46. Westphal, D.; Dewson, G.; Czabotar, P.E.; Kluck, R.M. Molecular biology of Bax and Bak activation and action. *BBA-Mol. Cell Res.* **2011**, *1813*, 521–531. [CrossRef]
47. Tobiume, K.; Matsuzawa, A.; Takahashi, T.; Nishitoh, H.; Morita, K.; Takeda, K.; Minowa, O.; Miyazono, K.; Noda, T.; Ichijo, H. ASK1 is required for sustained activations of JNK/p38 MAP kinases and apoptosis. *EMBO Rep.* **2001**, *2*, 222–228. [CrossRef]
48. Sun, P.; Zeng, Q.; Cheng, D.; Zhang, K.; Zheng, J.; Liu, Y.; Yuan, Y.F.; Tang, Y.D. Caspase Recruitment Domain Protein 6 protects against hepatic steatosis and insulin resistance by suppressing Ask1. *Hepatology* **2018**, *68*, 2212–2229. [CrossRef]
49. Ye, P.; Xiang, M.; Liao, H.; Liu, J.; Luo, H.; Wang, Y.; Huang, L.; Chen, M.; Xia, J. Dual-specificity Phosphatase 9 Protects Against Non-alcoholic Fatty Liver Disease in Mice via ASK1 Suppression. *Hepatology* **2018**, *69*, 76–93. [CrossRef]
50. Lawan, A.; Zhang, L.; Gatzke, F.; Min, K.; Jurczak, M.J.; Al-Mutairi, M.; Richter, P.; Camporez, J.P.; Couvillon, A.; Pesta, D. Hepatic mitogen-activated protein kinase phosphatase 1 selectively regulates glucose metabolism and energy homeostasis. *Mol. Cell. Biol.* **2015**, *35*, 26. [CrossRef]
51. Cingolani, F.; Czaja, M.J. Oxidized Albumin—A Trojan Horse for p38 MAPK-Mediated Inflammation in Decompensated Cirrhosis. *Hepatology* **2018**, *68*, 1678–1680. [CrossRef] [PubMed]
52. Loomba, R.; Lawitz, E.; Mantry, P.S.; Jayakumar, S.; Caldwell, S.H.; Arnold, H.; Diehl, A.M.; Djedjos, C.S.; Han, L.; Myers, R.P.; et al. The ASK1 inhibitor selonsertib in patients with nonalcoholic steatohepatitis: A randomized, phase 2 trial. *Hepatology* **2018**, *67*, 549–559. [CrossRef] [PubMed]
53. Nakagawa, H.; Umemura, A.; Taniguchi, K.; Font-Burgada, J.; Dhar, D.; Ogata, H.; Zhong, Z.Y.; Valasek, M.A.; Seki, E.; Hidalgo, J.; et al. ER Stress Cooperates with Hypernutrition to Trigger TNF-Dependent Spontaneous HCC Development. *Cancer Cell* **2014**, *26*, 331–343. [CrossRef] [PubMed]
54. Ohki, T.; Tateishi, R.; Shiina, S.; Goto, E.; Sato, T.; Nakagawa, H.; Masuzaki, R.; Goto, T.; Hamamura, K.; Kanai, F.; et al. Visceral fat accumulation is an independent risk factor for hepatocellular carcinoma recurrence after curative treatment in patients with suspected NASH. *Gut* **2009**, *58*, 839–844. [CrossRef] [PubMed]
55. Le, T.T.; Huff, T.B.; Cheng, J.X. Coherent anti-Stokes Raman scattering imaging of lipids in cancer metastasis. *BMC Cancer* **2009**, *9*, 42. [CrossRef] [PubMed]
56. Ramos, C.V.; Taylor, H.B. Lipid-rich carcinoma of the breast. A clinicopathologic analysis of 13 examples. *Cancer* **1974**, *33*, 812–819. [CrossRef]
57. de los Monteros, A.E.; Hellmen, E.; Ramirez, G.A.; Herraez, P.; Rodriguez, F.; Ordas, J.; Millán, Y.; Lara, A.; de las Mulas, J.M. Lipid-rich Carcinomas of the Mammary Gland in Seven Dogs: Clinicopathologic and Immunohistochemical Features. *Vet. Pathol.* **2003**, *40*, 718–723. [CrossRef] [PubMed]
58. Lv, Y.; Jin, Y.; Zhou, Y.; Jin, J.; Ma, Z.; Ren, Z. Deep sequencing of transcriptome profiling of GSTM2 knock-down in swine testis cells. *Sci. Rep.* **2016**, *6*, 38254. [CrossRef]
59. Tang, Z.; Li, C.; Kang, B.; Gao, G.; Li, C.; Zhang, Z. GEPIA: A web server for cancer and normal gene expression profiling and interactive analyses. *Nucleic Acids Res.* **2017**, *45*, W98–W102. [CrossRef]

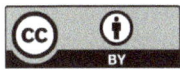

© 2019 by the authors. Licensee MDPI, Basel, Switzerland. This article is an open access article distributed under the terms and conditions of the Creative Commons Attribution (CC BY) license (http://creativecommons.org/licenses/by/4.0/).

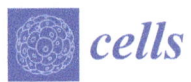

Article

Low VDAC1 Expression Is Associated with an Aggressive Phenotype and Reduced Overall Patient Survival in Cholangiocellular Carcinoma

René Günther Feichtinger [1,2,*,†], Daniel Neureiter [3,†], Ralf Kemmerling [3], Johannes Adalbert Mayr [2], Tobias Kiesslich [4] and Barbara Kofler [1,2,†]

1. Research Program for Receptor Biochemistry and Tumor Metabolism, Department of Pediatrics, University Hospital Salzburg of the Paracelsus Medical University, 5020 Salzburg, Austria; b.kofler@salk.at
2. Department of Pediatrics, University Hospital Salzburg of the Paracelsus Medical University, 5020 Salzburg, Austria; h.mayr@salk.at
3. Institute of Pathology, University Hospital Salzburg of the Paracelsus Medical University, 5020 Salzburg, Austria; d.neureiter@salk.at (D.N.); ralf.kemmerling@web.de (R.K.)
4. Laboratory for Tumor Biology and Experimental Therapies (TREAT), Institute of Physiology and Pathophysiology, Paracelsus Medical University, 5020 Salzburg, Austria; tobias.kiesslich@pmu.ac.at
* Correspondence: r.feichtinger@salk.at; Tel.: +43-5-7255-26276
† These authors contributed equally to the work.

Received: 17 May 2019; Accepted: 4 June 2019; Published: 4 June 2019

Abstract: Cancer cells frequently exhibit dysfunctional oxidative phosphorylation (OXPHOS) and a concomitant increase in glycolytic flux. We investigated the expression of OXPHOS complex subunits and mitochondrial mass in 34 human cholangiocellular carcinomas (CCCs) and adjacent normal tissue by using tissue microarrays. In the tumor periphery, all OXPHOS complexes were reduced except complex I. In addition, significantly lower levels of complex IV were found at the tumor center ($p < 0.0001$). Mitochondrial mass, as indicated by VDAC1 expression, was significantly increased in CCCs compared to corresponding normal tissue ($p < 0.0001$). VDAC1 levels were inversely correlated with UICC (Union Internationale Contre le Cancer) cancer stage classification ($p = 0.0065$). Furthermore, significantly lower VDAC1 was present in patients with lymph node involvement ($p = 0.02$). Consistent with this, patients whose carcinomas expressed VDAC1 at low to moderate levels had significantly reduced survival compared to high expressors ($p < 0.05$). Therefore, low mitochondrial mass is associated with more aggressive CCC. These metabolic features are indicative of a Warburg phenotype in CCCs. This metabolic signature has potential therapeutic implications because tumors with low mitochondrial function may be targeted by metabolic therapies such as a high-fat, low-carbohydrate ketogenic diet.

Keywords: cholangiocellular carcinoma; mitochondria; energy metabolism; oxidative phosphorylation

1. Introduction

Cholangiocellular carcinomas (CCCs) are rare but aggressive tumors that display features of biliary differentiation. CCCs comprise approximately 3% of gastrointestinal tumors and have an overall incidence of less than two per 100,000 [1]. According to their anatomical location, CCCs are commonly classified as intrahepatic and extrahepatic tumors, the latter entity being further subdivided into perihilar and distal tumors. In Germany, mortality from intrahepatic CCCs more than tripled between 1998 and 2008 [2]. In line with the increased mortality data, the number of reported cases of intrahepatic CCC also increased between 1970 and 2006 [3]. CCC is one of the most fatal cancers: the median overall survival is 20–28 months and five-year survival rates are about 25% [4,5]. In the United States, the number of CCC-related deaths per annum increased dramatically in the past two decades, surpassing 7000 by 2013 [6]. CCC mortality for those aged 25+ increased 36% between 1999 and 2014 [6]. The only curative option for CCC is surgical resection, but most patients develop a recurrence after resection.

Increased glucose metabolism and uptake is a hallmark of aggressive cancer. Accordingly, elevated ^{18}Fluorodesoxyglucose (FDG) uptake was present in 92% of CCCs [7]. This phenomenon, also called the Warburg effect, indicates that cancer cells generate energy predominantly via glycolysis even if sufficient oxygen is present. At first, it seems paradoxical that tumors use 'inefficient' glycolysis instead of OXPHOS for energy production. However, there are several explanations for why ATP generation is reprogrammed in cancer cells. First, aerobic glycolysis is not as inefficient as is often reported. Although it is correct that the amount of ATP generated per molecule of glucose is low, the rate of glucose metabolism is high in cancer cells. The production of lactate from glucose occurs 10–100 times faster than the complete oxidation in mitochondria, and the level of ATP production is similar [8]. Thus, rewiring energy metabolism toward glycolysis causes increased generation of lactate. Several studies suggested that lactate facilitates metastasis via production of a microenvironment toxic to normal cells and stimulation of tissue lysis [9,10]. Lactate dehydrogenase A (LDHA) catalyzes the inter-conversion of pyruvate and L-lactate with concomitant inter-conversion of nicotinamide adenine dinucleotide (NADH) and NAD$^+$ [11]. Secondly, the Warburg effect has been proposed to be an adaptive mechanism to support the biosynthetic requirements of uncontrolled proliferation. Glucose metabolites serve as carbon sources for anabolic processes. The excess carbon is diverted into branching pathways emanating from glycolysis and is used for the generation of cellular building blocks such as nucleotides, lipids, and proteins [12–15]. Another theory proposes that tumors shut down OXPHOS to reduce the reactive oxygen species (ROS) burden on their own biomolecules, while maintaining a level necessary for cell signaling [14]. The respiratory chain complexes are the main production sites of ROS, although their individual contributions to this process likely differ, with complex I being the most important in this vicious circle [16].

Immunohistochemical (IHC) staining of OXPHOS complexes of homogeneous tissue samples correlates well with enzymatic analysis, as the OXPHOS system is mainly regulated via the protein amount [17–19]. In the present study, we used IHC for technical reasons, foremost because it is nearly impossible to obtain sufficient amounts of frozen CCC tissue for functional evaluation of OXPHOS enzymes. In addition, substantial cellular heterogeneity is present within single tumors. Furthermore, a tumor cell content of over 80% is needed to generate reliable functional data on OXPHOS enzyme activity. IHC staining of heterogeneous samples is the method of choice because it reliably reflects the in vivo situation at the cellular level [18,19].

Therefore, the aim of the present study was to characterize the OXPHOS phenotype of CCC by IHC using tissue microarrays.

2. Materials and Methods

2.1. Ethics

Human tumors were obtained from the Institute of Pathology, University Hospital Salzburg. The study was performed according to the Austrian Gene Technology Act. Experiments were conducted in accordance with the Helsinki Declaration of 1975 (revised 2013) and the guidelines of the local ethics committee, being no clinical drug trial or epidemiological investigation. All patients signed an informed consent document concerning the surgical intervention. Furthermore, the study did not extend to the examination of individual case records. Patient anonymity was ensured at all times. All analyses on human CCC samples were approved by the local ethics committee (415-EP/73/37-2011).

2.2. Samples

To evaluate differences in expression between malignant and corresponding normal tissue, we constructed a tissue microarray (TMA) of formalin-fixed, paraffin-embedded (FFPE) tissue blocks from 34 individuals with CCC. Three punches of each individual were analyzed: the tumor center, the tumor periphery, and the adjacent normal tissue. Samples were analyzed by two professional pathologists and the mean values were taken for statistics.

2.3. Clinical Parameters

The following clinical parameters were evaluated: age, sex, overall survival from the day of diagnosis, localization (intrahepatic, perihilar, extrahepatic), growth type (mass forming, periductal, intraductal), tumor size, TNM (tumor, node, metastasis) classification, metastasis, UICC (Union Internationale Contre le Cancer), grading, etiology (Table S1).

2.4. Immunohistochemical Staining of OXPHOS Complex Subunits and VDAC1 (Porin) of FFPE Tissues

All primary antibodies (Table 1) were diluted in Dako antibody diluent with background-reducing components (Dako, Glostrup, Denmark). Immunohistochemistry was performed as described previously [20]. For antigen retrieval, the sections were immersed for 45 min in 1 mM EDTA, 0.05% Tween-20, pH 8, at 95 °C. Tissue sections were incubated for 30 min with the above-listed primary antibodies (Table 1).

Table 1. Antibodies used for immunohistochemical (IHC) staining.

Target Structure/Antigen Specificity (Species)	Vendor	Catalogue No.	Dilution
VDAC1	Abcam	Ab14734	1:2000
NDUFS4 (Complex I)	Abcam	Ab55540	1:1000
SDHA (Complex II)	Abcam	Ab14715	1:2000
UQCRC2 (Complex III)	Abcam	Ab14745	1:1500
MT-CO1 (Complex IV)	Abcam	Ab14705	1:1000
ATP5F1A (Complex V)	Abcam	Ab14748	1:2000
Ck7	Novocastra Laboratories	NCL-L-CK7-OVTL	1:100
Ck19	DakoCytomation	NCL-CK19	1:100
Vimentin	DakoCytomation	M0725	1:2000
Ki67	DakoCytomation	M7249	1:500
p16	mtm laboratories AG	9511	[a]
p27	DakoCytomation	M7203	1:100
p53	DakoCytomation	M7001	1:200

[a] according to the manufacturer's instructions.

2.5. Statistical Analysis

For comparison of tumors and normal adjacent tissue, a t-test was applied. For multiple comparisons, one-way ANOVA and Bonferroni correction were applied. The Pearson correlation was applied to analyze potential associations between the evaluated parameters. For analysis of survival, Kaplan–Meier curves were used.

3. Results

3.1. IHC Scoring

Staining intensities were rated using a scoring system ranging from 0 to 3, with 0 indicating no staining, 1 being mild, 2 moderate, and 3 strong staining. Score values were obtained by multiplying the staining intensity by the percentage of positive cells. The percentage of positive cells was analyzed with 10% increments. For 10–20% of positive cells a median value of 15% was used for statistics. Examples for immunohistochemical scorings are shown in Figure 1.

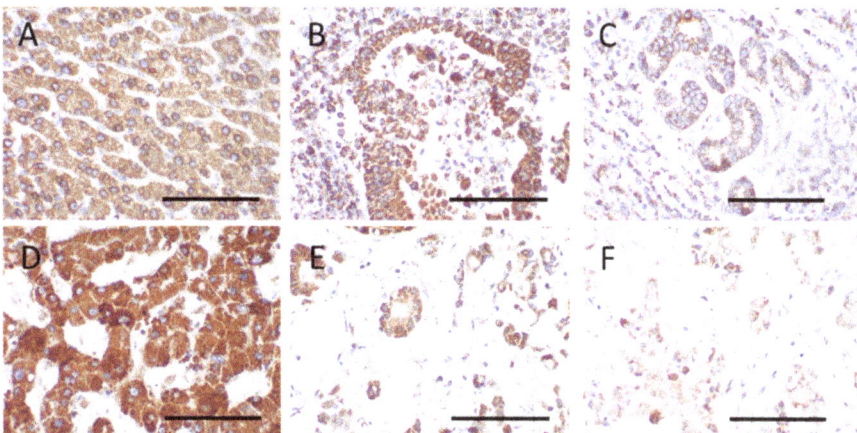

Figure 1. Immunohistochemical staining of VDAC1 and SDHA in the tumor center and periphery and normal adjacent tissue. (**A–C**) VDAC1 (case 28); (**D–F**) SDHA (case 4); (**A,D**) normal tissue; (**B,E**) tumor center; (**C,F**) tumor periphery. The following score values were evaluated for the images: Score value = intensity × percent positive cells; (**A**) 150 = 2 × 75; (**B**) 295 = 3 × 85; (**C**) 97.5 = 1.5 × 65; (**D**) 255 = 3 × 85; (**E**) 187.5 = 2.5 × 75; (**F**) 130 = 2 × 65. Magnification = 400×. Scale bar = 100 µm.

3.2. Expression of VDAC1 and Subunits of the Five OXPHOS Complexes

VDAC1 was used as a marker for the mitochondrial mass. It is highly expressed in the outer mitochondrial membrane which is otherwise relatively sparse of proteins. Therefore it represents the gold standard for determination of the mitochondrial amount. Protein complexes of the OXPHOS are localized in the inner mitochondrial membrane where they transport electrons to generate a proton gradient used by the ATP synthase (complex V) to make ATP. Subunits for each of the five OXPHOS complexes were analyzed in CCCs. Complex I (NADH coenzyme Q oxidoreductase) is the largest multisubunit complex of the OXPHOS system with a molecular mass of 970 kDa consisting of 45 subunits [21,22]. NDUFS4 is an iron–sulfur cluster-containing subunit incorporated during a very late stage of complex I assembly essential for complex I function. Complex II (succinate dehydrogenase) is the smallest complex consisting of four subunits and the only complex exclusively encoded by the nuclear DNA. Complex III (coenzyme Q: cytochrome c-oxidoreductase) consists of 22 subunits. Cytochrome b is the only mtDNA-encoded subunit of complex III [23]. Complex IV (cytochrome c oxidase) represents the last complex of the respiratory chain catalyzing the terminal step in reduction O_2. Three complex IV subunits are encoded by mtDNA. Complex V (ATP synthase) uses the protons translocated by the respiratory chain enzymes for production of ATP [23,24]. Complex I, complex III, and complex IV are furthermore organized in even bigger protein complexes, of which the most abundant one is termed respirasome [25].

Significantly higher VDAC1 expression was observed in the tumor center compared to adjacent normal tissue ($p < 0.0001$) (Figure 1A–C, Figure 2A,C and Figure 3A).

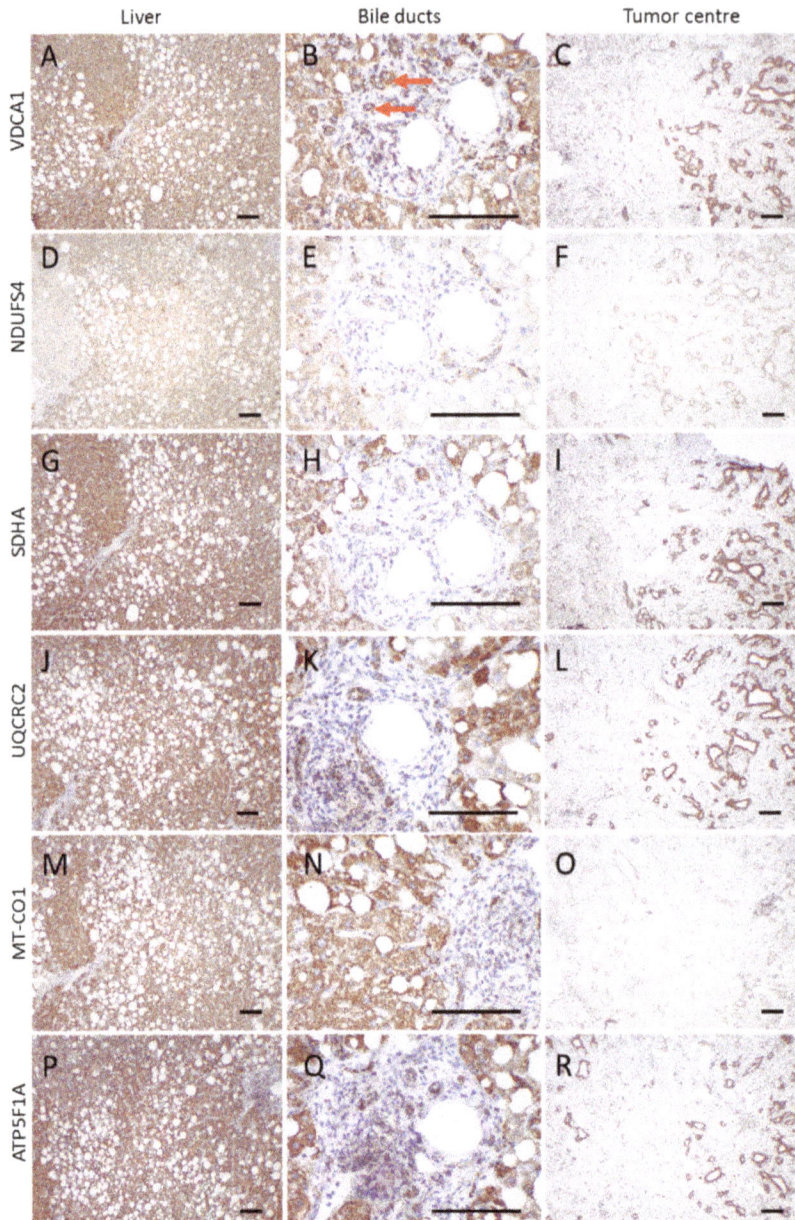

Figure 2. Immunohistochemical staining of a CCC and adjacent control tissue. (**A,D,G,J,M,P**) liver control tissue; (**B,E,H,K,N,O**) control bile duct tumor; (**C,F,I,L,O,R**) tumor center; (**A–C**) VDAC1; (**D–F**) NDUFS4; (**G–I**) SDHA; (**J–L**) UQCRC2; (**M–O**) MT-CO1; (**P–R**) ATP5F1A. Images of the liver and tumor center were taken at 100× magnification. For bile ducts a 400× magnification is shown. Scale bars = 100 µm. Red arrows highlight bile ducts. Case 11, a 59-year-old man, is shown.

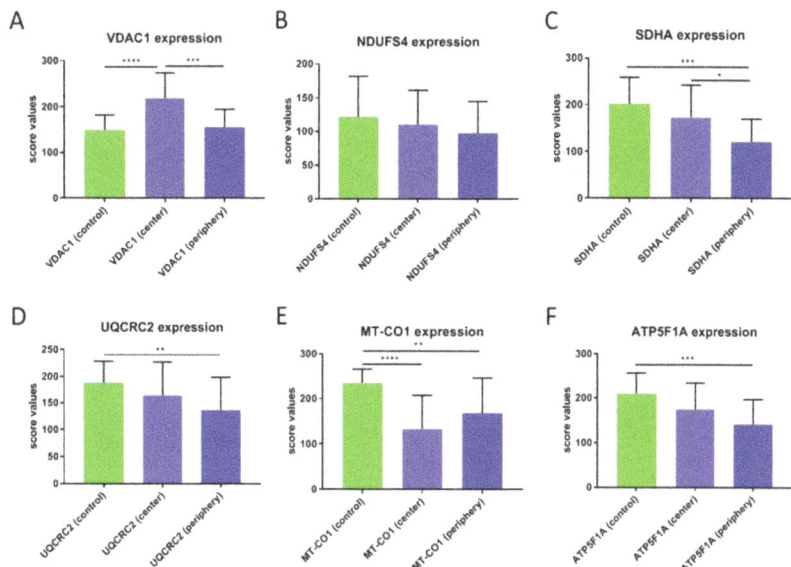

Figure 3. Score values of staining of the OXPHOS complexes and VDAC1 in CCCs. (**A**) VDAC1, (**B**) NDUFS4, (**C**) SDHA, (**D**) UQCRC2, (**E**) MT-CO1, (**F**) ATP5F1A. The mean score values ± SD of the staining of control tissues, tumor center, tumor periphery, and the average of center and periphery are given. **** $p < 0.0001$, *** $p < 0.001$, ** $p < 0.01$, * $p < 0.05$.

VDAC1 levels in the tumor periphery were similar to those in normal tissue and significantly lower than in the tumor center ($p < 0.001$) (Figure 1A–C and Figure 3A). NDUFS4 (subunit of complex I) expression did not differ between normal tissue and the tumor center or the periphery (Figures 2 and 3B). SDHA (subunit of complex II) levels were significantly lower in the tumor periphery than in the tumor center ($p < 0.05$) and in adjacent normal tissue ($p < 0.001$) (Figure 1D–F and Figure 3C). No significant difference was detected between the tumor center and normal tissue (Figure 1D,E). UQCRC2 (subunit of complex III) expression was lower in the periphery compared to the control tissue ($p < 0.01$) (Figure 3D). MT-CO1 (subunit of complex IV) protein levels were significantly reduced in both the center ($p < 0.0001$) and periphery ($p < 0.001$) of the tumors compared to normal tissue (Figure 3E). Finally, ATP5F1A (subunit of complex V/ATP synthase) was significantly diminished in the tumor periphery ($p < 0.001$) and showed a trend to lower levels in the center, compared to controls (Figure 3F).

Areas with cells negative for one or more OXPHOS subunits were found in both tumors and normal tissue (Figure 2D–F,M–O): 3% (tumor center), 21% (tumor periphery), and 25% (normal tissue) of the cases showed a loss of VDAC1 in more than 30% of the analyzed cells; 43% (tumor center), 60% (tumor periphery), and 35% (normal tissue) of the cases showed a loss of NDUFS4 (Figure 2F); 30% (tumor center), 54% (tumor periphery), and 11% (normal tissue) showed a loss of SDHA; 34% (tumor center), 54% (tumor periphery), and 10% (normal tissue) showed a loss of UQCRC2; 45% (tumor center) (Figure 2O), 41% (tumor periphery), 0% (normal tissue) showed a loss of MT-CO1; and 23% (tumor center), 30% (tumor periphery), and 0% (normal tissue) showed a loss of ATP5F1A.

3.3. Associations between OXPHOS Subunit and VDAC1 Expression and Clinical Outcome

A significant inverse correlation between the percentage of VDAC1-positive cells and MT-CO1-negative cells was detected ($p = 0.0093$). A significant inverse correlation was found between VDAC1 score values and UICC stage ($p = 0.0065$; $R = -0.4855$) (Table 2).

Table 2. Correlations of OXPHOS subunits and VDAC1 with respect to clinical parameters.

	VDAC1		NDUFS4		SDHA		UQCRC2		MT-CO1		ATP5F1A	
	p Value	R Value	p Value	R Value	p Value	R Value	p Value	R Value	p Value	R Value	p Value	R Value
Age at Diagnosis	0.4683	0.1376	0.6647	−0.0825	0.8635	0.0328	0.2555	−0.2182	0.2166	−0.2366	0.8365	−0.0394
Tumor Size	0.5292	0.1196	0.2929	0.1986	0.3501	0.1768	0.0833	0.3271	0.5767	0.1081	0.6339	−0.0906
TMN Stage	0.1458	−0.2721	0.5047	−0.1267	0.5106	−0.125	0.9133	0.0211	0.8660	0.0328	0.9418	−0.0139
UICC	0.0065	−0.4855	0.3039	−0.1941	0.3659	−0.1711	0.9702	−0.0073	0.5931	−0.1035	0.1066	−0.3005

VDAC1 levels in the tumor center were lower in cases with lymph node involvement ($p = 0.0201$). The tumor periphery showed a similar trend (mean score values N0 = 162 ± 31 versus N1 = 147 ± 46). The same trend was present when metastasis occurred in the tumor center (mean score value for M0 = 229 ± 54; mean score value for M1 = 186 ± 48) (Table 3). No differences were observed in the tumor periphery with respect to M stage. Significantly lower NDUFS4 levels were present in males compared to females ($p = 0.0454$).

Table 3. Mean staining scores of OXPHOS subunits and VDAC1 with respect to clinical parameters.

		VDAC1	p Value	NDUFS4	p Value	SDHA	UQCRC2	MT-CO1	ATP5F1A
Female	n = 9	215 ± 61		135 ± 51	0.0454	152 ± 84	154 ± 66	141 ± 84	179 ± 57
Male	n = 21	221 ± 54		103 ± 47		185 ± 61	166 ± 65	130 ± 71	175 ± 62
Intrahepatic	n = 16	224 ± 48		122 ± 50		182 ± 66	174 ± 61	148 ± 79	178 ± 54
Perihilar	n = 11	209 ± 64		104 ± 33		154 ± 77	141 ± 68	114 ± 74	170 ± 75
Extrahepatic	n = 3	224 ± 68		93 ± 103		221 ± 14	187 ± 68	123 ± 31	192 ± 36
Mass forming	n = 15	228 ± 49		116 ± 48		180 ± 61	178 ± 62	140 ± 81	172 ± 45
Periductal	n = 15	210 ± 61		109 ± 53		171 ± 77	148 ± 65	127 ± 67	181 ± 73
N stage 0	n = 18	240 ± 44	0.0201	115 ± 61		190 ± 63	177 ± 63	152 ± 76	187 ± 46
N stage 1	n = 12	187 ± 57		108 ± 29		153 ± 73	139 ± 62	104 ± 62	160 ± 75
M stage 0	n = 23	229 ± 54		116 ± 51		176 ± 71	161 ± 67	130 ± 82	175 ± 64
M stage 1	n = 7	186 ± 48		99 ± 45		174 ± 67	167 ± 59	147 ± 27	180 ± 49
Grade 2	n = 17	205 ± 63		105 ± 45		162 ± 62	150 ± 66	108 ± 67	160 ± 56
Grade 3	n = 11	239 ± 39		117 ± 53		179 ± 74	171 ± 65	164 ± 78	198 ± 51
R-status 0	n = 19	226 ± 52		106 ± 42		182 ± 62	176 ± 54	131 ± 60	167 ± 51
R-status 1	n = 11	207 ± 60		124 ± 62		164 ± 82	140 ± 76	140 ± 98	192 ± 73

The non-parametric Mann–Whitney test was used for analysis.

We divided the cases into high/moderate and low expressors. High expressors were defined as having staining intensities above 2. Since, in general, the staining intensities were lower for NDUFS4 and MT-CO1, high expressors for these subunits were defined by staining intensities above 1.5. A significant difference ($p < 0.05$) in survival was observed between these groups (high/moderate vs. low expressors) for VDAC1 expression (Figures 4 and 5).

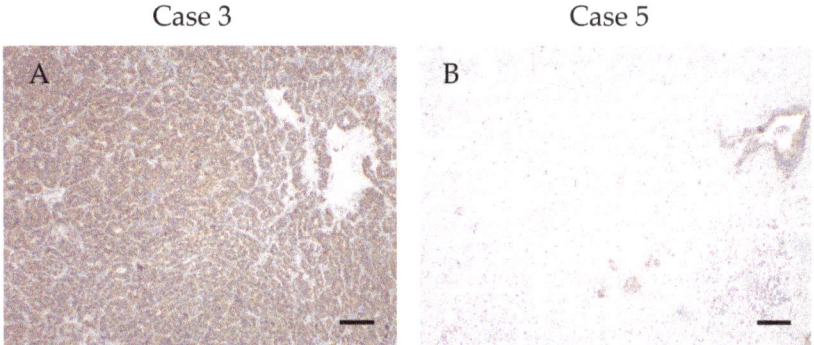

Figure 4. High and low VDAC1 expressors with low and high survival times. (**A**) High VDAC1 expression in case 3 with a survival time of 0.49 months. (**B**) Low VDAC1 expression in case 5 with a survival time of 30.05 months. Magnification 100×. Scale bar = 100 µm.

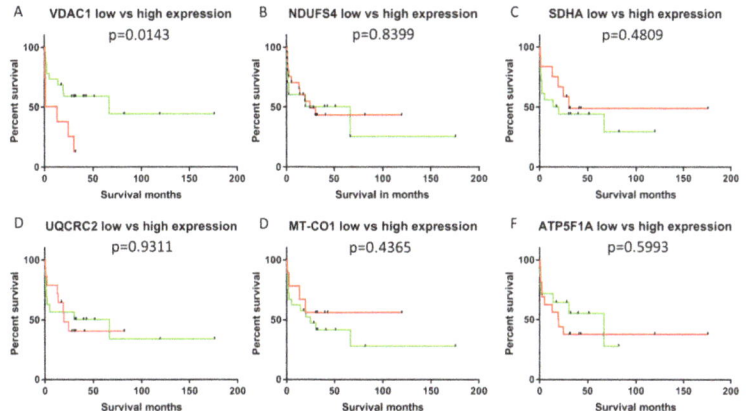

Figure 5. Kaplan–Meier plot of patients with cholangiocellular carcinomas exhibiting low/moderate or high VDAC1 staining intensity. High expressors are shown in red and low expressors in green. (**A**) VDAC1; (**B**) NDUFS4; (**C**) SDHA; (**D**) UQCRC2; (**E**) MT-CO1; (**F**) ATP5F1A. Significantly shorter survival was present in low/moderate expressors ($p < 0.05$).

No correlations were found between survival and expression of any of the markers of differentiation (epithelial: CK7, CK19; mesenchymal: vimentin), cell cycle proteins (p16, p27, p53 and Ki67) and OXPHOS subunits. Kaplan–Meier analysis revealed that individuals with tumors with high VDAC1 expression (staining intensity > 2) had significantly reduced overall survival ($p < 0.05$) compared to low expressors (staining intensity ≤ 2). None of the OXPHOS complexes was significantly associated with survival. Score values, extensities (percent positive/negative cells) and the intensities were used for the overall survival analysis. However, only the intensity of VDAC1 staining was associated with survival. Therefore, we suppose that the staining intensity might be an independent prognostic factor for CCCs indicating more an on–off-phenomenon than a gradient mechanism.

4. Discussion

The analysis of the mutational landscape revealed that TP53, KRAS (Kirsten rat sarcoma viral oncogene), IDH1 (Isocitrate dehydrogenase 1), and PTEN (Phosphatidylinositol 3,4,5-trisphosphate 3-phosphatase and dual-specificity protein phosphatase) are the most frequently mutated genes in intrahepatic CCCs [26]. Numerous studies have shown that p53 is involved in the regulation of many reactions in energy metabolism. p53 can be regarded as a master regulator of energy metabolism since it influences glycolysis, gluconeogenesis, the pentose-phosphate pathway, mitochondrial OXPHOS, and glutamine metabolism [27,28]. Mutations in the oncogene KRAS drive metabolic reprogramming through enhanced glucose uptake and regulation of glutamine metabolism [29]. Additionally, PTEN was shown to regulate several aspects of energy metabolism [30]. IDH1 catalyzes the reversible oxidative decarboxylation of isocitrate to yield α-ketoglutarate (α-KG). Under hypoxic conditions, IDH1 catalyzes the reverse reaction of α-KG to isocitrate, which contributes to citrate production via glutaminolysis [31,32]. In the present study, the levels of SDHA, UQCRC2, MT-CO1 and ATP5F1A were significantly reduced in the tumor periphery compared to the control tissue. Thus, genetic alterations of proteins influencing energy metabolism are clearly central to the pathogenesis of CCC.

Large areas of NDUFS4 negative cells were found in tumors and control tissue, suggesting that this is an early event in tumorigenesis. No patient had large negative regions of MT-CO1 or ATP5F1A in normal tissue. In addition, SDHA and UQCRC2 were affected in only 11% and 10% of the cases, respectively. Mitochondrial DNA was reported to be significantly mutated in CCCs [26,33]. This can partially explain the observed OXPHOS defects in our sample cohort. Moreover, the heteroplasmy of mtDNA mutations might explain the heterogeneity of the OXPHOS subunit expression [34]. According to the COSMIC database, potentially pathogenic mutations in nuclear-encoded OXPHOS subunits are very rare events in CCCs. Therefore, it would be interesting to analyze the mutational landscape (TP53, KRAS, IDH1, PTEN) in relation to the expression of OXPHOS subunits. However, it was not possible to perform a detailed genetic analysis because this was a retrospective study using formalin-fixed paraffin-embedded (FFPE) tissue.

As we found differences in the expression levels between the tumor center and periphery, we hypothesize that within CCCs, several modes of energy generation coexist. Tumor cells at the margin might be more dependent on glucose than tumor cells at the center, as indicated by the lower levels of OXPHOS subunits in the latter. This could be attributable to the fact that newly generated tumor cells at the growth front might not be sufficiently supplied with oxygen, because the generation of new blood vessels requires time. However, this hypothesis is controversial because necrosis is often seen in the tumor center, which is at least partially attributed (in the literature) to low oxygen supply.

Mitochondrial mass was increased in the tumor center compared to adjacent normal tissue, as indicated by VDAC1 staining. A significant inverse correlation found between the percentage of VDAC1-positive cells and MT-CO1-negative cells suggests there may be compensatory upregulation of mitochondrial mass. This phenomenon is well described in individuals with mitochondrial disorders, who frequently have increased mitochondrial content, as indicated by citrate synthase activity, VDAC1 levels, and mtDNA copy number [35]. In addition, oncocytic tumors, which are characterized by complex I defects caused by pathogenic mutations in mtDNA-encoded subunits, show a very pronounced increase in mitochondrial mass [19,36]. In addition, mtDNA content and mass increase in the tumorigenic progression of normal endometrial tissue to hyperplastic tissue to cancerous tissue [37]. MtDNA mutations and deletions have been reported in endometrial tumors [38].

Another possibility is that tumor cells at the periphery might express different sets of proteins compared to tumor cells in the center. The intercellular or cell–cell lactate shuttle hypothesis proposes that lactate is generated and exported from one cell and taken up and utilized by another cell. This mechanism has been described for neurons and astrocytes [39].

A significant inverse correlation was found between VDAC1 expression and UICC tumor stage. This agrees with findings in the literature, and may be explained as follows: aggressive tumors that are highly dependent on glucose should potentially exhibit low mitochondrial mass. In support, we found that VDAC1 levels were lower in cases with lymph node involvement. The same trend to lower VDAC1 levels was also present if metastasis occurred. Significantly lower survival was observed for low/moderate VDAC1 expressors compared to high expressors. That is, lower mitochondrial mass was associated with shorter survival.

The clear association between energy metabolism and CCC development has important therapeutic implications. CCCs might be susceptible to metabolic therapies such as the ketogenic (high-fat, low-carbohydrate) diet, which was recently shown to significantly inhibit tumor growth in numerous xenograft models and patients [40–43].

Supplementary Materials: The supplementary materials are available online at http://www.mdpi.com/2073-4409/8/6/539/s1.

Author Contributions: R.G.F. stained samples, analyzed data and wrote the first draft of the manuscript. D.N. and R.K. analyzed the IHC staining, prepared the tissue array and critically reviewed the manuscript. T.K. analyzed the IHC staining and provided material. B.K. and J.A.M. supervised the project. All authors discussed the results and commented on the manuscript.

Funding: This research was supported by grants from the "Vereinigung zur Förderung der pädiatrischen Forschung und Fortbildung Salzburg" and the Austrian Research Promotion Agency (822782/THERAPEP).

Conflicts of Interest: The authors declare no conflict of interest.

References

1. Bergquist, A.; von Seth, E. Epidemiology of cholangiocarcinoma. *Best Pr. Res. Clin. Gastroenterol.* **2015**, *29*, 221–232. [CrossRef] [PubMed]
2. Vogel, A.; Saborowski, A. Cholangiocellular Carcinoma. *Digestion* **2017**, *95*, 181–185. [CrossRef] [PubMed]
3. Von Hahn, T.; Ciesek, S.; Wegener, G.; Plentz, R.R.; Weismuller, T.J.; Wedemeyer, H.; Manns, M.P.; Greten, T.F.; Malek, N.P. Epidemiological trends in incidence and mortality of hepatobiliary cancers in Germany. *Scand. J. Gastroenterol.* **2011**, *46*, 1092–1098. [CrossRef] [PubMed]
4. Mavros, M.N.; Economopoulos, K.P.; Alexiou, V.G.; Pawlik, T.M. Treatment and Prognosis for Patients with Intrahepatic Cholangiocarcinoma: Systematic Review and Meta-analysis. *JAMA Surg.* **2014**, *149*, 565–574. [CrossRef]
5. Nathan, H.; Pawlik, T.M.; Wolfgang, C.L.; Choti, M.A.; Cameron, J.L.; Schulick, R.D. Trends in survival after surgery for cholangiocarcinoma: a 30-year population-based SEER database analysis. *J. Gastrointest. Surg.* **2007**, *11*, 1488–1496. [CrossRef]
6. Yao, K.J.; Jabbour, S.; Parekh, N.; Lin, Y.; Moss, R.A. Increasing mortality in the United States from cholangiocarcinoma: an analysis of the National Center for Health Statistics Database. *BMC Gastroenterol.* **2016**, *16*, 117. [CrossRef] [PubMed]
7. Jiang, L.; Tan, H.; Panje, C.M.; Yu, H.; Xiu, Y.; Shi, H. Role of 18F-FDG PET/CT Imaging in Intrahepatic Cholangiocarcinoma. *Clin. Nucl. Med.* **2016**, *41*, 1–7. [CrossRef]
8. Shestov, A.A.; Liu, X.; Ser, Z.; Cluntun, A.A.; Hung, Y.P.; Huang, L.; Kim, D.; Le, A.; Yellen, G.; Albeck, J.G.; et al. Quantitative determinants of aerobic glycolysis identify flux through the enzyme GAPDH as a limiting step. *Elife* **2014**, *3*, 03342. [CrossRef]
9. Estrella, V.; Chen, T.; Lloyd, M.; Wojtkowiak, J.; Cornnell, H.H.; Ibrahim-Hashim, A.; Bailey, K.; Balagurunathan, Y.; Rothberg, J.M.; Sloane, B.F.; et al. Acidity generated by the tumor microenvironment drives local invasion. *Cancer Res.* **2013**, *73*, 1524–1535. [CrossRef]
10. Gatenby, R.A.; Gawlinski, E.T. A reaction-diffusion model of cancer invasion. *Cancer Res.* **1996**, *56*, 5745–5753.
11. Hirschhaeuser, F.; Sattler, U.G.; Mueller-Klieser, W. Lactate: A metabolic key player in cancer. *Cancer Res.* **2011**, *71*, 6921–6925. [CrossRef]
12. Boroughs, L.K.; DeBerardinis, R.J. Metabolic pathways promoting cancer cell survival and growth. *Nat. Cell Biol.* **2015**, *17*, 351–359. [CrossRef]
13. Levine, A.J.; Puzio-Kuter, A.M. The control of the metabolic switch in cancers by oncogenes and tumor suppressor genes. *Science* **2010**, *330*, 1340–1344. [CrossRef]
14. Liberti, M.V.; Locasale, J.W. The Warburg Effect: How Does it Benefit Cancer Cells? *Trends Biochem. Sci.* **2016**, *41*, 211–218. [CrossRef]
15. Vander Heiden, M.G.; Cantley, L.C.; Thompson, C.B. Understanding the Warburg effect: The metabolic requirements of cell proliferation. *Science* **2009**, *324*, 1029–1033. [CrossRef]
16. Hirst, J.; King, M.S.; Pryde, K.R. The production of reactive oxygen species by complex I. *Biochem. Soc. Trans.* **2008**, *36*, 976–980. [CrossRef]

17. Feichtinger, R.G.; Neureiter, D.; Mayr, J.A.; Zimmermann, F.A.; Berthold, F.; Jones, N.; Sperl, W.; Kofler, B. Loss of mitochondria in ganglioneuromas. *Front. Biosci.* **2011**, *3*, 179–186.
18. Feichtinger, R.G.; Zimmermann, F.; Mayr, J.A.; Neureiter, D.; Hauser-Kronberger, C.; Schilling, F.H.; Jones, N.; Sperl, W.; Kofler, B. Low aerobic mitochondrial energy metabolism in poorly- or undifferentiated neuroblastoma. *BMC Cancer* **2010**, *10*, 149. [CrossRef]
19. Mayr, J.A.; Meierhofer, D.; Zimmermann, F.; Feichtinger, R.; Kogler, C.; Ratschek, M.; Schmeller, N.; Sperl, W.; Kofler, B. Loss of complex I due to mitochondrial DNA mutations in renal oncocytoma. *Clin. Cancer Res.* **2008**, *14*, 2270–2275. [CrossRef]
20. Zimmermann, F.A.; Mayr, J.A.; Neureiter, D.; Feichtinger, R.; Alinger, B.; Jones, N.D.; Eder, W.; Sperl, W.; Kofler, B. Lack of complex I is associated with oncocytic thyroid tumours. *Br. J. Cancer* **2009**, *100*, 1434–1437. [CrossRef]
21. Fiedorczuk, K.; Letts, J.A.; Degliesposti, G.; Kaszuba, K.; Skehel, M.; Sazanov, L.A. Atomic structure of the entire mammalian mitochondrial complex I. *Nature* **2016**, *538*, 406–410. [CrossRef]
22. Letts, J.A.; Sazanov, L.A. Gaining mass: The structure of respiratory complex I-from bacterial towards mitochondrial versions. *Curr. Opin. Struct. Biol.* **2015**, *33*, 135–145. [CrossRef]
23. Guo, R.; Gu, J.; Zong, S.; Wu, M.; Yang, M. Structure and mechanism of mitochondrial electron transport chain. *Biomed. J.* **2018**, *41*, 9–20. [CrossRef]
24. Song, J.; Pfanner, N.; Becker, T. Assembling the mitochondrial ATP synthase. *Proc. Natl. Acad. Sci. USA* **2018**, *115*, 2850–2852. [CrossRef]
25. Gu, J.; Wu, M.; Guo, R.; Yan, K.; Lei, J.; Gao, N.; Yang, M. The architecture of the mammalian respirasome. *Nature* **2016**, *537*, 639–643. [CrossRef]
26. Zou, S.; Li, J.; Zhou, H.; Frech, C.; Jiang, X.; Chu, J.S.; Zhao, X.; Li, Y.; Li, Q.; Wang, H.; et al. Mutational landscape of intrahepatic cholangiocarcinoma. *Nat. Commun.* **2014**, *5*, 5696. [CrossRef]
27. Itahana, Y.; Itahana, K. Emerging Roles of p53 Family Members in Glucose Metabolism. *Int. J. Mol. Sci.* **2018**, *19*, 776. [CrossRef]
28. Liang, Y.; Liu, J.; Feng, Z. The regulation of cellular metabolism by tumor suppressor p53. *Cell Biosci.* **2013**, *3*, 9. [CrossRef]
29. Hutton, J.E.; Wang, X.; Zimmerman, L.J.; Slebos, R.J.; Trenary, I.A.; Young, J.D.; Li, M.; Liebler, D.C. Oncogenic KRAS and BRAF Drive Metabolic Reprogramming in Colorectal Cancer. *Mol. Cell Proteom.* **2016**, *15*, 2924–2938. [CrossRef]
30. Liu, J.; Feng, Z. PTEN, energy metabolism and tumor suppression. *ACTA Biochim. Biophys. Sin.* **2012**, *44*, 629–631. [CrossRef]
31. Dimitrov, L.; Hong, C.S.; Yang, C.; Zhuang, Z.; Heiss, J.D. New developments in the pathogenesis and therapeutic targeting of the IDH1 mutation in glioma. *Int. J. Med. Sci.* **2015**, *12*, 201–213. [CrossRef]
32. Molenaar, R.J.; Radivoyevitch, T.; Maciejewski, J.P.; van Noorden, C.J.; Bleeker, F.E. The driver and passenger effects of isocitrate dehydrogenase 1 and 2 mutations in oncogenesis and survival prolongation. *Biochim. Et Biophys. ACTA* **2014**, *1846*, 326–341. [CrossRef]
33. Muisuk, K.; Silsirivanit, A.; Imtawil, K.; Bunthot, S.; Pukhem, A.; Pairojkul, C.; Wongkham, S.; Wongkham, C. Novel mutations in cholangiocarcinoma with low frequencies revealed by whole mitochondrial genome sequencing. *Asian Pac. J. Cancer Prev.* **2015**, *16*, 1737–1742. [CrossRef]
34. Wallace, D.C.; Chalkia, D. Mitochondrial DNA genetics and the heteroplasmy conundrum in evolution and disease. *Cold Spring Harb. Perspect. Biol.* **2013**, *5*, a021220. [CrossRef]
35. Picard, M.; Vincent, A.E.; Turnbull, D.M. Expanding Our Understanding of mtDNA Deletions. *Cell Metab.* **2016**, *24*, 3–4. [CrossRef]
36. Gasparre, G.; Porcelli, A.M.; Bonora, E.; Pennisi, L.F.; Toller, M.; Iommarini, L.; Ghelli, A.; Moretti, M.; Betts, C.M.; Martinelli, G.N.; et al. Disruptive mitochondrial DNA mutations in complex I subunits are markers of oncocytic phenotype in thyroid tumors. *Proc. Natl. Acad. Sci. USA* **2007**, *104*, 9001–9006. [CrossRef]
37. Cormio, A.; Guerra, F.; Cormio, G.; Pesce, V.; Fracasso, F.; Loizzi, V.; Resta, L.; Putignano, G.; Cantatore, P.; Selvaggi, L.E.; et al. Mitochondrial DNA content and mass increase in progression from normal to hyperplastic to cancer endometrium. *BMC Res. Notes* **2012**, *5*, 279. [CrossRef]

38. Guerra, F.; Kurelac, I.; Cormio, A.; Zuntini, R.; Amato, L.B.; Ceccarelli, C.; Santini, D.; Cormio, G.; Fracasso, F.; Selvaggi, L.; et al. Placing mitochondrial DNA mutations within the progression model of type I endometrial carcinoma. *Hum. Mol. Genet.* **2011**, *20*, 2394–2405. [CrossRef]
39. Genc, S.; Kurnaz, I.A.; Ozilgen, M. Astrocyte-neuron lactate shuttle may boost more ATP supply to the neuron under hypoxic conditions–in silico study supported by in vitro expression data. *BMC Syst. Biol.* **2011**, *5*, 162. [CrossRef]
40. Aminzadeh-Gohari, S.; Feichtinger, R.G.; Vidali, S.; Locker, F.; Rutherford, T.; O'Donnel, M.; Stoger-Kleiber, A.; Mayr, J.A.; Sperl, W.; Kofler, B. A ketogenic diet supplemented with medium-chain triglycerides enhances the anti-tumor and anti-angiogenic efficacy of chemotherapy on neuroblastoma xenografts in a CD1-nu mouse model. *Oncotarget* **2017**, *8*, 64728–64744. [CrossRef]
41. Liu, Y.M. Medium-chain triglyceride (MCT) ketogenic therapy. *Epilepsia* **2008**, *49*, 33–36. [CrossRef]
42. Zhou, W.; Mukherjee, P.; Kiebish, M.A.; Markis, W.T.; Mantis, J.G.; Seyfried, T.N. The calorically restricted ketogenic diet, an effective alternative therapy for malignant brain cancer. *Nutr. Metab.* **2007**, *4*, 5. [CrossRef]
43. Zuccoli, G.; Marcello, N.; Pisanello, A.; Servadei, F.; Vaccaro, S.; Mukherjee, P.; Seyfried, T.N. Metabolic management of glioblastoma multiforme using standard therapy together with a restricted ketogenic diet: Case Report. *Nutr. Metab.* **2010**, *7*, 33. [CrossRef]

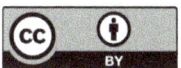

© 2019 by the authors. Licensee MDPI, Basel, Switzerland. This article is an open access article distributed under the terms and conditions of the Creative Commons Attribution (CC BY) license (http://creativecommons.org/licenses/by/4.0/).

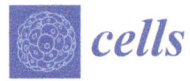

Review

Mitochondrial Involvement in the Adaptive Response to Chronic Exposure to Environmental Pollutants and High-Fat Feeding in a Rat Liver and Testis

Vincenzo Migliaccio [1,2,*], Ilaria Di Gregorio [1], Rosalba Putti [2] and Lillà Lionetti [1,*]

1. Department of Chemistry and Biology "Adolfo Zambelli", University of Salerno, 84084 Fisciano, Italy
2. Department of Biology, University of Naples, Federico II, 80126 Naples, Italy
* Correspondence: vincenzo.migliaccio@unina.it (V.M.); llionetti@unisa.it (L.L.); Tel.: +39-089-969-592 (L.L.)

Received: 11 June 2019; Accepted: 3 August 2019; Published: 5 August 2019

Abstract: In our modern society, exposure to stressful environmental stimuli, such as pollutants and/or chronic high-fat feeding, continuously induce tissular/organ metabolic adaptation to promote cellular survival. In extreme conditions, cellular death and tissular/organ damage occur. Mitochondria, as a cellular energy source, seem to play an important role in facing cellular stress induced by these environmental stimuli. On the other hand, mitochondrial dysfunction and oxidative stress play a key role in environmental stress-induced metabolic diseases. However, little is known about the combined effect of simultaneous exposure to chronic high-fat feeding and environmental pollutants on metabolic alterations at a tissular and cellular level, including mitochondrial dysfunction and oxidative stress induction. Our research group recently addressed this topic by analysing the effect of chronic exposure to a non-toxic dose of the environmental pollutant dichlorodiphenyldichloroethylene (DDE) associated with high-fat feeding in male Wistar rats. In this review, we mainly summarize our recent findings on mitochondrial adaptive response and oxidative stress induction in the liver, the main tissue involved in fat metabolism and pollutant detoxification, and in male gonads, the main targets of endocrine disruption induced by both high-fat feeding and environmental pollutants.

Keywords: DDE; high-fat diet; mitochondrial UCP2; ROS; antioxidant system

---

1. Introduction

Mitochondria are the main organelles involved in cellular energy production and play a key role in facing cellular needs in response to external stimuli. Environmental stimuli, such as pollutants and/or chronic high-fat overnutrition, are very frequent in modern society and may induce metabolic diseases by acting on the mitochondrial function and oxidative stress induction.

Several recent scientific studies have highlighted that environmental pollutants generate cellular toxicity in different animal species, including humans. It is well-known that hydrophobic chemicals, such as polychlorinated biphenyl compounds (PCBs), persist in the environment for a long time and are also detectable across the world at a long distance from the utilization site [1–3]. Dichlorodiphenyltrichloroethane (DDT) represents one of the well-known and most used organochlorines (OC) belonging to the PCBs family. This chemical was synthesized for the first time in 1874 by Othmar Zeidle, but it became famous in 1939, when the chemist Paul Hermann Müller discovered DDT's proprieties as poisonous against arthropod vectors of parasites [4]. In the last century, DDT was used during the second World War and post-World War period to control the extension of malaria cases. The massive and uncontrolled use of DDT briefly produced negative effects on the environment, such as the thinning of eggshells in birds [5,6] and reduction of hatching [7]. Moreover, negative implications were also observed in reproduction in higher animals [8]. Therefore, DDT use was banned in many countries and restricted to equatorial zones where malaria is still endemic [9]. However, DDT and its metabolites, as other persistent organic pollutants (POPs), can migrate through the atmosphere as gases and aerosols moving thousands of kilometers from the point of release [10]. Moreover, given their liposolubility, these substances undergo bioaccumulation and biomagnification phenomena, with an increase in concentration for the species at the top of the food chain [11]. Several recent studies underlined that DDT and its metabolites are able to induce metabolic alterations and dysfunction in different organs and tissues. For example, it has been shown that DDT and its major metabolite dichlorodiphenyldichloroethylene (DDE) promote diabetes, hepatic morphological alterations in terms of toxicant-associated steatohepatitis (TASH), and endocrine disorders that compromise reproductive efficiency [12–14]. In addition, DDT and DDE were found to be directly implicated in reactive oxygen species (ROS) over-production, cellular oxidative stress, and apoptosis onset in vivo and in vitro by modulating the mitochondrial function [15,16]. It is noteworthy that fat-soluble chemicals are easily introduced in organisms through contaminated food and their intake may increase during high-fat feeding. Fats represent a further point of interest for scientific research. It is well-known that high lipid consumption induces metabolic alterations, leading to the development of obesity and its related metabolic diseases, such as cardiovascular diseases, hepatic steatosis, and insulin resistance/diabetes [17–23]. It is noteworthy that a high-fat diet (HFD) elicits several metabolic disorders, including mitochondrial dysfunction and oxidative damage [24–30]. Mitochondrial function and its adaptation to dietary components represent a key point in metabolic research. In fact, HFD has been suggested to increase ROS production and induce mitochondrial dysfunction, generating metabolic alterations that, in turn, could lead to the development of HFD-induced insulin resistance [31,32]. However, little is known about the combined effect of simultaneous chronic high-fat feeding and environmental pollutant exposure on metabolic alterations at a tissular and cellular level, including mitochondrial dysfunction. This aspect could clarify whether dietary fat could act as a vehicle for the pesticide, suggesting a possible synergistic effect of the two different stimuli. Our research group recently addressed this topic by analysing the effect of chronic exposure to a non-toxic dose of the environmental pollutant DDE combined with a low-fat or high-fat diet in male Wistar rats, focusing in particular on the liver and testis function, as well as on the mitochondrial adaptive response [33,34]. In this mini review, we summarize our findings on metabolic responses in the liver, which represents the main tissue involved in energetic metabolism and detoxification, as well as in male gonads, which represent one of the principal targets of endocrine disrupter chemicals [35]. It is interesting to analyse how different organs respond to both overfeeding and environmental pollutant exposure, in order to observe whether common cellular mechanisms are involved. Our experimental design utilized adult male Wistar rats subdivided into four different groups: control animals, fed a standard laboratory diet (N group); DDE-treated animals, fed a standard diet associated with DDE administration (N + DDE group); high-fat-fed animals that received HFD (45% fat, D group); high-fat + DDE-treated animals that received simultaneous exposure to HFD and DDE (D + DDE group). Pesticide (10 mg/Kg b.w.) was administrated every day, orally, during a period of 28 days. In liver samples we analysed lipid accumulation, antioxidant system activity, mitochondrial function and cellular detoxification markers [34]. At a testicle level, we mainly focused our attention on seminiferous tubules, spermatogenesis compromising, oxidative stress, apoptosis and cellular proliferation [33].

In the first part of the present review, we introduce the role of mitochondria and oxidative stress in cellular homoeostasis. Then, we focus on the effect of HFD and DDE to a single exposure or a simultaneous exposure on hepatic metabolism and mitochondrial involvement. In the last part of the review, we focus on testis adaptation to HFD and DDE, as single exposure or simultaneous exposure. No-synergic effect of HFD and DDE was found in either the liver or testis.

2. Mitochondria and Oxidative Stress Generation in Biological Systems

Mitochondria are important organelles involved in different metabolic processes in cells. They play a key role in energy production, regulating several cellular physiological pathways, such as differentiation, proliferation, and programmed death [36]. These mechanisms are regulated by both mitochondrial and nuclear gene expression [37]. It is known that several mitochondrial proteins and subunits are encoded by nuclear genes, known as nuclear-encoded mitochondrial genes (NEMG). Moreover, accumulative evidence suggests that mitochondrial factors act as signals to regulate the expression of nuclear genes. The factors produced by nuclear activity regulate mitochondrial function, creating a crosstalk mechanism between mitochondria and the nucleus [37]. In this context, mitochondria–nucleus crosstalk represents an important physiological process that, if altered, permits mitochondrial dysfunction and/or cellular damage to take over. These two communication pathways are able to promptly satisfy cellular requests in response to metabolism alterations and exposure to environmental factors [38]. Moreover, mitochondrial-generated ROS and metabolites act as signaling molecules and cofactors that regulate fundamental nuclear processes. Excessive ROS production can induce cellular oxidative stress and damage cellular components and macromolecules, including DNA [39].

Oxidative stress represents a condition observed in biological systems due to the imbalance between ROS production and endogenous antioxidant systems useful to counteract oxidative damage. ROS are produced in different cellular districts and include radical and non-radical chemical species: (a) superoxide anion ($^\bullet O_2^-$), which is mainly produced at a mitochondrial level; (b) peroxyl radicals (R-OO$^\bullet$), which derive from the oxidative damage in membrane lipids; and (c) hydrogen peroxide (H_2O_2), which is produced as a consequence of superoxide-catalyzed dismutation by superoxide dismutase activity (SODs). Several studies have shown that the main source of ROS production is represented by mitochondria [40–42], where different sites of superoxide/hydrogen peroxide generation have been identified [43]. Most of these sites deliver their superoxide/hydrogen peroxide product exclusively to the mitochondrial matrix, but at least two of the sites (Complex III of the electron transport chain and mitochondrial glycerol 3-phosphate dehydrogenase) deliver superoxide to both the matrix and the cytosolic face of the inner membrane, because they are situated on the outer side of the mitochondrial inner membrane [44–47]. These different site-specific topologies in the delivery of superoxide/hydrogen peroxide to different compartments have been suggested to be of great importance in redox signaling. Indeed, ROS have also been shown to act as signaling molecules [48]. It has been hypothesized that redox signaling by the superoxide generated by complex III in the cytosol will be very different from redox signaling by the superoxide generated in the mitochondrial matrix by other sites [47]. It is interesting to underline that recent works have shown that increasing levels of superoxide, through treatment with the pesticide paraquat, result in an increased lifespan, and that ROS have a compartment-specific effect on the lifespan [49,50]: elevated ROS in the mitochondria act to increase the lifespan, whereas elevated ROS in the cytoplasm decrease the lifespan [51]. A further ROS source is represented by cytochrome P450 (CYP450) activity in mammalian species [52]. CYP enzymes catalyze the oxygenation of an organic substrate with the simultaneous reduction of molecular oxygen. This mechanism is involved in the xenobiotics-induced cellular detoxification process. ROS can be released by the P450 reaction cycle under conditions in which the transfer of oxygen to a substrate is not tightly controlled [52]. High ROS production induces oxidative damage in lipids and other macromolecules, generating metabolic alterations and cellular diseases. In physiological conditions, ROS levels can be regulated by antioxidant enzymes or antioxidant molecules which are able to quench radical species to limit oxidant process propagation. In this way, ROS levels remain low in cells, playing a key role in regulating cellular metabolism, proliferation, and death [53,54]. On the other hand, increased ROS levels are associated with metabolic dysfunction [55,56] and inflammation. Noteworthy, metabolic dysfunction and inflammation have also been suggested to be associated with xenobiotics exposure [57–59]. At a mitochondrial level, the superoxide may be reduced using antioxidant activity. In fact, superoxide released in the matrix or in the mitochondrial inner membrane space is converted into H_2O_2 by superoxide dismutases (SODs). In the mitochondrial matrix, GPx reduces H_2O_2 in a canalized-reaction consuming glutathione, producing H_2O. This system correctly balances ROS production under physiological conditions. However, the imbalance between ROS and antioxidant defense in favour of ROS overproduction generates oxidative stress. A metabolic state able to produce oxidative stress in different organs and typically observed in developed societies is represented by overfeeding, especially in terms of a high consumption of saturated lipids. Several research groups, including our group, have shown that HFD induces alterations in the serum lipid profile, as well as increasing both the body weight and lipid depots in adipose tissue and ectopic sites [17,29,60,61]. It is noteworthy that a high dietary fat intake has been shown to be associated with oxidative stress induction in different experimental models and tissues [29,31,32,62,63], suggesting that fatty acids represent a critical point in the development of metabolic disorders associated with obesity. Moreover, as stated above, another environmental condition that may induce oxidative stress in different tissues and organs is the exposure to environmental pollutants [15,16]. Our experimental results have shown that DDE induces oxidative damage, cellular death, and tissular injury [33,34]. In the following sections, we focus on the HFD and/or environmental pollutant, mainly DDE, effect on mitochondrial dysfunction and oxidative stress in the liver and testis.

3. Physiological Adaption to HFD and DDE in the Liver

3.1. HFD Induces Hepatic Fat Accumulation and Cellular Stress Targeting Mitochondria

It is well-known that HFD induces obesity and alters the serum lipid profile [64]. The excess fatty depots positively correlate with adipose tissue inflammation, insulin resistance and metabolic disorders, such as hepatic steatosis [65,66]. Fat depots in the adipose tissue remain unchanged over time under conditions of adequate nutritional intake. On the other hand, an imbalance in macronutrient percentage towards lipid intake elicits an increase in lipid depots and metabolic changes in energetic substrates utilization in both adipose tissue and ectopic fat depots, such as the liver. In fact, literature data reported that HFD increases the cellular capacity to utilize fatty acids by activating a pool of genes directly involved in the storage, mobilization, transport, and oxidation of fats [67–70]. In accordance, several studies have suggested that HFD-fed animals adapt their cellular metabolism, modulating the expression of nuclear genes mainly involved in lipid oxidation, such as the peroxisome proliferator-activated receptor (PPAR). PPAR family members (α, δ, γ) act as metabolic regulators in cells. PPARα has been shown to be involved in liver fatty acid metabolism [71]. It was found that PPARα regulates hepatic fatty acid transporters and carnitine palmitoyltransferase 1 and 2 (CPT-1 and -2) activity, increasing fatty acid utilization by mitochondria [72,73]. In fact, PPARα targets genes coding β-oxidative enzymes to regulate fatty acid utilization, [72]. This mechanism represents an important point of metabolic adaptation particularly used in a fasting condition, where fatty acid utilization generates ketone bodies used by tissues to produce energy [74]. Several researchers have also evidenced a role of PPARα in non-alcoholic fatty liver disease (NAFLD) models [29,75–77]. Lipid deposition and body mass increased in HFD-fed animals, resulting in increased plasma fatty free acids levels and hepatic PPARα expression [75]. Indeed, it has been shown that HFD increased hepatic PPARα levels and its nuclear localization [29]. It has also been reported that PPARs are able to induce mitochondrial uncoupling by stimulating mitochondrial UCPs in different organs [29,76,77], with a resulting increase in mitochondrial energy expenditure not coupled with ATP formation.

Under the condition of change in lipid metabolism towards fatty acid oxidation, ketone bodies (β-hydroxybutyrate and acetoacetate) are significantly increased in the serum [78], suggesting that ketogenesis represents a metabolic adaptation under conditions of high-fat feeding, as well as in insulin resistance and fasting [79]. Moreover, it was recently reported that ketogenesis could represent an important adaptive mechanism to prevent NAFLD in an animal model [74]. In fact, in mice with induced-insufficient ketogenesis, HFD produced severe hepatic injury, inflammation, impaired hepatic gluconeogenesis, and deranged hepatic tricarboxylic acid (TCA) cycle intermediate concentrations, suggesting that ketone bodies function as hepatic metabolic regulators, playing a possible central role in fatty liver disease prevention [80].

Several studies have suggested that alterations in mitochondrial function and oxidative stress play a key role in the onset of diet-induced hepatic steatosis [26,81–84]. In our recent works, we analysed mitochondrial fatty acid oxidation, oxidative stress, and antioxidant defenses in HFD-fed rats [34,85]. The results showed that HFD increased the beta-oxidation (β-ox) rate and carnitine palmitoyl-CoA transferase (CPT) activity, confirming that the liver increased the utilization of lipids as energetic substrates during overfeeding [34]. In addition, the excess fats introduced with food elicited lipid accumulation in the hepatocytes and increased oxidative damage in terms of the accumulation of both malondialdehyde (MDA) and oxidized glutathione (GSSG) in the tissue [34]. This cellular stress is probably due to the excess ROS produced at a mitochondrial level by increased hepatic lipid catabolism. It is noteworthy that the analyses of the antioxidant system suggested that the liver adapts its metabolism, at least in part, by stimulating both SODs and GPx protein levels and activities [34]. Therefore, the stimulation of antioxidant systems may play a key role in the control of the oxidative stress level. In addition, our study of the antioxidant system was extended to other classes of proteins with non-specific antioxidant activity, such as the small intracellular proteins known as metallothioneins (MTs) [85]. Experimental studies have shown that MTs quench hydroxyl radicals in vitro [86]. Unexpectedly, we found a reduction in MTs gene expression and protein synthesis in diet-induced hepatic steatosis and oxidative stress [85]. However, histochemical experiments highlighted increases in the nuclear localization of MTs, which was also confirmed by western blot analysis of a liver nuclear fraction [85]. These data, according to the literature, suggested a possible role of MTs at a nuclear level in oxidative stress conditions. MTs may play a key role in protecting DNA from hydroxyl radicals, in donating metals for several enzymes, or in chelating zinc from transcription factors such as zinc finger proteins [85,87–91]. In order to limit cellular stress, hepatocytes use an additional strategy to directly control ROS generation at a mitochondrial level through the uncoupling of mitochondrial respiration from the oxidative phosphorylation process. This mechanism is controlled by a family of protein carriers known as uncoupling proteins (UCPs), which are composed of different members that are expressed in different tissues: UCP1 (mainly in brown adipose tissue), UCP3 (mainly in muscle), and UCP4-5 (mainly in the brain) [92–94]. We analysed the member of the UCPs family that was found to be ubiquitously expressed: UCP2 [95]. This protein is essentially involved in the control of ROS production [96,97], representing the isoform that mainly differs in function compared to the other UCP isoforms. In our experimental conditions, HFD induced UCP2 gene expression and protein synthesis, suggesting its possible involvement in fatty liver metabolism [34]. Nevertheless, all the activated mechanisms seemed to be unable to completely counteract hepatic oxidative damage induced by fats. The liver seemed to fail to properly balance the excess ROS due to the large amount of lipids. Therefore, the liver accumulated fat and proceeded towards oxidative damage and steatosis, as also shown by the increase in serum levels of transaminase, markers of hepatic injury [34]. We have summarized the observed effects induced by HFD in hepatocytes in Figure 1.

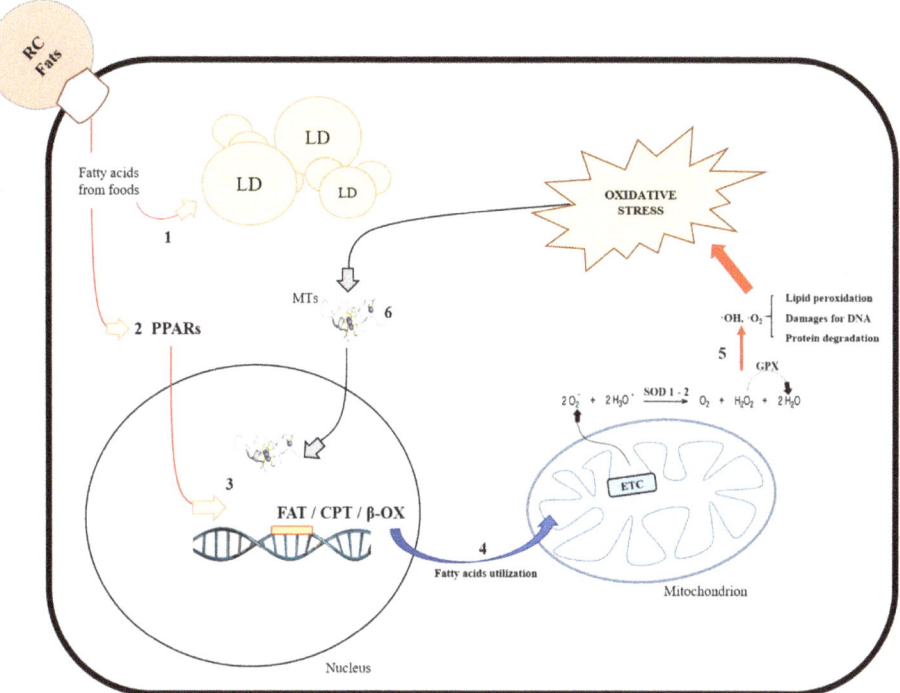

Figure 1. Effect of a high-fat diet (HFD) in hepatocytes. Dietary fats reach the liver from the blood vessels by remnant chylomicrons (RC) and enter the hepatocytes. In cell cytosol, elongated fatty acids can be in part accumulated in the form of lipid droplets (1) or used as energetic substrates. PPAR family members (2) play a key role in lipid catabolism activation by inducing the expression of genes (3) involved in the transport and use of fatty acids by mitochondria (4). As a consequence, increased mitochondrial activity produces elevated reactive oxygen species (ROS) levels that, if not adequately counterbalanced by endogenous antioxidant defenses, induce oxidative damage on lipids, proteins, and DNA (5), with negative consequences on the mitochondrial function. Under these metabolic conditions, nuclear transcriptional activity increases to adapt cellular metabolism. Then, MTs localize in the nucleus (6) to donate or chelate metals or to protect DNA from oxidative damage. RC: remnant chylomicrons; Fats: fatty acids; LD: lipid droplets; PPARs: peroxisome proliferator-activated receptors; FAT: fatty acid transporters; CPT: carnitine palmitoyl-transferase; β-OX: beta oxidation; ETC: electron transport chain; H_2O_2: hydrogen peroxide; $OH^\bullet$, $O_2^{\bullet-}$: reactive oxygen species; SOD1-2: superoxide dismutase; GPX: glutathione peroxidase; MTs: metallothioneins.

3.2. DDE Exposure: Hepatic Mechanisms Used to Counteract Liver Damage

In recent years, experimental evidence showed that environmental contaminants are also involved in inducing TASH, eliciting fatty liver injury in non-obese people exposed to chemicals and/or xenobiotics [98,99]. In fact, several environmental pollutants induce metabolic disorders in the cells [100]. Phthalates, organochlorines, and other environmental chemicals have been shown to be involved in ROS accumulation and apoptosis onset [15,101]. Under a stress condition, cells activate compensatory mechanisms that include the modulation of gene expression. In particular, phthalates can induce hepatic toxicity through PPARs transactivation, causing uncontrolled proliferation and hepatic tumorigenesis development [102]. In addition, PPARs have been shown to be directly involved in the regulation of cellular toxicity induced by air, water, and food pollutants [103]. Air pollutant exposure reduced PPARs levels, producing tissular injury in terms of hepatic inflammation, endoplasmic reticulum stress [104], and steatosis. In fact, PPARs not only regulate cellular proliferation, but also play an anti-inflammatory role and maintain lipid homeostasis in Kupffer cells, hepatocytes, and stellate cells [105]. Moreover, the induction of PPARγ gene expression in the presence of DDT has been seen in human mesenchymal stem cells, [106] suggesting that PPARs, as well as other nuclear receptors, are involved in the cellular response to toxicant.

In addition, chronic exposure to environmental toxic substances, including DDT and DDE, has been shown to induce DNA damage in different models in vivo and in vitro [107–109]. However, cells adapt their metabolic state under a stress condition by activating a series of signals that include the expression of genes involved in metabolic homeostasis, such as the up-regulation of antioxidant systems [110] and the increase in mitochondrial activity to produce the additional ATP required by the cellular function [111,112]. However, the increased mitochondrial activity is associated with increased ROS levels that, if not correctly balanced, generate oxidative stress that in turn elicits damage to macromolecules, genomic instability, and mitochondrial/cellular dysfunction [40].

Recent scientific findings showed that DDE induces oxidative stress, mitochondrial impairment, and cellular oxidative damage [15,16,34,35]. In our study, chronic exposure to a non-toxic DDE dose, associated with a standard diet regimen (N + DDE group), did not produce changes in terms of the serum lipid profile and fatty acid deposition in the tissues compared to the control group [34]. However, hepatic morphological alterations were histologically detected in terms of eosinophilic cells around the principal vessels, perivascular cellular vacuolization, and inflammation [34,85]. These morphological changes were probably due to oxidative stress induced by exposure to pesticides, which produce cellular modification typically associated with the onset of TASH [98]. Experimental data showed increased hepatic levels of MDA and GSSG, confirming the role of DDE in oxidative stress generation [34]. However, the mechanisms by which DDE induces ROS incrementation are not yet clear, but the main effects of DDE on hepatic cells involve the cytochrome P450 (CYP450) activity, used in the detoxification path [113]. It has been shown that DDE activates CYP450 gene family transcription, mainly CYP450 2B and 3A, by interacting with the constitutive androstane receptor (CAR) and pregnane X receptor (PXR) [114]. It has also been shown that pesticide can directly affect the mitochondrial electron transport chain inducing functional impairment [115,116]. In our experimental model, we found increases in both mitochondrial β-ox and CPT system activity [34]. These findings suggest that mitochondria play a pivotal role in the adaptation to DDE exposure by increasing fat catabolism to face the increased cellular energy needs for the hepatic detoxification processes. Together with hepatic oxidative damage, the principal antioxidant enzymes, namely SODs and GPx, were found to be stimulated in terms of protein synthesis and enzymatic activity [34]. In particular, also in this context, mitochondria played a central metabolic role in controlling the cellular oxidative balance. In fact, a strong stimulation of the mitochondrial SOD isoform (Mn-SOD, well-known as SOD2), was found that represents one of the most important mitochondrial defenses against ROS [34]. In addition, a reduction in MT levels was found in DDE-treated rats, as was found in a similar way in HFD-treated rats [85].

Moreover, we also demonstrated strong MTs nuclear localization in the DDE-treated liver, confirming a physiological nuclear role of MTs in an oxidative stress condition [85]. The mitochondrial role in the hepatic adaptation to pesticide-induced oxidative stress has become increasingly evident during research. In fact, alongside the high SOD2 level, hepatocytes from DDE-treated rats showed high UCP2 gene expression and protein synthesis [34]. Probably, both SOD2 and UCP2 play a cooperative role in response to DDE at a mitochondrial level. The electron transport chain produces a superoxide anion, which is rapidly converted into H_2O_2 by SOD2. However, to avoid an excessive accumulation of H_2O_2 at a mitochondrial and cellular level, mitochondrial uncoupling is induced in order to reduce superoxide production by mitochondrial activity. This effect, associated with the increase in GPx activity observed in the liver, probably contributes to not exacerbating the oxidative damage and hepatic injury, that, in terms of the serum transaminases level, is comparable to that induced by HFD treatment [34]. The hepatocyte response to OCs, namely DDE, has been summarized in Figure 2.

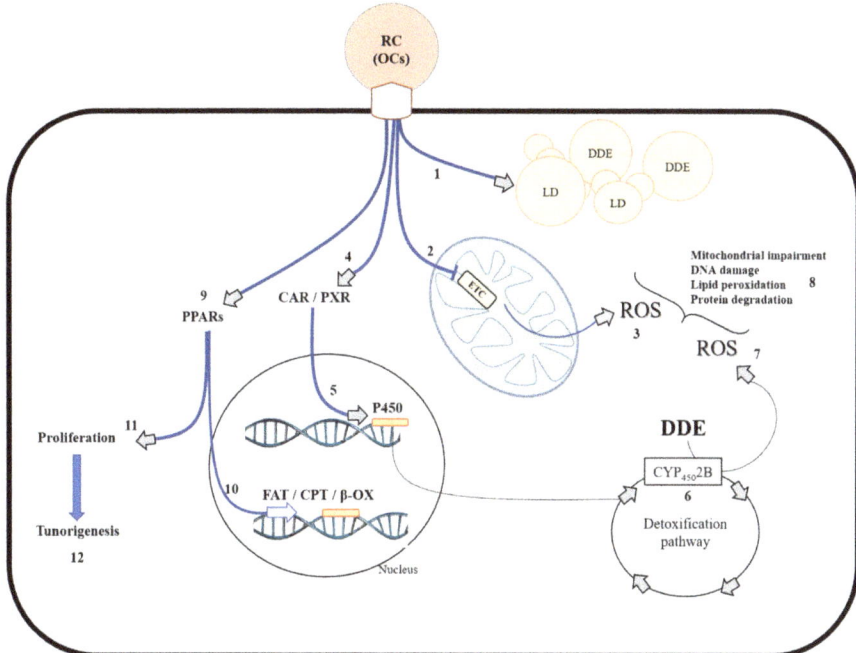

Figure 2. Principal mechanisms stimulated by organochlorinated compounds. Organochlorinated compounds (OCs), including DDE accumulated in contaminated foods, reach the liver from the blood vessels by remnant chylomicrons. In the cells, OCs can be, in part, stored in the lipid droplets (1). In addition, OCs can act on mitochondria, partially inhibiting the electron transport chain (2) and inducing mitochondrial ROS production (3). Moreover, OCs such as DDE can interact with CAR and PXR receptors (4), inducing expression of the P450 gene family (5) for detoxification (6). However, the detoxification path augments ROS levels (7). These mechanisms, if not effectively controlled by antioxidant defenses, produce oxidative damage in macromolecules (8). In addition, OCs can modulate transcriptional activity through PPAR family members (9), modulating fatty acid metabolism (10) and cellular proliferation (11). Uncontrolled proliferative mechanisms induced by OCs can lead to tumorigenesis (12). RC: remnant chylomicrons; OCs: organochlorinated compounds; DDE: Dichlorodiphenyldichloroethylene; LD: lipid droplets; ETC: electron transport chain; CAR: constitutive androstane receptor; PXR: pregnane X receptor; PPARs: peroxisome proliferator-activated receptors; FAT: fatty acid transporters; CPT: carnitine palmitoyl-transferase; β-OX: beta oxidation; P450: cytochrome P450; ROS: reactive oxygen species.

3.3. Dietary Fats and DDE Showed No Synergic Effect in Hepatic Stress Generation and Damage

The simultaneous exposure to HFD and the environmental pollutant DDE (D + DDE group), represents a very interesting topic to be addressed and we showed that pesticide affects hepatic metabolism differently, depending on the different dietary treatment (low-fat or high-fat diet) [34]. At a systemic level, D + DDE animals presented alterations in the serum lipid profile in terms of triglycerides and cholesterol levels, but serum triglyceride levels were found to be lower compared to the levels in D animals. In line with this result, hepatic lipid depots were found to be lower in D + DDE than in the D group. Moreover, mitochondrial β-ox and CPT system activities were increased to the same extent as in N + DDE-treated animals [34]. It can be suggested that the lower levels in serum triglycerides and hepatic lipid depots could be at least in part due to the increased hepatic fatty acid utilization required to produce energy to cope with the increase in the detoxification pathway. In fact, CYP450 2B protein content was found to be increased in the D + DDE and N + DDE groups [34]. Hepatic morphological changes showed several inflammatory foci, eosinophilic cells, and hepatocytes vacuolization around blood vessels [34]. Oxidative stress occurred in D + DDE animals with the accumulation of MDA and GSSG in the liver, as was found in the N + DDE animal group. We did not observe any additional oxidative damage in the D + DDE group compared to both the N + DDE and D group, as it can be expected by potential additional pro-oxidant effects due to the simultaneous exposure to two different pro-oxidant stimuli, namely HFD and DDE [34]. Therefore, it can be suggested that no synergic effects on hepatic stress and damage occurred, when pesticide exposure was simultaneous to high-fat diet treatment. Considering the hydrophobic nature of this pesticide, in the condition of lipid accumulation in adipose tissue and in ectopic sites observed in D and D + DDE groups, it can be hypothesized that a part of DDE remains stored in lipid depots in an inert form. Therefore, the adaptive metabolic responses in the D + DDE group were mainly induced by dietary fats and only in part by the pesticide, and no synergic effect of dietary fat and pesticide on oxidative stress was observed in D + DDE. Increased SOD and GPx activities and reduced MT levels were also found in the D + DDE group [34,85]. However, in this case, MTs maintained nuclear localization in the hepatocytes as in D group [85], whereas SOD2 activity was found to be intermediate between D and N + DDE [34], suggesting that dietary fats limit, at least in part, DDE activity. Moreover, mitochondrial levels of UCP2 in terms of gene expression and protein synthesis in the D + DDE group were intermediate between D and N + DDE groups. Finally, serum transaminase levels were found to be increased, as in D and N + DDE groups, indicating no further liver damage in the D + DDE group as a consequence of the sum of the responses to the two different stimuli [34].

4. Physiological Adaption to HFD and DDE in the Testis

4.1. HFD Alters Testicular Function and Affects Hormonal Homeostasis

Different analyses were conducted to evaluate the effects of dietary fats on testicular function and morphology [33]. The results showed that HFD alters the antioxidant system and induces oxidative damage. In fact, GPx activity reduction and lipid peroxidation induction with MDA accumulation were observed in the tissue [33]. Moreover, as observed in the liver, a reduction in MTs gene expression and protein synthesis occurred [85]. As a consequence of oxidative injury, morphological alterations were detected in the seminiferous epithelium [33]. Large spaces among germinal cells as well as cytoplasmic vacuolization in germinal and Sertoli cells were observed [33], probably due to lipid and/or fluid accumulation [117]. Activation of apoptotic stimuli was observed under the condition of oxidative stress [33]. Normally, testicular germ cell apoptosis represents a physiological process playing a key role in removing abnormal spermatozoa during spermatogenesis [118,119]. On the other hand, in a non-physiological metabolic state, such as an oxidative stress condition, the high apoptotic rate could be associated with male subfertility. In obese subjects, the onset of male subfertility with changes in sperm parameters, motility and counting, can occur due to the high-fat induced cellular oxidative stress [120–122]. In our study, we showed an increase in Bcl2 associated with X protein (BAX) levels and activated caspase 3 (casp-3) cell immunoreactivity in HFD-fed animals, where an apoptosis trigger was observed [33]. Moreover, HFD was also found to be involved in hormonal disorder generation, which probably represents a key point in testis functional alteration [123]. In fact, HFD-fed animals showed a reduction in testicular androgen receptor (AR) and serum testosterone (T) levels [33]. Noteworthy, we also found a stimulation of cellular proliferation through the increase in the content of proliferating cell nuclear antigen (PCNA). This increase may be involved in cellular mechanisms useful to counteract oxidative stress-induced cellular death in the testis. We have summarized the effect of HFD in the testis in Figure 3.

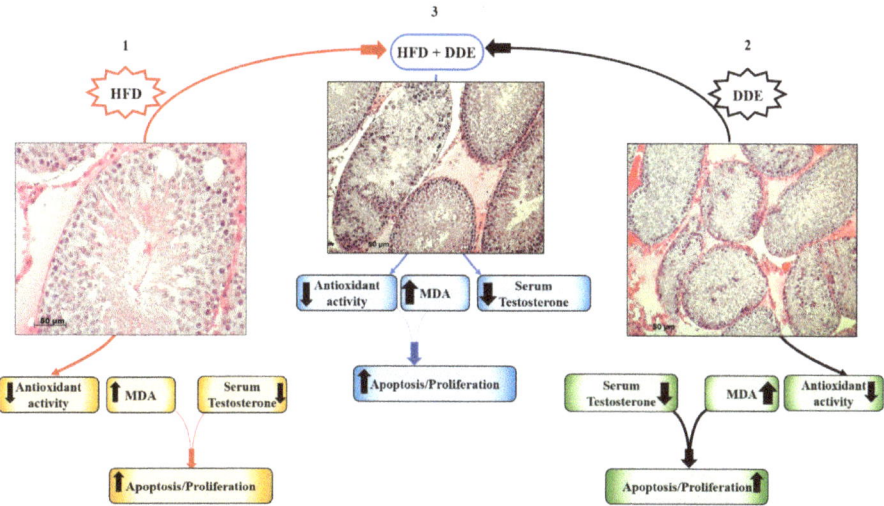

Figure 3. Effects of singular and simultaneous exposure to a high-fat diet (HFD) and/or dichlorodiphenyldichloroethylene (DDE) in testis. HFD (1) reduced antioxidant activity and generated oxidative stress. Increases in the apoptotic rate were found. In addition, dietary fats reduced serum testosterone levels, altering the hormonal balance. Both DDE exposure (2) and simultaneous HFD and DDE exposure (3) affected antioxidant system activity, which was strongly reduced. Oxidative damage further increased, and to a much greater extent in DDE-treated animals (2). Moreover, a trigger of apoptosis, tubular damage, and a reduction of testosterone levels were detected. To counteract cellular death, proliferation was stimulated in a similar way in HFD (1) and HFD + DDE (3), and was further increased in DDE (2), suggesting the different effects of pesticides at a cellular level.

4.2. DDE Negatively Affects Spermatogenesis and Testicular Function

It is well-known the effect of PCBs on the male reproductive system [124,125]. DDE acts as antiandrogenic chemical by interacting with androgen receptors [12]. In our work, we analysed the effect of DDE on the testicular function to evaluate the in vivo adaptive mechanisms during chronical exposure to a non-toxic dose [33]. We confirmed the pro-oxidant role of the pesticides with a reduction in both total SODs and GPx activities, as well as in MTs gene expression and protein synthesis [33], in accordance with previous finding [16]. In our study, antioxidant impairment in DDE-treated rats induced the highest MDA levels compared to the other experimental groups [33]. As a consequence, morphological alterations were detected at different levels. A strong disorganization of the seminiferous epithelium was observed in some tubules, where it was no longer possible to detect the typical cell–cell associations. Moreover, eosinophilic cells with pyknotic nuclei were detected. The lumen of severely altered tubules was rich in non-differentiated cells [33]. This observation suggested that cell-cell adhesion was lost, and non-differentiated cells were released in the lumen without completing spermatogenesis. A similar finding was also reported in further in vivo animal models with exposure to other toxic chemical species [126–128]. In DDE-treated rats, the highest BAX protein levels and casp-3 cell immunoreactivity were detected compared to N and D animals, associated with the induction of hormonal disorders in terms of reduced testicle AR protein levels and serum T [33]. Noteworthy, a stimulation of cell proliferation was observed in association with increases in the apoptotic rate, as also observed in HFD-fed group [33]. The highest PCNA levels observed in DDE-treated group [33] was in line with previous findings showing that DDE is able to induce cellular proliferation through oxidative stress [129] (Figure 3).

4.3. Simultaneous Exposure to HFD + DDE did not Show a Synergic Effect on Testicular Function

In the experimental group exposed to both HFD and DDE, the effects of DDE in the testis did not show synergistic effects with HFD [33], as described for the liver above [34]. The results obtained in D + DDE group showed a very similar effect to that of DDE-treated animals in terms of morphological alterations, antioxidant impairment, apoptosis, and hormonal changes [33]. On the other hand, MDA levels were found to be intermediate between D and N + DDE groups. According to the lower oxidative damage vs. N + DDE, we showed a reduced MTs gene expression and protein synthesis in D + DDE animals, as in the D group, suggesting the transcriptional regulation of MTs, depending on the tissular oxidative stress level. Moreover, cellular-induced proliferation didn't seem to be stimulated as observed in N + DDE, but the response was more similar to that observed in the D group [33]. These findings suggested that DDE has less impact when administrated together with HFD, in accordance with the lipid dissolving theory which hypothesizes that DDE storage in body fat deposits induces a decrease in DDE effects In Figure 3, we have schematized the responses to HFD and/or DDE in the testis.

5. Conclusions

In conclusion, our research confirmed the literature on HFD and DDE effects in terms of oxidative stress associated with changes in lipid metabolism, mainly in the liver.

Hepatic adaptations to dietary fats and pesticides induced a general control of hepatic injury in which mitochondrial function and cellular metabolism were directly involved. Antioxidant system stimulation and mitochondrial UCP2 up-regulation seemed to play a potential protective role in counteracting ROS overproduction, mainly in the presence of environmental pollutants.

In the testis, HFD altered the oxidative balance and induced lipotoxicity, cellular death and apoptosis. On the other hand, DDE generated the highest tissular alterations and dysfunctions with impairment of spermatogenesis under the conditions of both individual or simultaneous exposure to pesticide and dietary fats, with a worse redox state when pesticide exposure was not associated with a high fat consumption.

With the limitation that further studies are needed to better identify the mitochondrial role in response to environmental stimuli, such as pollutants and chronic high-fat feeding, our experimental research summarized in the present review was the first to address the topic of mitochondrial and oxidative stress responses to chronic simultaneous exposure to both environmental stimuli in different organs. Given that, in modern obesogenic society, we are frequently exposed to both a high-fat diet and several environmental pollutants with consequently increased risks of related metabolic disease, studies on mitochondrial involvement in the cellular response to these environmental stimuli can be useful in understanding the adaptive mitochondrial response required to maintain a healthy condition and, therefore, to target mitochondria in the prevention and therapy of environmental stimuli-induced metabolic diseases.

Funding: This work was supported by University of Salerno (Fondi FARB 2018, 300389FRB18LIONE).

Conflicts of Interest: The authors declare no conflict of interest.

References

1. Kannan, K.; Tanabe, S.; Williams, R.J.; Tatsukawa, R. Persistent organochlorine residues in foodstuffs from Australia, Papua New Guinea and the Solomon Islands: Contamination levels and human dietary exposure. *Sci. Total Environ.* **1994**, *153*, 29–49. [CrossRef]
2. Grimalt, J.O.; van Drooge, B.L.; Ribes, A.; Vilanova, R.M.; Fernandez, P.; Appleby, P. Persistent organochlorine compounds in soils and sediments of European high altitude mountain lakes. *Chemosphere* **2004**, *54*, 1549–1561. [CrossRef] [PubMed]
3. Carrera, G.; Fernández, P.; Vilanova, R.M.; Grimalt, J.O. Persistent organic pollutants in snow from European high mountain areas. *Sci. Total Environ.* **1994**, *153*, 29–49. [CrossRef]

4. Bishopp, F.C. Insect Problems in World War II with Special References to the Insecticide DDT. *Am. J. Public Health Nations Health* **1945**, *35*, 373–378. [CrossRef] [PubMed]
5. Davison, K.L.; Sell, J.L. DDT thins shells of eggs from mallard ducks maintained on ad libitum or controlled-feeding regimens. *Arch. Environ. Contam. Toxicol.* **1974**, *2*, 222–232. [CrossRef] [PubMed]
6. Speich, S.M.; Calambokidas, J.; Shea, D.W.; Peard, J.; Witter, M.; Fry, D.M. Eggshell Thinning and Organochlorine Contaminants in Western Washington Waterbirds. *Colon. Waterbirds* **1992**, *15*, 103–112. [CrossRef]
7. Fry, D.M. Reproductive effects in birds exposed to pesticides and industrial chemicals. *Environ. Health Perspect.* **1995**, *103*, 165–171. [CrossRef] [PubMed]
8. Ware, G.W. Effects of DDT on reproduction in higher animals. *Residue Rev.* **1975**, *59*, 119–140. [PubMed]
9. Rehwagen, R. WHO recommends DDT to control malaria. *BMJ* **2006**, *333*, 622. [CrossRef] [PubMed]
10. Wania, F.; Mackay, D. Tracking the Distribution of Persistent Organic Pollutants Control strategies for these contaminants will require a better understanding of how they move around the globe. *Environ. Sci. Technol.* **1996**, *30*, 390A–396A. [CrossRef] [PubMed]
11. Streit, B. Bioaccumulation processes in ecosystems. *Cell. Mol. Life Sci.* **1992**, *48*, 955–970. [CrossRef] [PubMed]
12. Kelce, W.R.; Stone, C.R.; Laws, S.C.; Gray, L.E.; Kemppainen, J.A.; Wilson, E.M. Persistent DDT metabolite p,p'–DDE is a potent androgen receptor antagonist. *Nature* **1995**, *375*, 581–585. [CrossRef] [PubMed]
13. Patisaul, H.B.; Adewale, H.B. Long-Term Effects of Environmental Endocrine Disruptors on Reproductive Physiology and Behavior. *Front. Behav. Neurosci.* **2009**, *3*, 10. [CrossRef] [PubMed]
14. Heindel, J.J.; Blumberg, B.; Cave, M.; Machtinger, R.; Mantovani, A.; Mendez, M.A.; Nadal, A.; Palanza, P.; Panzica, G.; Sargis, R.; et al. Metabolism disrupting chemicals and metabolic disorders. *Reprod. Toxicol.* **2017**, *68*, 3–33. [CrossRef] [PubMed]
15. Song, Y.; Liang, X.; Hu, Y.; Wang, Y.; Yu, H.; Yang, K. p,p'-DDE induces mitochondria-mediated apoptosis of cultured rat Sertoli cells. *Toxicology* **2008**, *253*, 53–61. [CrossRef] [PubMed]
16. Marouani, N.; Hallegue, D.; Sakly, M.; Benkhalifa, M.; Rhouma, K.B.; Tebourbi, O. p,p'-DDT induces testicular oxidative stress-induced apoptosis in adult rats. *Reprod. Biol. Endocrinol.* **2017**, *15*, 40. [CrossRef] [PubMed]
17. Hariri, N.; Thibault, L. High-fat diet-induced obesity in animal models. *Nutr. Res. Rev.* **2010**, *23*, 270–299. [CrossRef] [PubMed]
18. Han, Q.; Yeung, S.C.; Ip, M.S.M.; Mak, J.C.W. Dysregulation of cardiac lipid parameters in high-fat high-cholesterol diet-induced rat model. *Lipids Health Dis.* **2018**, *17*, 255. [CrossRef] [PubMed]
19. Mollica, M.P.; Lionetti, L.; Putti, R.; Cavaliere, G.; Gaita, M.; Barletta, A. From chronic overfeeding to hepatic injury: Role of endoplasmic reticulum stress and inflammation. *Nutr. Metab. Cardiovasc. Dis.* **2011**, *21*, 222–230. [CrossRef] [PubMed]
20. Lionetti, L.; Mollica, M.P.; Lombardi, A.; Cavaliere, G.; Gifuni, G.; Barletta, A. From chronic overnutrition to insulin resistance: The role of fat-storing capacity and inflammation. *Nutr. Metab. Cardiovasc. Dis.* **2009**, *19*, 146–152. [CrossRef] [PubMed]
21. Pataky, M.W.; Wang, H.; Yu, C.S.; Arias, E.B.; Ploutz-Snyder, R.J.; Zheng, X.; Cartee, G.D. High-Fat Diet-Induced Insulin Resistance in Single Skeletal Muscle Fibers is Fiber Type Selective. *Sci. Rep.* **2017**, *7*, 13642. [CrossRef] [PubMed]
22. Liu, Z.; Patil, I.Y.; Jiang, T.; Sancheti, H.; Walsh, J.P.; Stiles, B.L.; Yin, F.; Cadenas, E. High-fat diet induces hepatic insulin resistance and impairment of synaptic plasticity. *PLoS ONE* **2015**, *10*, e0128274. [CrossRef] [PubMed]
23. Soltis, A.R.; Kennedy, N.J.; Xin, X.; Zhou, F.; Ficarro, S.B.; Yap, Y.S.; Matthews, B.J.; Lauffenburger, D.A.; White, F.M.; Marto, J.A.; et al. Hepatic Dysfunction Caused by Consumption of a High-Fat Diet. *Cell Rep.* **2017**, *21*, 3317–3328. [CrossRef] [PubMed]
24. Koek, G.H.; Liedorp, P.R.; Bast, A. The role of oxidative stress in non-alcoholic steatohepatitis. *Clin. Chim. Acta* **2011**, *412*, 1297–1305. [CrossRef] [PubMed]
25. Nassir, F.; Ibdah, J.A. Role of mitochondria in non-alcoholic fatty liver disease. *Int. J. Mol. Sci.* **2014**, *15*, 8713–8742. [CrossRef] [PubMed]
26. Iossa, S.; Lionetti, L.; Mollica, M.P.; Crescenzo, R.; Botta, M.; Barletta, A.; Liverini, G. Effect of high-fat feeding on metabolic efficiency and mitochondrial oxidative capacity in adult rats. *Br. J. Nutr.* **2003**, *90*, 953–960. [CrossRef] [PubMed]

27. Lionetti, L.; Mollica, M.P.; Crescenzo, R.; D'Andrea, E.; Ferraro, M.; Bianco, F.; Liverini, G.; Iossa, S. Skeletal muscle subsarcolemmal mitochondrial dysfunction in high-fat fed rats exhibiting impaired glucose homeostasis. *Int. J. Obes. (Lond.)* **2007**, *31*, 1596–1604. [CrossRef]
28. Iossa, S.; Mollica, M.P.; Lionetti, L.; Crescenzo, R.; Botta, M.; Liverini, G. Skeletal muscle oxidative capacity in rats fed high-fat diet. *Int. J. Obes. Relat. Metab. Disord.* **2002**, *26*, 65–72. [CrossRef] [PubMed]
29. Lionetti, L.; Mollica, M.P.; Donizzetti, I.; Gifuni, G.; Sica, R.; Pignalosa, A.; Cavaliere, G.; Gaita, M.; De Filippo, C.; Zorzano, A.; et al. High-lard and high-fish-oil diets differ in their effects on function and dynamic behaviour of rat hepatic mitochondria. *PLoS ONE* **2014**, *9*, e92753. [CrossRef] [PubMed]
30. Putti, R.; Sica, R.; Migliaccio, V.; Lionetti, L. Diet impact on mitochondrial bioenergetics and dynamics. *Front. Physiol.* **2015**, *6*, 109. [CrossRef]
31. Matsuzawa-Nagata, N.; Takamura, T.; Ando, H.; Nakamura, S.; Kurita, S.; Misu, H.; Ota, T.; Yokoyama, M.; Honda, M.; Miyamoto, K.; et al. Increased oxidative stress precedes the onset of high-fat diet-induced insulin resistance and obesity. *Metabolism* **2008**, *57*, 1071–1077. [CrossRef]
32. Sergi, D.; Naumovski, N.; Heilbronn, L.K.; Abeywardena, M.; O'Callaghan, N.; Lionetti, L.; Luscombe-Marsh, N. Mitochondrial (Dys)function and Insulin Resistance: From Pathophysiological Molecular Mechanisms to the Impact of Diet. *Front. Physiol.* **2019**, *10*, 532. [CrossRef]
33. Migliaccio, V.; Sica, R.; Scudiero, R.; Simoniello, P.; Putti, R.; Lionetti, L. Physiological Adaptation to Simultaneous Chronic Exposure to High-Fat Diet and Dichlorodiphenyletylhene (DDE) in Wistar Rat Testis. *Cells* **2019**, *8*, 443. [CrossRef]
34. Migliaccio, V.; Scudiero, R.; Sica, R.; Lionetti, L.; Putti, R. Oxidative stress and mitochondrial uncoupling protein 2 expression in hepatic steatosis induced by exposure to xenobiotic DDE and high fat diet in male Wistar rats. *PLoS ONE* **2019**, *14*, e0215955. [CrossRef]
35. Yeung, B.H.; Wan, H.T.; Law, A.Y.; Wong, C.K. Endocrine disrupting chemicals: Multiple effects on testicular signaling and spermatogenesis. *Spermatogenesis* **2011**, *1*, 231–239. [CrossRef]
36. Nunnari, J.; Suomalainen, A. Mitochondria: In sickness and in health. *Cell* **2012**, *148*, 1145–1159. [CrossRef]
37. Grivell, L.A. Nucleo-mitochondrial interactions in mitochondrial gene expression. *Crit. Rev. Biochem. Mol. Biol.* **1995**, *30*, 121–164. [CrossRef]
38. Poyton, R.O.; McEwen, J.E. Crosstalk between nuclear and mitochondrial genomes. *Annu. Rev. Biochem.* **1996**, *65*, 563–607. [CrossRef]
39. Fakouri, N.B.; Hansen, T.L.; Desler, C.; Anugula, S.; Rasmussen, L.J. From Powerhouse to Perpetrator-Mitochondria in Health and Disease. *Biology* **2019**, *8*, 35. [CrossRef]
40. Lesnefsky, E.J.; Moghaddas, S.; Tandler, B.; Kerner, J.; Hoppel, C.L. Mitochondrial dysfunction in cardiac disease: Ischemia–reperfusion, aging, and heart failure. *J. Mol. Cell. Cardiol.* **2001**, *33*, 1065–1089. [CrossRef]
41. Wallace, D.C. Mitochondrial defects in cardiomyopathy and neuromuscular disease. *Am. Heart J. (Suppl.)* **2000**, *139*, 70–85. [CrossRef]
42. Barja, G. Mitochondrial oxygen radical generation and leak: Sites of production in states 4 and 3, organ specificity, and relation to aging and longevity. *J. Bioenerg. Biomembr.* **1999**, *31*, 347–366. [CrossRef]
43. Wong, H.S.; Dighe, P.A.; Mezera, V.; Monternier, P.A.; Brand, M.D. Production of superoxide and hydrogen peroxide from specific mitochondrial sites under different bioenergetic conditions. *J. Biol. Chem.* **2017**, *292*, 16804–16809. [CrossRef]
44. Chen, Q.; Vazquez, E.J.; Moghaddas, S.; Hoppel, C.L.; Lesnefsky, E.J. Production of reactive oxygen species by mitochondria: Central role of complex III. *J. Biol. Chem.* **2003**, *278*, 36027–36031. [CrossRef]
45. Muller, F.L.; Liu, Y.; Van Remmen, H. Complex III releases superoxide to both sides of the inner mitochondrial membrane. *J. Biol. Chem.* **2004**, *279*, 49064–49073. [CrossRef]
46. Bleier, L.; Dröse, S. Superoxide generation by complex III: From mechanistic rationales to functional consequences. *Biochim. Biophys. Acta* **2013**, *1827*, 1320–1331. [CrossRef]
47. Brand, M.D. Mitochondrial generation of superoxide and hydrogen peroxide as the source of mitochondrial redox signaling. *Free Radic. Biol. Med.* **2016**, *100*, 14–31. [CrossRef]
48. D'Autréaux, B.; Toledano, M.B. ROS as signalling molecules: Mechanisms that generate specificity in ROS homeostasis. *Nat. Rev. Mol. Cell Biol.* **2007**, *8*, 813–824. [CrossRef]
49. Yang, W.; Hekimi, S. A mitochondrial superoxide signal triggers increased longevity in *Caenorhabditis elegans*. *PLoS Biol.* **2010**, *8*, e1000556. [CrossRef]

50. Lee, S.J.; Hwang, A.B.; Kenyon, C. Inhibition of respiration extends C. elegans life span via reactive oxygen species that increase HIF-1 activity. *Curr. Biol.* **2010**, *20*, 2131–2136. [CrossRef]
51. Schaar, C.E.; Dues, D.J.; Spielbauer, K.K.; Machiela, E.; Cooper, J.F.; Senchuk, M.; Hekimi, S.; Van Raamsdonk, J.M. Mitochondrial and cytoplasmic ROS have opposing effects on lifespan. *PLoS Genet.* **2015**, *11*, e1004972. [CrossRef]
52. Hrycay, E.G.; Bandiera, S.M. Involvement of Cytochrome P450 in Reactive Oxygen Species Formation and Cancer. *Adv. Pharmacol.* **2015**, *74*, 35–84. [CrossRef]
53. Hamanaka, R.B.; Chandel, N.S. Mitochondrial reactive oxygen species regulate cellular signaling and dictate biological outcomes. *Trends Biochem. Sci.* **2010**, *35*, 505–513. [CrossRef]
54. Day, R.M.; Suzuki, Y.J. Cell proliferation, reactive oxygen and cellular glutathione. *Dose Response* **2006**, *3*, 425–442. [CrossRef]
55. Roberts, C.K.; Sindhu, K.K. Oxidative stress and metabolic syndrome. *Life Sci.* **2009**, *84*, 705–712. [CrossRef]
56. Mahjoub, S.; Masrour-Roudsari, J. Role of oxidative stress in pathogenesis of metabolic syndrome. *Casp. J. Intern. Med.* **2012**, *3*, 386–396.
57. Renaud, H.J.; Rutter, A.; Winn, L.M. Assessment of xenobiotic biotransformation including reactive oxygen species generation in the embryo using benzene as an example. *Methods Mol. Biol.* **2012**, *889*, 253–263. [CrossRef]
58. Turrens, J.F. Mitochondrial formation of reactive oxygen species. *J. Physiol.* **2003**, *552*, 335–344. [CrossRef]
59. Klotz, L.O.; Steinbrenner, H. Cellular adaptation to xenobiotics: Interplay between xenosensors, reactive oxygen species and FOXO transcription factors. *Redox Biol.* **2017**, *13*, 646–654. [CrossRef]
60. Kesh, S.B.; Sarkar, D.; Manna, K. High-fat diet-induced oxidative stress and its impact on metabolic syndrome: A review. *Asian J. Pharm. Clin. Res.* **2016**, *9*, 47–52.
61. Terra, L.F.; Lobba, A.R. High-fat diet and fish oil affect adipocyte metabolism in a depot-specific manner. *J. Physiol.* **2017**, *595*, 1859–1860. [CrossRef]
62. Du, Z.; Yang, Y.; Hu, Y.; Sun, Y.; Zhang, S.; Peng, W.; Zhong, Y.; Huang, X.; Kong, W. A long-term high-fat diet increases oxidative stress, mitochondrial damage and apoptosis in the inner ear of D-galactose-induced aging rats. *Hear Res.* **2012**, *287*, 15–24. [CrossRef]
63. Migliaccio, V.; Sica, R.; Di Gregorio, I.; Putti, R.; Lionetti, L. High-Fish Oil and High-Lard Diets Differently Affect Testicular Antioxidant Defense and Mitochondrial Fusion/Fission Balance in Male Wistar Rats: Potential Protective Effect of ω3 Polyunsaturated Fatty Acids Targeting Mitochondria Dynamics. *Int. J. Mol. Sci.* **2019**, *20*, 3110. [CrossRef]
64. Klop, B.; Elte, J.W.; Cabezas, M.C. Dyslipidemia in Obesity: Mechanisms and Potential Targets. *Nutrients* **2013**, *5*, 1218–1240. [CrossRef]
65. Lionetti, L.; Mollica, M.P.; Sica, R.; Donizzetti, I.; Gifuni, G.; Pignalosa, A.; Cavaliere, G.; Putti, R. Differential effects of high-fish oil and high-lard diets on cells and cytokines involved in the inflammatory process in rat insulin-sensitive tissues. *Int. J. Mol. Sci.* **2014**, *15*, 3040–3063. [CrossRef]
66. Shimobayashi, M.; Albert, V.; Woelnerhanssen, B.; Frei, I.C.; Weissenberger, D.; Meyer-Gerspach, A.C.; Clement, N.; Moes, S.; Colombi, M.; Meier, J.A.; et al. Insulin resistance causes inflammation in adipose tissue. *J. Clin. Investig.* **2018**, *128*, 1538–1550. [CrossRef]
67. Jeukendrup, A.E. Modulation of carbohydrate and fat utilization by diet, exercise and environment. *Biochem. Soc. Trans.* **2003**, *31*, 1270–1273. [CrossRef]
68. Fisher, E.C.; Evans, W.J.; Phinney, S.D.; Blackburn, G.L.; Bistrian, B.R.; Young, V.R. Changes in skeletal muscle metabolism induced by a eucaloric ketogenic diet. In *Biochemistry of Exercise*; Knuttgen, H.G., Vogel, J.A., Poortmans, J., Eds.; Human Kinetics Publishers Inc.: Champaign, IL, USA, 1983; pp. 497–507.
69. Kiens, B.; Helge, J.W. Effect of high-fat diets on exercise performance. *Proc. Nutr. Soc.* **1998**, *57*, 73–75. [CrossRef]
70. Samuel, V.T.; Liu, Z.X.; Qu, X.; Elder, B.D.; Bilz, S.; Befroy, D.; Romanelli, A.J.; Shulman, G.I. Mechanism of hepatic insulin resistance in non-alcoholic fatty liver disease. *J. Biol. Chem.* **2004**, *279*, 32345–32353. [CrossRef]
71. Szalowska, E.; Tesfay, H.A.; van Hijum, S.A.; Kersten, S. Transcriptomic signatures of peroxisome proliferator-activated receptor alpha (PPARalpha) in different mouse liver models identify novel aspects of its biology. *BMC Genom.* **2014**, *15*, 1106. [CrossRef]
72. Rakhshandehroo, M.; Knoch, B.; Muller, M.; Kersten, S. Peroxisome proliferator-activated receptor alpha target genes. *PPAR Res.* **2010**, *2010*, 612089. [CrossRef]

73. Kersten, S.; Seydoux, J.; Peters, J.M.; Gonzalez, F.J.; Desvergne, B.; Wahli, W. Peroxisome proliferator-activated receptor alpha mediates the adaptive response to fasting. *J. Clin. Investig.* **1999**, *103*, 1489–1498. [CrossRef]
74. Cotter, D.G.; Ercal, B.; Huang, X.; Leid, J.M.; d'Avignon, D.A.; Graham, M.J.; Dietzen, D.J.; Brunt, E.M.; Patti, G.J.; Crawford, P.A. Ketogenesis prevents diet-induced fatty liver injury and hyperglycemia. *J. Clin. Investig.* **2014**, *124*, 5175–5190. [CrossRef]
75. Liss, K.H.; Finck, B.N. PPARs and nonalcoholic fatty liver disease. *Biochimie* **2017**, *136*, 65–74. [CrossRef]
76. Villarroya, F.; Iglesias, R.; Giralt, M. PPARs in the Control of Uncoupling Proteins Gene Expression. *PPAR Res.* **2007**, *2007*, 74364. [CrossRef]
77. Nakatani, T.; Tsuboyama-Kasaoka, N.; Takahashi, M.; Miura, S.; Ezaki, O. Mechanism for Peroxisome Proliferator-activated Receptor-Activator-induced Up-regulation of UCP2 mRNA in Rodent Hepatocytes. *J. Biol. Chem.* **2002**, *277*, 9562–9569. [CrossRef]
78. Auestad, N.; Korsak, R.A.; Morrow, J.W.; Edmond, J. Fatty acid oxidation and ketogenesis by astrocytes in primary culture. *J. Neurochem.* **1991**, *56*, 1376–1386. [CrossRef]
79. Yamasaki, M.; Hasegawa, S.; Imai, M.; Takahashi, N.; Fukui, T. High-fat diet-induced obesity stimulates ketone body utilization in osteoclasts of the mouse bone. *Biochem. Biophys. Res. Commun.* **2016**, *473*, 654–661. [CrossRef]
80. Sunny, N.E.; Satapati, S.; Fu, X.; He, T.; Mehdibeigi, R.; Spring-Robinson, C.; Duarte, J.; Potthoff, M.J.; Browning, J.D.; Burgess, S.C. Progressive adaptation of hepatic ketogenesis in mice fed a high-fat diet. *Am. J. Physiol. Endocrinol. Metab.* **2010**, *298*, E1226–E1235. [CrossRef]
81. García-Ruiz, C.; Fernández-Checa, J.C. Mitochondrial Oxidative Stress and Antioxidants Balance in Fatty Liver Disease. *Hepatol. Commun.* **2018**, *2*, 1425–1439. [CrossRef]
82. Mollica, M.P.; Lionetti, L.; Moreno, M.; Lombardi, A.; De Lange, P.; Antonelli, A.; Lanni, A.; Cavaliere, G.; Barletta, A.; Goglia, F. 3,5-diiodo-l-thyronine, by modulating mitochondrial functions, reverses hepatic fat accumulation in rats fed a high-fat diet. *J. Hepatol.* **2009**, *51*, 363–370. [CrossRef]
83. Iossa, S.; Lionetti, L.; Mollica, M.P.; Crescenzo, R.; Barletta, A.; Liverini, G. Effect of long-term high-fat feeding on energy balance and liver oxidative activity in rats. *Br. J. Nutr.* **2000**, *84*, 377–385. [CrossRef]
84. Lionetti, L.; Iossa, S.; Brand, M.D.; Liverini, G. Relationship between membrane potential and respiration rate in isolated liver mitochondria from rats fed an energy dense diet. *Mol. Cell. Biochem.* **1996**, *158*, 133–138.
85. Migliaccio, V.; Lionetti, L.; Putti, R.; Sica, R.; Scudiero, R. Combined effects of DDE and hyperlipidic diet on metallothionein expression and synthesis in rat tissues. *Environ. Toxicol.* **2019**, *34*, 283–293. [CrossRef]
86. Viarengo, A.; Burlando, B.; Ceratto, N.; Panfoli, I. Antioxidant role of metallothioneins: A comparative overview. *Cell. Mol. Biol. (Noisy-le-Grand)* **2000**, *46*, 407–417.
87. Takahashi, Y.; Ogra, Y.; Suzuki, K.T. Nuclear trafficking of metallothionein requires oxidation of a cytosolic partner. *J. Cell. Physiol.* **2005**, *202*, 563–569. [CrossRef]
88. Chubatsu, L.S.; Meneghini, R. Metallothionein protects DNA from oxidative damage. *Biochem. J.* **1993**, *291*, 193–198. [CrossRef]
89. Vukovic, V.; Pheng, S.R.; Stewart, A.; Vik, C.H.; Hedley, D.W. Protection from radiation-induced DNA single-strand breaks by induction of nuclear Metallothionein. *Int. J. Radiat. Biol.* **2000**, *76*, 757–762. [CrossRef]
90. Abel, J.; de Ruiter, N. Inhibition of hydroxyl-radical-generated DNA degradation by metallothionein. *Toxicol. Lett.* **1989**, *47*, 191–196. [CrossRef]
91. Chiaverini, N.; De Ley, M. Protective effect of metallothionein on oxidative stress-induced DNA damage. *Free Radic. Res.* **2010**, *44*, 605–613. [CrossRef]
92. Ledesma, A.; de Lacoba, M.G.; Rial, E. The mitochondrial uncoupling proteins. *Genome Biol. Prot. Fam. Rev.* **2002**, *3*, 1–9.
93. Boss, O.; Samec, S.; Paoloni-Giacobino, A.; Rossier, C.; Dulloo, A.; Seydoux, J.; Muzzin, P.; Giacobino, J.P. Uncoupling protein-3: A new member of the mitochondrial carrier family with tissue specific expression. *FEBS Lett.* **1997**, *408*, 39–42. [CrossRef]
94. Ramsden, D.B.; Ho, P.W.L.; Ho, J.W.M.; Liu, H.F.; So, D.H.F.; Tse, H.M.; Chan, K.H.; Ho, S.L. Human neuronal uncoupling proteins 4 and 5 (UCP4 and UCP5): Structural properties, regulation, and physiological role in protection against oxidative stress and mitochondrial dysfunction. *Brain Behav.* **2012**, *2*, 468–478. [CrossRef]
95. Sreedhar, A.; Zhao, Y. Uncoupling Protein 2 and Metabolic Diseases. *Mitochondrion* **2017**, *34*, 135–140. [CrossRef]

96. Negre-Salvayre, A.; Hirtz, C.; Carrera, G.; Cazenave, R.; Troly, M.; Salvayre, R.; Pénicaud, L.; Casteilla, L. A role for uncoupling protein-2 as a regulator of mitochondrial hydrogen peroxide generation. *FASEB J.* **1999**, *11*, 809–815. [CrossRef]
97. Horimoto, M.; Fulop, P.; Derdak, Z.; Resnick, M.; Wands, J.R.; Baffy, G. Uncoupling protein-2 deficiency promotes oxidant stress and delays liver regeneration in mice. *Hepatology* **2004**, *39*, 386–392. [CrossRef]
98. Wahlang, B.; Beier, J.I.; Clair, H.B.; Bellis-Jones, H.J.; Falkner, K.C.; McClain, C.J.; Cave, M.C. Toxicant-associated steatohepatitis. *Toxicol. Pathol.* **2013**, *41*, 343–360. [CrossRef]
99. Schwingel, P.A.; Cotrim, H.P.; Salles, B.R.; Almeida, C.E.; dos Santos, C.R., Jr.; Nachef, B.; Andrade, A.R.; Zoppi, C.C. Anabolic-androgenic steroids: A possible new risk factor of toxicant-associated fatty liver disease. *Liver Int.* **2011**, *31*, 348–353. [CrossRef]
100. Le Magueresse-Battistoni, B.; Vidal, H.; Naville, D. Environmental Pollutants and Metabolic Disorders: The Multi-Exposure Scenario of Life. *Front. Endocrinol. (Lausanne)* **2018**, *9*, 582. [CrossRef]
101. Kourouma, A.; Quan, C.; Duan, P.; Qi, S.; Yu, T.; Wang, Y.; Yang, K. Bisphenol A Induces Apoptosis in Liver Cells through Induction of ROS. *Adv. Toxicol.* **2015**, *2015*, 901983. [CrossRef]
102. Yavaşoğlu, N.Ü.; Köksal, C.; Dağdeviren, M.; Aktuğ, H.; Yavaşoğlu, A. Induction of oxidative stress and histological changes in liver by subacute doses of butyl cyclohexyl phthalate. *Environ. Toxicol.* **2014**, *29*, 345–353. [CrossRef]
103. Arciello, M.; Gori, M.; Maggio, R.; Barbaro, B.; Tarocchi, M.; Galli, A.; Balsano, C. Environmental pollution: A tangible risk for NAFLD pathogenesis. *Int. J. Mol. Sci.* **2013**, *14*, 22052–22066. [CrossRef]
104. Laing, S.; Wang, G.; Briazova, T.; Zhang, C.; Wang, A.; Zheng, Z.; Gow, A.; Chen, A.F.; Rajagopalan, S.; Chen, L.C.; et al. Airborne particulate matter selectively activates endoplasmic reticulum stress response in the lung and liver tissues. *Am. J. Physiol. Cell Physiol.* **2010**, *299*, C736–C749. [CrossRef]
105. Tan, H.-H.; Fiel, M.I.; Sun, Q.; Guo, J.; Gordon, R.E.; Chen, L.C.; Friedman, S.L.; Odin, J.A.; Allina, J. Kupffer cell activation by ambient air particulate matter exposure may exacerbate non-alcoholic fatty liver disease. *J. Immunotoxicol.* **2009**, *6*, 266–275. [CrossRef]
106. Huang, Q.; Chen, Q. Mediating Roles of PPARs in the Effects of Environmental Chemicals on Sex Steroids. *PPAR Res.* **2017**, *2017*, 3203161. [CrossRef]
107. Yáñez, L.; Borja-Aburto, V.H.; Rojas, E.; de la Fuente, H.; González-Amaro, R.; Gómez, H.; Jongitud, A.A.; Díaz-Barriga, F. DDT induces DNA damage in blood cells. Studies in vitro and in women chronically exposed to this insecticide. *Environ. Res.* **2004**, *94*, 18–24. [CrossRef]
108. Binelli, A.; Riva, C.; Cogni, D.; Provini, A. Genotoxic effects of p,p'-DDT (1,1,1-trichloro-2,2-bis-(chlorophenyl)ethane) and its metabolites in *Zebra mussel* (*D. polymorpha*) by SCGE assay and micronucleus test. *Environ. Mol. Mutagen.* **2008**, *49*, 406–415. [CrossRef]
109. Song, Y.; Yang, K.D. Effect of p, p'-DDE on DNA damage and expression of FasL gene of rat Sertoli cell in vitro. *Wei Sheng Yan Jiu* **2006**, *35*, 261–263.
110. Espinosa-Diez, C.; Miguel, V.; Mennerich, D.; Kietzmann, T.; Sánchez-Pérez, P.; Cadenas, S.; Lamas, S. Antioxidant responses and cellular adjustments to oxidative stress. *Redox Biol.* **2015**, *6*, 183–197. [CrossRef]
111. Qin, L.; Fan, M.; Candas, D.; Jiang, G.; Papadopoulos, S.; Tian, L.; Woloschak, G.; Grdina, D.J.; Li, J.J. CDK1 Enhances Mitochondrial Bioenergetics for Radiation-Induced DNA Repair. *Cell Rep.* **2015**, *13*, 2056–2063. [CrossRef]
112. Brace, L.E.; Vose, S.C.; Stanya, K.; Gathungu, R.M.; Marur, V.R.; Longchamp, A.; Treviño-Villarreal, H.; Mejia, P.; Vargas, D.; Inouye, K.; et al. Increased oxidative phosphorylation in response to acute and chronic DNA damage. *NPJ Aging Mech. Dis.* **2016**, *2*, 16022. [CrossRef]
113. Nims, R.W.; Lubet, R.A. Induction of cytochrome P-450 in the Norway rat, Rattus norvegicus, following exposure to potential environmental contaminants. *J. Toxicol. Environ. Health* **1995**, *46*, 271–292. [CrossRef]
114. Wyde, M.E.; Bartolucci, E.; Ueda, A.; Zhang, H.; Yan, B.; Negishi, M.; You, L. The environmental pollutant 1,1-dichloro-2,2-bis (p-chlorophenyl) ethylene induces rat hepatic cytochrome P450 2B and 3A expression through the constitutive androstane receptor and pregnane X receptor. *Mol. Pharmacol.* **2003**, *64*, 474–481. [CrossRef]
115. Mota, P.C.; Cordeiro, M.; Pereira, S.P.; Oliveira, P.J.; Moreno, A.J.; Ramalho-Santos, J. Differential effects of p,p'-DDE on testis and liver mitochondria: Implications for reproductive toxicology. *Reprod. Toxicol.* **2011**, *31*, 80–85. [CrossRef]

116. Ferreira, F.M.; Madeira, V.M.; Moreno, A.J. Interactions of 2,2-bis(p-chlorophenyl)-1,1-dichloroethylene with mitochondrial oxidative phosphorylation. *Biochem. Pharmacol.* **1997**, *53*, 299–308. [CrossRef]
117. Vidal, J.D.; Whitney, K.M. Morphologic manifestations of testicular and epididymal toxicity. *Spermatogenesis* **2014**, *4*, 1–17. [CrossRef]
118. Siddighi, S.; Patton, W.C.; Jacobson, J.D.; King, A.; Chan, P.J. Correlation of sperm parameters with apoptosis assessed by dual fluorescence dna integrity assay. *Arch. Androl.* **2009**, *50*, 311–314. [CrossRef]
119. França, L.R.; Avelar, G.F.; Almeida, F.F. Spermatogenesis and sperm transit through the epididymis in mammals with emphasis on pigs. *Theriogenology* **2005**, *63*, 300–318. [CrossRef]
120. Palmer, N.O.; Bakos, H.W.; Fullston, T.; Lane, M. Impact of obesity on male fertility, sperm function and molecular composition. *Spermatogenesis* **2012**, *2*, 253–263. [CrossRef]
121. Katib, A. Mechanisms linking obesity to male infertility. *Cent. Eur. J. Urol.* **2015**, *68*, 79–85. [CrossRef]
122. Kort, H.I.; Massey, J.B.; Elsner, C.W.; Mitchell-Leef, D.; Shapiro, D.B.; Witt, M.A.; Roudebush, W.E. Impact of body mass index values on sperm quantity and quality. *J. Androl.* **2006**, *27*, 450–452. [CrossRef]
123. MacDonald, A.A.; Herbison, G.P.; Showell, M.; Farquhar, C.M. The impact of body mass index on semen parameters and reproductive hormones in human males: A systematic review with meta-analysis. *Hum. Reprod. Update* **2010**, *16*, 293–311. [CrossRef]
124. Vested, A.; Giwercman, A.; Bonde, J.P.; Toft, G. Persistent organic pollutants and male reproductive health. *Asian J. Androl.* **2014**, *16*, 71–80. [CrossRef]
125. Bonefeld-Jørgensen, E.C.; Andersen, H.R.; Rasmussen, T.H.; Vinggaard, A.M. Effect of highly bioaccumulated polychlorinated biphenyl congeners on estrogen and androgen receptor activity. *Toxicology* **2001**, *158*, 141–153. [CrossRef]
126. Penna-Videau, S.; Bustos-Obregon, E.; Cermeno-Vivas, J.R.; Chirino, D. Malathion affects spermatogenic proliferation in mouse. *Int. J. Morphol.* **2012**, *30*, 1399–1407. [CrossRef]
127. Lebda, M.; Gad, S.; Gaafar, H. Effects of lipoic acid on acrylamide induced testicular damage. *Mater. Sociomed.* **2014**, *26*, 208–212. [CrossRef]
128. Türedi, S.; Yuluğ, E.; Alver, A.; Kutlu, O.; Kahraman, C. Effects of resveratrol on doxorubicin induced testicular damage in rats. *Exp. Toxicol. Pathol.* **2015**, *67*, 229–235. [CrossRef]
129. Song, L.; Liu, J.; Jin, X.; Li, Z.; Zhao, M.; Liu, W. p,p'-Dichlorodiphenyldichloroethylene induces colorectal adenocarcinoma cell proliferation through oxidative stress. *PLoS ONE* **2014**, *9*, e112700. [CrossRef]

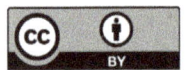

© 2019 by the authors. Licensee MDPI, Basel, Switzerland. This article is an open access article distributed under the terms and conditions of the Creative Commons Attribution (CC BY) license (http://creativecommons.org/licenses/by/4.0/).

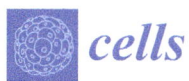

Article

Hypoxic Adaptation of Mitochondrial Metabolism in Rat Cerebellum Decreases in Pregnancy

Anastasia Graf [1,2], Lidia Trofimova [1], Alexander Ksenofontov [3], Lyudmila Baratova [3] and Victoria Bunik [3,4,5,*]

1. Faculty of Biology, Lomonosov Moscow State University, 119234 Moscow, Russia; nastjushka@gmail.com (A.G.); lidtrof@gmail.com (L.T.)
2. Faculty of Nano-, Bio-, Informational and Cognitive and Socio-humanistic Sciences and Technologies at Moscow Institute of Physics and Technology, 123098 Moscow, Russia
3. A.N. Belozersky Institute of Physicochemical Biology, Lomonosov Moscow State University, 119992 Moscow, Russia; alexksenofon@gmail.com (A.K.); kukarino@yandex.ru (L.B.)
4. Faculty of Bioengineering and Bioinformatics, Lomonosov Moscow State University, 119234 Moscow, Russia
5. Biochemistry Department, Sechenov University, 119048 Moscow, Russia
* Correspondence: bunik@belozersky.msu.ru; Tel.: +7-495-939-4484; Fax: +7-495-939-3181

Received: 29 November 2019; Accepted: 2 January 2020; Published: 7 January 2020

Abstract: Function of brain amino acids as neurotransmitters or their precursors implies changes in the amino acid levels and/or metabolism in response to physiological and environmental challenges. Modelling such challenges by pregnancy and/or hypoxia, we characterize the amino acid pool in the rat cerebellum, quantifying the levels and correlations of 15 amino acids and activity of 2-oxoglutarate dehydrogenase complex (OGDHC). The parameters are systemic indicators of metabolism because OGDHC limits the flux through mitochondrial TCA cycle, where amino acids are degraded and their precursors synthesized. Compared to non-pregnant state, pregnancy increases the cerebellar content of glutamate and tryptophan, decreasing interdependence between the quantified components of amino acid metabolism. In response to hypoxia, the dependence of cerebellar amino acid pool on OGDHC and the average levels of arginine, glutamate, lysine, methionine, serine, phenylalanine, and tryptophan increase in non-pregnant rats only. This is accompanied by a higher hypoxic resistance of the non-pregnant vs. pregnant rats, pointing to adaptive significance of the hypoxia-induced changes in the cerebellar amino acid metabolism. These adaptive mechanisms are not effective in the pregnancy-changed metabolic network. Thus, the cerebellar amino acid levels and OGDHC activity provide sensitive markers of the physiology-dependent organization of metabolic network and its stress adaptations.

Keywords: amino acid neurotransmitter; cerebellar amino acid metabolism; hypoxia; 2-oxoglutarate dehydrogenase; tricarboxylic acid cycle

1. Introduction

Many amino acids and/or their derivatives are neurotransmitters. Hence, metabolic perturbations in the brain, affecting the levels of amino acids, often have neurological consequences, and vice versa. However, systemic consequences of changed levels of specific amino acids or related enzymes are not easily predictable. For instance, administration of arginine or nitric oxide synthase inhibitors at cerebral infarction may cause opposite physiological outcomes [1]. The glutamate-induced excitotoxicity could be either aggravated [2] or alleviated [1] by nitric oxide signaling. Obviously, one should take into account that generation of nitric oxide involves an intercept between metabolism of lysine and arginine [3], which, in their turn, are tightly linked to other amino acids through multiple intercepts in the amino acid metabolism. In particular, the transporters for the amino acid influx are usually common for a group of amino acids which thus compete for their intracellular transport.

This work is dedicated to elaboration of systemic markers of the changed metabolism of amino acids, resulting from the brain response to the physiological or pathological challenges. To achieve this goal, we consider the two important features of the amino acid metabolism. First, mitochondrial tricarboxylic acid (TCA) cycle actively participates both in the amino acid degradation and de novo biosynthesis of the amino acid precursors, such as 2-oxoglutarate and oxaloacetate. Under maximal energy demands, the flux through the cycle is limited by the highly regulated multienzyme complex of 2-oxoglutarate dehydrogenase (OGDHC) [4–6], which strongly impacts on the amino acid metabolism in the brain and cerebellar neuronal cells in culture [7–10]. Based on the tight interconnection between the 2-oxo and amino acids, which may contribute to the common neurological symptoms upon the impaired degradation of 2-oxo acids [4,6], we consider dependence of the brain amino acid levels on the OGDHC activity as a systemic marker of mitochondrial metabolism. Second, specific (patho) physiological settings may strongly contribute to different systemic outcomes of the same treatment, because organization of metabolism under these settings may vary. Indeed, the tissue-specific expression of enzymes in a pathway is an important factor in predicting the metabolic changes in health and disease [11], and the expression pattern may vary even in the same tissue in different (patho) physiological states. Indeed, inhibition of 2-oxoglutarate-dehydrogenase, through which glutamate is degraded in the TCA cycle, may increase or decrease the glutamate levels in the rat brain cortex, dependent on pregnancy, which in turn defines the level of OGDHC activity [7,8,12]. Levels of another amino acid of signaling importance, homoarginine, are also affected in pregnancy [13]. Thus, pregnant rats provide a good model of physiological differences in organization of metabolic networks, important for central nervous system functions. On the other hand, influence of specific inhibition of the brain OGDHC on biochemical, physiological, and behavioral parameters of experimental animals strongly depend on the pathological conditions, such as acute hypoxia or ethanol intoxication [12,14]. Because hypoxia is the most common pathogenic factor known to perturb the high-impact signaling by glutamate, (homo) arginine/nitric oxide, and their interaction, we use our well-established model of acute hypobaric hypoxia to study the changes in the brain amino acid metabolism under pathological conditions.

Because of the significant regional heterogeneity of the brain metabolism and signaling, we focus our investigation on the easily isolated brain structure, cerebellum, which is also well-characterized regarding its physiological functions. In particular, cerebellum is involved in compensatory responses of brain to impaired movement control [15], which also occurs in rats exposed to acute hypobaric hypoxia. The movement disorders in Parkinson disease affecting cerebellum [16,17] have been associated with perturbations in cerebellar pool of amino acids and their signaling [18]. These biochemical changes in cerebellum may be further translated into behavioral changes because of high interconnectivity in the brain [16,19].

In our analysis of systemic response in the healthy and hypoxia-affected brain, we take into account that correlated changes of certain metabolites may provide more information on biosystems than single markers [20–23]. As a result, the present study demonstrates that the metabolic interdependence of the brain amino acids and OGDHC provides systemic markers of different physiological and pathological states, which complement the information based on analysis of traditional metabolic markers, such as average levels of metabolites or enzymatic activities. Even when single indicators do not significantly change because of homeostatic mechanisms employed by biosystems, the patterns of metabolic correlations reliably estimate systemic changes, helping to suggest the affected pathways.

2. Materials and Method

2.1. Animal Experiments

All animal experiments were performed according to the Guide for the Care and Use of Laboratory Animals published by the European Union Directives 86/609/EEC and 2010/63/EU, and were approved by Bioethics Committee of Lomonosov Moscow State University (protocol number 69-o from 09.06.2016). Animals were kept at 21 ± 2 °C and relative humidity 53 ± 5% with the 12/12 h light/dark cycle (lights on 9:00 = ZT 0, lights off 21:00 = ZT 12).

Wistar female rats, pregnant and non-pregnant ones, of about 250–300 g were used in the experiment. To obtain pregnant rats, two virgin female rats were located in a cage with one male. After 24 h, vaginal smears were examined. When sperm was found in the vaginal smear, it was considered as the first day of pregnancy, and the male rat was separated. The rats were purchased from the State Research Center of the Russian Federation—Institute for Biomedical Problems, Russian Academy of Sciences, and were kept at our conditions for two weeks prior to the experiments. T/4K cages (555/4K, 580 × 375 × 200 mm) were used. Five to six animals were kept in each cage. Standard rodent pellet food (laboratorkorm.ru) and tap water were available ad libitum.

Four groups of female rats were used: (1) normoxic control non-pregnant group; (2) hypoxic treatment non-pregnant group; (3) normoxic control pregnant group; (4) pregnant group exposed to hypoxia at the 9–10th day of pregnancy, which in rats is roughly correspondent to the first trimester of human pregnancy [24]. Total number of animals in an experimental group, n, comprised animals from several independent experiments and is indicated in the figures and tables. On the second day after the treatment, when the physiological assessment was completed, animals were sacrificed for further biochemical analyses by decapitation. At this stage, the number of pups (10 ± 2) did not significantly differ between the control and hypoxic rats, although independent long-term physiological monitoring indicated that the pregnancy failures occurred more often in the latter than former rats.

Cerebella were quickly excised from animal brains on ice, frozen in liquid nitrogen, and stored at −70 °C prior to biochemical analyses. A half of each thawed cerebellum was used to prepare the homogenates for enzymatic assays, the other half—to make extracts for the amino acid quantification.

2.2. Acute Hypobaric Hypoxia

Female rats were exposed to hypobaric hypoxia at 5% O_2 (11500 m altitude, 145 mm Hg) in a decompression (altitude) chamber "Mez Mohelnice" (Mohelnice, Czech Republic) of 3.3 L volume, as described previously [25,26]. Briefly, after closing the chamber, air pressure inside the chamber was progressively decreased during 1 min (200 m/sec) by the vacuum pump connected to the chamber. The pressure was controlled using the pressure gauge. Overall response of an organism to hypoxia at subcritical lack of oxygen is defined by the lifetime (LT) which is evaluated from the moment of reaching the target height (i.e., 11,500 m altitude, 5% O_2, 145 mm Hg) to the second agonal breath. LT characterizes the ability of animals to mobilize their protective mechanisms for survival under life-incompatible extreme conditions. The pressure and oxygen in the chamber returned to the nominal values after the second agonal breath. According to LT, the rats were divided into groups of high resistance (HR, LT ≥ 10 min), middle resistance (MR, LT within 5–10 min), and low resistance (LR, LT within 1–5 min). These types of animals are known to demonstrate different functional and metabolic patterns, including differences in the CNS activity and neurohumoral regulation, stress-responsive systems, oxygen transport by the blood, and tissue respiration [27–29].

2.3. Enzyme Assays

Homogenization of cerebella and assays of the overall OGDHC activity of brain homogenates were performed as described earlier [30] with 20% glycerol added to the homogenization buffer and sonication as in [12].

2.4. Ninhydrine Quantification of Amino Acids

Preparation of the acetic acid/methanol extracts of cerebella and quantification of their amino acids was done as described in [31], using L-8800 amino acid analyzer (Hitachi, Tokyo, Japan) in the standard mode according to the manufacturer's User Manual (Hitachi High-Technologies Corporation, Tokyo, Japan, 1998). The samples were stored at −70 °C. Briefly, the extracts were subjected to an ion-exchange column 2622SC (PH) (Hitachi, Ltd., Tokyo, Japan, P/N 855-3508, 4.6 × 80 mm), eluted by step gradient of four sodium-acetate buffers at a flow rate of 0.4 mL/min at 57 °C. A total of 20 µL of a 25-fold diluted amino acid standard mix (AA-S-18 −5 ML analytical standard, SIGMA, or standard of basic amino acids, Type B, Hitachi, 016-08641) or 50 µL of cerebellar extracts were injected to the column. Fifteen amino acids eluted as separate peaks in this procedure were quantified. Post-column derivatization (136 °C, flow rate 0.35 mL/min) was performed using the mix of equal volumes of ninhydrin buffer R2 and ninhydrin solution R1 (Wako Pure Chemical Industries, P/N 298-69601). Colored products were detected by absorption at 570 nm. Data were processed using MultiChrom for Windows software (Ampersand Ltd., Moscow, Russia).

2.5. Data Acquisition and Statistics

Statistical analysis was performed using Statistica 10.0 (StatSoft Inc., Tulsa, OK, USA). Averaged values are presented as means ± SEM. Comparison between the two experimental groups was done using non-parametric Mann–Whitney U-test. The Pearson's correlations between the levels of different amino acids or between the levels of amino acids and OGDHC activity were characterized by the correlation coefficients and p-values of the correlation. Statistical significance of differences in the parameters characterizing metabolic interactions between the levels of OGDHC activity and/or amino acids were assessed by the Wilcoxon signed rank test. Differences with $p \leq 0.05$ were considered significant.

3. Results

3.1. Pregnancy-Induced Changes in Cerebellar Levels of Amino Acids and OGDHC Activity

Table 1 compares the average levels of the OGDHC activity and 15 quantified amino acids in cerebella of the non-pregnant and pregnant rats.

Table 1. Influence of pregnancy on the levels of cerebellar amino acids and 2-oxoglutarate dehydrogenase complex (OGDHC) activity.

Parameter	Rats		
	Non-Pregnant	Pregnant	p Values
OGDHC	1.13 ± 0.13	1.21 ± 0.15	0.61
ALA	0.59 ± 0.05	0.62 ± 0.04	0.67
ARG	0.15 ± 0.03	0.15 ± 0.02	0.22
ASP	1.96 ± 0.09	2.01 ± 0.11	0.32
GABA	1.72 ± 0.18	1.63 ± 0.16	0.67
GLU	*9.11 ± 0.36*	*11.00 ± 0.39*	*0.02↑*
GLY	0.82 ± 0.10	0.75 ± 0.10	0.47
HIS	0.06 ± 0.01	0.07 ± 0.01	0.19
ILE	0.03 ± 0.01	0.03 ± 0.01	1.00
LEU	0.08 ± 0.02	0.07 ± 0.01	0.71
LYS	0.35 ± 0.02	0.37 ± 0.02	0.24
MET	0.05 ± 0.00	0.06 ± 0.01	0.59
PHE	0.06 ± 0.01	0.08 ± 0.02	0.16
SER	0.61 ± 0.03	0.56 ± 0.03	0.24
TRP	*0.07 ± 0.00*	*0.11 ± 0.03*	*0.02↑*
TYR	0.07 ± 0.01	0.07 ± 0.01	0.89

Amino acids are given in alphabetical order. Proteinogenic amino acids are indicated by their standard abbreviations, GABA-γ-aminobutyric acid. Levels of the amino acids and OGDHC activity are presented as mean ± SEM in µmol and µmol per min, correspondingly, per g of the tissue fresh weight. p values indicate significance of the differences between the two groups, estimated by the Mann-Whitney U-test. Significant ($p \leq 0.05$) differences are indicated in bold italics. Seventeen non-pregnant and eight pregnant rats were used in the comparison.

The data presented in Table 1 show that most of the differences between the amino acid pools in cerebella of the non-pregnant and pregnant rats are within the quantification errors. However, pregnancy increases the levels of cerebellar glutamate and tryptophan by 22 and 57%, respectively.

3.2. Hypoxia-Induced Changes in Cerebellar Pool of Amino Acids Depend on Physiological State

Table 2 shows that hypoxia induces significant changes in the cerebellar pool of amino acids of non-pregnant female rats. Half of the quantified amino acids (Arg, Glu. Lys, Met, Phe, Ser, Trp) undergo statistically significant increases.

Table 2. Influence of acute hypobaric hypoxia on the OGDHC activity and amino acid pool in cerebella of the non-pregnant and pregnant rats.

Groups / Parameters	Non-Pregnant Rats			Pregnant Rats		
	Control	Hypoxia	p Values	Control	Hypoxia	p Values
OGDH	1.13 ± 0.13	1.11 ± 0.18	0.561	1.21 ± 0.15	1.24 ± 0.18	0.875
ALA	0.59 ± 0.05	0.73 ± 0.06	0.081	0.62 ± 0.04	0.60 ± 0.04	0.633
ARG	*0.15 ± 0.03*	*0.23 ± 0.04*	*0.048↑*	0.15 ± 0.02	0.16 ± 0.02	0.762
ASP	1.96 ± 0.09	2.30 ± 0.19	0.180	2.01 ± 0.11	2.08 ± 0.09	0.573
GABA	1.72 ± 0.18	2.22 ± 0.25	0.091	1.63 ± 0.16	1.54 ± 0.11	0.460
Glu	*9.11 ± 0.36*	*10.93 ±0.61*	*0.027↑*	11.00 ± 0.01	10.56 ± 0.42	0.274
GLY	0.82 ± 0.10	1.03 ± 0.14	0.180	0.75 ± 0.10	0.77 ± 0.08	1.000
HIS	0.06 ± 0.01	0.08 ± 0.01	0.055	0.07 ± 0.01	0.07 ± 0.01	0.696
ILE	0.03 ± 0.01	0.05 ± 0.01	0.162	0.03 ± 0.01	0.04 ± 0.01	0.696
LEU	0.08± 0.02	0.12 ±0.02	0.116	0.07 ±0.01	0.10 ± 0.02	0.829
LYS	*0.35 ± 0.02*	*0.42 ± 0.03*	*0.048↑*	0.37 ± 0.02	0.39 ± 0.03	0.515
MET	*0.05 ± 0.00*	*0.09 ± 0.00*	*0.014↑*	0.06 ± 0.01	0.07 ± 0.01	0.573
PHE	*0.06 ± 0.01*	*0.13 ± 0.02*	*0.004↑*	0.08 ± 0.02	0.09 ± 0.01	0.829
SER	*0.51 ± 0.03*	*0.61 ± 0.02*	*0.036↑*	0.56 ± 0.03	0.56 ± 0.05	0.274
TRP	*0.07 ± 0.00*	*0.10 ± 0.01*	*0.048↑*	0.11 ± 0.03	0.09 ± 0.01	0.083
TYR	0.07 ± 0.01	0.08 ± 0.01	0.351	0.07 ± 0.01	0.07 ± 0.01	1.000

Amino acids are abbreviated as in Table 1. Levels of amino acids and OGDHC activity are presented as mean ± SEM in μmol and μmol per min, correspondingly, per g of the tissue fresh weight. p values indicate significance of the differences between the two groups, estimated by the Mann-Whitney U-test. Significant ($p \leq 0.05$) differences are shown in bold italics. Number of animals in the groups: 17 control non-pregnant, 8 hypoxic non-pregnant, 8 control pregnant and 10 hypoxic pregnant.

In contrast, under the same metabolic stress of pregnant rats, their cerebellar levels of amino acids remain unaffected (Table 2). Remarkably, the tryptophan level, which is increased by pregnancy, exhibits a trend (0.08) to decrease (from 0.11 to 0.09 μmol per g FW) after exposure of the pregnant rats to hypoxia, while in the non-pregnant rats hypoxia induces an opposite change in the tryptophan level, which increases from 0.07 to 0.12 μmol per g FW (Table 2).

3.3. Interdependence of Cerebellar Levels of OGDHC Activity and/or Amino Acids Varies under Different Physiological Settings

Metabolic pathways of amino acids have not only common transporters for certain groups of amino acids, but also many common substrates. For instance, transaminase reactions link the levels of the corresponding pairs of the amino acids (aspartate and glutamate in the aspartate transaminase reaction), GABA is produced from glutamate etc. As noted in the introduction section, the amino acid metabolism in general is tightly coupled to the TCA cycle, whose metabolic flux is limited by the activity of OGDHC [4]. As a result, OGDHC inhibition strongly affects the amino acid pool in cerebellar granule neurons in culture [9] and amino acids levels in animal brain in vivo (reviewed in [6]). These metabolic features should cause interdependence of the tissue levels of amino acids. The interdependence is manifested in the correlated variations in the levels of amino acids and OGDHC activity in different animals, because the interindividual variability in the biochemical parameters is contributed by minor variations in the metabolic network organization. Indeed, such correlation analysis of the levels of the cerebellar OGDHC activity and 15 quantified amino acids in a sample of the non-pregnant and pregnant (Table 3) rats reveals a number of highly significant correlations between the studied biochemical parameters, pointing to a strongly interdependent content of different amino acids in rat cerebellum, imposed by intercepts in their metabolism.

Visual inspection indicates that the correlation patterns change along with physiological settings (Table 3, the lower left triangles in A and B). The sets of strongly interacting parameters differ between the non-pregnant and pregnant rats. For instance, pregnancy drastically decreases the interdependences of Glu, Phe, Met with other amino acids and OGDHC, compared to those manifested in the cerebellum of non-pregnant rats. On the other hand, some features of the metabolic network are preserved in both the non-pregnant and pregnant rats. That is, lysine and tryptophan show a low number of interactions in both physiological states (Table 3). Independent of pregnancy, none of the cerebellar amino acids show statistically significant correlation with OGDHC activity, although cerebellar tryptophan tends to positively correlate with OGDHC in both non-pregnant (R = 0.79, 0.061) and pregnant (R = 0.85, 0.07) rats (Table 3).

In our previous work [23], an approach to quantify subtle physiological shifts in metabolic networks, based on the data of correlation analysis, has been developed. It employs reduction of the correlation matrix dimension, resulting in a small number of easily comparable parameters presented in Table 4. The parameters are: the summarized and averaged correlation coefficients for each element of the matrix, which characterize an overall degree of interdependence of the elements in a specific (patho) physiological state, and the total number of significant ($p < 0.05$) correlations (positive or negative) in the matrix, which indicates how many strong and very strong interdependences of the studied elements are inherent in a metabolic network. According to the data presented in Table 4, the summarized and averaged correlation coefficients are significantly lower in the pregnant rats, compared to the non-pregnant ones, pointing to generally lower interdependences in the amino acid levels in the former than the latter. The lower interdependence is consistent with the lower number of statistically significant correlations in the pregnant vs. non-pregnant rats (38 vs. 62 for the positive correlations and 0 vs. 4 for the negative correlations, Table 4), although this difference does not reach statistical significance.

Table 3. Correlation matrices characterizing interdependence between the amino acid levels and OGDHC activity in the cerebella of the non-pregnant and pregnant rats from the control (C) and hypoxia-exposed (H) groups.

(A) Non-Pregnant Rats

H / C	OGDHC	ALA	ARG	ASP	GABA	GLU	GLY	HIS	ILE	LEU	LYS	MET	PHE	SER	TRP	TYR
OGDHC		−0.94 0.001	−0.94 0.001	−0.90 0.002	−0.95 0.000	−0.84 0.009	−0.95 0.000	−0.94 0.000	−0.95 0.000	−0.95 0.000	−0.69 0.059	−0.65 0.084	−0.95 0.000	−0.19 0.649	0.53 0.181	−0.89 0.003
ALA	−0.42 0.407		0.99 0.000	0.86 0.006	0.97 0.000	0.82 0.013	0.96 0.000	0.94 0.000	0.97 0.000	0.98 0.000	0.81 0.015	0.71 0.046	0.99 0.000	0.31 0.452	−0.68 0.065	0.93 0.001
ARG	−0.62 0.187	0.87 0.025		0.85 0.008	0.98 0.000	0.83 0.010	0.99 0.000	0.94 0.000	0.98 0.000	0.98 0.000	0.78 0.022	0.62 0.103	0.97 0.000	0.27 0.518	−0.66 0.078	0.97 0.000
ASP	−0.68 0.135	0.78 0.068	0.97 0.001		0.91 0.001	0.94 0.001	0.87 0.005	0.91 0.002	0.89 0.003	0.88 0.004	0.80 0.017	0.71 0.050	0.86 0.007	0.56 0.147	−0.33 0.422	0.86 0.006
GABA	−0.63 0.178	0.91 0.011	0.92 0.009	0.93 0.008		0.92 0.001	0.99 0.000	0.94 0.000	0.97 0.000	0.96 0.000	0.80 0.017	0.60 0.116	0.97 0.000	0.35 0.397	−0.56 0.152	0.97 0.000
GLU	−0.42 0.402	0.76 0.081	0.84 0.036	0.90 0.014	0.90 0.014		0.89 0.003	0.90 0.003	0.85 0.007	0.84 0.009	0.84 0.009	0.46 0.246	0.83 0.011	0.53 0.176	−0.39 0.340	0.90 0.002
GLY	−0.64 0.170	0.86 0.027	0.98 0.000	0.96 0.002	0.94 0.005	0.83 0.040		0.95 0.000	0.98 0.000	0.97 0.000	0.76 0.030	0.53 0.172	0.97 0.000	0.25 0.546	−0.56 0.148	0.96 0.000
HIS	0.03 0.955	−0.05 0.918	0.12 0.814	0.06 0.911	−0.05 0.932	−0.17 0.750	0.22 0.671		0.02 0.970	−0.04 0.940	0.85 0.008	0.64 0.085	0.93 0.001	0.39 0.340	−0.58 0.132	0.93 0.001
ILE	−0.72 0.106	0.93 0.008	0.91 0.011	0.87 0.025	0.95 0.003	0.74 0.093	0.93 0.007			0.97 0.000	0.78 0.024	0.64 0.091	0.97 0.000	0.30 0.468	−0.56 0.151	0.94 0.000
LEU	−0.70 0.125	0.94 0.005	0.90 0.015	0.86 0.028	0.96 0.002	0.76 0.078	0.91 0.011	−0.32 0.543	0.99 0.000		0.80 0.018	0.66 0.073	0.97 0.000	0.31 0.455	−0.60 0.117	0.93 0.001
LYS	−0.56 0.251	0.67 0.142	0.60 0.206	0.69 0.127	0.85 0.031	0.81 0.049	0.65 0.159	−0.32 0.543	0.74 0.096	0.77 0.071		0.64 0.090	0.74 0.034	0.72 0.043	−0.67 0.068	0.84 0.009
MET	0.67 0.144	−0.65 0.158	−0.48 0.341	−0.38 0.454	−0.57 0.240	−0.19 0.726	−0.50 0.311	0.09 0.859	−0.77 0.075	−0.76 0.079	−0.46 0.356		0.65 0.081	0.53 0.179	−0.43 0.284	0.54 0.172
PHE	−0.64 0.174	0.75 0.089	0.90 0.014	0.96 0.002	0.91 0.011	0.96 0.003	0.88 0.022	−0.18 0.730	0.81 0.050	0.82 0.047	0.78 0.068	−0.32 0.541		0.23 0.580	−0.60 0.116	0.91 0.002
SER	0.32 0.531	−0.63 0.181	−0.72 0.104	−0.79 0.059	−0.75 0.086	−0.93 0.006	−0.66 0.158	0.42 0.403	−0.57 0.234	−0.61 0.203	−0.68 0.134	0.05 0.924	−0.91 0.011		−0.11 0.789	0.40 0.329
TRP	0.79 0.061	−0.17 0.745	−0.51 0.305	−0.54 0.272	−0.38 0.458	−0.17 0.744	−0.57 0.239	−0.56 0.246	−0.49 0.327	−0.43 0.400	−0.17 0.753	0.39 0.446	−0.36 0.483	−0.02 0.965		−0.63 0.097
TYR	−0.06 0.906	0.87 0.025	0.79 0.062	0.699 0.126	0.76 0.078	0.74 0.095	0.79 0.059	0.23 0.666	0.70 0.120	0.71 0.115	0.46 0.357	−0.25 0.629	0.63 0.182	−0.59 0.221	−0.06 0.912	

Table 3. Cont.

(B) Pregnant Rats

H \ C	OGDHC	ALA	ARG	ASP	GABA	GLU	GLY	HIS	ILE	LEU	LYS	MET	PHE	SER	TRP	TYR
OGDHC		−0.17 0.629	−0.03 0.931	−0.06 0.864	−0.12 0.748	−0.22 0.532	−0.15 0.670	0.03 0.944	0.14 0.708	0.19 0.602	0.24 0.506	**0.63** **0.050**	0.08 0.832	0.44 0.201	0.05 0.891	0.13 0.725
ALA	−0.35 0.569		**0.76** **0.010**	0.28 0.439	0.61 0.062	0.10 0.791	**0.77** **0.009**	0.60 0.069	**0.83** **0.003**	**0.79** **0.006**	0.40 0.255	0.40 0.248	0.60 0.067	**0.67** **0.034**	−0.02 0.949	**0.73** **0.016**
ARG	−0.33 0.582	0.86 0.063		**0.03** **0.926**	**0.84** **0.002**	−0.42 0.226	**0.94** **0.000**	0.30 0.406	**0.77** **0.009**	**0.64** **0.048**	−0.07 0.838	0.46 0.180	**0.91** **0.000**	0.36 0.313	−0.52 0.122	0.37 0.298
ASP	−0.04 0.953	0.85 0.066	0.85 0.067		0.35 0.323	**0.75** **0.012**	0.22 0.548	**0.65** **0.042**	−0.11 0.769	−0.10 0.777	0.16 0.653	−0.22 0.544	−0.05 0.885	0.10 0.787	0.58 0.081	0.25 0.478
GABA	−0.55 0.340	**0.88** **0.052**	**0.96** **0.010**	0.82 0.087		−0.17 0.631	**0.96** **0.000**	0.44 0.204	0.53 0.118	0.37 0.291	−0.24 0.510	0.16 0.650	**0.80** **0.005**	0.14 0.704	−0.45 0.189	0.22 0.548
GLU	0.33 0.588	0.49 0.398	0.21 0.732	0.68 0.205	0.23 0.710		−0.25 0.480	0.45 0.192	−0.36 0.306	−0.28 0.432	0.23 0.522	−0.49 0.152	−0.55 0.100	0.02 0.947	**0.89** **0.000**	0.11 0.769
GLY	−0.51 0.380	0.78 0.118	**0.96** **0.010**	0.80 0.104	**0.98** **0.003**	0.15 0.808		0.44 0.203	**0.72** **0.020**	0.58 0.081	−0.08 0.818	0.32 0.375	**0.87** **0.001**	0.31 0.390	−0.49 0.153	0.38 0.274
HIS	0.76 0.136	0.24 0.700	0.27 0.660	0.39 0.519	0.01 0.990	0.34 0.576	0.01 0.989		0.30 0.393	0.34 0.341	0.49 0.150	0.27 0.452	0.38 0.279	0.54 0.104	0.30 0.405	0.59 0.075
ILE	−0.44 0.456	**0.93** **0.022**	**0.98** **0.003**	0.85 0.071	**0.98** **0.003**	0.26 0.672	**0.95** **0.015**	0.17 0.780		**0.98** **0.000**	0.46 0.184	**0.74** **0.015**	**0.69** **0.028**	**0.77** **0.010**	−0.39 0.268	**0.77** **0.009**
LEU	−0.42 0.479	**0.90** **0.036**	**0.99** **0.001**	**0.84** **0.076**	**0.98** **0.004**	0.22 0.724	**0.96** **0.011**	0.20 0.752	**0.99** **0.000**		0.62 0.054	**0.78** **0.008**	0.57 0.084	**0.96** **0.001**	−0.27 0.450	**0.86** **0.001**
LYS	0.07 0.910	0.80 0.106	0.81 0.095	0.71 0.177	0.66 0.230	0.26 0.670	0.61 0.275	0.70 0.191	0.79 0.112	0.80 0.106		0.60 0.068	−0.05 0.898	**0.81** **0.005**	0.33 0.353	**0.87** **0.001**
MET	−0.15 0.812	0.00 0.994	0.39 0.518	−0.08 0.893	0.24 0.698	−0.74 0.156	0.33 0.585	0.21 0.740	0.28 0.651	0.34 0.578	0.39 0.512		0.54 0.111	**0.78** **0.007**	−0.31 0.377	**0.66** **0.039**
PHE	−0.04 0.951	0.50 0.396	0.84 0.077	0.58 0.310	0.67 0.213	−0.14 0.827	0.74 0.149	0.49 0.402	0.72 0.166	0.77 0.125	0.78 0.123	0.76 0.137		0.36 0.307	**−0.64** **0.046**	0.34 0.340
SER	0.36 0.549	0.43 0.466	0.60 0.288	0.45 0.446	0.35 0.565	0.02 0.978	0.36 0.546	0.86 0.065	0.50 0.393	0.53 0.353	**0.89** **0.045**	0.61 0.272	0.82 0.086		0.12 0.739	**0.90** **0.000**
TRP	0.85 0.070	−0.21 0.740	−0.45 0.444	0.01 0.988	−0.55 0.339	0.64 0.242	−0.59 0.295	0.53 0.358	−0.46 0.433	−0.48 0.409	−0.08 0.903	−0.63 0.255	−0.43 0.470	0.02 0.979		0.09 0.815
TYR	−0.08 0.900	0.81 0.097	**0.96** **0.008**	0.86 0.061	0.85 0.068	0.27 0.663	0.86 0.064	0.52 0.373	**0.91** **0.031**	**0.93** **0.022**	**0.90** **0.035**	0.42 0.482	**0.89** **0.041**	0.77 0.129	−0.26 0.669	

Pearson's correlation coefficient (upper value) and p-value of the correlation (lower value) are shown. Statistically significant ($p < 0.05$) positive (light grey) and negative (dark grey) correlations are marked. The lower left and upper right triangles refer to the control (C) rats ($n = 6$ in both cases) and the hypoxia-exposed (H) rats ($n = 8$ in A and $n = 10$ in B).

Table 4. Analysis of the hypoxia-induced changes in interdependence of the levels of amino acids and OGDHC activity in cerebella of the non-pregnant and pregnant rats.

Groups	Non-Pregnant Rats								Pregnant Rats							
	Σ		$\overline{X}$		+		−		Σ		$\overline{X}$		+		−	
Parameter	Control	Hypoxia	Control	Hypoxia	Control	Hypoxia	Control	Hypoxia	Control	Hypoxia	Control	Hypoxia	Control	Hypoxia	Control	Hypoxia
OGDHC	7.90	12.26	0.53	0.82	0	0	0	11	5.28	2.68	0.35	0.18	0	1	0	0
ALA	10.26	12.86	0.68	0.86	5	12	0	1	9.03	7.73	0.60	0.52	3	6	0	0
ARG	11.13	12.75	0.74	0.85	8	11	0	1	10.46	7.42	0.70	0.49	5	7	0	0
ASP	11.06	12.13	0.74	0.81	7	12	0	1	8.81	3.91	0.59	0.26	0	2	0	0
GABA	11.41	12.84	0.76	0.86	8	11	0	1	9.71	6.4	0.65	0.43	5	3	0	0
GLU	10.12	11.78	0.67	0.79	6	11	1	1	4.98	5.29	0.33	0.35	0	2	0	0
GLY	11.32	12.58	0.75	0.84	8	11	0	1	9.59	7.48	0.64	0.50	4	5	0	0
HIS	2.56	12.79	0.17	0.85	0	11	0	1	5.7	6.12	0.38	0.41	0	1	0	0
ILE	11.14	12.74	0.74	0.85	6	11	0	1	10.21	8.56	0.68	0.57	6	8	0	0
LEU	11.16	12.8	0.74	0.85	6	11	0	1	10.35	8.23	0.69	0.55	6	6	0	0
LYS	9.21	11.52	0.61	0.77	0	12	0	1	9.25	5.65	0.62	0.38	2	2	0	0
MET	6.53	9.01	0.44	0.60	0	0	0	0	5.57	7.36	0.37	0.49	0	3	0	0
PHE	10.81	12.54	0.72	0.84	7	11	1	1	9.17	7.43	0.61	0.50	1	4	0	1
SER	8.65	5.45	0.58	0.36	0	1	2	0	7.57	7.18	0.50	0.48	1	6	0	0
TRP	5.61	7.89	0.37	0.53	0	0	0	0	6.19	5.45	0.41	0.36	0	1	0	1
TYR	8.33	12.6	0.56	0.84	1	11	0	1	10.29	7.27	0.69	0.48	5	6	0	0
Sum or Average	147.20	184.54	0.61	0.77	62	136	4	22	132.16 #	104.16#	0.55 #	0.43 #	38	63 #	0	2 #
p value of the difference	0.004		0.004		0.002		0.04		0.004		0.004		0.005			0.18

For the OGDHC activity (OGDHC) and each of the amino acids, the sum of its correlation coefficients (absolute values) to other amino acids (Σ), average correlation coefficient ($\overline{X}$), and total number of statistically significant positive (+) and negative (−) correlations are shown. At the bottom, the sum (Σs, positive and negative correlations) or average (Xs) of all the values in the row and p values of the differences between the parameters in the control and hypoxia groups, estimated by the Wilcoxon signed rank test, are shown, with the statistically significant differences between the control and hypoxia groups in bold. # Significant ($p \leq 0.05$) differences between the parameters of the corresponding non-pregnant and pregnant groups.

3.4. Concerted Hypoxia-Induced Shift to the Negative Correlations between the Levels of Amino Acids and OGDHC Activity Is not Observed in Pregnancy

Exposure of rats to an environmental challenge, such as acute hypobaric hypoxia, strongly changes the correlation matrices (Table 3, the upper right triangles) and their overall parameters (Table 4). Moreover, the hypoxia-induced changes in the interdependences are well-detectable in both the non-pregnant and pregnant rats (Tables 3 and 4), in contrast to the changes in the average levels of amino acids and OGDHC activity, which are detectable in the non-pregnant rats only (Table 2). That said, the correlation analysis reveals a very different response to hypoxia of the interdependences between OGDHC activity and/or amino acids in the non-pregnant and pregnant rats. Thus, not only the control correlation matrices, but also those after exposure of animals to hypoxia are very different in non-pregnant and pregnant rats (Table 3, the upper right triangles). As shown in Table 3 hypoxia induces a high number of negative correlations of amino acids with OGDHC in non-pregnant rats. Induction by hypoxia of the negative correlations between the amino acid levels and OGDHC activity exclusively in non-pregnant rats (Table 3, the upper right triangle) thus coincides with the hypoxic reactivity of the average levels of amino acids in non-pregnant rats only (Table 2). In contrast, in pregnant rats hypoxia induces one positive correlation between OGDHC and methionine and one negative correlation between the amino acids tryptophan and phenylalanine (Table 3, the upper right triangle).

The overall interdependence parameters (Table 4) point to statistically significant differences in the hypoxic responses of cerebellum in both the non-pregnant and pregnant rats. This finding indicates that analysis of the correlation matrices (Table 4) detects the responses to hypoxic stress with a much higher sensitivity, compared to the average levels of amino acids, which did not reveal any changes in the cerebellum of pregnant rats after hypoxia (Table 2). Yet both markers of hypoxic stress point to different responses to hypoxia in the different physiological states. The strong negative correlations between the levels of amino acids and OGDHC activity after hypoxic exposure of non-pregnant rats (Table 3) coincide with the hypoxia-increased levels of the amino acids in these rats (Table 2) and with the overall increase in the interdependence between the OGDHC activity and/or amino acid levels, indicted by the summarized and averaged correlation coefficients and number of statistically significant correlations (Table 4). Contrary, in pregnant rats, demonstrating no changes in the average levels of amino acids after hypoxia (Table 2), no negative correlations of the amino acid levels with OGDHC activity are induced by hypoxia (Table 3), and the overall interdependence is diminished, based on the summarized and averaged correlation coefficients between the studied parameters (Table 4). Remarkably, the number of statistically significant positive correlations between the parameters is increased by hypoxia in pregnant rats too (from 38 to 63, Table 4). However, in accordance with a generally decreased interdependence, evident from the decreased correlation coefficients (summarized and average, Table 4), the increased number of statistically significant positive correlations is expressed less than in non-pregnant rats (Table 4). The most significant contribution to increases in the positive correlations is provided by different amino acids; in non-pregnant rats they are histidine, lysine, and tyrosine, whereas in pregnant rats they are methionine, serine, and phenylalanine (Tables 3 and 4). Thus, hypoxia affects different metabolic pathways in the cerebella of pregnant and non-pregnant rats.

3.5. Physiological Consequences of the Hypoxia-Induced Changes in the Interdependent Levels of OGDHC Activity and/or Amino Acids in Cerebellum

In hypoxic experiments, rats are exposed to acute hypobaric hypoxia until they collapse, which is registered as apnea. As described in the methods section, the time between the established hypoxic condition (5% O_2) and apnea, i.e., the life time (LT), characterizes individual and/or group differences in the resistance to hypoxia according to the arbitrary intervals of the LT, indicated in the legend to Figure 1. Figure 1 shows that distribution of a sample of the rats into the animals with varied resistance to hypoxia differs dependent on the physiological state. Pregnant rats are characterized by decreased fraction of the animals with high resistance to hypoxia, with the corresponding increase in the fraction of the low resistant rats. The difference is also manifested in a higher average value of LT for non-pregnant rats (369 ± 45.1 s), compared to LT of the pregnant rats (277 ± 37 s) (n = 41; 0.048, according to Mann-Whitney test). Thus, the reactivity to hypoxia is higher (Figure 1) when no significant changes in the OGDHC activity or amino acid levels, neither any negative correlations between these parameters occur in the cerebellum, as observed in the pregnant rats (Tables 2–4).

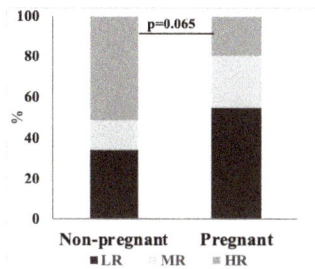

Figure 1. Distribution of the non-pregnant (n = 41) and pregnant (n =31) rats according to their relative resistance to acute hypobaric hypoxia. HR—highly resistant rats (dark-grey), spent under hypoxia ≥10 min; MR—medium resistant rats (light-grey), spent under hypoxia between 5 and 10 min; LR—low resistant rats (middle-grey), spent under hypoxia ≤5 min. % of each sub-group to total number of animals in the group is shown in shades of grey. The indicated p value is estimated using Fisher exact test.

Accordingly, the hypoxia-induced changes in the average levels (Table 2) and/or interdependence (Tables 3 and 4) of cerebellar OGDHC activity and amino acids, which are observed in the non-pregnant rats, are of compensatory significance. That is, the changes in the amino acid pool (Table 2) and its dependence on OGDHC activity (Table 3), observed in the non-pregnant rats and absent in the pregnant ones, obviously enable the former to resist hypoxia better than the latter (Figure 1).

4. Discussion

In this work, cerebellar metabolism of amino acids and its dependence on the TCA-cycle-limiting OGDHC are shown to be affected by physiological settings (pregnancy) and metabolic stress (acute hypobaric hypoxia). Pregnancy increases cerebellar levels of glutamate and tryptophan (Table 1) and decreases overall interdependence of the studied components of amino acid metabolism, compared to their interdependence in non-pregnant rats (Table 4).

Hormonal changes during pregnancy are known to coordinate a broad range of physiological adaptations, from the supply of nutrients and oxygen for the fetus growth in utero to specific patterns of parental behavior [32,33]. Changed metabolism of amino acids in the brain of the pregnant females may be involved in these adaptations, as many of amino acids are neurotransmitters or their precursors. The increases in cerebellar glutamate and tryptophan in pregnant rats, observed in this work, are consistent with independent studies on the pregnancy-imposed changes in glutamatergic and serotonergic signaling. In fact, pregnancy is known to change expression of glutamate receptors to address specific physiological challenges faced by pregnant females [34,35]. Our data on the pregnancy-increased cerebellar content of tryptophan are in line with the activation of serotonergic signaling observed during pregnancy, because tryptophan is the serotonin precursor [36]. The interaction between the levels of serotonin and estrogens also underlies sex-dimorphic prevalence of the serotonin-linked diseases, including migraine, depression, eating disorders and pregnancy-associated pathologies [36,37].

Our previous studies pointed to certain relationship between the amino acid levels in the blood plasma and brain [23], which may be used for translation of findings on the brain samples in animal models to human studies. For instance, increased content of tryptophan in cerebellum of pregnant rats, shown in our study (Table 1) corresponds to the findings in humans, which indicate that in maternal plasma, tryptophan catabolites and related compounds change in pregnancy [38,39]. This study suggests the neurotransmitters-dependent adaptation of maternal body to the fetus growth. As considered above, such adaptation is obvious also from our findings (Table 1). Biomarker significance of the amino acid levels in human plasma and urine has also been explored in other studies [40–42]. Their findings point to the potential diagnostic significance of the changes in multivariate metabolic profiles, including amino acids, for prediction of gestational diabetes [42]. Besides, the pregnancy-dependent changes in the content of amino acids and their metabolites in plasma and urine point to variation of these parameters, dependent on the increased amino acid demands for the growing fetus [40,41].

The pregnancy-induced changes in cerebellar pool of amino acids (Table 1) are associated with different responses of cerebellar amino acid metabolism to hypoxia in the pregnant and non-pregnant rats (Tables 2–4). Strong negative correlations between the amino acid levels and OGDHC activity, which are a hallmark of cerebellar metabolism after hypoxia of non-pregnant rats, are not induced by hypoxia in the pregnant rats (Tables 3 and 4). Simultaneously, hypoxia significantly increases average levels of cerebellar amino acids in the non-pregnant rats only (Table 2). Because the observed biochemical changes in the cerebellar metabolism of amino acids are associated with a higher resistance to hypoxia in the non-pregnant vs. pregnant rats (Figure 1), the metabolic rearrangement in the cerebellum of non-pregnant rats is of adaptive significance. In particular, increased flux of the amino acids degraded through OGDHC (Glu, Gln, Arg, His, Pro) and of the branched-chain amino acids Val and Ile may generate succinyl-CoA for the substrate level phosphorylation in mitochondria. Generation of ATP at the expense of succinyl-CoA may help overcoming energy deficits upon hypoxia which impairs oxidative phosphorylation. Increased degradation of amino acids in the TCA cycle whose flux is limited by OGDHC, is in good accordance with the negative correlations between the OGDHC activity and the levels of cerebellar amino acids after hypoxia, in contrast to normal metabolism (Table 3). It is worth noting in this regard that hypoxic tolerance is associated with the mTOR-dependent autophagy [43]. Increased autophagy may generate the higher amino acid levels after hypoxia (Table 2) to use them for the substrate-level ADP phosphorylation in the hypoxic brain of non-pregnant rats. Autophagy is also coupled to pro-survival function of mitochondrial fission under energy stress [44–47]. However, the homeostatic and pro-survival functions of mTOR, autophagy and mitochondrial fission are highly conditional, with overactivation of these processes also mediating the brain damage by hypoxia [48–50].

Different levels of activation of mTOR, autophagy and mitochondrial fission may be required for their pro-survival and death-inducing outcomes in different physiological states. In this regard, no increase in the brain amino acid levels by hypoxic exposure of pregnant rats (Table 2) was due to a higher damaging potential of the autophagy stimulation in this physiological state. No adaptation to hypoxia by increased degradation of amino acids through OGDHC in pregnant rats is also evident from the hypoxia-induced decrease in the interdependences between the levels of OGDHC activity and/or amino acids, whereas in the non-pregnant rats hypoxia increases these interdependences (Table 4). The different action of hypoxia in the two physiological states is obvious from comparison of the hypoxia-induced changes in the summarized and average correlation coefficients or in the number of significant correlations in the pregnant and non-pregnant rats (Table 4). In view of the increased sensitivity of pregnant vs. non-pregnant rats to hypoxia (Figure 1), the stability of the biochemical parameters in the cerebellum of the pregnant rats exposed to hypoxia (Table 2) along with the absence of negative correlations between the OGDHC activity and levels of amino acids (Tables 3 and 4) manifest limitations of the hypoxic adaptation through increased degradation of amino acids in the pregnant vs. non-pregnant rats. These findings indicate that the pregnancy-imposed changes in the cerebellar amino acid pool (Table 2) and metabolism (Tables 3 and 4) are associated with decreased stress adaptability, in line with other studies showing decreased perception of stress in pregnant females [51–53].

It is worth noting that the response of the metabolic network of pregnant rats to hypoxia, undetectable from the average levels of amino acids (Table 2), is evident from the correlation analysis (Table 4). Hence, average levels of cerebellar amino acids are not as sensitive indicators of metabolic changes, as the cumulative parameters characterizing the interdependence of components of the corresponding metabolic network.

It has been noted previously that correlating metabolites may not only be of diagnostic significance [23], but also help deciphering the yet unknown or poorly characterized synthetic and regulatory pathways [20]. In this regard, the pregnancy-induced changes in metabolic correlations of cerebellar lysine are of interest, because gestational diabetes is associated with plasma levels of lysine and tyrosine [54], both of them correlating to each other much stronger in cerebellum of the pregnant than non-pregnant rats (Table 3). Besides, lysine catabolism is related to biosynthesis of homoarginine which is elevated in normal pregnancy [13], with some studies linking its elevation to pregnancy disorders, including preeclampsia [55]. Physiological manifestations of pre-eclampsia and eclampsia, associated with nearly one-tenth of all maternal deaths [56], involve changed cerebral hemodynamics and hypertensive encephalopathy [57–59], potentially linked to impaired signaling by homoarginine, known as a predictor of cardiovascular risk and mortality [3]. Alternatively, homoarginine is synthesized from arginine and glycine. Because these amino acids are highly correlated independent of pregnancy and/or hypoxia (Table 3), metabolism of cerebellar lysine appears to be a more likely contributor to specific adaptations imposed by pregnancy. This is further supported by the fact that lysine is known as an antagonist of a serotonin receptor [60], with serotonergic signaling increased in pregnancy [36,37] and depressed upon increased synthesis of homoarginine from lysine [61].

5. Conclusions

Markers of systemic changes in the cerebellar metabolism of amino acids were introduced, showing decreased reactivity of the pregnancy-changed amino acids network to metabolic stress, such as acute hypobaric hypoxia.

Author Contributions: A.G.: methodology, investigation (animal experiments), data curation, formal analysis, writing–review & editing; L.T.: investigation (animal experiments, sample preparation, enzyme assay), methodology; A.K.: investigation (ninhydrin quantification of amino acids), methodology; L.B.: methodology; V.B.: investigation (combining animal experiments with biochemical assays), methodology, formal analysis, writing–original draft, review & editing, supervision, project administration, funding acquisition. All authors have read and agreed to the published version of the manuscript.

Funding: This research was funded by Russian Science Foundation grant number N 18-14-00116 to Victoria I Bunik.

Acknowledgments: We thank E. Kulakovskaya (Faculty of Biology, Moscow Lomonosov State University) and G. Mkrtchyan (Faculty of Bioengineering and Bioinformatics, Moscow Lomonosov State University, currently at University of Copenhagen, Denmark) for technical assistance with sample preparation.

Conflicts of Interest: The authors declare no conflict of interest.

References

1. Kondoh, T.; Kameishi, M.; Mallick, H.N.; Ono, T.; Torii, K. Lysine and Arginine Reduce the Effects of Cerebral Ischemic Insults and Inhibit Glutamate-Induced Neuronal Activity in Rats. *Front. Integr. Neurosci.* **2010**, *4*, 1–10. [CrossRef] [PubMed]
2. Khandare, A.L.; Ankulu, M.; Aparna, N. Role of Glutamate and Nitric Oxide in Onset of Motor Neuron Degeneration in Neurolathyrism. *Neurotoxicology* **2013**, *34*, 269–274. [CrossRef] [PubMed]
3. März, W.; Meinitzer, A.; Drechsler, C.; Pilz, S.; Krane, V.; Kleber, M.E.; Fischer, J.; Winkelmann, B.R.; Böhm, B.O.; Ritz, E.; et al. Homoarginine, Cardiovascular Risk, and Mortality. *Circulation* **2010**, *122*, 967–975. [CrossRef] [PubMed]
4. Bunik, V.I.; Fernie, A.R. Metabolic Control Exerted by the 2-Oxoglutarate Dehydrogenase Reaction: A Cross-Kingdom Comparison of the Crossroad between Energy Production and Nitrogen Assimilation. *Biochem. J.* **2009**, *422*, 405–421. [CrossRef] [PubMed]
5. Bunik, V.I.; Raddatz, G.; Strumilo, S. Translating Enzymology into Metabolic Regulation: The Case of the 2-Oxoglutarate Dehydrogenase Multienzyme Complex. *Curr. Chem. Biol.* **2013**, *7*, 74–93. [CrossRef]

6. Bunik, V.I.; Tylicki, A.; Lukashev, N.V. Thiamin Diphosphate-Dependent Enzymes: From Enzymology to Metabolic Regulation, Drug Design and Disease Models. *FEBS J.* **2013**, *280*, 6412–6442. [CrossRef]
7. Mkrtchyan, G.V.; Graf, A.; Trofimova, L.; Ksenofontov, A.; Baratova, L.; Bunik, V. Positive Correlation between Rat Brain Glutamate Concentrations and Mitochondrial 2-Oxoglutarate Dehydrogenase Activity. *Anal. Biochem.* **2018**, *552*, 100–109. [CrossRef]
8. Araújo, W.L.; Trofimova, L.; Mkrtchyan, G.; Steinhauser, D.; Krall, L.; Graf, A.; Fernie, A.R.; Bunik, V.I. On the Role of the Mitochondrial 2-Oxoglutarate Dehydrogenase Complex in Amino Acid Metabolism. *Amino Acids* **2013**, *44*, 683–700. [CrossRef]
9. Trofimova, L.; Araujo, W.; Strokina, A.; Fernie, A.; Bettendorff, L.; Bunik, V. Consequences of the α-Ketoglutarate Dehydrogenase Inhibition for Neuronal Metabolism and Survival: Implications for Neurodegenerative Diseases. *Curr. Med. Chem.* **2012**, *19*, 5895–5906. [CrossRef]
10. Santos, S.S.; Gibson, G.E.; Cooper, A.J.L.; Denton, T.T.; Thompson, C.M.; Bunik, V.I.; Alves, P.M.; Sonnewald, U. Inhibitors of the α-Ketoglutarate Dehydrogenase Complex Alter [1-13C] Glucose and [U-13C] Glutamate Metabolism in Cerebellar Granule Neurons. *J. Neurosci. Res.* **2006**, *83*, 450–458. [CrossRef]
11. Stavrum, A.-K.; Heiland, I.; Schuster, S.; Puntervoll, P.; Ziegler, M. Model of Tryptophan Metabolism, Readily Scalable Using Tissue-Specific Gene Expression Data. *J. Biol. Chem.* **2013**, *288*, 34555–34566. [CrossRef] [PubMed]
12. Graf, A.; Trofimova, L.; Loshinskaja, A.; Mkrtchyan, G.; Strokina, A.; Lovat, M.; Tylicky, A.; Strumilo, S.; Bettendorff, L.; Bunik, V.I. Up-Regulation of 2-Oxoglutarate Dehydrogenase as a Stress Response. *Int. J. Biochem. Cell Biol.* **2013**, *45*, 175–189. [CrossRef] [PubMed]
13. Valtonen, P.; Laitinen, T.; Lyyra-Laitinen, T.; Raitakari, O.T.; Juonala, M.; Viikari, J.S.A.; Heiskanen, N.; Vanninen, E.; Punnonen, K.; Heinonen, S. Serum L-Homoarginine Concentration Is Elevated during Normal Pregnancy and Is Related to Flow-Mediated Vasodilatation. *Circ. J.* **2008**, *72*, 1879–1884. [CrossRef] [PubMed]
14. Trofimova, L.; Lovat, M.; Groznaya, A.; Efimova, E.; Dunaeva, T.; Maslova, M.; Graf, A.; Bunik, V. Behavioral Impact of the Regulation of the Brain 2-Oxoglutarate Dehydrogenase Complex by Synthetic Phosphonate Analog of 2-Oxoglutarate: Implications into the Role of the Complex in Neurodegenerative Diseases. *Int. J. Alzheimer's Dis.* **2010**, *3*, 1–8. [CrossRef]
15. Wu, T.; Hallett, M. Reply: The Cerebellum in Parkinson's Disease and Parkinsonism in Cerebellar Disorders. *Brain* **2013**, *136*, e249. [CrossRef]
16. O'Callaghan, C.; Hornberger, M.; Balsters, J.H.; Halliday, G.M.; Lewis, S.J.G.; Shine, J.M. Cerebellar Atrophy in Parkinson's Disease and Its Implication for Network Connectivity. *Brain* **2016**, *139*, 845–855. [CrossRef]
17. Mirdamadi, J.L. Cerebellar Role in Parkinson's Disease. *J. Neurophysiol.* **2016**, *116*, 917–919. [CrossRef]
18. Khadrawy, Y.A.; Mourad, I.M.; Mohammed, H.S.; Noor, N.A.; Aboul, H.S. Cerebellar Neurochemical and Histopathological Changes in Rat Model of Parkinson's Disease Induced by Intrastriatal Injection of Rotenone. *Gen. Physiol. Biophys.* **2017**, *36*, 99–108. [CrossRef]
19. Kishore, A.; Meunier, S.; Popa, T. Cerebellar Influence on Motor Cortex Plasticity: Behavioral Implications for Parkinson's Disease. *Front. Neurol.* **2014**, *5*, 1–8. [CrossRef]
20. Roessner, U.; Luedemann, A.; Brust, D.; Fiehn, O.; Linke, T.; Willmitzer, L.; Fernie, A.R. Metabolic Profiling Allows Comprehensive Phenotyping of Genetically or Environmentally Modified Plant Systems. *Plant Cell* **2001**, *13*, 11–29. [CrossRef]
21. Szymanski, J.; Jozefczuk, S.; Nikoloski, Z.; Selbig, J.; Nikiforova, V.; Catchpole, G.; Willmitzer, L. Stability of Metabolic Correlations under Changing Environmental Conditions in Escherichia Coli—A Systems Approach. *PLoS ONE* **2009**, *4*, e7441. [CrossRef] [PubMed]
22. Endrőczi, E. *Neuropeptides and Psychosomatic Processes*; Taylor & Francis: London, UK, 1983.
23. Tsepkova, P.M.; Artiukhov, A.V.; Boyko, A.I.; Aleshin, V.A.; Mkrtchyan, G.V.; Zvyagintseva, M.A.; Ryabov, S.I.; Ksenofontov, A.L.; Baratova, L.A.; Graf, A.V.; et al. Thiamine Induces Long-Term Changes in Amino Acid Profiles and Activities of 2-Oxoglutarate and 2-Oxoadipate Dehydrogenases in Rat Brain. *Biochemistry (Moscow)* **2017**, *82*, 723–736. [CrossRef] [PubMed]
24. Rothberg, H. Effects of Cytotoxic Agents on the Fetus. *JAMA* **1960**, *173*, 1616. [CrossRef]
25. Maslova, M.V.; Graf, A.V.; Maklakova, A.S.; Krushinskaya, Y.V.; Sokolova, N.A.; Koshelev, V.B. Acute Hypoxia during Organogenesis Affects Cardiac Autonomic Balance in Pregnant Rats. *Bull. Exp. Biol. Med.* **2005**, *139*, 180–182. [CrossRef] [PubMed]

26. Lukyanova, L.D.; Germanova, E.L.; Kopaladze, R.A. Development of Resistance of an Organism under Various Conditions of Hypoxic Preconditioning: Role of the Hypoxic Period and Reoxygenation. *Bull. Exp. Biol. Med.* **2009**, *147*, 400. [CrossRef]
27. Malyshev, A.Y.; Luk'yanova, L.D.; Krapivin, S.V. Effect of Hypoxia of Increasing Severity on the Dynamics of Cerebral Cortex EEGs in Rats with Different Resistance to Acute Oxygen Deficiency. *Bull. Exp. Biol. Med.* **1996**, *122*, 879–884. [CrossRef]
28. Bondarenko, N.A.; Germanova, E.L.; Luk'yanova, L.D. Behavioral Peculiarities and Reactions of Brain Dopaminergic Systems in Rats with Different Resistance to Acute Hypobaric Hypoxia. *Bull. Exp. Biol. Med.* **2000**, *130*, 849–851. [CrossRef]
29. Luk'yanova, L.D.; Romanova, V.E.; Chernobaeva, G.N. Oxidative Phosphorylation in Brain Mitochondria of Rats Differing in Their Sensitivity to Hypoxia. *Bull. Exp. Biol. Med.* **1991**, *112*, 962–965. [CrossRef]
30. Graf, A.; Kabysheva, M.; Klimuk, E.; Trofimova, L.; Dunaeva, T.; Zündorf, G.; Kahlert, S.; Reiser, G.; Storozhevykh, T.; Pinelis, V.; et al. Role of 2-Oxoglutarate Dehydrogenase in Brain Pathologies Involving Glutamate Neurotoxicity. *J. Mol. Catal. B Enzym.* **2009**, *61*, 80–87. [CrossRef]
31. Ksenofontov, A.L.; Boyko, A.I.; Mkrtchyan, G.V.; Tashlitsky, V.N.; Timofeeva, A.V.; Graf, A.V.; Bunik, V.I.; Baratova, L.A. Analysis of Free Amino Acids in Mammalian Brain Extracts. *Biochemistry (Moscow)* **2017**, *82*, 1183–1192. [CrossRef]
32. Smiley, K.O.; Ladyman, S.R.; Gustafson, P.; Grattan, D.R.; Brown, R.S.E. Neuroendocrinology and Adaptive Physiology of Maternal Care. *Curr. Top Behav. Neurosci.* **2019**. [CrossRef]
33. Napso, T.; Yong, H.E.J.; Lopez-Tello, J.; Sferruzzi-Perri, A.N. The Role of Placental Hormones in Mediating Maternal Adaptations to Support Pregnancy and Lactation. *Front. Physiol.* **2018**, *9*, 1091. [CrossRef] [PubMed]
34. Ghosh, C.; Storey-Workley, M.; Usip, S.; Hafemeister, J.; Miller, K.E.; Papka, R.E. Glutamate and Metabotropic Glutamate Receptors Associated with Innervation of the Uterine Cervix during Pregnancy: Receptor Antagonism Inhibits c-Fos Expression in Rat Lumbosacral Spinal Cord at Parturition. *J. Neurosci. Res.* **2007**, *85*, 1318–1335. [CrossRef] [PubMed]
35. Bhandage, A.K.; Jin, Z.; Hellgren, C.; Korol, S.V.; Nowak, K.; Williamsson, L.; Sundström-Poromaa, I.; Birnir, B. AMPA, NMDA and Kainate Glutamate Receptor Subunits Are Expressed in Human Peripheral Blood Mononuclear Cells (PBMCs) Where the Expression of GluK4 Is Altered by Pregnancy and GluN2D by Depression in Pregnant Women. *J. Neuroimmunol.* **2017**, *305*, 51–58. [CrossRef] [PubMed]
36. Cengiz, H.; Dagdeviren, H.; Caypinar, S.S.; Kanawati, A.; Yildiz, S.; Ekin, M. Plasma Serotonin Levels Are Elevated in Pregnant Women with Hyperemesis Gravidarum. *Arch. Gynecol. Obstet.* **2015**, *291*, 1271–1276. [CrossRef]
37. Thibeault, A.-A.H.; Sanderson, J.T.; Vaillancourt, C. Serotonin-Estrogen Interactions: What Can We Learn from Pregnancy? *Biochimie* **2019**, *161*, 88–108. [CrossRef]
38. Luan, H.; Meng, N.; Liu, P.; Feng, Q.; Lin, S.; Fu, J.; Davidson, R.; Chen, X.; Rao, W.; Chen, F.; et al. Pregnancy-Induced Metabolic Phenotype Variations in Maternal Plasma. *J. Proteome Res.* **2014**, *13*, 1527–1536. [CrossRef]
39. Di Giulio, A.M.; Carelli, S.; Castoldi, R.E.; Gorio, A.; Taricco, E.; Cetin, I. Plasma Amino Acid Concentrations throughout Normal Pregnancy and Early Stages of Intrauterine Growth Restricted Pregnancy. *J. Matern. Neonatal Med.* **2004**, *15*, 356–362. [CrossRef]
40. Diaz, S.O.; Barros, A.S.; Goodfellow, B.J.; Duarte, I.F.; Carreira, I.M.; Galhano, E.; Pita, C.; do Céu Almeida, M.; Gil, A.M. Following Healthy Pregnancy by Nuclear Magnetic Resonance (NMR) Metabolic Profiling of Human Urine. *J. Proteome Res.* **2012**, *12*, 969–979. [CrossRef]
41. Pinto, J.; Barros, A.S.; Domingues, M.R.M.; Goodfellow, B.J.; Galhano, E.; Pita, C.; Almeida, M.D.C.; Carreira, I.M.; Gil, A.M. Following Healthy Pregnancy by NMR Metabolomics of Plasma and Correlation to Urine. *J. Proteome Res.* **2015**, *14*, 1263–1274. [CrossRef]
42. Pinto, J.; Almeida, L.M.; Martins, A.S.; Duarte, D.; Barros, A.S.; Galhano, E.; Pita, C.; Almeida, M.d.C.; Carreira, I.M.; Gil, A.M. Prediction of Gestational Diabetes through NMR Metabolomics of Maternal Blood. *J. Proteome Res.* **2015**, *14*, 2696–2706. [CrossRef] [PubMed]
43. Qi, R.; Zhang, X.; Xie, Y.; Jiang, S.; Liu, Y.; Liu, X.; Xie, W.; Jia, X.; Bade, R.; Shi, R.; et al. 5-Aza-2′-Deoxycytidine Increases Hypoxia Tolerance-Dependent Autophagy in Mouse Neuronal Cells by Initiating the TSC1/MTOR Pathway. *Biomed. Pharmacother.* **2019**, *118*, 109219. [CrossRef]

44. Huang, Q.; Zhan, L.; Cao, H.; Li, J.; Lyu, Y.; Guo, X.; Zhang, J.; Ji, L.; Ren, T.; An, J.; et al. Increased Mitochondrial Fission Promotes Autophagy and Hepatocellular Carcinoma Cell Survival through the ROS-Modulated Coordinated Regulation of the NFKB and TP53 Pathways. *Autophagy* **2016**, *12*, 999–1014. [CrossRef] [PubMed]
45. Bae, J.-E.; Kang, G.M.; Min, S.H.; Jo, D.S.; Jung, Y.-K.; Kim, K.; Kim, M.-S.; Cho, D.-H. Primary Cilia Mediate Mitochondrial Stress Responses to Promote Dopamine Neuron Survival in a Parkinson's Disease Model. *Cell Death Dis.* **2019**, *10*, 1–15. [CrossRef] [PubMed]
46. Wang, R.; Wang, G. Autophagy in Mitochondrial Quality Control. In *Autophagy: Biology and Diseases*; Springer: Berlin, Germany, 2019; pp. 421–434.
47. Toyama, E.Q.; Herzig, S.; Courchet, J.; Lewis, T.L.; Losón, O.C.; Hellberg, K.; Young, N.P.; Chen, H.; Polleux, F.; Chan, D.C.; et al. AMP-Activated Protein Kinase Mediates Mitochondrial Fission in Response to Energy Stress. *Science* **2016**, *351*, 275–281. [CrossRef]
48. Guo, X.; Liu, Y.; Zhao, Y.; Fan, R.; Bai, Y.; Guo, X.; Li, J.; Chen, C. Role of the PI3K-MTOR Autophagy Pathway in Nerve Damage in Rats with Intermittent Hypoxia-Aggravated Whole Brain Ischemia. *Mol. Med. Rep.* **2019**, *20*, 1411–1417. [CrossRef]
49. Tang, T.; Gao, D.; Yang, X.; Hua, X.; Li, S.; Sun, H. Exogenous Netrin-1 Inhibits Autophagy of Ischemic Brain Tissues and Hypoxic Neurons via PI3K/MTOR Pathway in Ischemic Stroke. *J. Stroke Cerebrovasc. Dis.* **2019**, *28*, 1338–1345. [CrossRef]
50. Sun, B.; Ou, H.; Ren, F.; Huan, Y.; Zhong, T.; Gao, M.; Cai, H. Propofol Inhibited Autophagy through Ca 2+/CaMKKβ/AMPK/MTOR Pathway in OGD/R-Induced Neuron Injury. *Mol. Med.* **2018**, *24*, 58. [CrossRef]
51. Lübke, K.T.; Busch, A.; Hoenen, M.; Schaal, B.; Pause, B.M. Pregnancy Reduces the Perception of Anxiety. *Sci. Rep.* **2017**, *7*, 9213. [CrossRef]
52. Entringer, S.; Buss, C.; Shirtcliff, E.A.; Cammack, A.L.; Yim, I.S.; Chicz-DeMet, A.; Sandman, C.A.; Wadhwa, P.D. Attenuation of Maternal Psychophysiological Stress Responses and the Maternal Cortisol Awakening Response over the Course of Human Pregnancy. *Stress* **2010**, *13*, 258–268. [CrossRef]
53. Klinkenberg, A.V.; Nater, U.M.; Nierop, A.; Bratsikas, A.; Zimmermann, R.; Ehlert, U. Heart Rate Variability Changes in Pregnant and Non-Pregnant Women during Standardized Psychosocial Stress 1. *Acta Obstet. Gynecol. Scand.* **2009**, *88*, 77–82. [CrossRef] [PubMed]
54. Park, S.; Park, J.Y.; Lee, J.H.; Kim, S.-H. Plasma Levels of Lysine, Tyrosine, and Valine during Pregnancy Are Independent Risk Factors of Insulin Resistance and Gestational Diabetes. *Metab. Syndr. Relat. Disord.* **2015**, *13*, 64–70. [CrossRef] [PubMed]
55. Adams, S.; Che, D.; Qin, G.; Farouk, M.H.; Hailong, J.; Rui, H. Novel Biosynthesis, Metabolism and Physiological Functions of L-Homoarginine. *Curr. Protein Pept. Sci.* **2019**, *20*, 184–193. [CrossRef] [PubMed]
56. Matsubara, K. Hypoxia in the Pathogenesis of Preeclampsia. *Hypertens. Res. Pregnancy* **2018**, *5*, 46–51. [CrossRef]
57. Logue, O.C.; George, E.M.; Bidwell, G.L., III. Preeclampsia and the Brain: Neural Control of Cardiovascular Changes during Pregnancy and Neurological Outcomes of Preeclampsia. *Clin. Sci.* **2016**, *130*, 1417–1434. [CrossRef]
58. Siepmann, T.; Boardman, H.; Bilderbeck, A.; Griffanti, L.; Kenworthy, Y.; Zwager, C.; McKean, D.; Francis, J.; Neubauer, S.; Grace, Z.Y.; et al. Long-Term Cerebral White and Gray Matter Changes after Preeclampsia. *Neurology* **2017**, *88*, 1256–1264. [CrossRef]
59. Junewar, V.; Verma, R.; Sankhwar, P.L.; Garg, R.K.; Singh, M.K.; Malhotra, H.S.; Sharma, P.K.; Parihar, A. Neuroimaging Features and Predictors of Outcome in Eclamptic Encephalopathy: A Prospective Observational Study. *Am. J. Neuroradiol.* **2014**, *35*, 1728–1734. [CrossRef]
60. Smriga, M.; Torii, K. L-Lysine Acts like a Partial Serotonin Receptor 4 Antagonist and Inhibits Serotonin-Mediated Intestinal Pathologies and Anxiety in Rats. *Proc. Natl. Acad. Sci. USA* **2003**, *100*, 15370–15375. [CrossRef]
61. Hiramatsu, M. A Role for Guanidino Compounds in the Brain. *Mol. Cell. Biochem.* **2003**, *244*, 57–62. [CrossRef]

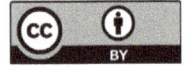

© 2020 by the authors. Licensee MDPI, Basel, Switzerland. This article is an open access article distributed under the terms and conditions of the Creative Commons Attribution (CC BY) license (http://creativecommons.org/licenses/by/4.0/).

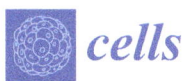

Review

Myocardial Adaptation in Pseudohypoxia: Signaling and Regulation of mPTP via Mitochondrial Connexin 43 and Cardiolipin

Miroslav Ferko *, Natália Andelová, Barbara Szeiffová Bačová and Magdaléna Jašová

Center of Experimental Medicine, Slovak Academy of Sciences, Institute for Heart Research, Dúbravská cesta 9, 841 04 Bratislava, Slovakia; nat.andelova@gmail.com (N.A.); usrdbaca@savba.sk (B.S.B.); jasovam@gmail.com (M.J.)
* Correspondence: usrdmife@savba.sk; Tel.: +421-907065665

Received: 7 November 2019; Accepted: 15 November 2019; Published: 17 November 2019

Abstract: Therapies intended to mitigate cardiovascular complications cannot be applied in practice without detailed knowledge of molecular mechanisms. Mitochondria, as the end-effector of cardioprotection, represent one of the possible therapeutic approaches. The present review provides an overview of factors affecting the regulation processes of mitochondria at the level of mitochondrial permeability transition pores (mPTP) resulting in comprehensive myocardial protection. The regulation of mPTP seems to be an important part of the mechanisms for maintaining the energy equilibrium of the heart under pathological conditions. Mitochondrial connexin 43 is involved in the regulation process by inhibition of mPTP opening. These individual cardioprotective mechanisms can be interconnected in the process of mitochondrial oxidative phosphorylation resulting in the maintenance of adenosine triphosphate (ATP) production. In this context, the degree of mitochondrial membrane fluidity appears to be a key factor in the preservation of ATP synthase rotation required for ATP formation. Moreover, changes in the composition of the cardiolipin's structure in the mitochondrial membrane can significantly affect the energy system under unfavorable conditions. This review aims to elucidate functional and structural changes of cardiac mitochondria subjected to preconditioning, with an emphasis on signaling pathways leading to mitochondrial energy maintenance during partial oxygen deprivation.

Keywords: cardioprotection; mitochondria; mitochondrial permeability transition pores; mitochondrial connexin 43; cardiolipin

---

1. Introduction

Mitochondria are considered to be one of the most important organelles, not only in terms of their ability to control apoptosis [1] or necrosis [2], but also for their important participation in cardioprotection [3]. Mitochondria can cope with energy demanding situations due to their adaptability. The adaptation mechanisms of mitochondria are very important especially in the heart [4]. Cardiac mitochondria provide more than 90% of the total energy required for the cell [5]. Moreover, mitochondria are able to adapt to new conditions through signaling pathways affecting membrane remodeling, mitochondrial dynamics, or energy production [6,7].

Currently, many studies suggest that regulation of mitochondrial permeability transition pore (mPTP) opening plays a key role in the induction of cardioprotection [8–11]. Modulation of mitochondrial membrane fluidity through its major component, cardiolipin, or signalization via mitochondrial connexin 43 (mtCx43) leads to myocardial energy maintenance under the conditions of reduced oxygen utilization.

The common denominator of cardioprotection induction seems to be the exposure of the organism to oxygen limiting conditions [12]. The partial or complete absence of oxygen (hypoxia, anoxia) or damage of the respiratory chain affect the changes of biochemical and metabolic processes and induce remodeling of membrane systems [13]. A limited supply or damage in oxygen processing activates signaling pathways that result in structural and functional changes involved in the adaptation of myocardium to pathological conditions.

The mPTP, cardiolipin, and mtCx43 signaling pathways are calcium associated. Calcium (Ca^{2+}) ions as major inducers of mPTP opening show a high affinity to cardiolipin [14,15]. The process of hypoxia and subsequent reoxygenation also affect mPTP opening coupled with regulation of Ca^{2+} handling and cardiolipin oxidation [16]. Similarly, mtCx43 forms Ca^{2+} permeable hemichannels allowing Ca^{2+} entry and triggering a permeable transition leading to cell death [17]. In the following parts of this review, we discuss the signaling pathways through mPTP regulation in cooperation with cardiolipin and mtCx43 leading to myocardial adaptation in pseudohypoxia.

2. Cardioprotection and Mitochondrial Energetics

Myocardium is highly dependent on sufficient oxygen supply. For this reason, cardiac mitochondria must maintain adequate oxygen to continue oxidative phosphorylation [18–20]. Mitochondrial biogenesis is increased at the metabolically active site of the cell where the consumption of adenosine triphosphate (ATP) is increased [21,22]. Therefore, mitochondria occupy up to 35% of the cell volume of cardiomyocytes of heart ventricles [23–25]. The oxygen consumption varies depending on the physiological state of the organism [26]. Insufficient oxygen supply, characteristic of pathological situations, is reflected in the reduction of energy production in cardiac mitochondria [22,27,28]. Although cardiac mitochondria are the main energy source of cells, their dysfunction contributes to the development of a wide range of diseases [29,30]. The most common diseases, such as ischemic heart disease [31] or diabetes mellitus [32,33], create conditions in which the organism is exposed to a significant lack of oxygen. Partial (hypoxia) or complete (anoxia) absence of oxygen or the inability to use available oxygen due to damage of the mitochondrial respiratory chain (pseudohypoxia) well characterizes the disease of diabetes mellitus [34] and changes of several biochemical and metabolic processes [32]. Therefore, attention is required to develop new therapeutic approaches directed to mitochondria as target organelles triggering cardioprotection.

The principle of the new cardioprotective models is based on controlled oxygen restriction [35]. One of the first well known phenomena of cardioprotection is ischemic preconditioning (IPC), consisting of several repetitions of short ischemic and subsequent reperfusion episodes that reduce myocardial sensitivity before the next prolonged ischemic episode of the heart [36]. The duration of ischemia is crucial for the rate of myocardial damage [37]. While the early phase of ischemia causes reversible changes of cardiomyocyte and decreases the contractility of myocardium, prolonged ischemia (more than 20 to 30 min) leads to irreversible changes in the metabolism, function, and ultrastructure of the heart [30].

Although many studies have confirmed the efficacy of the classical form of IPC [38–40], attention is drawn to an alternative method of controlled induction of short term non-lethal series of ischemic and subsequent reperfusion impulses on specific organs or tissues remote from the heart, known as remote ischemic preconditioning (RPC) [41]. This phenomenon provides protection of myocardium against lethal ischemic damage [42].

An insufficient oxygen supply and nutrients in cardiomyocytes is the main cause of heart ischemia/reperfusion (I/R) injury [43,44]. In a situation with a continuous lack of oxygen, anaerobic glycolysis is preferred [45]. A change in substrate preference used for energy production seems to be the key mechanism favorable for cells with a limited oxygen supply. This is one of the reasons why partial oxygen deprivation is the main factor used in experimental models for the induction of cardioprotection [46].

3. Cardiac Mitochondrial Energetics in Partial Oxygen Deprivation

Oxygen deprivation is reflected in specific metabolic changes that result in a balance disorder between fatty acids and glucose oxidation. The restriction of oxygen supply is reflected in changes in preferences for substrates used for energy production [47,48]. In comparison with fatty acid oxidation, a higher amount of ATP is produced by aerobic oxidation of glucose in relation to oxygen consumption [49]. Therefore, glucose is the preferred energy substrate. Despite the fact that fatty acids are less efficient energy substrates compared to glucose, fatty acids are the preferred source of energy in situations associated with impaired mitochondrial function, reduced respiration, and decreased ATP production, such as ischemia of the heart or diabetes mellitus [50].

Increasing oxidation of fatty acids in the heart reduces oxidation of glucose and vice versa. The oxidation of fatty acids increases nicotinamide adenine dinucleotide (NADH) and acetyl-CoA levels, which inhibit pyruvate dehydrogenase (PDH) associated glucose metabolism reduction [51,52]. The process of mutual regulation of glucose and fatty acid metabolism is called the Randle cycle [53]. However, the predominance of fatty acid oxidation during reperfusion versus glucose oxidation negatively affects the activity of the heart [48,54]. Consequently, manipulating heart metabolism to redirect fatty acid oxidation during reperfusion to glucose utilization may constitute a proof-of-concept on how to preserve heart function after ischemia or hypoxia [55,56].

When a sufficient supply of oxygen is ensured, glucose is metabolized by aerobic oxidation [57]. The PDH complex metabolizes glucose to acetyl-CoA, which then enters into the Krebs cycle [58]. A limited supply of oxygen causes phosphorylation of PDH subunits, i.e., PDH inactivation, which is reflected in the inability to metabolize glucose to pyruvate and acetyl-CoA. Then, glucose is metabolized by anaerobic glycolysis to lactate [59,60]. This process is used mainly by cancer cells that are permanently in anaerobic conditions [61]. Oxygen deprivation stimulates the overexpression of hypoxia-inducible factor 1α (HIF-1α) and inactivation of PDH through pyruvate dehydrogenase kinase 1, resulting in the preference of anaerobic glucose oxidation [62–64]. This process in which the glucose metabolism is reprogrammed from aerobic to anaerobic is known as the Warburg effect [65]. Despite the fact that ATP production in anaerobic glycolysis is much lower, i.e., two molecules of ATP are produced by anaerobic glycolysis, but up to 36 molecules of ATP by the oxidative phosphorylation of one glucose molecule, anaerobic glycolysis is preferred due to low oxygen consumption [66]. Deletion of HIF-1α affects heart function under normoxic conditions, despite the fact that the heart is protected by HIF-1 against hypoxia [32]. Since PDH and the electron transport chain of mitochondria are the major sources of reactive oxygen species (ROS), a preference for anaerobic glycolysis prevents the apoptosis of cancer cells [67,68]. Moreover, continuous production of ATP is ensured by constant glucose supply (malignancy or hyperglycemia) [69]. In addition, the process of anaerobic glycolysis is 100-times faster than oxidative phosphorylation [70]. A constant supply of small amounts of energy with a low oxygen consumption is advantageous for immediate energy supply [71,72]. Besides that, the function of mitochondria is considerably limited in affected cells; therefore, anaerobic glycolysis is the major mechanism of energy production. Since cancer cells are capable of increased proliferation even under these restricted conditions, we can consider that preference for anaerobic glycolysis is beneficial for cells exposed to hypoxia [66,73]. According to the above, we can suppose that cardiomyocytes from diabetic myocardium could be used to describe metabolic processes such as those of cancer cells [63]. Diabetic myocardium is characterized by a state of pseudohypoxia, as a result of electron transport chain damage associated with a limitation of oxidative phosphorylation and impairment of HIF-1 activation [32]. Pseudohypoxia is described as impaired cellular oxygen utilization capacity due to reduced levels of NAD, which may cause NADH accumulation with NADH/NAD redox imbalances [74,75]. Therefore, anaerobic glycolysis could also be advantageous for the cells of diabetic organisms [34,76]. Despite the known side effects of PDH inhibition, such as diabetes mellitus [58,77–79], metabolic syndrome [80], heart failure [81], and fatty liver [82], we can assume that cells of diabetic hearts use similar adaptation mechanisms to increase their survival. A sufficient supply of glucose ensures a prompt and continuous production of energy. These facts explain the advantage of anaerobic glycolysis in a diabetic heart [52]. Another important factor is age, which leads to dysregulation of molecular pathways linked to mitochondria. Increased apoptosis, declined autophagy, increased disruption of mPTP, and worsened injury after hypoxic-ischemic insults are the results of aging. The age related decrease in NAD+ contributes to substrate starvation leading to a pseudohypoxic state [83].

4. Metabolic Preconditioning

Adaptation of the heart to altered metabolic conditions allows the maintenance of its function. It allows the heart to meet the requirements of the body effectively [84]. One of the most commonly used experimental models for the induction of metabolic preconditioning (MPC) is streptozotocin-induced diabetes mellitus with positive structural and metabolic changes present during its acute phase [84–88]. The acute stage of diabetes is characterized by the inhibition of insulin secretion and decreased signaling of insulin receptors in target cells [89]. After the seven days following streptozotocin administration, changes induced by diabetes mellitus are fully developed, without side complication characteristics for the chronic stage of the disease [90]. The acute phase of diabetes mellitus persists for the next three weeks [89].

The chronic phase of streptozotocin diabetes mellitus can be induced by a longer administration of streptozotocin, i.e., for more than 60 days. It is characterized by many complications, such as neuropathy, retinopathy, nephropathy, microangiopathy, etc. [91].

Despite the fact that diabetes mellitus causes extensive changes in the structure and function of cardiomyocytes, its impact is not necessarily entirely harmful. A short-term exposure of the heart to a high glucose concentration or diabetes mellitus has proven beneficial effects against ischemic insult [92,93]. The first evidence of a compensation effect due to diabetes was presented by a study pointing out a better recovery of contractility of a diabetic heart after an I/R injury [94].

The acute phase of MPC induced by diabetes is characterized not only by metabolic changes [84], but also by positively affecting the heart efficiency and its sensitivity to pathological stimuli, remodeling the cardiomyocyte membrane, as well as cardiac mitochondria [95,96]. Indeed, remodeling has a central role in maintaining or repairing the heart tissue [97].

5. Involvement of Mitochondrial Connexin 43 in Cardioprotection

It has been well established that the modulation of membrane channel protein "connexin 43" (Cx43), the most abundant connexin in the heart [98], could have various cardioprotective effects [99–102]. The association of six subunits of Cx43 results in the formation of hemichannel "connexon" [103]. After transportation in secretory vesicles to the plasma membrane, two opposing connexons from adjacent cells create the "Cx channel". Thousands of Cx43 channels aggregate into gap junction plaques at the intercalated disks [104,105]. This direct connection between two adjacent cells provides electrical and metabolic cell-to-cell coupling [106]. Cx43 hemichannels are not only precursors for Cx43 channels, but can also exist as non-junctional hemichannels at the plasma membrane and can contribute to volume regulation, to the release of ATP and NAD+ from the cytosol, and the activation of cell survival pathways [107]. In addition to predominantly localized Cx43 at the intercalated disks, 4% Cx43 is present in mitochondria due to translocation from cardiomyocytes [108,109].

MtCx43 in the cardiomyocytes is situated in the inner mitochondrial membrane (IMM) of subsarcolemmal mitochondria (SSM) where it forms an mtCx43 hemichannel [110,111]. MtCx43 import to the IMM of SSM is mediated by the interaction between Cx43 with the heat shock protein 90 (HSP90) and translocase of the outer membrane 20 [109]. The physiological role of mtCx43 is not fully clarified, but some studies support its involvement in the regulation of K$^+$ fluxes [112], mitochondrial respiration [113], oxygen consumption [111,112], mitochondrial redox state [114], and in mitochondrial Ca^{2+} homeostasis [115] (Figure 1). In this context, it is understandable that mtCx43 is attributed to cardioprotection.

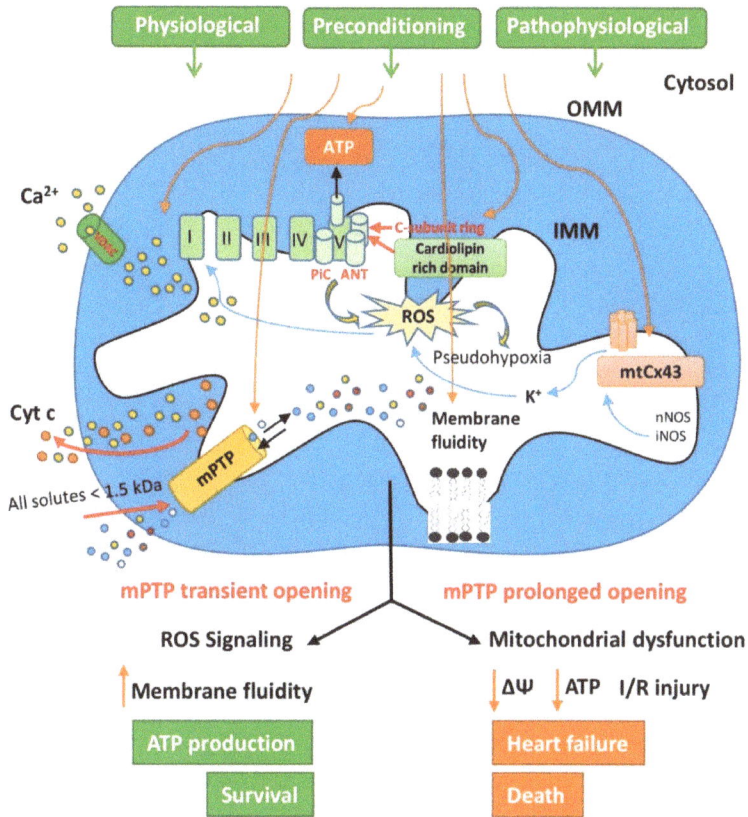

Figure 1. Diagram of signaling pathways affecting mitochondrial permeability transition pores (mPTP) regulation in preconditioned and pathological myocardium. For details, see the text.

The implication of mtCx43 in the cardioprotective pathway of IPC has been mostly elucidated [109,111,116]. The protein level of mtCx43 very rapidly increased in response to IPC and was maintained for at least 90 min in a pig model of IPC [108], whereas attenuation of mtCx43 was associated with lost IPC cardioprotection [108]. Evidence that mtCx43 is implicated in this mechanism was also demonstrated in an experiment by Heinzel et al. in 2015, where pharmacological preconditioning by diazoxide mediated by gating of mitochondrial ATP sensitive potassium channels (KATP) and protein kinase C activation [117] was repealed in cardiomyocytes isolated from mice with a reduced Cx43 level. Mitochondrial KATP channels have also a key role in mitochondrial physiology and potential effects on several pathological processes, thanks to their involvement in cellular energetic status by regulation of organelle volume and function [118].

Indeed, diazoxide affects the generation of ROS necessary in low amounts as trigger molecules of IPC [119]. In the experimental model of Cx43-deficient mice, nitric oxide (NO) production was significantly lower compared to wild type control mice [120]. Increased S-nitrosation of mtCx43 by IPC elevated mitochondrial permeability and subsequently ROS formation [121]. Moreover, diazoxide modulates the opening of the mPTP [122]. The relationship between mtCx43 and mPTP has been elucidated. In this study, pharmacological inhibition of mtCx43 induced opening of mPTP in SSM by increased levels of Ca^{2+} [123]. Another study with IPC abolishment in which reduction of mtCx43 was induced by geldanamycin (which prevents translocation of Cx43 to mitochondria by blocking the HSP90 dependent pathway) confirmed that only mtCx43 is implicated in this cardioprotection [124].

MtCx43 can also be implicated in cardioprotection by interaction with proteins related to mitochondrial fraction and metabolism. MtCx43 interacts with the apoptosis inducing factor (AIF) involved in oxidative phosphorylation and redox control. Interestingly, AIF deficient mice had the same pattern of changes in ROS generation and mitochondrial complex 1 activity as Cx43 deficient mice [113]. In cardiomyocytes with overexpression of Cx43, only complex I respiration was increased, while complex II remained unchanged [113]. A close relationship between mtCx43 and with anti- and pro-apoptosis markers Bcl-2 and Bax was observed. In this experiment, elevated levels of mtCx43 were accompanied by the upregulation of Bcl-2 and inhibition of Bax in the cardiac mitochondria after hypoxic postconditioning [125].

6. The Role of Cardiolipin in Heart Mitochondrial Signaling

Cardiolipin, as a unique phospholipid, is an important component of the IMM [126,127]. It is a relevant indicator of mitochondrial membrane fluidity damage [128]. Due to the localization of respiratory enzymes and oxidative phosphorylation in the IMM, maintaining a positive membrane fluidity remodeling is essential to ensure the bioenergetic processes of the cell [95,129–131] (Figure 1). The fluidity of the mitochondrial membrane is an important part of endogenous protective mechanisms, especially in pathological conditions such as diabetes mellitus [34], ischemia-reperfusion damage [132,133], and hypercholesterolemia [130]. Maintaining membrane fluidity under load conditions at the control level improves ATP transport from the mitochondrial matrix to the cytosol of cardiomyocytes [130]. The sustainability of phospholipid composition in the mitochondrial membrane results in the proper mitochondrial function and structure, phospholipid metabolism, and energy transport [134].

Changes in the composition of the cardiolipin structure, content, and acyl chain are associated with mitochondrial dysfunction in the tissues of certain pathophysiological conditions, including apoptosis [125], ischemia [135], I/R [136], in various stages of thyroid disease [137,138], diabetes mellitus [139], aging [140], and heart failure [135,141].

Cardiolipin is an oxidatively sensitive phospholipid, particularly to ROS [142], due to a high content of unsaturated fatty acids [143]. Oxidative damage of cardiolipin negatively affects the biochemical function of mitochondrial membranes [127], which is reflected in the alteration of the membrane fluidity, ion permeability, as well as the structure and function of the electron transport chain. These alterations lead to a reduced oxidative phosphorylation efficacy of mitochondria [144,145].

Cardiolipin contributes to the protein function in the IMM and maintains the integrity and flow of the electron transport chain, including anionic carriers and respiratory chain complexes [146,147]. Cardiolipin is specifically required for electron transfer in mitochondria respiratory chain complex I [136]. Respiratory complex III of the mammalian chain contains bound cardiolipin molecules that are essential for the enzyme activity [148]. ROS induced oxidative damage of cardiolipin in mitochondria may be responsible for the observed defect in the activity of complex III [149]. Similarly, complex IV contains tightly bound cardiolipin whose removal results in a change of its structure and function [150].

Today, many diseases in which mitochondrial dysfunction has been associated with cardiolipin peroxidation have been described [151]. It seems that a high concentration of Ca^{2+} has a negative impact on mitochondrial function related to the cardiolipin peroxidation. A high concentration of Ca^{2+} together with cardiolipin peroxidation participates in mPTP opening [127]. It has been suggested the cardiolipin associated with the adenine nucleotide translocator (ANT) may be the site at which Ca^{2+} binds and activates mPTP opening. Binding of Ca^{2+} to ANT surrounding cardiolipins enhances the mobility of ANT-Cys^{56}, which could be a potential pathway of Ca^{2+} for induction of mPTP opening [152] (Figure 1).

The accumulation of oxidized cardiolipin in the outer mitochondrial membrane (OMM) contributes to mPTP opening, which is also accompanied by the release of cytochrome c (Cyt c) from mitochondria into the cytosol [153]. The role of cardiolipin in Cyt c releasing from mitochondria seems to be very important in the process of apoptosis [154,155].

Cardiolipin is required to maintain the proper function of ATP synthase and facilitate its rotation, which is supported by the transmembrane proton gradient [156,157]. Cardiolipin is involved in mPTP control via affecting the function of ATP synthase [158,159]. Positive mitochondrial membrane remodeling is associated with an increased membrane fluidity, as well as increased mitochondrial ATP synthase activity in streptozotocin induced pseudohypoxic acute diabetic conditions [160].

7. The Role of Mitochondrial Permeability Transition Pores in Signaling Processes of Cardioprotection

Substantial evidence has revealed that the mPTP are associated with the signaling pathway of cardioprotective models and seem to be an end-effector of cardioprotection [161,162]. It has been shown that the inhibition of mPTP opening not only provides a protective strategy against reperfusion injury [163], but is also a key point in cardioprotective mechanisms such as IPC or MPC [164–166] (Figure 1). The cardioprotective effect of RPC has been associated with the inhibition of mPTP formation [44]. Transient mPTP opening, which allows the release of Ca^{2+} from the mitochondria into the matrix, appears to be a key mechanism in MPC [167].

Under physiological conditions, the mPTP are closed or not present. Their opening is associated with postischemic reperfusion, when the perturbations in intracellular Ca^{2+} homeostasis, ROS accumulation, and a reduction of mitochondrial membrane potential ($\Delta\psi$) are characteristic [168,169]. The massive opening of mPTP results in an increase in IMM permeability and the entry of metabolites into the mitochondrial matrix, which leads to mitochondrial swelling, collapse of $\Delta\psi$, reduction in the efficiency of ATP production by uncoupling the electron transport system from oxidative phosphorylation [170–172], and cell death [10,168]. mPTP remain closed due to low intracellular pH (<7.0) during ischemia, but they are opened during the first minutes of reperfusion associated with the normalization of pH, which causes irreversible heart damage [162,173,174]. Although mPTP are associated with mitochondrial damage and cell death, transient mPTP opening represents one of the physiological processes that is used in the mitochondria of healthy cells [170]. In the heart, transient mPTP opening during preconditioning could be a protective tool that ensures a physiological role during damage [175]. It is believed that transient mPTP opening releases Ca^{2+} from the mitochondrial matrix to maintain mitochondrial homeostasis. Transient mPTP opening is also associated with a temporary increase in ROS as signaling molecules [176].

Increased mPTP production has also been reported in the experimental model of acute diabetes mellitus [177]. The increased formation of mPTP is presented as a compensating mechanism that facilitates the transfer of ATP molecules from the mitochondria into the cytosol, where energy supply is currently needed. Residual mitochondrial ATP production due to its increased cytosolic transfer has been shown to be adequate to maintain sufficient levels of adenine nucleotides in acute diabetic myocardium [34]. The inhibition of mPTP opening may also be achieved by pharmacological drugs. The development of inhibitors, except of a prototype compound such as cyclosporine A (CsA), is limited by side effects and a low therapeutic efficacy [178]. Similarly, there is evidence of a protective mechanism of mPTP inhibition against cancer cell survival and proliferation. mPTP has become a promising strategy for improving cancer therapies [179].

In studies by Heather et al., SSM was adapted to hypoxic conditions and thus mitochondria acquired increased resistance to oxidative damage under conditions of limited oxygen supply. These hypoxia mediated changes induced functional adaptation of mitochondria to a certain dose of stress, resembling the mechanism of the preconditioning effect [180].

mPTP represent a protein complex whose molecular composition remains unexplained. The new knowledge about the structure and regulation of this mitochondrial pore comes annually. The hypothesis about the nature of mPTP suggests that their number is increasing after a conformational change in ATP synthase after binding of Ca^{2+} [181,182]. This change should lead to the opening of the hidden megachannel. It has been discussed whether the role of ATP synthase can be changed from a key energy producing enzyme to an energy dissipating channel that leads to cell death [182]. ATP synthase, together with a phosphate carrier protein (PiC) and ANT, is organized into supramolecular units called synthasomes, which increases the efficiency of ATP production [14,183]. Cyclophilin D (CypD) regulates mPTP, as well as the dynamics of the synthasome, depending on the bioenergy state of mitochondria [184]. Cardiolipin oxidation can disrupt the interactions between the components of the ATP synthasome, which can cause destabilization in this supercomplex, thereby promoting mPTP opening [185].

However, a study by Carroll et al. denied the idea of ATP synthase as the main structural component of mPTP. mPTP opening also occurred after deletion of selected ATP synthase subunits after Ca^{2+} overload. Based on these findings, the authors unlikely considered that ATP synthase and its subunits are involved in the mPTP structure [186]. Interestingly, new findings confirmed the participation of ANT in the mPTP structure. Results achieved by Karch et al. supported the idea about ANT dependent mPTP activity, which is regulated by CypD. ANT dependent mPTP is activated in response to higher mitochondrial matrix Ca^{2+} levels, which means independently of CypD [187]. Many question marks hang over the mPTP structure, again.

8. Unregulated Mitochondrial Permeability Transition Pore Opening

The prolonged mPTP opening results in disruption of the mitochondrial ultrastructure, halting of mitochondrial energy, and ATP synthesis, resulting in a variety of diseases, currently without successful treatment [188]. The unregulated mPTP opening and the consequent oxidative damage are considered as the major mechanisms of mitochondrial energetic dysfunction, which ultimately lead to cell death [8,189]. mPTP opening has an impact on the release of Cyt c from mitochondria, which is associated with pathophysiological situations such as I/R injury, aging, and other degenerative diseases [127]. One of the independent risk factors that may cause structural, molecular, and biochemical changes is aging. Aging increases CypD expression and its interaction with ATP synthase leading to a higher risk of mPTP opening. Thus, mPTP are important factors controlling mitochondrial function affected by aging [190]. Cardioprotective mechanisms, such as preconditioning, could be also impaired by aging and lead to defects in protective cell signaling. In a study by Griecsova et al., the efficacy of preconditioning was attenuated in mature adult rats in contrast with younger animals. Increasing age caused the decrease of heart ischemic tolerance, as well as changes in cellular expression of proteins involved in the protective signaling [191]. Age related disorders are also associated with increased ROS production and dysregulation of intracellular Ca^{2+} levels, resulting in mPTP opening [192]. mPTP are opened during reperfusion after previous ischemic injury of the heart, leading to myocardial damage [193]. Likewise, disruption of Ca^{2+} homeostasis in addition to myocardial I/R injury also occur in neurodegenerative diseases that lead to mPTP opening [194]. Chronic diseases such as diabetes or hypertension cause changes in mitochondrial bioenergetics manifested by inhibition of respiratory chain complex activity, increased proton leakage from the IMM, increased ROS production, and Ca^{2+} overload resulting in mPTP opening [8,172,195]. It has been found that the prevention of mPTP opening by mPTP inhibitors would be beneficial in a wide range of therapeutically challenging diseases. Therefore, significant effort is being made to develop mPTP specific inhibitors that would overcome the major disadvantages of CsA. Further studies are needed to progress from research to therapeutics [188,196].

9. Conclusions

In conclusion, here we emphasize the necessity of maintaining a proper function of cardiac mitochondria even in situations with limited oxygen supply, such as heart ischemic disease. Since it is known that mitochondria have a crucial role in the adaptation process of the heart in unfavorable conditions, the idea of a positive effect of partial oxygen deprivation was studied in new therapeutic approaches. The expression of hypoxic genes and the preference of anaerobic glycolysis associated with the regulation of mPTP are considered as the key mechanisms. The previous findings suggest that not only functional, but also structural changes in cardiac mitochondria are involved in the adaptation process. This knowledge is supported by the relation of mitochondrial membrane composition and functional properties of the heart. The composition of the cardiolipin structure, the amount of mtCx43, and the degree of mitochondrial membrane fluidity affect the formation and opening of mPTP, which is reflected in ATP synthase activity and mitochondrial survival.

Author Contributions: Conceptualization, M.F. and M.J.; resources, M.F., M.J., N.A., and B.S.B.; writing, review and editing, M.F., M.J., N.A., and B.S.B.; visualization, M.F.; supervision, M.F.; project administration, M.F.; funding acquisition, M.F.

Funding: This research was supported by the Scientific Grant Agency of the Ministry of Education, Science Research and Sport of the Slovak Republic VEGA 2/0121/18, VEGA 2/0158/19 and the Slovak Research and Development Agency APVV 15-0119; as well as projects of Structural Funds ITMS 26230120009.

Conflicts of Interest: The authors declare no conflict of interest.

Abbreviations

AIF, apoptosis-inducing factor; ANT, adenine nucleotide translocator; ATP, adenosine triphosphate; Ca^{2+}, calcium; CsA, cyclosporine A; CypD, cyclophilin D; Cyt c, cytochrome c; Cx43, connexin 43; HIF-1α, hypoxia-inducible factor 1α; HSP90, heat shock protein 90; I/R, ischemia/reperfusion; IMM, inner mitochondrial membrane; IPC, ischemic preconditioning; KATP, ATP-sensitive potassium channel; MPC, metabolic preconditioning; mPTP, mitochondrial permeability transition pores; mtCx43, mitochondrial connexin 43; NADH, nicotinamide adenine dinucleotide; NO, nitric oxide; OMM, outer mitochondrial membrane; PDH, pyruvate dehydrogenase; PiC, phosphate carrier protein; ROS, reactive oxygen species; RPC, remote ischemic preconditioning; SSM, subsarcolemmal mitochondria; Δψ, mitochondrial membrane potential.

References

1. Wang, X. The expanding role of mitochondria in apoptosis. *Genes Dev.* **2001**, *15*, 2922–2933. [PubMed]
2. Karch, J.; Molkentin, J.D. Regulated necrotic cell death. *Circ. Res.* **2015**, *116*, 1800–1809. [CrossRef] [PubMed]
3. Siasos, G.; Tsigkou, V.; Kosmopoulos, M.; Theodosiadis, D.; Simantiris, S.; Tagkou, N.M.; Tsimpiktsioglou, A.; Stampouloglou, P.K.; Oikonomou, E.; Mourouzis, K.; et al. Mitochondria and cardiovascular diseases—From pathophysiology to treatment. *Ann. Transl. Med.* **2018**, *6*, 256. [CrossRef] [PubMed]
4. Meerson, F.Z.; Malyshev, I.Y.; Zamotrinsky, A.V. Adaptive protection of the heart and stabilization of myocardial structures. *Basic Res. Cardiol.* **1991**, *86*, 87–98. [CrossRef]
5. Wallace, D.C. A mitochondrial paradigm of metabolic and degenerative diseases, aging, and cancer: A dawn for evolutionary medicine. *Annu. Rev. Genet.* **2005**, *39*, 359–407. [CrossRef]
6. Ferree, A.; Shirihai, O. Mitochondrial dynamics: The intersection of form and function. In *Advances in Experimental Medicine and Biology*; Springer: Berlin, Germany, 2012; Volume 748, pp. 13–40.
7. Picard, M.; McEwen, B.S.; Epel, E.S.; Sandi, C. An energetic view of stress: Focus on mitochondria. *Front. Neuroendocrinol.* **2018**, *49*, 72–85. [CrossRef]
8. Kwong, J.Q.; Molkentin, J.D. Physiological and pathological roles of the mitochondrial permeability transition pore in the heart. *Cell Metab.* **2015**, *21*, 206–214. [CrossRef]
9. Ferdinandy, P.; Schulz, R.; Baxter, G.F. Interaction of cardiovascular risk factors with myocardial ischemia/reperfusion injury, preconditioning, and postconditioning. *Pharmacol. Rev.* **2007**, *59*, 418–458. [CrossRef]
10. Halestrap, A.P. What is the mitochondrial permeability transition pore? *J. Mol. Cell. Cardiol.* **2009**, *46*, 821–831. [CrossRef]
11. Perrelli, M.-G. Ischemia/reperfusion injury and cardioprotective mechanisms: Role of mitochondria and reactive oxygen species. *World J. Cardiol.* **2011**, *3*, 186. [CrossRef]
12. Giaccia, A.J. The biology of hypoxia: The role of oxygen sensing in development, normal function, and disease. *Genes Dev.* **2004**, *18*, 2183–2194. [CrossRef] [PubMed]
13. Fuhrmann, D.C.; Brüne, B. Mitochondrial composition and function under the control of hypoxia. *Redox Biol.* **2017**, *12*, 208–215. [CrossRef] [PubMed]
14. Paradies, G.; Paradies, V.; Ruggiero, F.M.; Petrosillo, G. Role of cardiolipin in mitochondrial function and dynamics in health and disease: Molecular and pharmacological aspects. *Cells* **2019**, *8*, 728. [CrossRef] [PubMed]

15. Paradies, G.; Petrosillo, G.; Paradies, V.; Ruggiero, F.M. Role of cardiolipin peroxidation and Ca^{2+} in mitochondrial dysfunction and disease. *Cell Calcium* **2009**, *45*, 643–650. [CrossRef]
16. Assaly, R.; de Tassigny, A.D.A.; Paradis, S.; Jacquin, S.; Berdeaux, A.; Morin, D. Oxidative stress, mitochondrial permeability transition pore opening and cell death during hypoxia–reoxygenation in adult cardiomyocytes. *Eur. J. Pharmacol.* **2012**, *675*, 6–14. [CrossRef]
17. Gadicherla, A.K.; Wang, N.; Bulic, M.; Agullo-Pascual, E.; Lissoni, A.; De Smet, M.; Delmar, M.; Bultynck, G.; Krysko, D.V.; Camara, A.; et al. Mitochondrial Cx43 hemichannels contribute to mitochondrial calcium entry and cell death in the heart. *Basic Res. Cardiol.* **2017**, *112*, 27. [CrossRef]
18. Ardehali, A.; Ports, T.A. Myocardial Oxygen Supply and Demand* *Cardiovascular Research Institute, and Division of Cardiology, Department of Medicine, University of California, San Francisco. *Chest* **1990**, *98*, 699–705. [CrossRef]
19. Manneschi, L.; Federico, A. Polarographic analyses of subsarcolemmal and intermyofibrillar mitochondria from rat skeletal and cardiac muscle. *J. Neurol. Sci.* **1995**, *128*, 151–156. [CrossRef]
20. Kueh, H.Y.; Niethammer, P.; Mitchison, T.J. Maintenance of mitochondrial oxygen homeostasis by cosubstrate compensation. *Biophys. J.* **2013**, *104*, 1338–1348. [CrossRef]
21. Riva, A.; Tandler, B.; Loffredo, F.; Vazquez, E.; Hoppel, C. Structural differences in two biochemically defined populations of cardiac mitochondria. *Am. J. Physiol. Circ. Physiol.* **2005**, *289*, H868–H872. [CrossRef]
22. Huss, J.M.; Kelly, D.P. Mitochondrial energy metabolism in heart failure: A question of balance. *J. Clin. Investig.* **2005**, *115*, 547–555. [CrossRef] [PubMed]
23. Barth, E. Ultrastructural quantitation of mitochondria and myofilaments in cardiac muscle from 10 different animal species including man. *J. Mol. Cell. Cardiol.* **1992**, *24*, 669–681. [CrossRef]
24. Ferrari, R.; Cargnoni, A.; Ceconi, C. Anti-ischaemic effect of ivabradine. *Pharmacol. Res.* **2006**, *53*, 435–439. [CrossRef] [PubMed]
25. Dedkova, E.N.; Blatter, L.A. Measuring mitochondrial function in intact cardiac myocytes. *J. Mol. Cell. Cardiol.* **2012**, *52*, 48–61. [CrossRef]
26. Saks, V.; Favier, R.; Guzun, R.; Schlattner, U.; Wallimann, T. Molecular system bioenergetics: Regulation of substrate supply in response to heart energy demands. *J. Physiol.* **2006**, *577*, 769–777. [CrossRef]
27. Kojić, Z.; Kojić, Z.; Kojić, Z.; Šćepanović, L.; Šćepanović, L.; Šćepanović, L.; Popović, N.; Popović, N.; Popović, N. Myocardial oxygen consumption regulation in isolated mouse heart: Assessment by intracoronary administration of exogenous nitric oxide. *Acta Physiol. Hung.* **2006**, *93*, 263–270. [CrossRef]
28. Ventura-Clapier, R.; Garnier, A.; Veksler, V.; Joubert, F. Bioenergetics of the failing heart. *Biochim. Biophys. Acta Mol. Cell Res.* **2011**, *1813*, 1360–1372. [CrossRef]
29. Stanley, W.C.; Recchia, F.A.; Lopaschuk, G.D. Myocardial substrate metabolism in the normal and failing heart. *Physiol. Rev.* **2005**, *85*, 1093–1129. [CrossRef]
30. Hoppel, C.L.; Tandler, B.; Fujioka, H.; Riva, A. Dynamic organization of mitochondria in human heart and in myocardial disease. *Int. J. Biochem. Cell Biol.* **2009**, *41*, 1949–1956. [CrossRef]
31. Schanze, N.; Bode, C.; Duerschmied, D. Platelet contributions to myocardial ischemia/reperfusion injury. *Front. Immunol.* **2019**, *10*, 1260. [CrossRef]
32. Cerychova, R.; Pavlinkova, G. HIF-1, metabolism, and diabetes in the embryonic and adult heart. *Front. Endocrinol.* **2018**, *9*, 460. [CrossRef] [PubMed]
33. Nyengaard, J.R.; Ido, Y.; Kilo, C.; Williamson, J.R. Interactions between hyperglycemia and hypoxia: Implications for diabetic retinopathy. *Diabetes* **2004**, *53*, 2931–2938. [CrossRef] [PubMed]
34. Ziegelhöffer, A.; Waczulíková, I.; Ferko, M.; Kincelová, D.; Ziegelhöffer, B.; Ravingerová, T.; Cagalinec, M.; Schönburg, M.; Ziegelhoeffer, T.; Šikurová, L.; et al. Calcium signaling-mediated endogenous protection of cell energetics in the acutely diabetic myocardiumThis article is one of a selection of papers published in a special issue on Advances in Cardiovascular Research. *Can. J. Physiol. Pharmacol.* **2009**, *87*, 1083–1094. [CrossRef] [PubMed]
35. Forini, F.; Nicolini, G.; Iervasi, G. Mitochondria as key targets of cardioprotection in cardiac ischemic disease: Role of thyroid hormone triiodothyronine. *Int. J. Mol. Sci.* **2015**, *16*, 6312–6336. [CrossRef]
36. Murry, C.E.; Jennings, R.B.; Reimer, K.A. Preconditioning with ischemia: A delay of lethal cell injury in ischemic myocardium. *Circulation* **1986**, *74*, 1124–1136. [CrossRef]
37. Honda, H.M.; Korge, P.; Weiss, J.N. Mitochondria and Ischemia/Reperfusion Injury. *Ann. N. Y. Acad. Sci.* **2005**, *1047*, 248–258. [CrossRef]

38. Ravingerová, T.; Pancza, D.; Ziegelhoffer, A.; Styk, J. Preconditioning modulates susceptibility to ischemia-induced arrhythmias in the rat heart: The role of α-adrenergic stimulation and K(ATP) channels. *Physiol. Res.* **2002**, *51*, 101–119.
39. Waldow, T.; Alexiou, K.; Witt, W.; Albrecht, S.; Wagner, F.; Knaut, M.; Matschke, K. Protection against acute porcine lung ischemia/reperfusion injury by systemic preconditioning via hind limb ischemia. *Transpl. Int.* **2005**, *18*, 198–205. [CrossRef]
40. Chen, Q.; Camara, A.K.S.; Stowe, D.F.; Hoppel, C.L.; Lesnefsky, E.J. Modulation of electron transport protects cardiac mitochondria and decreases myocardial injury during ischemia and reperfusion. *Am. J. Physiol. Physiol.* **2007**, *292*, C137–C147. [CrossRef]
41. Przyklenk, K.; Bauer, B.; Ovize, M.; Kloner, R.A.; Whittaker, P. Regional ischemic "preconditioning" protects remote virgin myocardium from subsequent sustained coronary occlusion. *Circulation* **1993**, *87*, 893–899. [CrossRef]
42. Kharbanda, R.K.; Peters, M.; Walton, B.; Kattenhorn, M.; Mullen, M.; Klein, N.; Vallance, P.; Deanfield, J.; MacAllister, R. Ischemic preconditioning prevents endothelial injury and systemic neutrophil activation during ischemia-reperfusion in humans In Vivo. *Circulation* **2001**, *103*, 1624–1630. [CrossRef] [PubMed]
43. Ravingerova, T.; Farkasova, V.; Griecsova, L.; Carnicka, S.; Murarikova, M.; Barlaka, E.; Kolar, F.; Bartekova, M.; Lonek, L.; Slezak, J.; et al. Remote preconditioning as a novel " conditioning" approach to repair the broken heart: Potential mechanisms and clinical applications. *Physiol. Res.* **2016**, *65*, S55–S64. [PubMed]
44. Hausenloy, D.J.; Yellon, D.M. Remote ischaemic preconditioning: Underlying mechanisms and clinical application. *Cardiovasc. Res.* **2008**, *79*, 377–386. [CrossRef] [PubMed]
45. Raedschelders, K.; Ansley, D.M.; Chen, D.D.Y. The cellular and molecular origin of reactive oxygen species generation during myocardial ischemia and reperfusion. *Pharmacol. Ther.* **2012**, *133*, 230–255. [CrossRef] [PubMed]
46. Consolini, A.E.; Ragone, M.I.; Bonazzola, P.; Colareda, G.A. Mitochondrial bioenergetics during ischemia and reperfusion. In *Advances in Experimental Medicine and Biology*; Springer: Berlin, Germany, 2017; Volume 982, pp. 141–167.
47. Liu, Y.; Silverstein, F.S.; Skoff, R.; Barks, J.D.E. Hypoxic-ischemic oligodendroglial injury in neonatal rat brain. *Pediatr. Res.* **2002**, *51*, 25–33. [CrossRef]
48. Lopaschuk, G.D.; Ussher, J.R.; Folmes, C.D.L.; Jaswal, J.S.; Stanley, W.C. Myocardial fatty acid metabolism in health and disease. *Physiol. Rev.* **2010**, *90*, 207–258. [CrossRef]
49. Navarro, A.; Boveris, A. The mitochondrial energy transduction system and the aging process. *Am. J. Physiol. Physiol.* **2007**, *292*, C670–C686. [CrossRef]
50. Peterson, L.R.; McKenzie, C.R.; Schaffer, J.E. Diabetic cardiovascular disease: Getting to the heart of the matter. *J. Cardiovasc. Transl. Res.* **2012**, *5*, 436–445. [CrossRef]
51. Sugden, M.C.; Holness, M.J. Recent advances in mechanisms regulating glucose oxidation at the level of the pyruvate dehydrogenase complex by PDKs. *Am. J. Physiol. Endocrinol. Metab.* **2003**, *284*, E855–E862. [CrossRef]
52. Heather, L.C.; Clarke, K. Metabolism, hypoxia and the diabetic heart. *J. Mol. Cell. Cardiol.* **2011**, *50*, 598–605. [CrossRef]
53. Randle, P.J.; Garland, P.B.; Hales, C.N.; Newsholme, E.A. The glucose fatty-acid cycle its role in insulin sensitivity and the metabolic disturbances of diabetes mellitus. *Lancet* **1963**, *281*, 785–789. [CrossRef]
54. Jaswal, J.S.; Keung, W.; Wang, W.; Ussher, J.R.; Lopaschuk, G.D. Targeting fatty acid and carbohydrate oxidation—A novel therapeutic intervention in the ischemic and failing heart. *Biochim. Biophys. Acta Mol. Cell Res.* **2011**, *1813*, 1333–1350. [CrossRef] [PubMed]
55. Zhou, L.; Huang, H.; McElfresh, T.A.; Prosdocimo, D.A.; Stanley, W.C. Impact of anaerobic glycolysis and oxidative substrate selection on contractile function and mechanical efficiency during moderate severity ischemia. *Am. J. Physiol. Circ. Physiol.* **2008**, *295*, H939–H945. [CrossRef] [PubMed]
56. Johannsen, D.L.; Ravussin, E. The role of mitochondria in health and disease. *Curr. Opin. Pharmacol.* **2009**, *9*, 780–786. [CrossRef] [PubMed]
57. Giordano, F.J. Oxygen, oxidative stress, hypoxia, and heart failure. *J. Clin. Investig.* **2005**, *115*, 500–508. [CrossRef] [PubMed]
58. Jeoung, N.H. Pyruvate dehydrogenase kinases: Therapeutic targets for diabetes and cancers. *Diabetes Metab. J.* **2015**, *39*, 188. [CrossRef] [PubMed]

59. Smolle, M.; Lindsay, J.G. Molecular architecture of the pyruvate dehydrogenase complex: Bridging the gap. *Biochem. Soc. Trans.* **2006**, *34*, 815–818. [CrossRef]
60. Jeoung, N.H.; Harris, C.R.; Harris, R.A. Regulation of pyruvate metabolism in metabolic-related diseases. *Rev. Endocr. Metab. Disord.* **2014**, *15*, 99–110. [CrossRef]
61. Zheng, J. Energy metabolism of cancer: Glycolysis versus oxidative phosphorylation (Review). *Oncol. Lett.* **2012**, *4*, 1151–1157. [CrossRef]
62. Kim, J.; Tchernyshyov, I.; Semenza, G.L.; Dang, C.V. HIF-1-mediated expression of pyruvate dehydrogenase kinase: A metabolic switch required for cellular adaptation to hypoxia. *Cell Metab.* **2006**, *3*, 177–185. [CrossRef]
63. Courtnay, R.; Ngo, D.C.; Malik, N.; Ververis, K.; Tortorella, S.M.; Karagiannis, T.C. Cancer metabolism and the Warburg effect: The role of HIF-1 and PI3K. *Mol. Biol. Rep.* **2015**, *42*, 841–851. [CrossRef] [PubMed]
64. Dodd, M.S.; da Sousa Fialho, M.L.; Montes Aparicio, C.N.; Kerr, M.; Timm, K.N.; Griffin, J.L.; Luiken, J.J.F.P.; Glatz, J.F.C.; Tyler, D.J.; Heather, L.C. Fatty acids prevent hypoxia-inducible Factor-1α signaling through decreased succinate in diabetes. *JACC Basic Transl. Sci.* **2018**, *3*, 485–498. [CrossRef] [PubMed]
65. Warburg, O. On the origin of cancer cells. *Science* **1956**, *123*, 309–314. [CrossRef] [PubMed]
66. Denko, N.C. Hypoxia, HIF1 and glucose metabolism in the solid tumour. *Nat. Rev. Cancer* **2008**, *8*, 705–713. [CrossRef]
67. Papandreou, I.; Cairns, R.A.; Fontana, L.; Lim, A.L.; Denko, N.C. HIF-1 mediates adaptation to hypoxia by actively downregulating mitochondrial oxygen consumption. *Cell Metab.* **2006**, *3*, 187–197. [CrossRef]
68. Vander Heiden, M.G.; Cantley, L.C.; Thompson, C.B. Understanding the warburg effect: The metabolic requirements of cell proliferation. *Science* **2009**, *324*, 1029–1033. [CrossRef]
69. Wittig, R.; Coy, J.F. The role of glucose metabolism and glucose-associated signalling in cancer. *Perspect. Medicin. Chem.* **2007**, *1*. [CrossRef]
70. Liberti, M.V.; Locasale, J.W. The warburg effect: How does it benefit cancer cells? *Trends Biochem. Sci.* **2016**, *41*, 211–218. [CrossRef]
71. Gunaydin, B.; Çakici, I.; Soncul, H.; Kalaycioglu, S.; Çevik, C.; Sancak, B.; Kanzik, I.; Karadenizli, Y. Does remote organ ischemia trigger cardiac preconditioning during coronary artery surgery? *Pharmacol. Res.* **2000**, *41*, 493–496. [CrossRef]
72. Doenst, T.; Nguyen, T.D.; Abel, E.D. Cardiac metabolism in heart failure. *Circ. Res.* **2013**, *113*, 709–724. [CrossRef]
73. Daşu, A.; Toma-Daşu, I.; Karlsson, M. Theoretical simulation of tumour oxygenation and results from acute and chronic hypoxia. *Phys. Med. Biol.* **2003**, *48*, 2829–2842. [PubMed]
74. Yan, L.-J.; Wu, J.; Jin, Z.; Zheng, H. Sources and implications of NADH/NAD+ redox imbalance in diabetes and its complications. *Diabetes Metab. Syndr. Obes. Targets Ther.* **2016**, *9*, 145–153. [CrossRef] [PubMed]
75. Williamson, J.R.; Chang, K.; Frangos, M.; Hasan, K.S.; Ido, Y.; Kawamura, T.; Nyengaard, J.R.; van Den Enden, M.; Kilo, C.; Tilton, R.G. Hyperglycemic pseudohypoxia and diabetic complications. *Diabetes* **1993**, *42*, 801–813. [CrossRef] [PubMed]
76. Sivitz, W.I.; Yorek, M.A. Mitochondrial dysfunction in diabetes: From molecular mechanisms to functional significance and therapeutic opportunities. *Antioxid. Redox Signal.* **2010**, *12*, 537–577. [CrossRef] [PubMed]
77. McFate, T.; Mohyeldin, A.; Lu, H.; Thakar, J.; Henriques, J.; Halim, N.D.; Wu, H.; Schell, M.J.; Tsang, T.M.; Teahan, O.; et al. Pyruvate dehydrogenase complex activity controls metabolic and malignant phenotype in cancer cells. *J. Biol. Chem.* **2008**, *283*, 22700–22708. [CrossRef] [PubMed]
78. Peters, S.J.; Harris, R.A.; Wu, P.; Pehleman, T.L.; Heigenhauser, G.J.F.; Spriet, L.L. Human skeletal muscle PDH kinase activity and isoform expression during a 3-day high-fat/low-carbohydrate diet. *Am. J. Physiol. Endocrinol. Metab.* **2001**, *281*, E1151–E1158. [CrossRef] [PubMed]
79. Park, S.; Jeon, J.-H.; Min, B.-K.; Ha, C.-M.; Thoudam, T.; Park, B.-Y.; Lee, I.-K. Role of the pyruvate dehydrogenase complex in metabolic remodeling: Differential pyruvate dehydrogenase complex functions in metabolism. *Diabetes Metab. J.* **2018**, *42*, 270. [CrossRef]
80. Lee, I.-K. The role of pyruvate dehydrogenase kinase in diabetes and obesity. *Diabetes Metab. J.* **2014**, *38*, 181. [CrossRef]
81. Sun, W.; Liu, Q.; Leng, J.; Zheng, Y.; Li, J. The role of Pyruvate Dehydrogenase Complex in cardiovascular diseases. *Life Sci.* **2015**, *121*, 97–103. [CrossRef]

82. Hwang, S.; Lee, S.-G.; Belghiti, J. Liver transplantation for HCC: Its role. *J. Hepatobiliary Pancreat. Sci.* **2010**, *17*, 443–448. [CrossRef]
83. Ham, P.B.; Raju, R. Mitochondrial function in hypoxic ischemic injury and influence of aging. *Prog. Neurobiol.* **2017**, *157*, 92–116. [CrossRef] [PubMed]
84. Malfitano, C.; de Souza Junior, A.L.; Carbonaro, M.; Bolsoni-Lopes, A.; Figueroa, D.; de Souza, L.E.; Silva, K.A.S.; Consolim-Colombo, F.; Curi, R.; Irigoyen, M.C. Glucose and fatty acid metabolism in infarcted heart from streptozotocin-induced diabetic rats after 2 weeks of tissue remodeling. *Cardiovasc. Diabetol.* **2015**, *14*, 149. [CrossRef] [PubMed]
85. Xu, G.; Takashi, E.; Kudo, M.; Ishiwata, T.; Naito, Z. Contradictory effects of short-and long-term hyperglycemias on ischemic injury of myocardium via intracellular signaling pathway. *Exp. Mol. Pathol.* **2004**, *76*, 57–65. [CrossRef] [PubMed]
86. Ferko, M.; Habodászová, D.; Waczulíková, I.; Mujkošová, J.; Kucharská, J.; Šikurová, L.; Ziegelhoffer, B.; Styk, J.; Ziegelhffer, A. Endogenous protective mechanisms in remodeling of rat heart mitochondrial membranes in the acute phase of streptozotocin-induced diabetes. *Physiol. Res.* **2008**, *57*, S67–S73. [PubMed]
87. Zhu, X.-H.; Yuan, H.-J.; Wu, Y.-N.; Kang, Y.; Jiao, J.-J.; Gao, W.-Z.; Liu, Y.-X.; Lou, J.-S.; Xia, Z. Non-invasive limb ischemic pre-conditioning reduces oxidative stress and attenuates myocardium ischemia-reperfusion injury in diabetic rats. *Free Radic. Res.* **2011**, *45*, 201–210. [CrossRef] [PubMed]
88. King, A.J.F. The use of animal models in diabetes research. *Br. J. Pharmacol.* **2012**, *166*, 877–894. [CrossRef]
89. Kadowaki, T.; Kasuga, M.; Akanuma, Y.; Ezaki, O.; Takaku, F. Decreased autophosphorylation of the insulin receptor-kinase in streptozotocin-diabetic rats. *J. Biol. Chem.* **1984**, *259*, 14208–14216.
90. Ziegelhöffer, A.; Ravingerová, T.; Styk, J.; Tribulová, N.; Volkovová, K.; Šeboková, J.; Breier, A. Diabetic cardiomyopathy in rats: Biochemical mechanisms of increased tolerance to calcium overload. *Diabetes Res. Clin. Pract.* **1996**, *31*, S93–S103. [CrossRef]
91. Oliveira, P.J.; Seiça, R.; Coxito, P.M.; Rolo, A.P.; Palmeira, C.M.; Santos, M.S.; Moreno, A.J.M. Enhanced permeability transition explains the reduced calcium uptake in cardiac mitochondria from streptozotocin-induced diabetic rats. *FEBS Lett.* **2003**, *554*, 511–514. [CrossRef]
92. Rodrigues, B.; Figueroa, D.M.T.; Fang, J.; Rosa, K.T.; Llesuy, S.; De Angelis, K.; Irigoyen, M.C. Short-term diabetes attenuates left ventricular dysfunction and mortality rates after myocardial infarction in rodents. *Clinics* **2011**, *66*, 1437–1442. [CrossRef]
93. Malfitano, C.; Barboza, C.A.; Mostarda, C.; da Palma, R.K.; dos Santos, C.P.; Rodrigues, B.; Freitas, S.C.F.; Belló-Klein, A.; Llesuy, S.; Irigoyen, M.-C.; et al. Diabetic hyperglycemia attenuates sympathetic dysfunction and oxidative stress after myocardial infarction in rats. *Cardiovasc. Diabetol.* **2014**, *13*, 131. [CrossRef] [PubMed]
94. Tani, M.; Neely, J.R. Hearts from diabetic rats are more resistant to in vitro ischemia: Possible role of altered Ca^{2+} metabolism. *Circ. Res.* **1988**, *62*, 931–940. [CrossRef] [PubMed]
95. Kancirová, I.; Jašová, M.; Muráriková, M.; Sumbalová, Z.; Uličná, O.; Ravingerová, T.; Waczulíková, I.; Ziegelhöffer, A.; Ferko, M. Cardioprotection induced by remote ischemic preconditioning preserves the mitochondrial respiratory function in acute diabetic myocardium. *Physiol. Res.* **2016**, *65*, S611–S619. [PubMed]
96. Ferko, M.; Gvozdjaková, A.; Kucharská, J.; Mujkošová, J.; Waczulíková, I.; Styk, J.; Ravingerová, T.; Ziegelhöffer-Mihalovičová, B.; Ziegelhöffer, A. Functional remodeling of heart mitochondria in acute diabetes: Interrelationships between damage endogenous protection and adaptation. *Gen. Physiol. Biophys.* **2006**, *25*, 397–413.
97. Mapanga, R.F.; Rajamani, U.; Dlamini, N.; Zungu-Edmondson, M.; Kelly-Laubscher, R.; Shafiullah, M.; Wahab, A.; Hasan, M.Y.; Fahim, M.A.; Rondeau, P.; et al. Oleanolic acid: A novel cardioprotective agent that blunts hyperglycemia-induced contractile dysfunction. *PLoS ONE* **2012**, *7*, e47322. [CrossRef]
98. Severs, N.J.; Bruce, A.F.; Dupont, E.; Rothery, S. Remodelling of gap junctions and connexin expression in diseased myocardium. *Cardiovasc. Res.* **2008**, *80*, 9–19. [CrossRef]
99. Tribulova, N.; Szeiffova Bacova, B.; Egan Benova, T.; Knezl, V.; Barancik, M.; Slezak, J. Omega-3 index and anti-arrhythmic potential of omega-3 PUFAs. *Nutrients* **2017**, *9*, 1191. [CrossRef]
100. Katengua-Thamahane, E.; Szeiffova Bacova, B.; Bernatova, I.; Sykora, M.; Knezl, V.; Van Rooyen, J.; Tribulova, N. Effects of red palm oil on myocardial antioxidant enzymes, nitric oxide synthase and heart function in spontaneously hypertensive rats. *Int. J. Mol. Sci.* **2017**, *18*, 2476. [CrossRef]

101. Sykora, M.; Szeiffova Bacova, B.; Egan Benova, T.; Barancik, M.; Zurmanova, J.; Rauchova, H.; Weismann, P.; Pavelka, S.; Kurahara, L.H.; Slezak, J.; et al. Cardiac Cx43 and ECM Responses to Altered Thyroid Status Are Blunted in Spontaneously Hypertensive versus Normotensive Rats. *Int. J. Mol. Sci.* **2019**, *20*, 3758. [CrossRef]
102. Prado, N.J.; Egan Beňová, T.; Diez, E.R.; Knezl, V.; Lipták, B.; Ponce Zumino, A.Z.; Llamedo-Soria, M.; Szeiffová Bačová, B.; Miatello, R.M.; Tribulová, N. Melatonin receptor activation protects against low potassium-induced ventricular fibrillation by preserving action potentials and connexin-43 topology in isolated rat hearts. *J. Pineal Res.* **2019**, *67*. [CrossRef]
103. Laird, D.W. Life cycle of connexins in health and disease. *Biochem. J.* **2006**, *394*, 527–543. [CrossRef] [PubMed]
104. Veenstra, R.D.; Wang, H.-Z.; Beblo, D.A.; Chilton, M.G.; Harris, A.L.; Beyer, E.C.; Brink, P.R. Selectivity of connexin-specific gap junctions does not correlate with channel conductance. *Circ. Res.* **1995**, *77*, 1156–1165. [CrossRef] [PubMed]
105. Goodenough, D.A. Connexins, connexons, and intercellular communication. *Annu. Rev. Biochem.* **1996**, *65*, 475–502. [CrossRef] [PubMed]
106. Severs, N. Gap junction alterations in human cardiac disease. *Cardiovasc. Res.* **2004**, *62*, 368–377. [CrossRef]
107. Sáez, J.C.; Retamal, M.A.; Basilio, D.; Bukauskas, F.F.; Bennett, M.V.L. Connexin-based gap junction hemichannels: Gating mechanisms. *Biochim. Biophys. Acta Biomembr.* **2005**, *1711*, 215–224. [CrossRef]
108. Boengler, K.; Dodoni, G.; Rodriguezsinovas, A.; Cabestrero, A.; Ruizmeana, M.; Gres, P.; Konietzka, I.; Lopeziglesias, C.; Garciadorado, D.; Dilisa, F. Connexin 43 in cardiomyocyte mitochondria and its increase by ischemic preconditioning. *Cardiovasc. Res.* **2005**, *67*, 234–244. [CrossRef]
109. Ruiz-Meana, M.; Rodriguez-Sinovas, A.; Cabestrero, A.; Boengler, K.; Heusch, G.; Garcia-Dorado, D. Mitochondrial connexin43 as a new player in the pathophysiology of myocardial ischaemia-reperfusion injury. *Cardiovasc. Res.* **2007**, *77*, 325–333. [CrossRef]
110. Boengler, K.; Stahlhofen, S.; Sand, A.; Gres, P.; Ruiz-Meana, M.; Garcia-Dorado, D.; Heusch, G.; Schulz, R. Presence of connexin 43 in subsarcolemmal, but not in interfibrillar cardiomyocyte mitochondria. *Basic Res. Cardiol.* **2009**, *104*, 141–147. [CrossRef]
111. Rodríguez-Sinovas, A.; Ruiz-Meana, M.; Denuc, A.; García-Dorado, D. Mitochondrial Cx43, an important component of cardiac preconditioning. *Biochim. Biophys. Acta Biomembr.* **2018**, *1860*, 174–181. [CrossRef]
112. Boengler, K.; Schulz, R. Connexin 43 and mitochondria in cardiovascular health and disease. In *Advances in Experimental Medicine and Biology*; Springer: Berlin, Germany, 2017; Volume 982, pp. 227–246.
113. Boengler, K.; Ruiz-Meana, M.; Gent, S.; Ungefug, E.; Soetkamp, D.; Miro-Casas, E.; Cabestrero, A.; Fernandez-Sanz, C.; Semenzato, M.; Di Lisa, F.; et al. Mitochondrial connexin 43 impacts on respiratory complex I activity and mitochondrial oxygen consumption. *J. Cell. Mol. Med.* **2012**, *16*, 1649–1655. [CrossRef]
114. Denuc, A.; Núñez, E.; Calvo, E.; Loureiro, M.; Miro-Casas, E.; Guarás, A.; Vázquez, J.; Garcia-Dorado, D. New protein-protein interactions of mitochondrial connexin 43 in mouse heart. *J. Cell. Mol. Med.* **2016**, *20*, 794–803. [CrossRef] [PubMed]
115. Guo, R.; Si, R.; Scott, B.T.; Makino, A. Mitochondrial connexin40 regulates mitochondrial calcium uptake in coronary endothelial cells. *Am. J. Physiol. Physiol.* **2017**, *312*, C398–C406. [CrossRef] [PubMed]
116. Schulz, R.; Görge, P.M.; Görbe, A.; Ferdinandy, P.; Lampe, P.D.; Leybaert, L. Connexin 43 is an emerging therapeutic target in ischemia/reperfusion injury, cardioprotection and neuroprotection. *Pharmacol. Ther.* **2015**, *153*, 90–106. [CrossRef] [PubMed]
117. Heinzel, F.R.; Luo, Y.; Li, X.; Boengler, K.; Buechert, A.; García-Dorado, D.; Di Lisa, F.; Schulz, R.; Heusch, G. Impairment of diazoxide-induced formation of reactive oxygen species and loss of cardioprotection in connexin 43 deficient mice. *Circ. Res.* **2005**, *97*, 583–586. [CrossRef]
118. Paggio, A.; Checchetto, V.; Campo, A.; Menabò, R.; Di Marco, G.; Di Lisa, F.; Szabo, I.; Rizzuto, R.; De Stefani, D. Identification of an ATP-sensitive potassium channel in mitochondria. *Nature* **2019**, *572*, 609–613. [CrossRef]
119. Korge, P.; Honda, H.M.; Weiss, J.N. Protection of cardiac mitochondria by diazoxide and protein kinase C: Implications for ischemic preconditioning. *Proc. Natl. Acad. Sci. USA* **2002**, *99*, 3312–3317. [CrossRef]
120. Kirca, M.; Kleinbongard, P.; Soetkamp, D.; Heger, J.; Csonka, C.; Ferdinandy, P.; Schulz, R. Interaction between Connexin 43 and nitric oxide synthase in mice heart mitochondria. *J. Cell. Mol. Med.* **2015**, *19*, 815–825. [CrossRef]

121. Soetkamp, D.; Nguyen, T.T.; Menazza, S.; Hirschhäuser, C.; Hendgen-Cotta, U.B.; Rassaf, T.; Schlüter, K.D.; Boengler, K.; Murphy, E.; Schulz, R. S-nitrosation of mitochondrial connexin 43 regulates mitochondrial function. *Basic Res. Cardiol.* **2014**, *109*, 433. [CrossRef]
122. Katoh, H.; Nishigaki, N.; Hayashi, H. Diazoxide opens the mitochondrial permeability transition pore and alters Ca^{2+} transients in rat ventricular myocytes. *Circulation* **2002**, *105*, 2666–2671. [CrossRef]
123. Srisakuldee, W.; Makazan, Z.; Nickel, B.E.; Zhang, F.; Thliveris, J.A.; Pasumarthi, K.B.S.; Kardami, E. The FGF-2-triggered protection of cardiac subsarcolemmal mitochondria from calcium overload is mitochondrial connexin 43-dependent. *Cardiovasc. Res.* **2014**, *103*, 72–80. [CrossRef]
124. Rodriguez-Sinovas, A.; Boengler, K.; Cabestrero, A.; Gres, P.; Morente, M.; Ruiz-Meana, M.; Konietzka, I.; Miró, E.; Totzeck, A.; Heusch, G.; et al. Translocation of connexin 43 to the inner mitochondrial membrane of cardiomyocytes through the heat shock protein 90–dependent TOM pathway and its importance for cardioprotection. *Circ. Res.* **2006**, *99*, 93–101. [CrossRef] [PubMed]
125. Kagan, V.E.; Tyurin, V.A.; Jiang, J.; Tyurina, Y.Y.; Ritov, V.B.; Amoscato, A.A.; Osipov, A.N.; Belikova, N.A.; Kapralov, A.A.; Kini, V.; et al. Cytochrome c acts as a cardiolipin oxygenase required for release of proapoptotic factors. *Nat. Chem. Biol.* **2005**, *1*, 223–232. [CrossRef] [PubMed]
126. Houtkooper, R.H.; Vaz, F.M. Cardiolipin, the heart of mitochondrial metabolism. *Cell. Mol. Life Sci.* **2008**, *65*, 2493–2506. [CrossRef] [PubMed]
127. Paradies, G.; Paradies, V.; De Benedictis, V.; Ruggiero, F.M.; Petrosillo, G. Functional role of cardiolipin in mitochondrial bioenergetics. *Biochim. Biophys. Acta Bioenerg.* **2014**, *1837*, 408–417. [CrossRef]
128. Unsay, J.D.; Cosentino, K.; Subburaj, Y.; García-Sáez, A.J. Cardiolipin effects on membrane structure and dynamics. *Langmuir* **2013**, *29*, 15878–15887. [CrossRef]
129. Giorgio, V.; Guo, L.; Bassot, C.; Petronilli, V.; Bernardi, P. Calcium and regulation of the mitochondrial permeability transition. *Cell Calcium* **2018**, *70*, 56–63. [CrossRef]
130. Ferko, M.; Farkasova, V.; Jasova, M.; Kancirova, I.; Ravingerova, T.; Adameova, A.D.; Andelova, N.; Waczulikova, I. Hypercholesterolemia antagonized heart adaptation and functional remodeling of the mitochondria observed in acute diabetes mellitus subjected to ischemia/reperfusion injury. *J. Physiol. Pharmacol.* **2018**, *69*, 685–697.
131. Palovicova, V.; Bardelcikova, A.; Obernauerova, M. Absence of anionic phospholipids in Kluyveromyces lactis cells is fatal without F1-catalysed ATP hydrolysis. *Can. J. Microbiol.* **2012**, *58*, 694–702. [CrossRef]
132. Jones, R.M.; Bagchi, M.; Das, D.K. Preconditioning of heart by repeated stunning: Adaptive modification of myocardial lipid membrane. *Basic Res. Cardiol.* **1992**, *87*, 527–535. [CrossRef]
133. Muráriková, M.; Ferko, M.; Waczulíková, I.; Jašová, M.; Kancirová, I.; Murínová, J.; Ravingerová, T. Changes in mitochondrial properties may contribute to enhanced resistance to ischemia–reperfusion injury in the diabetic rat heart. *Can. J. Physiol. Pharmacol.* **2017**, *95*, 969–976. [CrossRef]
134. Schenkel, L.C.; Bakovic, M. Formation and regulation of mitochondrial membranes. *Int. J. Cell Biol.* **2014**, *2014*, 1–13. [CrossRef] [PubMed]
135. Lesnefsky, E.J.; Slabe, T.J.; Stoll, M.S.K.; Minkler, P.E.; Hoppel, C.L. Myocardial ischemia selectively depletes cardiolipin in rabbit heart subsarcolemmal mitochondria. *Am. J. Physiol. Hear Circ. Physiol.* **2001**, *280*, H2770–H2778. [CrossRef] [PubMed]
136. Paradies, G.; Petrosillo, G.; Pistolese, M.; Di Venosa, N.; Federici, A.; Ruggiero, F.M. Decrease in mitochondrial complex i activity in ischemic/reperfused rat heart. *Circ. Res.* **2004**, *94*, 53–59. [CrossRef] [PubMed]
137. Cao, S.G.; Cheng, P.; Angel, A.; Hatch, G.M. Thyroxine stimulates phosphatidylglycerolphosphate synthase activity in rat heart mitochondria. *Biochim. Biophys. Acta Lipids Lipid Metab.* **1995**, *1256*, 241–244. [CrossRef]
138. Hostetler, K.Y. Effect of thyroxine on the activity of mitochondrial cardiolipin synthase in rat liver. *Biochim. Biophys. Acta Lipids Lipid Metab.* **1991**, *1086*, 139–140. [CrossRef]
139. He, Q.; Han, X. Cardiolipin remodeling in diabetic heart. *Chem. Phys. Lipids* **2014**, *179*, 75–81. [CrossRef]
140. Lesnefsky, E.J.; Chen, Q.; Hoppel, C.L. Mitochondrial metabolism in aging heart. *Circ. Res.* **2016**, *118*, 1593–1611. [CrossRef]
141. Dolinsky, V.W.; Cole, L.K.; Sparagna, G.C.; Hatch, G.M. Cardiac mitochondrial energy metabolism in heart failure: Role of cardiolipin and sirtuins. *Biochim. Biophys. Acta Mol. Cell Biol. Lipids* **2016**, *1861*, 1544–1554. [CrossRef]
142. Yin, H.; Zhu, M. Free radical oxidation of cardiolipin: Chemical mechanisms, detection and implication in apoptosis, mitochondrial dysfunction and human diseases. *Free Radic. Res.* **2012**, *46*, 959–974. [CrossRef]

143. Fajardo, V.A.; Mikhaeil, J.S.; Leveille, C.F.; Saint, C.; LeBlanc, P.J. Cardiolipin content, linoleic acid composition, and tafazzin expression in response to skeletal muscle overload and unload stimuli. *Sci. Rep.* **2017**, *7*, 2060. [CrossRef]
144. Dudek, J. Role of cardiolipin in mitochondrial signaling pathways. *Front. Cell Dev. Biol.* **2017**, *5*, 90. [CrossRef] [PubMed]
145. Patil, V.A.; Greenberg, M.L. Cardiolipin-mediated cellular signaling. *Adv. Exp. Med. Biol.* **2013**, *991*, 195–213. [PubMed]
146. Sparagna, G.C.; Lesnefsky, E.J. Cardiolipin remodeling in the heart. *J. Cardiovasc. Pharmacol.* **2009**, *53*, 290–301. [CrossRef] [PubMed]
147. Zhang, M.; Mileykovskaya, E.; Dowhan, W. Gluing the respiratory chain together. *J. Biol. Chem.* **2002**, *277*, 43553–43556. [CrossRef]
148. Gomez, B.; Robinson, N.C. Phospholipase digestion of bound cardiolipin reversibly inactivates bovine cytochrome bc 1 †. *Biochemistry* **1999**, *38*, 9031–9038. [CrossRef]
149. Petrosillo, G.; Ruggiero, F.M.; Di Venosa, N.; Paradies, G. Decreased complex III activity in mitochondria isolated from rat heart subjected to ischemia and reperfusion: Role of reactive oxygen species and cardiolipin. *FASEB J.* **2003**, *7*, 714–716. [CrossRef]
150. Sedlák, E.; Robinson, N.C. Phospholipase A 2 digestion of cardiolipin bound to bovine cytochrome c oxidase alters both activity and quaternary structure †. *Biochemistry* **1999**, *38*, 14966–14972. [CrossRef]
151. Chicco, A.J.; Sparagna, G.C. Role of cardiolipin alterations in mitochondrial dysfunction and disease. *Am. J. Physiol. Physiol.* **2007**, *292*, C33–C44. [CrossRef]
152. Pestana, C.R.; Silva, C.H.T.P.; Pardo-Andreu, G.L.; Rodrigues, F.P.; Santos, A.C.; Uyemura, S.A.; Curti, C. Ca^{2+} binding to c-state of adenine nucleotide translocase (ANT)-surrounding cardiolipins enhances (ANT)-Cys56 relative mobility: A computational-based mitochondrial permeability transition study. *Biochim. Biophys. Acta Bioenerg.* **2009**, *1787*, 176–182. [CrossRef]
153. Ostrander, D.B.; Sparagna, G.C.; Amoscato, A.A.; McMillin, J.B.; Dowhan, W. Decreased cardiolipin synthesis corresponds with cytochrome c release in palmitate-induced cardiomyocyte apoptosis. *J. Biol. Chem.* **2001**, *276*, 38061–38067.
154. Ott, M.; Robertson, J.D.; Gogvadze, V.; Zhivotovsky, B.; Orrenius, S. Cytochrome c release from mitochondria proceeds by a two-step process. *Proc. Natl. Acad. Sci. USA* **2002**, *99*, 1259–1263. [CrossRef] [PubMed]
155. Ott, M.; Zhivotovsky, B.; Orrenius, S. Role of cardiolipin in cytochrome c release from mitochondria. *Cell Death Differ.* **2007**, *14*, 1243–1247. [CrossRef] [PubMed]
156. Smith Eble, K.; Coleman, W.B.; Hantgan, R.R.; Cunningham, C.C. Tightly associated cardiolipin in the bovine heart mitochondrial ATP synthase as analyzed by 31 P nuclear magnetic resonance spectroscopy. *J. Biol. Chem.* **1990**, *265*, 19434–19440.
157. Duncan, A.L.; Robinson, A.J.; Walker, J.E. Cardiolipin binds selectively but transiently to conserved lysine residues in the rotor of metazoan ATP synthases. *Proc. Natl. Acad. Sci. USA* **2016**, *113*, 8687–8692. [CrossRef]
158. Biasutto, L.; Azzolini, M.; Szabò, I.; Zoratti, M. The mitochondrial permeability transition pore in AD 2016: An update. *Biochim. Biophys. Acta Mol. Cell Res.* **2016**, *1863*, 2515–2530. [CrossRef]
159. Carraro, M.; Checchetto, V.; Szabó, I.; Bernardi, P. F-ATP synthase and the permeability transition pore: Fewer doubts, more certainties. *FEBS Lett.* **2019**, *593*, 1542–1553. [CrossRef]
160. Jašová, M.; Kancirová, I.; Waczulíková, I.; Ferko, M. Mitochondria as a target of cardioprotection in models of preconditioning. *J. Bioenerg. Biomembr.* **2017**, *49*, 357–368. [CrossRef]
161. Javadov, S.; Karmazyn, M.; Escobales, N. Mitochondrial permeability transition pore opening as a promising therapeutic target in cardiac diseases. *J. Pharmacol. Exp. Ther.* **2009**, *330*, 670–678. [CrossRef]
162. Bernardi, P.; Di Lisa, F. The mitochondrial permeability transition pore: Molecular nature and role as a target in cardioprotection. *J. Mol. Cell. Cardiol.* **2015**, *78*, 100–106. [CrossRef]
163. Szabo, I.; Zoratti, M. The mitochondrial megachannel is the permeability transition pore. *J. Bioenerg. Biomembr.* **1992**, *24*, 111–117. [CrossRef]
164. Javadov, S.; Karmazyn, M. Mitochondrial permeability transition pore opening as an endpoint to initiate cell death and as a putative target for cardioprotection. *Cell. Physiol. Biochem.* **2007**, *20*, 1–22. [CrossRef] [PubMed]

165. Nazari, A.; Sadr, S.S.; Faghihi, M.; Azizi, Y.; Hosseini, M.-J.; Mobarra, N.; Tavakoli, A.; Imani, A. Vasopressin attenuates ischemia–reperfusion injury via reduction of oxidative stress and inhibition of mitochondrial permeability transition pore opening in rat hearts. *Eur. J. Pharmacol.* **2015**, *760*, 96–102. [CrossRef] [PubMed]
166. Argaud, L. Preconditioning delays Ca^{2+}-induced mitochondrial permeability transition. *Cardiovasc. Res.* **2004**, *61*, 115–122. [CrossRef] [PubMed]
167. Ziegelhöffer-Mihalovičová, B.; Waczulíková, I.; Šikurová, L.; Styk, J.; Čársky, J.; Ziegelhöffer, A. Remodelling of the sarcolemma in diabetic rat hearts: The role of membrane fluidity. *Mol. Cell. Biochem.* **2003**, *249*, 175–182. [CrossRef] [PubMed]
168. Naderi, R.; Imani, A.; Faghihi, M.; Moghimian, M. Phenylephrine induces early and late cardioprotection through mitochondrial permeability transition pore in the isolated rat heart. *J. Surg. Res.* **2010**, *164*, e37–e42. [CrossRef] [PubMed]
169. Ong, S.-B.; Samangouei, P.; Kalkhoran, S.B.; Hausenloy, D.J. The mitochondrial permeability transition pore and its role in myocardial ischemia reperfusion injury. *J. Mol. Cell. Cardiol.* **2015**, *78*, 23–34. [CrossRef]
170. Elrod, J.W.; Molkentin, J.D. Physiologic functions of cyclophilin d and the mitochondrial permeability transition pore. *Circ. J.* **2013**, *77*, 1111–1122. [CrossRef]
171. Mnatsakanyan, N.; Beutner, G.; Porter, G.A.; Alavian, K.N.; Jonas, E.A. Physiological roles of the mitochondrial permeability transition pore. *J. Bioenerg. Biomembr.* **2017**, *49*, 13–25. [CrossRef]
172. Pérez, M.J.; Quintanilla, R.A. Development or disease: Duality of the mitochondrial permeability transition pore. *Dev. Biol.* **2017**, *426*, 1–7. [CrossRef]
173. Javadov, S.; Jang, S.; Parodi-Rullán, R.; Khuchua, Z.; Kuznetsov, A.V. Mitochondrial permeability transition in cardiac ischemia–reperfusion: Whether cyclophilin D is a viable target for cardioprotection? *Cell. Mol. Life Sci.* **2017**, *74*, 2795–2813. [CrossRef]
174. Halestrap, A.P.; Richardson, A.P. The mitochondrial permeability transition: A current perspective on its identity and role in ischaemia/reperfusion injury. *J. Mol. Cell. Cardiol.* **2015**, *78*, 129–141. [CrossRef] [PubMed]
175. Hou, Y.; Ghosh, P.; Wan, R.; Ouyang, X.; Cheng, H.; Mattson, M.P.; Cheng, A. Permeability transition pore-mediated mitochondrial superoxide flashes mediate an early inhibitory effect of amyloid beta1–42 on neural progenitor cell proliferation. *Neurobiol. Aging* **2014**, *35*, 975–989. [CrossRef] [PubMed]
176. Lu, X.; Kwong, J.Q.; Molkentin, J.D.; Bers, D.M. Individual cardiac mitochondria undergo rare transient permeability transition pore openings. *Circ. Res.* **2016**, *118*, 834–841. [CrossRef] [PubMed]
177. Ziegelhoffer-Mihalovicova, B.; Okruhlicová, L.; Tribulová, N.; Ravingerová, T.; Volkovová, K.; Šeboková, J.; Ziegelhöffer, A. Mitochondrial contact sites detected by creatine phosphokinase activity in the hearts of normal and diabetic rats: Is mitochondrial contact sites formation a calcium-dependent process? *Gen. Physiol. Biophys.* **1997**, *16*, 329–338.
178. Briston, T.; Selwood, D.L.; Szabadkai, G.; Duchen, M.R. Mitochondrial permeability transition: A molecular lesion with multiple drug targets. *Trends Pharmacol. Sci.* **2019**, *40*, 50–70. [CrossRef]
179. Bonora, M.; Pinton, P. The mitochondrial permeability transition pore and cancer: Molecular mechanisms involved in cell death. *Front. Oncol.* **2014**, *4*, 302. [CrossRef]
180. Heather, L.C.; Cole, M.A.; Tan, J.-J.; Ambrose, L.J.A.; Pope, S.; Abd-Jamil, A.H.; Carter, E.E.; Dodd, M.S.; Yeoh, K.K.; Schofield, C.J.; et al. Metabolic adaptation to chronic hypoxia in cardiac mitochondria. *Basic Res. Cardiol.* **2012**, *107*, 268. [CrossRef]
181. Jonckheere, A.I.; Smeitink, J.A.M.; Rodenburg, R.J.T. Mitochondrial ATP synthase: Architecture, function and pathology. *J. Inherit. Metab. Dis.* **2012**, *35*, 211–225. [CrossRef]
182. Bernardi, P. Why F-ATP Synthase remains a strong candidate as the mitochondrial permeability transition pore. *Front. Physiol.* **2018**, *9*, 1543. [CrossRef]
183. Karch, J.; Molkentin, J.D. Identifying the components of the elusive mitochondrial permeability transition pore. *Proc. Natl. Acad. Sci. USA* **2014**, *111*, 10396–10397. [CrossRef]
184. Beutner, G.; Alanzalon, R.E.; Porter, G.A. Cyclophilin D regulates the dynamic assembly of mitochondrial ATP synthase into synthasomes. *Sci. Rep.* **2017**, *7*, 14488. [CrossRef]
185. Claypool, S.M. Cardiolipin, a critical determinant of mitochondrial carrier protein assembly and function. *Biochim. Biophys. Acta Biomembr.* **2009**, *1788*, 2059–2068. [CrossRef] [PubMed]
186. Carroll, J.; He, J.; Ding, S.; Fearnley, I.M.; Walker, J.E. Persistence of the permeability transition pore in human mitochondria devoid of an assembled ATP synthase. *Proc. Natl. Acad. Sci. USA* **2019**, *116*, 12816–12821. [CrossRef] [PubMed]

187. Karch, J.; Bround, M.J.; Khalil, H.; Sargent, M.A.; Latchman, N.; Terada, N.; Peixoto, P.M.; Molkentin, J.D. Inhibition of mitochondrial permeability transition by deletion of the ANT family and CypD. *Sci. Adv.* **2019**, *5*, eaaw4597. [CrossRef]
188. Šileikytė, J.; Forte, M. The mitochondrial permeability transition in mitochondrial disorders. *Oxidative Med. Cell. Longev.* **2019**, *2019*, 11. [CrossRef]
189. Penna, C.; Perrelli, M.-G.; Pagliaro, P. Mitochondrial pathways, permeability transition pore, and redox signaling in cardioprotection: Therapeutic implications. *Antioxid. Redox Signal.* **2013**, *18*, 556–599. [CrossRef] [PubMed]
190. Gauba, E.; Guo, L.; Du, H. Cyclophilin D promotes brain mitochondrial F1FO ATP synthase dysfunction in aging mice. *J. Alzheimer Dis.* **2016**, *55*, 1351–1362. [CrossRef] [PubMed]
191. Griecsová, L.; Farkašová, V.; Gáblovskỳ, I.; Khandelwal, V.K.M.; Bernátová, I.; Tatarková, Z.; Kaplan, P.; Ravingerová, T. Effect of maturation on the resistance of rat hearts against ischemia. Study of potential molecular mechanisms. *Physiol. Res.* **2015**, *64*, S685–S696.
192. Müller, M.; Ahumada-Castro, U.; Sanhueza, M.; Gonzalez-Billault, C.; Court, F.A.; Cárdenas, C. Mitochondria and calcium regulation as basis of neurodegeneration associated with aging. *Front. Neurosci.* **2018**, *12*, 470. [CrossRef] [PubMed]
193. Griffiths, E.J.; Halestrap, A.P. Protection by cyclosporin a of ischemia/reperfusion-induced damage in isolated rat hearts. *J. Mol. Cell. Cardiol.* **1993**, *25*, 1461–1469. [CrossRef]
194. Abeti, R.; Abramov, A.Y. Mitochondrial Ca^{2+} in neurodegenerative disorders. *Pharmacol. Res.* **2015**, *99*, 377–381. [CrossRef] [PubMed]
195. Walters, A.M.; Porter, G.A.; Brookes, P.S. Mitochondria as a drug target in ischemic heart disease and cardiomyopathy. *Circ. Res.* **2012**, *111*, 1222–1236. [CrossRef] [PubMed]
196. Bhosale, G.; Duchen, M.R. Investigating the mitochondrial permeability transition pore in disease phenotypes and drug screening. *Curr. Protoc. Pharmacol.* **2019**, *85*, e59. [CrossRef] [PubMed]

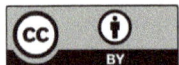

© 2019 by the authors. Licensee MDPI, Basel, Switzerland. This article is an open access article distributed under the terms and conditions of the Creative Commons Attribution (CC BY) license (http://creativecommons.org/licenses/by/4.0/).

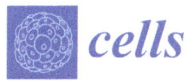

Article

Mitochondrial DNA Variation of Leber's Hereditary Optic Neuropathy in Western Siberia

Elena Starikovskaya [1,*], Sofia Shalaurova [1], Stanislav Dryomov [1], Azhar Nazhmidenova [1], Natalia Volodko [2], Igor Bychkov [3], Ilia Mazunin [4,*] and Rem Sukernik [1]

1. Laboratory of Human Molecular Genetics, Institute of Molecular and Cellular Biology, SBRAS, Novosibirsk 630090, Russia; sofigold@listu.ru (S.S.); stasundr@gmail.com (S.D.); deviliona@yandex.ru (A.N.); sukernik@gmail.com (R.S.)
2. Department of Pediatrics, University of Alberta, Edmonton, AB T6G 2R3, Canada; michael.brown@ualberta.ca
3. Novosibirsk Branch of S.N. Fedorov NMRC "MNTK Eye Microsurgery", Moscow 127486, Russia; fgu@mntk.ru
4. Center of Life Sciences, Skolkovo Institute of Science and Technology, Skolkovo 121205, Russia
* Correspondence: estariko18@gmail.com (E.S.); I.Mazunin@skoltech.ru (I.M.)

Received: 23 October 2019; Accepted: 2 December 2019; Published: 4 December 2019

Abstract: Our data first represent the variety of Leber's hereditary optic neuropathy (LHON) mutations in Western Siberia. LHON is a disorder caused by pathogenic mutations in the mitochondrial DNA (mtDNA), inherited maternally and presents mainly in young adults, predominantly males. Clinically, LHON manifests itself as painless central vision loss, resulting in early onset of disability. The epidemiology of LHON has not been fully investigated yet. In this study, we report 44 genetically unrelated families with LHON manifestation. We performed whole mtDNA genome sequencing and provided genealogical and molecular genetic data on mutations and haplogroup background of LHON patients. Known "primary" pathogenic mtDNA mutations (MITOMAP) were found in 32 families: m.11778G>A represents 53.10% (17/32), m.3460G>A—21.90% (7/32), m.14484T>C–18.75% (6/32), and rare m.10663T>C and m.3635G>A represent 6.25% (2/32). We describe potentially pathogenic m.4659G>A in one subject without known pathogenic mutations, and potentially pathogenic m.6261G>A, m.8412T>C, m.8551T>C, m.9444C>T, m.9921G>A, and m.15077G>A in families with known pathogenic mutations confirmed. We suppose these mutations could contribute to the pathogenesis of optic neuropathy development. Our results indicate that haplogroup affiliation and mutational spectrum of the Western Siberian LHON cohort substantially deviate from those of European populations.

Keywords: LHON; Siberian population; ancient mutation; specific genetic background

1. Introduction

Leber's hereditary optic neuropathy (LHON) is a form of hereditary disorder caused by pathogenic mutations in mitochondrial DNA. These mutations are non-synonymous, and affect genes coding for different subunits of complex I of the mitochondrial respiratory chain. The occurrence of such kinds of mutations in mtDNA subunits leads to dysfunction of the electron transport, increased reactive oxygen species production, and defective ATP synthesis [1–3]. Retinal ganglion cells are highly susceptible to death during LHON progression, because of their high sensibility to disrupted ATP production and oxidative stress [4]. Therefore, LHON is usually painless, acute, or subacute, central visual loss of one or both eyes, which results in early onset of disability. The onset of Leber's hereditary optic neuropathy is relatively rare and has better visual prognosis. The peak age of onset of visual loss among LHON carriers is 20–30 years old [5]. In some cases, LHON patients have been reported as having additional neurologic, cardiac, and endocrine disorders [6–8]. Leber's disease is maternally inherited and manifests itself in youth predominantly (~50% of man and ~10% of women). Interestingly, this sex predilection cannot be explained by the principles of mitochondrial inheritance [4].

At the present time, a number of mtDNA point mutations have been described, but the most prevalent are m.3460G>A, m.11778G>A, and m.14484T>C, accounting for about 90% of cases of LHON worldwide. The prevalence of each mutation varies among different populations, but the average is 69–92% for m.11778G>A, and 3–19% for m.14484T>C and m.3460G>A [9–14]. However, there are significant deviations from the average in some populations, for example, among French Canadians 87% of cases are due to m.14484T>C as a result of a founder effect [15]. Moreover, phenotypic expression of these primary mutations has been found to vary in different populations and different pedigrees. This incomplete penetrance suggests that other factors, such as mtDNA haplogroup background, nuclear genetic background, and environmental factors, may influence the modulation of phenotypic expression and severity of the disease [16–18].

Consequently, the worldwide prevalence of LHON varies in different populations and is unknown for the majority of them. This prevalence is estimated to range between 1:30,000 and 1:50,000 [19,20]. The epidemiology of LHON has not been fully investigated in Russian Federation, and our previous studies included the description of isolated cases [21–23]. Hence, in the present study, we report 44 genetically unrelated LHON families, performed whole mtDNA sequencing, and provide molecular genetic data on mutations and the haplogroup background of LHON patients in the Western Siberian population.

2. Materials and Methods

2.1. Subjects

This study was approved by the Ethics Committee IRB 00001360 affiliated with Vector State Research Center of Virology and Biotechnology (SRC VB Vector), Novosibirsk, Russian Federation. The total number of subjects in the study is 168 individuals from 44 unrelated families (85 affected and 83 healthy carriers), including 17 cases from our previous studies [21–23]. The clinical follow-up of LHON patients has been carried out by the Novosibirsk Branch of Federal Eye Microsurgery Department since 1997, conducted by one of the authors. The clinical diagnosis was based on a combination of symptoms and signs: painless acute or subacute central vision loss; fundus changes; and visual field abnormality, such as pseudopapilledema, optic nerve atrophy, and central or centrocecal scotoma. All the individuals made an informed decision to take part in the study and provided written consent. Family history was taken in each case to identify maternal inheritance of symptoms. The complete mtDNA genomes were sequenced for the family's probands, and for the other individuals the certain mutations were confirmed by sequencing of associated mtDNA regions.

2.2. MtDNA Analysis

Whole peripheral blood samples were collected from the donors in 10 mL Vacutech EDTA tubes. Total DNA was extracted from a buffy-coat layer using the SileksMagNA-G Blood DNA Isolation kit, according to the manufacturer's protocols. The complete sequencing procedure entailed PCR amplification of 22 overlapping mtDNA templates [24], which were sequenced in both directions with BigDye 3.1 terminator chemistry (PE Applied Biosystems, Foster City, CA, United States). The trace files were analyzed with Sequencher (version 4.5 GeneCode Corporation) software. To perform capillary electrophoresis on an ABI Prism 3130XL DNA Analyzer, we used core facilities of the "Genomika" Sequencing Center (SBRAS, Novosibirsk, Russian Federation). Variants were scored relative to the Reconstructed Sapiens Reference Sequence, RSRS [25]. MtDNA haplotypes were identified following the nomenclature suggested by the PhyloTree Build 17 [26]. Forty-two mitochondrial genomes obtained through this study were deposited in GenBank with accession numbers MN413201–MN413242. Two genomes, EU807741.1 and EU807742.1, had been deposited to the GenBank earlier [21].

2.3. Penetrance Analysis

We determined penetrance as the proportion of affected individuals from all maternally related family members using family pedigrees [19]. Values for both men and women were calculated separately.

2.4. Analysis of Pathogenicity for Non-Synonymous Mutations

To make sure that the revealed non-synonymous mtDNA mutations were not sequencing errors or to not point out to general population polymorphisms, and in turn to find out the disease-associated polymorphisms among those published earlier, we used several databases: MITOMAP [27]; mtDB (Human Mitochondrial Genome Database, containing 2704 human mitochondrial genomes) [28]; and HmtDB (Human Mitochondrial DataBase), which contains 32922 human mitochondrial genomes [29]. To assess the possible pathogenicity of these mutations, and to predict whether a protein sequence variation affects protein function, we used the following web applications: MutPred 1.2 [30], MutPred 2 [31], PolyPhen–2 [32], PROVEAN (Protein Variation Effect Analyzer) [33], and SIFT (Sorting Intolerant from Tolerant) [34]. All the sources are provided in the public domain.

3. Results

From 44 LHON families, 32 harbored a primary mutation; the results are shown in Table 1. Among families with a primary mutation, the m.11778G>A represented 53.10% (17/32), m.3460G>A was 21.90% (7/32), and m.14484T>C represented 18,75% (6/32). Rare m.10663T>C and m.3635G>A represented 6.25% (2/32) of the families.

Table 1. Summary data for examined Leber's hereditary optic neuropathy (LHON) and LHON-like (without primary mutations) families. Age of onset of visual loss vary between families/patients; the peak age of onset is ~20–30 years old. Some families were published previously * [23]; ** [22]; *** [21].

No.	Family Name	Ethnicity in Maternal Line	Number of Examined Individuals (Affected/Healthy)	Family History of Visual Loss	Primary LHON Mutation (MITOMAP)	mtDNA Haplogroup
1	L18 *	Altaian	4 (2/2)	No	m.3460G>A	D4p
2	L24 *	Tuvinian	19 (7/12)	Yes	m.3460G>A	C5d1
3	L25 ***	Russian	5 (3/2)	Yes	m.3460G>A	D5a2a2
4	L41	German	2 (1/1)	No	m.3460G>A	H40a
5	L57	-/-	1 (1/0)	Yes	m.3460G>A	V1a1
6	L58	-/-	2 (1/1)	Yes	m.3460G>A	J1c3
7	L61	-/-	4 (2/2)	Yes	m.3460G>A	H1b1
8	L30 ***	-/-	19 (11/8)	Yes	m.3635G>A	J2b1c1
9	L2 **	-/-	6 (2/4)	Yes	m.10663T>C	J1c4
10	L1 *	Russian	9 (1/8)	Yes	m.11778G>A	T2b
11	L3 *	-/-	4 (1/3)	Yes	m.11778G>A	T2d1b1
12	L5 *	-/-	1 (1/0)	Yes	m.11778G>A	J1c2i
13	L12 *	-/-	2 (1/1)	No	m.11778G>A	J2b1a1
14	L14 *	-/-	5 (2/3)	No	m.11778G>A	T2b28

Table 1. Cont.

No.	Family Name	Ethnicity in Maternal Line	Number of Examined Individuals (Affected/Healthy)	Family History of Visual Loss	Primary LHON Mutation (MITOMAP)	mtDNA Haplogroup
15	L23 *	Azerbaijani	1 (1/0)	Unknown	m.11778G>A	J2b1
16	L26 *	-/-	13 (8/5)	Yes	m.11778G>A	J1c7a
17	L27 ***	-/-	11 (2/9)	Yes	m.11778G>A	H2a5b
18	L28 ***	-/-	9 (2/7)	Yes	m.11778G>A	T2b8
19	L38	Ukrainian	2 (2/0)	Yes	m.11778G>A	J1c2c2a
20	L39	Unknown	2 (1/1)	No	m.11778G>A	V
21	L42	Belarusian	2 (1/1)	Yes	m.11778G>A	H1c
22	L43	Russian	3 (1/2)	No	m.11778G>A	H
23	L49	Unknown	1 (1/0)	No	m.11778G>A	K1c
24	L52	Russian	3 (1/2)	No	m.11778G>A	J1c2
25	L53	Unknown	3 (1/2)	Unknown	m.11778G>A	H1b2
26	L60	Russian	2 (1/1)	No	m.11778G>A	H1b2
27	L10 *	-/-	8 (3/5)	Yes	m.14484T>C	M9a1a1c1a
28	L17 *	-/-	8 (4/4)	Yes	m.14484T>C	J1c2c1
29	L32	Unknown	1 (1/0)	Unknown	m.14484T>C	V
30	L40	Albanian	1 (1/0)	Yes	m.14484T>C	H
31	L47	-/-	1 (1/0)	No	m.14484T>C	J1c5a1
32	L50	Unknown	1 (1/0)	Unknown	m.14484T>C	U5a2b1c
33	L6	-/-	2 (2/0)	No	-	U4a1d
34	L8	Unknown	1 (1/0)	No	-	U2e1
35	L9	Russian	2 (2/0)	Yes	-	U5a1b1c1
36	L20	-/-	3 (2/1)	Yes	-	U4b1b1
37	L31 ***	-/-	3 (2\1)	Yes	-	U3b1b
38	L45	-/-	2 (1/1)	No	-	U5a2e
39	L46	-/-	2 (1/1)	No	-	H13a1d
40	L51	Unknown	1 (1/0)	Unknown	-	U2c1b
41	L54	Russian	2 (1/1)	No	-	U4a2a
42	L56	-/-	2 (1/1)	No	-	J1c1b1
43	L59	Ukrainian	2 (1/1)	No	-	V7a
44	L62	-/-	1 (1/0)	Yes	-	H

According to the family pedigrees, only 50% (22/44) of cases had a family history of vision loss in the maternal lineage in more than one generation, among which m.11778G>A represented 36% (8/22), m.3460G>A covered 23% (5/22), and the m.14484T>C was 14% (3/22), as well as those without primary mutations (LHON-like cases), which represented 18% (4/22). Rare mutation cases (m.10663T>C and m.3635G>A) were family–inherited. In total, 39% (17/44) of cases were sporadic, among which 13 were cases with only one affected person diagnosed, and four were cases with two affected persons in one generation. Among the sporadic cases, m.11778G>A represented 41% (7/17), m.3460G>A was 12% (2/17), m.14484T>C was 6% (1/17), and the LHON-like cases represented 41% (7/17) of the total.

Summary information on penetrance is shown in Table 2. The penetrance is highly variable between separate families, even with the same primary mutation. The average penetrance among men was 32% (6–100%) and 12% among women (0–58%); these correlate with data previously published [4]. However, there are some families with higher penetrance among females than among males: L24, L26, and L28.

Table 2. Summary information about penetrance.

	m.11778G>A (n = 15)	m.14484T>C (n = 4)	m.3460G>A (n = 7)	Average
Males	34%	46%	15%	32%
Females	12%	12%	10%	12%

In 12 families with clear-cut LHON phenotypes, no pathogenic mtDNA mutations were found. Analysis of the mtDNA revealed non-synonymous mutations: m.4766A>G, m.13105A>G, m.14002A>G, which have not been noted as associated with LHON or other diseases in the MITOMAP database. All pathogenicity prediction tools indicated low probability that the amino acid substitutions are disease-associated for these mutations. Mutation m.4659G>A has been previously reported as being associated with Parkinson's disease [35], as well as in an Australian LHON pedigree that was heteroplasmic for the m.14484T>C [36]. Polyphen-2 predicted the pathogenicity for this mutation as benign and MutPed 2 showed low probability score, but MutPred 1.2, PROVEAN, and SIFT determined this mutation as deleterious. The results are shown in Table 3.

Table 3. Non-synonymous mutations revealed in LHON-like cases. Known primary mutations (m.3460G>A, m.3635G>, m.10663T>C, m.11778G>A, and m.14484T>C) are placed in bold to demonstrate distinction between different prediction algorithms and frequencies in general population for pathogenic mutations. A MutPred 1.2 score > 0.75 and a Mutpred 2 score > 0.50 would suggest pathogenicity.

Mutation	Protein-Coding Region of mtDNA	Amino Acid Substitution	PolyPhen – 2 Score	MutPred 1.2/2 Score (Cutoff 0.75/0.50)	PROVEAN/SIFT Pathogenicity Prediction	Frequency in General Population (as per mtDB)	Frequency in General Population (as per HmtDB)	Family
m.14002A>G	ND5	T556A	0.002 (benign)	0.387/0.059	Neutral/Tolerated	0.0037	0.00289	L45
m.4766A>G	ND2	M99I	0.001 (benign)	0.571/0.225	Neutral/Tolerated	0	0.00009	L46
m.4659G>A	ND2	A64T	0.029 (benign)	0.790/0.256	Deleterious/Damaging	0.0011	0.00161	L51
m.13105A>G	ND5	I257V	0.001 (benign)	0.198/0.032	Neutral/Tolerated	0.0612	0	L51
m.3460G>A	ND1	A52T	1.000 (probably damaging)	0.789/0.418	Neutral/Damaging	0.0097	0.00058	-
m.3635G>A	ND1	S110N	0.999 (probably damaging)	0.873/0.493	Deleterious/Damaging	0	0.00027	-
m.10663T>C	ND4L	V65A	0.946 (probably damaging)	0.604/0.694	Deleterious/Damaging	0	0.00003	-
m.11778G>A	ND4	R340H	0.999 (probably damaging)	0.919/0.494	Deleterious/Damaging	0.0097	0.0034	-
m.14484T>C	ND6	M64V	0.993 (probably damaging)	0.618/0.787	Neutral/Damaging	0.0026	0.00146	-

In several families with primary mutations (L01, L03, L12, L28, L30, L40, L43, and L50) we found out additional, non-synonymous mutations (Table 4). Mutations m.8875T>C, m.14582A>G, m.8400T>C, and m.4639T>C were neutral, and mutation m.9444C>T had a high probability of being pathogenic, according to data from all the pathogenicity prediction tools; for other mutations, we observed divergence of prediction results. Since prediction results for primary pathogenic mutations diverged too (see Table 3), novel non-synonymous nucleotide change was considered potentially pathogenic if it had extremely low frequency in the general population, and if it was predicted by at least three algorithms to have an effect on protein function. For mutations m.6261G>A and m.15468C>T, only PolyPhen2 predicted pathogenicity as probably damaging and possible damaging, respectively. However, mutation m.6261G>A had already been reported by Abu-Amero [37] in patients with optic neuropathy, and also as a somatic mutation associated with prostate cancer. Interestingly, the family (L01) with m.6261G>A and m.11778G>A has the same haplogroup, T2, as the case reported by Abu-Amero. Other mutations (m.8412T>C, m.8551T>C, m.9921G>A, m.15077G>A) were predicted as pathogenic by at least by three algorithms, but the first three of them have not been noted as associated with diseases in the MITOMAP database, and mutation m.15077G>A was reported as being associated with maternally-inherited isolated deafness [38].

Table 4. Additional, non-synonymous mutations revealed in LHON cases. All these mutations still have no the status of "primary LHON mutations". A MutPred 1.2 score > 0.75 and a Mutpred 2 score > 0.50 would suggest pathogenicity.

Mutation	Protein-Coding Region of mtDNA	Amino Acid Substitution	PolyPhen-2 Score	MutPred 1.2/2 Score (Cutoff 0,75/0,50)	PROVEAN /SIFT Prediction	Frequency in General Population (mtDB)	Frequency in General Population (HmtDB)	Family
m.6261G>A	CO1	A120T	0.998 (probably damaging)	0.491/0.324	Neutral/ Tolerated	0.0048	0.00553	L01
m.8875T>C	ATP6	F117L	0 (benign)	0.251/0.429	Neutral/ Tolerated	0.0007	0.001276	L03
m.9921G>A	CO3	A239T	0.009 (benign)	0.543/0.624	Deleterious/ Damaging	0.0011	0.00082	L12
m.15468C>T	CYB	T241M	0.890 (possible damaging)	0.245/0.079	Neutral/ Tolerated	0.0004	0.00043	L28
m.8551T>C	ATP6	F9L	0.976 (probably damaging)	0.676/0.418	Deleterious/ Damaging	0.0007	0	L30
m.14582A>G	ND6	V31A	0.003 (benign)	0.245/0.181	Neutral/ Tolerated	0.0086	0.00571	L40
m.8400T>C	ATP8	M12T	0 (benign)	0.504/0.118	Neutral/ Tolerated	0.0011	0.00052	L43
m.9444C>T	CO3	R80W	0.999 (probably damaging)	0.875/0.586	Deleterious/ Damaging	0	0	L43
m.4639T>C	ND2	I57T	0.001 (benign)	0.297/0.047	Neutral/ Tolerated	0.0082	0.00395	L43
m.8412T>C	ATP8	M16T	0.711 (possible damaging)	0.677/0.542	Deleterious/ Tolerated	0	0.00039	L50
m.15077G>A	CYB	E111K	0.992 (probably damaging)	0.684/0.331	Deleterious/ Damaging (low confidence)	0.0007	0.00213	L50

Phylogenetic analysis illustrates that Siberian carriers of pathogenic LHON mutations are unrelated and belong to different maternal lines. In rare cases (4/44), m.3460G>A and m.14484T>C belong to East Eurasian M8, M9, and D haploclusters (Figure 1). The classic (m.3460G>A, m.11778G>A, m.14484T>C) and rare LHON-causing mutations occur mostly in the mtDNA background of West Eurasian haploclusters H'V (Figure 2), J'T and U'K (Figure 3).

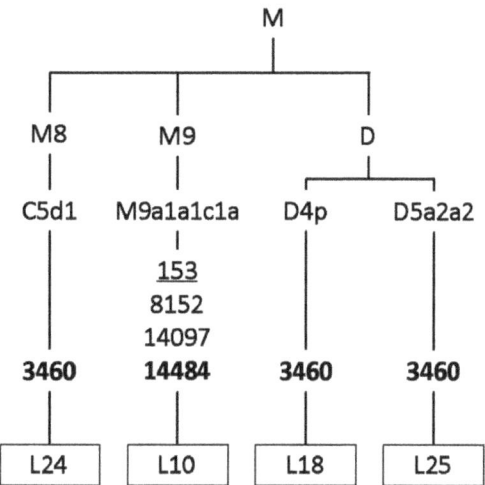

Figure 1. Phylogenetic tree based on the complete mtDNA genome sequences of pedigree probands with pathogenic LHON mutations (M8, M9, and D haploclusters). The non-synonymous coding region variants are denoted by "ns" (known pathogenic mutations designated in bold). Mutations are transitions unless a specific base change was specified; deletions are denoted by "del"; underlined mutations are recurrent.

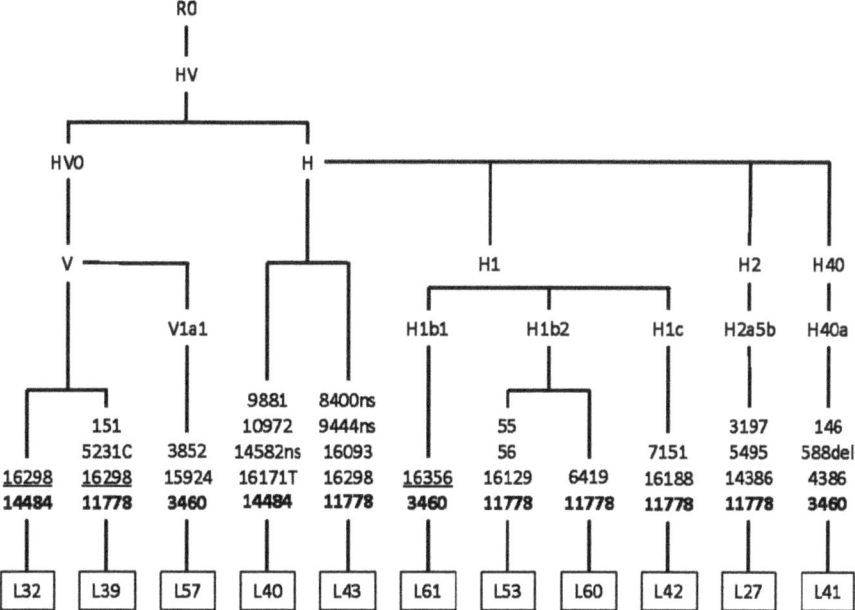

Figure 2. Phylogenetic tree based on the complete mtDNA genome sequences of pedigree probands with pathogenic LHON mutations (H'V haplocluster). The non-synonymous coding region variants are denoted by "ns" (known pathogenic mutations designated in bold). Mutations are transitions unless a specific base change was specified; deletions are denoted by "del"; underlined mutations are recurrent.

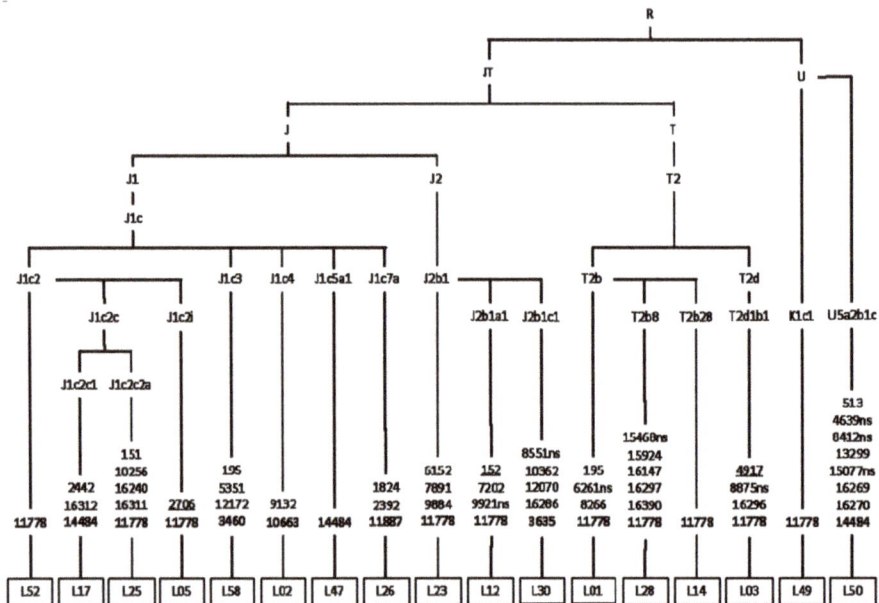

Figure 3. Phylogenetic tree based on the complete mtDNA genome sequences of pedigree probands with pathogenic LHON mutations (J'T, and U'K haploclusters). The non-synonymous coding region variants are denoted by "ns" (known pathogenic mutations designated in bold). Mutations are transitions unless a specific base change was specified; deletions are denoted by "del"; underlined mutations are recurrent.

4. Discussion

4.1. Leber's Hereditary Optic Neuropathy Primary Mutations

Regarding our preliminary data, the frequencies of primary mutations are different from frequencies reported for Europe and Asia. The most prevalent m.11778G>A (~55%) is less common in Western Siberia than in Europe, at ~69% [9]; as well as in China and Japan, at ~90% [10,13]. The prevalence of m.3460G>A (~24%) is twice as much as in Europe, but m.14484T>C (~14%) do not deviate from those of other European populations [9].

In 12 families with LHON-like manifestation, no known pathogenic mtDNA mutation was found. However, there are other elaborations in which the clinical diagnosis cannot be confirmed by molecular genetic analysis [37,39–41]. Definitively, mtDNA mutation-caused LHON is clinically indistinguishable from the other forms of optic neuropathy, such as a dominant optic neuropathy (DOA), especially when it is sporadic. Compared to LHON, DOA visual loss is detected between ages 4 and 6 in the majority of patients, and 58–84% of patients with DOA report visual impairment by age 11 [42]. In our 12 cases, the ages of onset were between 13–36 years. We will be studying these cases for the mutation spectrum of common pathogenic genes for DOA in future.

4.2. Penetrance

We suppose that relatively reduced incidence of LHON in Western Siberia is associated with incomplete penetrance and diagnostic difficulties of atypical (e.g., late-onset) and combined (e.g., multiple sclerosis) forms of LHON. Patients with LHON could have also been wrongly diagnosed as suffering from toxic amblyopia, tobacco–alcohol amblyopia, or optic neuritis [41]. On the other hand, the problem is that patients do not know their family history. Molecular testing for LHON is not routinely performed in patients with optic atrophy in Russian Federation. Identification and registration of unaffected carriers plays an important role for prevention of disease manifestation. For example, there is strong evidence that smoking is associated with an increased risk of visual failure among LHON carriers—93% penetrance of vision loss in male smokers versus 66% in male non-smokers [17].

Our observations highlight the importance of molecular genetic examination for unaffected carriers. The presence of pathogenic mutations should be tested not only for probands, but for all relatives in the maternal line, Since the proportion of sporadic cases is about 40% according to our published data [4].

4.3. Potentially Pathogenic Mutation m.4659G>A

We found m.4659G>A in one subject without any known primary mutations (L51). This sequence change is located at codon 64 in the functional domain of the ND2 gene and changes an alanine—a hydrophobic amino acid—into threonine—a neutral amino acid. Mutation m.4659G>A has been reported as being associated with LHON in an Australian pedigree that also had heteroplasmic mutations m.14484T>C and m.5460G>A [36]. This family had 10 maternally-related descendants, five of whom had vision loss. Unfortunately, our patient does not know his family history, and we could not confirm maternal inheritance for this mutation. However, m.4659G>A has very low frequency in the general population (0.0011–0.00161), and has a high probability of being pathogenic (Table 3).

4.4. Additional Non-Synonymous Mutations Revealed in LHON Cases

The phenomenon of co-existence of two pathogenic mutations in one family has already been described. The first case included m.4659G>A, m.5460G>A, and m.14484T>C in an Australian LHON pedigree, described above [36]. In the second case, a Polish family harboring two primary LHON mutations m.3460G>A and m.11778G>A occurred in a haplogroup H background [43]. In the third case, a family harbored two primary LHON mutations, m.11778G>A and m.14484T>C, and both mutations had a synergistic pathogenic effect on protein function, as well as a higher degree of heteroplasmy of the m.14484T>C, correlated with an earlier age at onset [44]. Finally, the fourth example is a unique double-mutant ND4L with two concurrent mutations (m.10609T>C and m.10663T>C) in an Arab pedigree from Kuwait [45].

We reported mutations m.6261G>A, m.8412T>C, m.8551T>C, m.9444C>T, m.9921G>A, and m.15077G>A, which could be potentially pathogenic because of their low frequency in the general population, and high probability of pathogenicity according to data from different prediction tools. Two of them, m.6261G>A and m.15077G>A, have already been reported in subjects with optic neuropathy and maternally-inherited isolated deafness, respectively. However, we suppose that additional non-synonymous mutations could either have a synergistically pathogenic or a protective effect. To demonstrate the full significance of novel mutations, a respiratory chain assay would need to be performed. An example is the study [38], where cybrids with m.15077G>A showed normal activities for mitochondrial electron chain enzymatic complexes.

4.5. Haplogroup Analysis

Our LHON cohort from the Western Siberia region is represented predominantly by West Eurasian haplogroups and includes several East Eurasian haplogroups, namely C5d1 (L24), D4p (L18), D5a2a2 (L25), and M9a1a1c1a (L10).

Rare LHON mutations m.10663T>C and m.3635G>A were found in Russian families from Kazakhstan (the first) and the Novosibirsk region (the second), associated with the European haplogroups J1c4 and J2b1c1, respectively [21,22]. Mutation m.10663T>C was also reported in the background of the haplogroups J1c2c, L2a1, L3'4, and L3f1b [37,45–47], and mutation m.3635G>A was reported in haplogroups R11a, D4g2b, M7b4, F1a, B5b, and M7b [48,49]. The presence of the same pathogenic mutations on the background of various mitochondrial haplogroups confirms that pathogenic LHON mutations arise de novo, independently from the mtDNA or ethnic backgrounds.

It is known that the clinical impact of mDNA mutations may be modulated by mitochondrial haplogroup background. For example, Hudson et al. performed a multicenter study of 3613 subjects from 159 different families, and showed that the risk of visual failure is greater when m.11778G>A or m.14484T>C mutations are present in specific subgroups of haplogroup J; the same as the m.3460G>A mutation is present in haplogroup K, and the risk of visual failure is significantly lower when m.11778G>A occurs in haplogroup H [50]. Romero et al. supposed that haplogroup D has a protective effect in carriers of LHON mutations. His hypothesis was based on the fact that there was a markedly decreased frequency of haplogroup D in Chilean subjects with LHON, as haplogroup D is one of the most common in the Chilean population [12]. Also, other experimental research serves as proof that cybrids and fibroblasts bearing LHON mutations have different response to neurotoxic agents, depending on haplogroup background [51].

It has been suggested that at the end of the last glaciation, phylogenetically more ancient mutations could have provided their carriers with adaptive advantages during the human population expansion. Today, those mutations contribute to the saving and expression of weakly pathogenic LHON mutations, which appear randomly in different region-specific genetic backgrounds [52,53]. The theory could be tested by further searching of pathogenic, LHON-causing mutations in relation to specific mtDNA backgrounds (phylogenetically ancient set of mutations).

New data collected from future studies regarding mtDNA variations of LHON in Western Siberia might be used to develop a LHON system registry in the Russian Federation. We intend to conduct consecutive experimental research, including the parameters of the pathogenicity of each novel substitution.

5. Limitations of the Study

The main limitation of the data presented is the absence of physiological tests as proof with respect to the pathogenicity of novel mtDNA substitutions. Additional tests should be done, such as oxygen consumption, ATP and ROS measuring, and electron microscopy study (for example, [54]). In addition, development of the newest editing systems [55] could give us more reliable instruments to test pathogenicity.

Author Contributions: Conceptualization, E.S. and R.S.; data curation, I.B., E.S., S.S., S.D., A.N., N.V., I.M., and R.S.; analysis and interpretation of data, E.S., S.S., S.D., A.N., and R.S., writing—review and editing, E.S., S.S., S.D., A.N., I.M., and R.S.

Funding: The research was supported by the Russian Science Foundation [No. 17-75-20015] and the Russian Foundation of Basic Research [No. 19-29-04101].

Conflicts of Interest: The authors declare no conflict of interest.

References

1. Baracca, A.; Solaini, G.; Sgarbi, G.; Lenaz, G.; Baruzzi, A.; Schapira, A.H.; Martinuzzi, A.; Carelli, V. Severe impairment of complex I-driven adenosine triphosphate synthesis in leber hereditary optic neuropathy cybrids. *Arch. Neurol.* **2005**, *62*, 730–736. [CrossRef] [PubMed]
2. Lin, C.S.; Sharpley, M.S.; Fan, W.; Waymire, K.G.; Sadun, A.A.; Carelli, V.; Ross-Cisneros, F.N.; Baciu, P.; Sung, E.; McManus, M.J.; et al. Mouse mtDNA mutant model of Leber hereditary optic neuropathy. *Proc Natl. Acad. Sci. USA* **2012**, *109*, 20065–20070. [CrossRef] [PubMed]
3. Kim, U.S.; Jurkute, N.; Yu-Wai-Man, P. Leber Hereditary Optic Neuropathy-Light at the End of the Tunnel? *Asia Pac. J. Opthalmol. (Phila)* **2018**, *7*, 242–245. [CrossRef]
4. Meyerson, C.; Van Stavern, G.; McClelland, C. Leber hereditary optic neuropathy: Current perspectives. *Clin. Ophthalmol.* **2015**, *9*, 1165–1176. [CrossRef] [PubMed]

5. Majander, A.; Bowman, R.; Poulton, J.; Antcliff, R.J.; Reddy, M.A.; Michaelides, M.; Webster, A.R.; Chinnery, P.F.; Votruba, M.; Moore, A.T.; et al. Childhood-onset Leber hereditary optic neuropathy. *Br. J. Ophthalmol.* **2017**, *101*, 1505–1509. [CrossRef]
6. Finsterer, J.; Zarrouk-Mahjoub, S. Leber's hereditary optic neuropathy is multiorgan not mono-organ. *Clin. Ophthalmol.* **2016**, *10*, 2187–2190. [CrossRef]
7. Haas, R.H. Mitochondrial Dysfunction in Aging and Diseases of Aging. *Biology* **2019**, *8*, 48. [CrossRef]
8. Barcelos, I.P.d.; Troxell, R.M.; Graves, J.S. Mitochondrial dysfunction and multiple sclerosis. *Biology* **2019**, *8*, 37. [CrossRef]
9. Mackey, D.A.; Oostra, R.J.; Rosenberg, T.; Nikoskelainen, E.; Bronte-Stewart, J.; Poulton, J.; Harding, A.E.; Govan, G.; Bolhuis, P.A.; Norby, S. Primary pathogenic mtDNA mutations in multigeneration pedigrees with Leber hereditary optic neuropathy. *Am. J. Hum. Genet.* **1996**, *59*, 481–485.
10. Mashima, Y.; Yamada, K.; Wakakura, M.; Kigasawa, K.; Kudoh, J.; Shimizu, N.; Oguchi, Y. Spectrum of pathogenic mitochondrial DNA mutations and clinical features in Japanese families with Leber's hereditary optic neuropathy. *Curr. Eye Res.* **1998**, *17*, 403–408. [CrossRef]
11. Kumar, M.; Kaur, P.; Kumar, M.; Saxena, R.; Sharma, P.; Dada, R. Clinical characterization and mitochondrial DNA sequence variations in Leber hereditary optic neuropathy. *Mol. Vis.* **2012**, *18*, 2687–2699. [PubMed]
12. Romero, P.; Fernandez, V.; Slabaugh, M.; Seleme, N.; Reyes, N.; Gallardo, P.; Herrera, L.; Pena, L.; Pezo, P.; Moraga, M. Pan-American mDNA haplogroups in Chilean patients with Leber's hereditary optic neuropathy. *Mol. Vis.* **2014**, *20*, 334–340. [PubMed]
13. Jiang, P.; Liang, M.; Zhang, J.; Gao, Y.; He, Z.; Yu, H.; Zhao, F.; Ji, Y.; Liu, X.; Zhang, M.; et al. Prevalence of Mitochondrial ND4 Mutations in 1281 Han Chinese Subjects With Leber's Hereditary Optic Neuropathy. *Invest Ophthalmol. Vis. Sci.* **2015**, *56*, 4778–4788. [CrossRef] [PubMed]
14. Khan, N.A.; Govindaraj, P.; Soumittra, N.; Sharma, S.; Srilekha, S.; Ambika, S.; Vanniarajan, A.; Meena, A.K.; Uppin, M.S.; Sundaram, C.; et al. Leber's hereditary optic neuropathy–specific mutation m.11778G>A exists on diverse mitochondrial haplogroups in India. *Invest. Ophthalmol. Vis. Sci.* **2017**, *58*, 3923–3930. [CrossRef] [PubMed]
15. Laberge, A.M.; Jomphe, M.; Houde, L.; Vezina, H.; Tremblay, M.; Desjardins, B.; Labuda, D.; St-Hilaire, M.; Macmillan, C.; Shoubridge, E.A.; et al. A "Fille du Roy" introduced the T14484C Leber hereditary optic neuropathy mutation in French Canadians. *Am. J. Hum. Genet.* **2005**, *77*, 313–317. [CrossRef] [PubMed]
16. Jacobi, F.K.; Leo-Kottler, B.; Mittelviefhaus, K.; Zrenner, E.; Meyer, J.; Pusch, C.M.; Wissinger, B. Segregation patterns and heteroplasmy prevalence in Leber's hereditary optic neuropathy. *Inves.t Ophthalmol. Vis. Sci.* **2001**, *42*, 1208–1214.
17. Kirkman, M.A.; Yu-Wai-Man, P.; Korsten, A.; Leonhardt, M.; Dimitriadis, K.; De Coo, I.F.; Klopstock, T.; Chinnery, P.F. Gene-environment interactions in Leber hereditary optic neuropathy. *Brain* **2009**, *132*, 2317–2326. [CrossRef]
18. Istikharah, R.; Tun, A.W.; Kaewsutthi, S.; Aryal, P.; Kunhapan, B.; Katanyoo, W.; Chuenkongkaew, W.; Lertrit, P. Identification of the variants in PARL, the nuclear modifier gene, responsible for the expression of LHON patients in Thailand. *Exp. Eye Res.* **2013**, *116*, 55–57. [CrossRef]
19. Puomila, A.; Hamalainen, P.; Kivioja, S.; Savontaus, M.L.; Koivumaki, S.; Huoponen, K.; Nikoskelainen, E. Epidemiology and penetrance of Leber hereditary optic neuropathy in Finland. *Eur. J. Hum. Genet.* **2007**, *15*, 1079–1089. [CrossRef]
20. Mascialino, B.; Leinonen, M.; Meier, T. Meta-analysis of the prevalence of Leber hereditary optic neuropathy mtDNA mutations in Europe. *Eur. J. Ophthalmol.* **2012**, *22*, 461–465. [CrossRef]
21. Brown, M.D.; Zhadanov, S.; Allen, J.C.; Hosseini, S.; Newman, N.J.; Atamonov, V.V.; Mikhailovskaya, I.E.; Sukernik, R.I.; Wallace, D.C. Novel mtDNA mutations and oxidative phosphorylation dysfunction in Russian LHON families. *Hum. Genet.* **2001**, *109*, 33–39. [CrossRef] [PubMed]
22. Brown, M.D.; Starikovskaya, E.; Derbeneva, O.; Hosseini, S.; Allen, J.C.; Mikhailovskaya, I.E.; Sukernik, R.I.; Wallace, D.C. The role of mtDNA background in disease expression: A new primary LHON mutation associated with Western Eurasian haplogroup. *J. Hum. Genet.* **2002**, *110*, 130–138. [CrossRef] [PubMed]
23. Volod'ko, N.V.; L'Vova, M.; Starikovskaia, E.B.; Derbeneva, O.A.; Bychkov, I.; Mikhailovskaia, I.E.; Pogozheva, I.V.; Fedotov, F.F.; Soyan, G.V.; Procaccio, V.; et al. Spectrum of pathogenic mtDNA mutations in Leber hereditary optic neuropathy families from Siberia. *Genetika* **2006**, *42*, 89–97. [PubMed]

24. Nochez, Y.; Arsene, S.; Gueguen, N.; Chevrollier, A.; Ferre, M.; Guillet, V.; Desquiret, V.; Toutain, A.; Bonneau, D.; Procaccio, V.; et al. Acute and late-onset optic atrophy due to a novel OPA1 mutation leading to a mitochondrial coupling defect. *Mol. Vis.* **2009**, *15*, 598–608. [PubMed]
25. Behar, D.M.; van Oven, M.; Rosset, S.; Metspalu, M.; Loogväli, E.L.; Silva, N.M.; Kivisild, T.; Torroni, A.; Villems, R. A "Copernican" reassessment of the human mitochondrial DNA tree from its root. *Am. J. Hum. Genet.* **2012**, *90*, 675–684. [CrossRef]
26. van Oven, M.; Kayser, M. Updated comprehensive phylogenetic tree of global human mitochondrial DNA variation. *Hum. Mutat.* **2009**, *30*, E386–E394. [CrossRef]
27. Brandon, M.C.; Lott, M.T.; Nguyen, K.C.; Spolim, S.; Navathe, S.B.; Baldi, P.; Wallace, D.C. MITOMAP: A human mitochondrial genome database-2004 update. *Nucleic Acids Res.* **2005**, *33*, D611–D613. [CrossRef]
28. Ingman, M.; Gyllensten, U. mtDB: Human Mitochondrial Genome Database, a resource for population genetics and medical sciences. *Nucleic Acids Res.* **2006**, *34*, D749–D751. [CrossRef]
29. Attimonelli, M.; Accetturo, M.; Santamaria, M.; Lascaro, D.; Scioscia, G.; Pappada, G.; Russo, L.; Zanchetta, L.; Tommaseo-Ponzetta, M. HmtDB, a human mitochondrial genomic resource based on variability studies supporting population genetics and biomedical research. *BMC Bioinformatics* **2005**. [CrossRef]
30. Li, B.; Krishnan, V.G.; Mort, M.E.; Xin, F.; Kamati, K.K.; Cooper, D.N.; Mooney, S.D.; Radivojac, P. Automated inference of molecular mechanisms of disease from amino acid substitutions. *Bioinformatics* **2009**, *25*, 2744–2750. [CrossRef]
31. Pejaver, V.; Urresti, J.; Lugo-Martinez, J.; Pagel, K.A.; Lin, G.N.; Nam, H.; Mort, M.; Cooper, D.N.; Sebat, J.; Iakoucheva, L.M.; et al. MutPred2: Inferring the molecular and phenotypic impact of amino acid variants. *bioRxiv* 134981. [CrossRef]
32. Adzhubei, I.A.; Schmidt, S.; Peshkin, L.; Ramensky, V.E.; Gerasimova, A.; Bork, P.; Kondrashov, A.S.; Sunyaev, S.R. A method and server for predicting damaging missense mutations. *Nat. Methods* **2010**, *7*, 248–249. [CrossRef] [PubMed]
33. Choi, Y.; Sims, G.E.; Murphy, S.; Miller, J.R.; Chan, A.P. Predicting the functional effect of amino acid substitutions and indels. *PLoS ONE* **2012**, *7*, e46688. [CrossRef] [PubMed]
34. Kumar, P.; Henikoff, S.; Ng, P.C. Predicting the effects of coding non-synonymous variants on protein function using the SIFT algorithm. *Nat. Protoc.* **2009**, *4*, 1073–1081. [CrossRef] [PubMed]
35. Khusnutdinova, E.; Gilyazova, I.; Ruiz-Pesini, E.; Derbeneva, O.; Khusainova, R.; Khidiyatova, I.; Magzhanov, R.; Wallace, D.C. A mitochondrial etiology of neurodegenerative diseases: Evidence from Parkinson's disease. *Ann. NY Acad. Sci.* **2008**, *1147*, 1–20. [CrossRef] [PubMed]
36. Mackey, D.; Howell, N. A variant of Leber hereditary optic neuropathy characterized by recovery of vision and by an unusual mitochondrial genetic etiology. *Am. J. Hum. Genet.* **1992**, *51*, 1218–1228. [PubMed]
37. Abu-Amero, K.K.; Bosley, T.M. Mitochondrial abnormalities in patients with LHON-like optic neuropathies. *Invest. Ophthalmol. Vis. Sci.* **2006**, *47*, 4211–4220. [CrossRef]
38. Gutierrez Cortes, N.; Pertuiset, C.; Dumon, E.; Borlin, M.; Hebert-Chatelain, E.; Pierron, D.; Feldmann, D.; Jonard, L.; Marlin, S.; Letellier, T.; et al. Novel mitochondrial DNA mutations responsible for maternally inherited nonsyndromic hearing loss. *Hum. Mutat.* **2012**, *33*, 681–689. [CrossRef]
39. Howell, N.; Oostra, R.J.; Bolhuis, P.A.; Spruijt, L.; Clarke, L.A.; Mackey, D.A.; Preston, G.; Herrnstadt, C. Sequence analysis of the mitochondrial genomes from Dutch pedigrees with Leber hereditary optic neuropathy. *Am. J. Hum. Genet.* **2003**, *72*, 1460–1469. [CrossRef]
40. Aitullina, A.; Baumane, K.; Zalite, S.; Ranka, R.; Zole, E.; Pole, I.; Sepetiene, S.; Laganovska, G.; Baumanis, V.; Pliss, L. Point mutations associated with Leber hereditary optic neuropathy in a Latvian population. *Mol. Vis.* **2013**, *19*, 2343–2351.
41. Rosenberg, T.; Norby, S.; Schwartz, M.; Saillard, J.; Magalhaes, P.J.; Leroy, D.; Kann, E.C.; Duno, M. Prevalence and Genetics of Leber Hereditary Optic Neuropathy in the Danish Population. *Invest. Ophthalmol. Vis. Sci.* **2016**, *57*, 1370–1375. [CrossRef]
42. Fraser, J.A.; Biousse, V.; Newman, N.J. The neuro-ophthalmology of mitochondrial disease. *Surv. Ophthalmol.* **2010**, *55*, 299–334. [CrossRef] [PubMed]
43. Tonska, K.; Kurzawa, M.; Ambroziak, A.M.; Korwin-Rujna, M.; Szaflik, J.P.; Grabowska, E.; Szaflik, J.; Bartnik, E. A family with 3460G>A and 11778G>A mutations and haplogroup analysis of Polish Leber hereditary optic neuropathy patients. *Mitochondrion* **2008**, *5-6*, 383–388. [CrossRef] [PubMed]

44. Catarino, C.B.; Ahting, U.; Gusic, M.; Iuso, A.; Repp, B.; Peters, K.; Biskup, S.; von Livonius, B.; Prokisch, H.; Klopstock, T. Characterization of a Leber's hereditary optic neuropathy (LHON) family harboring two primary LHON mutations m.11778G>A and m.14484T>C of the mitochondrial DNA. *Mitochondrion* **2016**, *36*, 15–20. [CrossRef] [PubMed]
45. Behbehani, R.; Melhem, M.; Alghanim, G.; Behbehani, K.; Alsmadi, O. ND4L gene concurrent 10609T>C and 10663T>C mutations are associated with Leber's hereditary optic neuropathy in a large pedigree from Kuwait. *Br. J. Ophthalmol.* **2014**, *98*, 826–831. [CrossRef]
46. Achilli, A.; Iommarini, L.; Olivieri, A.; Pala, M.; Hooshiar Kashani, B.; Reynier, P.; La Morgia, C.; Valentino, L.M.; Liguori, R.; Pizza, F.; et al. Rare primary mitochondrial DNA mutations and probable synergistic variants in Leber's hereditary optic neuropathy. *PLoS One* **2012**, *7*, e42242. [CrossRef]
47. Al-Kharashi, M.; Al-Kharashi, A.; Al-Obailan, M.; Kondkar, A.A.; Abu-Amero, K.K. Co-existence of m.10663T>C Mutation with Haplogroup L3f1b Background in a Patient with LHON. *Can. J. Neurol. Sci.* **2016**, *43*, 332–333. [CrossRef]
48. Yang, J.; Zhu, Y.; Tong, Y.; Chen, L.; Liu, L.; Zhang, Z.; Wang, X.; Huang, D.; Qiu, W.; Zhuang, S.; et al. Confirmation of the mitochondrial ND1 gene mutation G3635A as a primary LHON mutation. *Biochem. Biophys. Res. Commun.* **2006**, *386*, 50–54. [CrossRef]
49. Bi, R.; Zhang, A.M.; Jia, X.; Zhang, Q.; Yao, Y.G. Complete mitochondrial DNA genome sequence variation of Chinese families with mutation m.3635G>A and Leber hereditary optic neuropathy. *Mol. Vis.* **2012**, *18*, 3087–3094.
50. Hudson, G.; Carelli, V.; Spruijt, L.; Gerards, M.; Mowbray, C.; Achilli, A.; Pyle, A.; Elson, J.; Howell, N.; La Morgia, C.; et al. Clinical expression of Leber hereditary optic neuropathy is affected by the mitochondrial DNA-haplogroup background. *Am. J. Hum. Genet.* **2007**, *81*, 228–233. [CrossRef]
51. Ghelli, A.; Porcelli, A.M.; Zanna, C.; Vidoni, S.; Mattioli, S.; Barbieri, A.; Iommarini, L.; Pala, M.; Achilli, A.; Torroni, A.; et al. The background of mitochondrial DNA haplogroup J increases the sensitivity of Leber's hereditary optic neuropathy cells to 2,5-hexanedione toxicity. *PLoS ONE* **2009**, *4*, e7922. [CrossRef]
52. Wallace, D.C. The mitochondrial genome in human adaptive radiation and disease: On road to therapeutics and performance enhancement. *Gene* **2005**, *354*, 169–180. [CrossRef] [PubMed]
53. Wallace, D.C. Mitochondrial DNA Variation in Human Radiation and Disease. *Cell* **2015**, *163*, 33–38. [CrossRef] [PubMed]
54. Lui, Z.; Song, Y.; Li, D.; He, X.; Li, S.; Wu, B.; Wang, W.; Gu, S.; Zhu, X.; Wang, X.; et al. The novel mitochondrial 16S rRNA 2336T>C mutation is associated with hypertrophic cardiomyopathy. *J. Med. Genet.* **2014**, *51*, 176–184. [CrossRef]
55. Verechshagina, N.; Nikitchina, N.; Yamada, Y.; Harashima, H.; Tanaka, M.; Orishchenko, K.; Mazunin, I. Future of human mitochondrial DNA editing technologies. *Mitochondrial DNA A DNA Mapp. Seq. Anal.* **2019**, *30*, 214–221. [CrossRef]

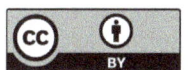

© 2019 by the authors. Licensee MDPI, Basel, Switzerland. This article is an open access article distributed under the terms and conditions of the Creative Commons Attribution (CC BY) license (http://creativecommons.org/licenses/by/4.0/).

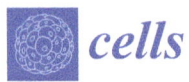

Article

PPARγ-Independent Side Effects of Thiazolidinediones on Mitochondrial Redox State in Rat Isolated Hearts

Matthias L. Riess [1,2,3,*], Reem Elorbany [4], Dorothee Weihrauch [5], David F. Stowe [5,6,7,8] and Amadou K.S. Camara [5,6]

1. Anesthesiology, TVHS VA Medical Center, Nashville, TN 37212, USA
2. Department of Anesthesiology, Vanderbilt University Medical Center, Nashville, TN 37232, USA
3. Department of Pharmacology, Vanderbilt University, Nashville, TN 37232, USA
4. Interdisciplinary Scientist Training Program, University of Chicago, Chicago, IL 60637, USA; reemelorbany@uchicago.edu
5. Department of Anesthesiology, Medical College of Wisconsin, Milwaukee, WI 53226, USA; dorothee@mcw.edu (D.W.); dfstowe@mcw.edu (D.F.S.); aksc@mcw.edu (A.K.S.C.)
6. Department of Physiology, Medical College of Wisconsin, Milwaukee, WI 53226, USA
7. Department of Biomedical Engineering, Medical College of Wisconsin, Milwaukee, WI 53226, USA
8. Clement J. Zablocki VA Medical Center, Milwaukee, WI 53295, USA
* Correspondence: matthias.riess@vanderbilt.edu; Tel.: +1-(615)-936-0277; Fax: +1-(615)-343-3916

Received: 16 December 2019; Accepted: 17 January 2020; Published: 20 January 2020

Abstract: The effect of anti-diabetic thiazolidinediones (TZDs) on contributing to heart failure and cardiac ischemia/reperfusion (IR) injury is controversial. In this study we investigated the effect of select TZDs on myocardial and mitochondrial function in Brown Norway rat isolated hearts. In a first set of experiments, the TZD rosiglitazone was given acutely before global myocardial IR, and pre- and post-IR function and infarct size were assessed. In a second set of experiments, different concentrations of rosiglitazone and pioglitazone were administered in the presence or absence of the specific PPARγ antagonist GW9662, and their effects on the mitochondrial redox state were measured by online NADH and FAD autofluorescence. The administration of rosiglitazone did not significantly affect myocardial function except for transiently increasing coronary flow, but it increased IR injury compared to the control hearts. Both TZDs resulted in dose-dependent, reversible increases in mitochondrial oxidation which was not attenuated by GW9662. Taken together, these data suggest that TZDs cause excessive mitochondrial uncoupling by a PPARγ-independent mechanism. Acute rosiglitazone administration before IR was associated with enhanced cardiac injury. If translated clinically, susceptible patients on PPARγ agonists may experience enhanced myocardial IR injury by mitochondrial dysfunction.

Keywords: GW9662; ischemia reperfusion injury; Langendorff; myocardial; pioglitazone; redox state; rosiglitazone; TZD; uncoupling

1. Introduction

Thiazolidinediones (TZDs) are a class of anti-diabetic drugs that sensitize fat cells to insulin [1] through activation of the peroxisome proliferator-activated receptor-gamma (PPARγ). PPARγ activation has been postulated to activate endothelial nitric oxide synthase, which plays a key role in cardioprotection [2,3]. Therefore, TZDs have cardioprotective effects in ischemia/reperfusion (IR) injury, as reported both in in- and ex-vivo models [4–10]. Moreover, since the PPARγ antagonist GW9662 abolishes both endogenous [11] and exogenous [11,12] cardioprotection against IR injury, the notion that TZDs could be beneficial indirectly through controlling diabetes and through direct cardioprotection against IR injury appears attractive.

However, reports about the deleterious cardiovascular side effects of one of the TZDs, rosiglitazone, first in animals [13–17] and later in humans [18,19] have dampened these hopes. As a result rosiglitazone was taken off the market in Europe and had been put under sales restriction in the USA for several years [20,21]. Pioglitazone, another popular TZD, has a better cardiovascular safety profile [22], but was subsequently taken off the market in several countries after reports of an increased incidence of bladder cancer [23–25]. Although rosiglitazone was subsequently not found to be associated with increased ischemic events [26] and the sales restrictions were lifted in the USA, both drugs remain contra-indicated in patients with heart failure [27,28].

One potential mechanism of this process may involve mitochondria, which play a key role in cell signaling and cell death, and can attenuate or aggravate IR injury [29]. The goal of our study was to investigate if TZDs affect the mitochondrial redox state in rat isolated hearts.

2. Material and Methods

Our isolated heart model has been described in detail [30–33]. All drugs were purchased from Sigma (St. Louis, MO, USA) unless otherwise indicated. Rosiglitazone, pioglitazone, and GW 9662 were dissolved in dimethyl sulfoxide (DMSO) and 1000-fold diluted in Krebs solution to yield the indicated final drug concentrations in 0.1% DMSO.

2.1. Animals

The investigation conformed to the Guide for the Care and Use of Laboratory Animals (Institute for Laboratory Animal Research, National Academy of Sciences, 8th edition, 2011) and was approved by the Institutional Animal Care and Use Committee (ACORP 7435-1, VA Medical Center, Milwaukee, WI, USA). We used 12 and 12 eight-week-old male Brown Norway (BN) rats [32–34] for the IR experiments and for dose-response experiments, respectively.

2.2. Heart Isolation

The animals were anesthetized by the intraperitoneal injection of 100 mg/kg ketamine along with 1000 U heparin to prevent blood clotting. After a negative response to a noxious stimulus, the animals were euthanized by decapitation followed by thoracotomy. The aorta was cannulated distal to the aortic valve, and the heart was perfused retrograde with oxygenated Krebs solution (4 °C) containing (in mM) 148 Na^+, 4.7 K^+, 1.2 Mg^{2+}, 1.6 Ca^{2+}, 127 Cl^-, 27.8 HCO_3^-, 1.2 $H_2PO_4^-$, 1.2 SO_4^{2-}, 5.5 glucose, 2 pyruvate, 0.026 EDTA, and 5 U/l insulin. Both the venae cavae were ligated, and the heart was rapidly placed into a Langendorff support system and perfused at a constant pressure of 70 mmHg at 37 °C. The perfusate was equilibrated with ~95% O_2 and ~5% CO_2 to maintain a constant pH of 7.40 and filtered in-line (5 µm pore size). The isovolumetric left ventricular pressure (LVP) was measured with a saline-filled latex balloon (Radnoti LLC, Monrovia, CA, USA) inserted into the left ventricle. The diastolic LVP was initially adjusted to 10 mmHg at baseline (bl) so that any subsequent pressure increases reflected diastolic contracture. Systolic, diastolic, and developed (systolic–diastolic) LVP, and its maximal and minimal first derivatives ($dLVP/dt_{max}$ and $dLVP/dt_{min}$) were calculated as indices of ventricular contractility and relaxation, respectively. Electrodes attached to the right atrial and ventricular walls monitored atrial and ventricular electrocardiograms to calculate the spontaneous heart rate (HR) and identify arrhythmias. The rate-pressure product (RPP) as the product of developed pressure and HR was calculated to correct for HR-dependent changes in developed pressure. The coronary flow was measured in-line with an ultrasonic flowmeter (model T106X; Transonic Systems, Ithaca, NY, USA). All the analog signals were digitized (PowerLab/16 SP, AD Instruments; Castle Hill, Australia) and recorded at 200 Hz (Chart & Scope version 5.6.6, AD Instruments) for later analysis.

2.3. Protocols

The experimental protocols are illustrated in Figure 1. The baseline readings were taken after 20 min stabilization.

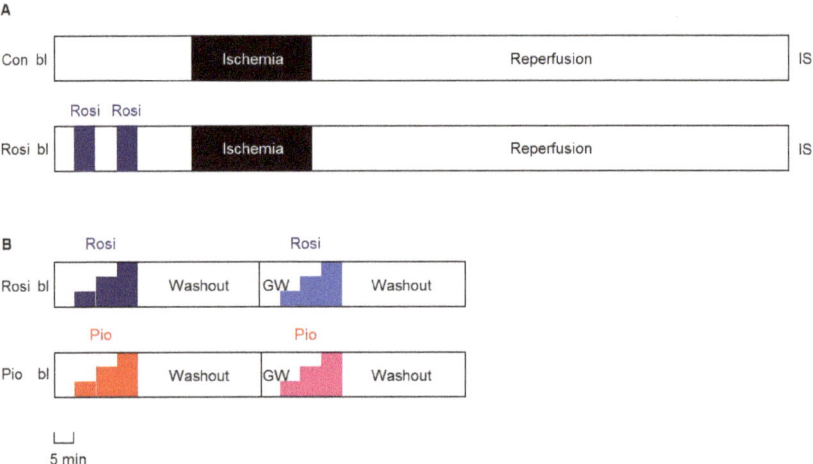

Figure 1. Shows the experimental protocols. The hearts were isolated from eight-week-old male Brown Norway rats and mounted in a Langendorff setup. After 20 min equilibration and a baseline (bl) reading, the hearts in the first set of experiments (n = 12; Panel (**A**)) were given rosiglitazone (Rosi, 50 µM) or a vehicle (Con) for two times, 5 min each with a 5 min washout period interspersed and followed by 15 min washout before 30 min of global no-flow ischemia and 120 min of reperfusion (IR) and subsequent infarct size (IS) determination. In a second set of experiments (Panel (**B**)), the hearts were given increasing concentrations (2, 10, and 50 µM) of either rosiglitazone (Rosi, blue colors; n = 6) or pioglitazone (Pio, red colors; n = 6) for 5 min each followed by 30 min washout. This series was repeated in the presence of 10 µM of the PPARγ antagonist GW9662 (GW, white). The hearts were not subject to IR or to IS determination.

2.3.1. IR Experiments

In this first set of experiments (n = 12; Figure 1, Panel A), rosiglitazone (Rosi, 50 µM) as a clinically used TZD was given as a preconditioning agent for two times, 5 min each with a 5 min washout period interspersed and followed by 15 min washout before 30 min of acute global no-flow ischemia and 120 min of reperfusion. This protocol was chosen to mimic our ischemic and other pharmacological preconditioning protocols [30,31,35,36] shown to be more effective than single exposure [31,37]. The control hearts (Con) received 0.1% DMSO as a vehicle only.

After removal of the hearts at the end of the experiments, the atria were discarded and the ventricles were cut into 2-mm transverse slices and incubated for 10 min in 1% 2,3,5-triphenyltetrazolium chloride in a 0.1 M KH_2PO_4 buffer (pH 7.4, 38°C) [38,39] which stains viable tissue red. The slices were digitally imaged on a green background, and the infarcted areas of each slice were measured automatically by planimetry using Image J 1.44i software (NIH, Bethesda, MD). The individual slice infarctions were weight-averaged to calculate the total ventricular infarct size (IS) per heart [32,40].

2.3.2. Dose-Response Experiments

In a second set of experiments (n = 12; Figure 1, Panel B), the hearts were given increasing concentrations (2, 10 and 50 µM) of either rosiglitazone (Rosi) or pioglitazone (Pio) for 5 min each, without intervening IR or IS determination. After a 30 min washout, this series was repeated in the presence of the PPARγ antagonist GW9662 [12] at a concentration of 10 µM [11,41,42].

2.4. Fluorescence Measurement of Mitochondrial Redox State

Autofluorescence is widely used to measure mitochondrial electron transport in myocardial tissue [30,43,44]. Thus, the experiments were conducted in a light-blocking Faraday cage to assess the online autofluorescence of reduced NADH and oxidized FAD. The distal end of a trifurcated fiberoptic cable was placed gently against the left anterior ventricular wall while the proximal ends were connected to a modified spectrophotometer (Horiba, Piscataway, NJ, USA). At selected times, the shutter for excitation was opened for 2.5 sec intervals. The NADH fluorescence was excited at 350 nm followed by FAD fluorescence excitation at 488 nm. The NADH emissions were filtered at 460 ± 10 nm (Chroma Technology Corp., Brattleboro, VT, USA), FAD emissions at 540 ± 10 nm, and their respective fluorescence intensities were measured by photomultipliers.

2.5. Statistical Analysis

Unless otherwise indicated, all the values are expressed as a mean ± standard error of the mean (SEM) as %bl, and compared by analysis of variance (SigmaStat 3.5, Systat Software Inc., San Jose, CA, USA). If the F values were significant, Student-Newman-Keuls (SNK) post-hoc tests were conducted. Comparisons of only two groups were conducted with unpaired Student t-tests. All the results were considered statistically significant at $P < 0.05$ (2-tailed): *vs. Con (0 μM TZD).

3. Results

3.1. IR Experiments

The rosiglitazone (50 μM for 2 × 5 min) given before IR did not have a significant effect on myocardial function during its administration except for reversibly increasing coronary flow (Table 1). The infarct size was significantly increased in the rosiglitazone-treated hearts, but there was no significant positive or negative difference in the functional outcome after IR between the rosiglitazone-treated and control hearts.

Table 1. Myocardial Function and Infarct Size. This table shows myocardial function during the application of the thiazolidinedione rosiglitazone (Rosi, 50 μM, n = 5), and myocardial function and infarct size at 120 min reperfusion following 30 min global no-flow ischemia compared to control (Con, n = 7) rat isolated hearts.

	During Application		120 min Reperfusion	
	Con	Rosi	Con	Rosi
sysLVP (%bl)	95.5 ± 2.0	101.9 ± 2.8	70.5 ± 4.9	60.3 ± 3.9
diaLVP (mmHg)	10.5 ± 2.1	9.9 ± 0.8	32.3 ± 4.3	31.8 ± 2.7
devLVP (%bl)	92.6 ± 3.8	102.4 ± 3.6	33.8 ± 3.7	29.7 ± 1.0
RPP (%bl)	96.4 ± 5.5	101.3 ± 4.4	33.5 ± 3.7	30.9 ± 0.7
dLVP/dt$_{max}$ (%bl)	94.4 ± 3.5	106.6 ± 4.7	35.9 ± 2.6	32.8 ± 1.3
dLVP/dt$_{min}$ (%bl)	97.2 ± 2.4	100.6 ± 4.5	38.9 ± 5.0	30.4 ± 1.1
HR (%bl)	105.3 ± 2.8	98.8 ± 2.2	98.4 ± 2.7	104.3 ± 1.6
CF (%bl)	100.0 ± 1.0	* 124.0 ± 6.1	64.6 ± 5.3	64.5 ± 3.0
IS (%)			36.2 ± 3.4	* 45.3 ± 0.7

bl = baseline; LVP = left ventricular pressure; sys = systolic; dia = diastolic; dev = developed; RPP = rate-pressure product; dLVP/dt$_{max}$ = contractility; dLVP/dt$_{min}$ = relaxation; HR = heart rate; CF = coronary flow; IS = ventricular infarct size. All values are mean ± standard error of the mean of %bl unless otherwise indicated. Statistics: unpaired student t-test with * $P < 0.05$ (two-tailed).

3.2. Dose-Response Experiments

Figure 2 shows the representative time courses of NADH and FAD fluorescence for an experiment with increasing doses of rosiglitazone (2, 10 and 50 μM) first in the absence and then, after a 30 min washout period, in the presence of the PPARγ antagonist GW9662 (10 μM). These dose-response experiments in the absence and presence of the PPARγ antagonist GW9662 revealed a PPARγ-independent increase in mitochondrial oxidation by rosiglitazone as evidenced by a dose-dependent decrease in NADH autofluorescence (Figures 2 and 3A) and a dose-dependent increase in FAD autofluorescence (Figures 2 and 3B). Neither of these was attenuated or abolished by GW9662 at a dose previously used to abolish endogenous and exogenous cardioprotection in the same [11] and in other models [41,42]. In order to test for a group- rather than a single drug-effect, the same dose-response curve was repeated with 2, 10, and 50 µM pioglitazone with essentially the same results (Figure 3).

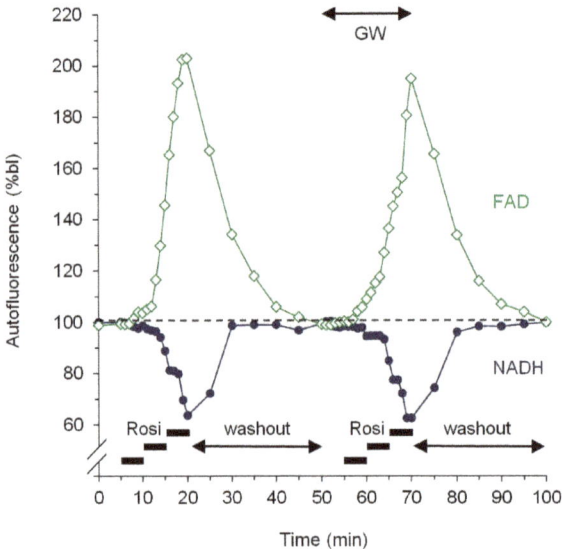

Figure 2. Shows representative time courses of NADH (closed blue circles) and FAD (open green diamonds) autofluorescence for an experiment with rosiglitazone (Rosi) in increasing doses from 0 to 50 µM (5 min each) first in the absence and then, after a 30 min washout period, in the presence of the PPARγ antagonist GW9662 (GW, 10 µM).

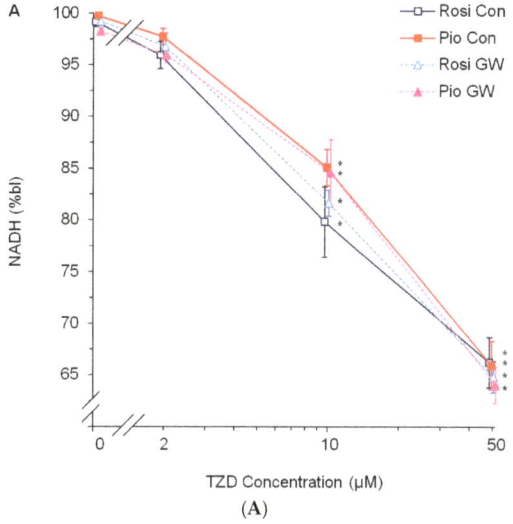

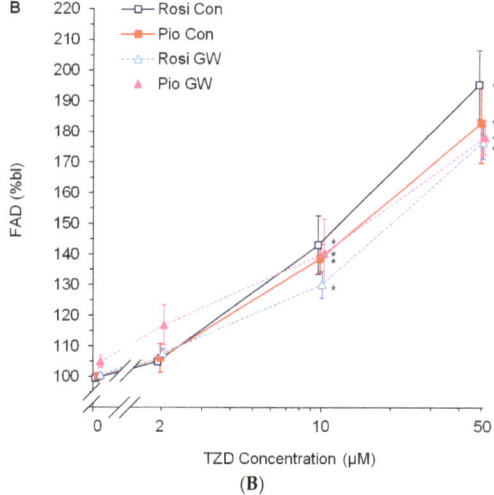

Figure 3. Shows a concentration-dependent decrease in autofluorescence of reduced NADH (Panel (**A**)) and a concomitant concentration-dependent increase in autofluorescence of oxidized FAD (Panel (**B**)) with administration of the thiazolidinediones (TZDs) rosiglitazone (Rosi, open dark-blue square) and pioglitazone (Pio, closed red square) compared to % baseline (bl). The PPARγ antagonist GW9662 (GW, 10 μM) did not alter the effect of rosiglitazone (open light-blue triangle) or pioglitazone (closed pink triangle) on NADH (Panel (**A**)) or FAD (Panel (**B**)) at any of the concentrations. Statistics: ANOVA followed by SNK post-hoc test with $P < 0.05$ (two-tailed) vs. * 0 μM TZD; n = 6 per group. Please note that the slight horizontal offset of curves for any given concentration is for visual purposes only.

4. Discussion

Our study has several key findings: In line with prior reports of cardiovascular side effects of TZDs [45,46], it confirms an increase in cardiac IR injury following the acute administration and washout of the TZD rosiglitazone in rat isolated hearts. A novel finding in this context however, is that in further dose-response experiments we found a considerable, rosiglitazone-induced, fully reversible increase in mitochondrial oxidation as assessed by decreased NADH and increased FAD autofluorescence. This finding was independent of PPARγ activation as it was not abolished by the PPARγ antagonist GW9662. Moreover, all the observed rosiglitazone effects on the mitochondrial redox state were replicated with another member of the TZD family, pioglitazone, which suggests a group- rather than a mere single drug-dependent side effect on mitochondrial function.

4.1. PPARγ Activation and Myocardial Protection: Friend or Foe?

Several options are available to investigate the specific aspects of a particular signaling pathway. For example, the expression, modification and/or activity of a certain protein/enzyme can be measured. An agonist can be used to activate a certain pathway. Or a specific antagonist can be used to attenuate or abolish a certain finding. Using the latter, we have previously shown in a consomic rat model of resistance against myocardial IR that the specific PPARγ antagonist GW9662 prevented endogenous and exogenous cardioprotection [11]. Thus, PPARγ activation is a critical part of cardioprotective pathways that can be initiated by different triggers upstream of PPARγ [12].

Conversely, administration of specific PPARγ agonists should be able to mimic the above phenotype and activate a cardioprotective pathway directly without the need for, e.g., ischemic or anesthetic preconditioning, and their acutely cardio-depressant and other side effects [12]. While numerous experiments with the PPARγ antagonist GW9662 have largely shown myocardial protection against IR injury by PPARγ activation [2,12,47–51], experiments with agonists like TZDs have revealed less clear results, particularly under pathological conditions [52]. To the contrary, but in line with our findings, the TZD-triggered aggravation of myocardial outcome was shown in animal studies [13–17] and in humans [18,19]. The apparently contradictory findings among some of these studies may be due to differences in the species and experimental models being used, the protocol and duration of TZD administration, co-morbidities, and/or related to the used dosage.

4.2. Specificity of TZDs for PPARγ Activation

Conclusions from experiments using agonists and/or antagonists generally rely on their respective specificity for any given pathway or receptor. Thus, it is possible that TZDs have PPARγ-independent binding sites [53] that can influence cardiovascular outcome directly or indirectly [54–56]. Reports about the deleterious effects of TZDs without their prevention by the use of a specific PPARγ-antagonist [13,15–17] may, therefore, be due to PPARγ-independent side effects as previously discussed by Feinstein and colleagues [54]. Moreover, these reports pose the question of whether those side effects are specific to individual members of the TZD group or side effects of the TZD group as a whole because of their chemical similarities [53]. The use of more than one member of the TZD group within the same study and demonstration of failure to abolish the observed effect with GW9662 can add clarification in these regards.

4.3. TZDs Affect Mitochondrial Function

Our knowledge about the cardiac mitochondrial side effects of TZDs is sketchy [54]. An in-vivo and in-vitro study in mice [57] reported rosiglitazone to cause dysfunction of cardiac mitochondria as evidenced by decreased mitochondrial respiration and substrate oxidation, as well as decreased complex I and IV activities. Rosiglitazone also increased superoxide production from complexes I and III. Neither genetic PPARγ deletion nor the PPARγ antagonist GW9662 prevented these effects. Moreover, these findings were associated with decreased ATP synthesis and increased cardiac dysfunction during rosiglitazone administration. The authors emphasize that, similarly to our findings, these were dose-dependent effects found at concentrations of 10 μM and higher.

Reactive oxygen species (ROS) are produced from different intracellular sources with mitochondria and different mitochondrial electron transport chain complexes being the major sources in cardiomyocytes [58]. While inhibition of the mitochondrial electron transport chain at specific sites of complex I and/or III [58] can lead to oxidative stress, the latter is not necessarily proof of a blockade but could also be caused by an increase in electron transport, as is the case with uncoupling [59]. Indeed, mitochondrial uncoupling makes oxidative phosphorylation less efficient, increases ROS, and—if not countered by increased delivery of the reducing equivalents, NADH and $FADH_2$, through the Krebs cycle—can lead to a decreased membrane potential and ATP synthesis. Thus, a decrease in membrane potential or ATP synthesis or an increase in ROS production cannot distinguish between the uncoupling and blockade of mitochondrial electron transport, unless the mitochondrial redox state is measured. In this context, our results suggest a dose-dependent and reversible mitochondrial oxidation by two different TZDs independent of PPARγ activation. Excessive mitochondrial oxidation can lead to decreased ATP synthesis and excessive ROS production, all of which can damage the myocardium and/or lead to increased sensitivity to subsequent IR.

4.4. Study Limitations and Summary

This study needs to be interpreted within its natural constraints. We used one species and an acute rather than chronic experimental IR injury model. Mitochondrial function was assessed by two different redox state measurements in intact hearts, but not by mitochondrial oxygen consumption in isolated mitochondria, and we did not assess ROS production, membrane potential or ATP synthesis, neither of which would have added to differentiating severe blockade of mitochondrial electron transport from uncoupling. The IR injury assessment was limited to one TZD and one dose given twice acutely and washed out before IR. On the other hand, rosiglitazone's effects on the redox state, with or without the PPARγ antagonist GW9662, were closely mimicked by pioglitazone; the NADH results mirrored the FAD measurements; and the GW9662 results were nearly identical to the ones in its absence, serving as internal controls. Although we have not conducted a formal dose-response study with the PPARγ antagonist GW9662 or Western blot analysis, we have chosen a dose (10 µM) commonly used to block PPARγ in the isolated heart [11] and isolated cardiomyocyte studies [41,42]. Demonstration of a change in infarct size remains the gold standard for in- and ex-vivo studies on cardioprotective or -toxic agents and strategies, even in the absence of significant functional changes. Within limits, compensatory mechanisms, such as e.g., mildly increased intracellular calcium in surviving cardiomyocytes, can make up for the loss of function in the infarcted myocardium. The infarct size is among the more sensitive parameters with earlier responses to IR than functional changes [36]. We exposed hearts from non-diabetic animals to an acute dose of rosiglitazone; chronic exposure in diabetic individuals would require the study of chronically diabetic and, thus, hyperglycemic hearts in the control group vs. normoglycemic hearts chronically exposed to a TZD which would complement but not replace the findings in the present study and add additional confounders to the study.

In summary, our study in rat isolated hearts suggests that the off-target effects of the TZDs, rosiglitazone and pioglitazone, include a significant degree of mitochondrial oxidation associated with aggravated myocardial IR injury that can help explain the reported increase in adverse cardiac events. Because of the large number of diabetic patients worldwide who are chronically treated with TZDs, it is important to unravel the mechanisms of these adverse effects and their clinical consequence in future studies, including diabetic IR models, in order to improve overall patient outcome while minimizing unwanted side effects.

Author Contributions: Study design by M.L.R., D.W., D.F.S. and A.K.S.C.; experiments conducted by M.L.R. and R.E.; data analysis and presentation by M.L.R. and R.E.; manuscript written by M.L.R. and A.K.S.C.; manuscript revised and approved by M.L.R., R.E., D.W., D.F.S. and A.K.S.C.; agreement to be accountable for all aspects of the work by M.L.R., R.E., D.W., D.F.S. and A.K.S.C. All authors have read and agreed to the published version of the manuscript.

Funding: This work was supported in part by the US Department of Veterans Affairs Biomedical Laboratory R&D Service (IK2BX001278 and I01 BX003482), the National Institutes of Health (5R01 HL123227), a Roizen Anesthesia Research Foundation New Investigator Grant from the Society of Cardiovascular Anesthesiologists, and by institutional funds to MLR.

Acknowledgments: The authors wish to thank Qunli Cheng, James S. Heisner (Department of Anesthesiology, Medical College of Wisconsin, Milwaukee, WI), Sushrut V. Shidham and Darren S. Nabor (formerly Medical College of Wisconsin Affiliated Hospitals, Milwaukee, WI) and William J. Cleveland (Department of Anesthesiology, Vanderbilt University Medical Center, Nashville, TN) for their valuable contributions to this study.

Conflicts of Interest: The authors declare no conflict of interest.

References

1. Eldor, R.; DeFronzo, R.A.; Abdul-Ghani, M. In vivo actions of peroxisome proliferator-activated receptors: Glycemic control, insulin sensitivity, and insulin secretion. *Diabetes Care* **2013**, *36*, S162–S174. [CrossRef]
2. Kobayashi, N.; Ohno, T.; Yoshida, K.; Fukushima, H.; Mamada, Y.; Nomura, M.; Hirata, H.; Machida, Y.; Shinoda, M.; Suzuki, N.; et al. Cardioprotective mechanism of telmisartan via PPAR-gamma-eNOS pathway in dahl salt-sensitive hypertensive rats. *Am. J. Hypertens.* **2008**, *21*, 576–581. [CrossRef]
3. Yasuda, S.; Kobayashi, H.; Iwasa, M.; Kawamura, I.; Sumi, S.; Narentuoya, B.; Yamaki, T.; Ushikoshi, H.; Nishigaki, K.; Nagashima, K.; et al. Antidiabetic drug pioglitazone protects the heart via activation of PPAR-gamma receptors, PI3-kinase, Akt, and eNOS pathway in a rabbit model of myocardial infarction. *Am. J. Physiol. Heart Circ. Physiol.* **2009**, *296*, H1558–H1565. [CrossRef]
4. Zhu, P.; Lu, L.; Xu, Y.; Schwartz, G.G. Troglitazone improves recovery of left ventricular function after regional ischemia in pigs. *Circulation* **2000**, *101*, 1165–1171. [CrossRef] [PubMed]
5. Yue, T.L.; Chen, J.; Bao, W.; Narayanan, P.K.; Bril, A.; Jiang, W.; Lysko, P.G.; Gu, J.L.; Boyce, R.; Zimmerman, D.M.; et al. In vivo myocardial protection from ischemia/reperfusion injury by the peroxisome proliferator-activated receptor-gamma agonist rosiglitazone. *Circulation* **2001**, *104*, 2588–2594. [CrossRef] [PubMed]
6. Khandoudi, N.; Delerive, P.; Berrebi-Bertrand, I.; Buckingham, R.E.; Staels, B.; Bril, A. Rosiglitazone, a peroxisome proliferator-activated receptor-gamma, inhibits the Jun NH(2)-terminal kinase/activating protein 1 pathway and protects the heart from ischemia/reperfusion injury. *Diabetes* **2002**, *51*, 1507–1514. [CrossRef] [PubMed]
7. Wayman, N.S.; Hattori, Y.; McDonald, M.C.; Mota-Filipe, H.; Cuzzocrea, S.; Pisano, B.; Chatterjee, P.K.; Thiemermann, C. Ligands of the peroxisome proliferator-activated receptors (PPAR-gamma and PPAR-alpha) reduce myocardial infarct size. *FASEB J.* **2002**, *16*, 1027–1040. [CrossRef]
8. Wynne, A.M.; Mocanu, M.M.; Yellon, D.M. Pioglitazone mimics preconditioning in the isolated perfused rat heart: A role for the prosurvival kinases PI3K and P42/44MAPK. *J. Cardiovasc. Pharmacol.* **2005**, *46*, 817–822. [CrossRef]
9. Li, J.; Lang, M.J.; Mao, X.B.; Tian, L.; Feng, Y.B. Antiapoptosis and mitochondrial effect of pioglitazone preconditioning in the ischemic/reperfused heart of rat. *Cardiovasc. Drugs Ther.* **2008**, *22*, 283–291. [CrossRef]
10. Hu, Q.; Chen, J.; Jiang, C.; Liu, H.F. Effect of peroxisome proliferator-activated receptor gamma agonist on heart of rabbits with acute myocardial ischemia/reperfusion injury. *Asian Pac. J. Trop. Med.* **2014**, *7*, 271–275. [CrossRef]
11. Nabor, D.; ElOrbany, R.; Cheng, Q.; Kersten, J.; Stowe, D.; Riess, M. PPARγ Mediates Endogenous and Exogenous Cardioprotection Associated with Rat Chromosome 6. *Anesth. Analg.* **2013**, *116*, S93.
12. Lotz, C.; Lange, M.; Redel, A.; Stumpner, J.; Schmidt, J.; Tischer-Zeitz, T.; Roewer, N.; Kehl, F. Peroxisome-proliferator-activated receptor gamma mediates the second window of anaesthetic-induced preconditioning. *Exp. Physiol.* **2011**, *96*, 317–324. [CrossRef]
13. Xu, Y.; Lu, L.; Greyson, C.; Lee, J.; Gen, M.; Kinugawa, K.; Long, C.S.; Schwartz, G.G. Deleterious effects of acute treatment with a peroxisome proliferator-activated receptor-gamma activator in myocardial ischemia and reperfusion in pigs. *Diabetes* **2003**, *52*, 1187–1194. [CrossRef] [PubMed]
14. Xu, Y.; Gen, M.; Lu, L.; Fox, J.; Weiss, S.O.; Brown, R.D.; Perlov, D.; Ahmad, H.; Zhu, P.; Greyson, C.; et al. PPAR-gamma activation fails to provide myocardial protection in ischemia and reperfusion in pigs. *Am. J. Physiol. Heart Circ. Physiol.* **2005**, *288*, H1314–H1323. [CrossRef] [PubMed]
15. Palee, S.; Weerateerangkul, P.; Surinkeaw, S.; Chattipakorn, S.; Chattipakorn, N. Effect of rosiglitazone on cardiac electrophysiology, infarct size and mitochondrial function in ischaemia and reperfusion of swine and rat heart. *Exp. Physiol.* **2011**, *96*, 778–789. [CrossRef]

16. Sarraf, M.; Lu, L.; Ye, S.; Reiter, M.J.; Greyson, C.R.; Schwartz, G.G. Thiazolidinedione drugs promote onset, alter characteristics, and increase mortality of ischemic ventricular fibrillation in pigs. *Cardiovasc. Drugs Ther.* **2012**, *26*, 195–204. [CrossRef]
17. Palee, S.; Weerateerangkul, P.; Chinda, K.; Chattipakorn, S.C.; Chattipakorn, N. Mechanisms responsible for beneficial and adverse effects of rosiglitazone in a rat model of acute cardiac ischaemia-reperfusion. *Exp. Physiol.* **2013**, *98*, 1028–1037. [CrossRef]
18. Nissen, S.E.; Wolski, K. Effect of rosiglitazone on the risk of myocardial infarction and death from cardiovascular causes. *N. Engl. J. Med.* **2007**, *356*, 2457–2471. [CrossRef]
19. Chen, X.; Yang, L.; Zhai, S.D. Risk of cardiovascular disease and all-cause mortality among diabetic patients prescribed rosiglitazone or pioglitazone: A meta-analysis of retrospective cohort studies. *Chin. Med. J.* **2012**, *125*, 4301–4306.
20. Nissen, S.E. Rosiglitazone: A case of regulatory hubris. *BMJ* **2013**, *347*, f7428. [CrossRef]
21. Hickson, R.P.; Cole, A.L.; Dusetzina, S.B. Implications of Removing Rosiglitazone's Black Box Warning and Restricted Access Program on the Uptake of Thiazolidinediones and Dipeptidyl Peptidase-4 Inhibitors Among Patients with Type 2 Diabetes. *J. Manag. Care Spec. Pharm.* **2019**, *25*, 72–79. [CrossRef] [PubMed]
22. Lincoff, A.M.; Wolski, K.; Nicholls, S.J.; Nissen, S.E. Pioglitazone and risk of cardiovascular events in patients with type 2 diabetes mellitus: A meta-analysis of randomized trials. *JAMA* **2007**, *298*, 1180–1188. [CrossRef] [PubMed]
23. Colmers, I.N.; Bowker, S.L.; Majumdar, S.R.; Johnson, J.A. Use of thiazolidinediones and the risk of bladder cancer among people with type 2 diabetes: A meta-analysis. *CMAJ* **2012**, *184*, E675–E683. [CrossRef] [PubMed]
24. Turner, R.M.; Kwok, C.S.; Chen-Turner, C.; Maduakor, C.A.; Singh, S.; Loke, Y.K. Thiazolidinediones and associated risk of bladder cancer: A systematic review and meta-analysis. *Br. J. Clin. Pharmacol.* **2014**, *78*, 258–273. [CrossRef]
25. Tang, H.; Shi, W.; Fu, S.; Wang, T.; Zhai, S.; Song, Y.; Han, J. Pioglitazone and bladder cancer risk: A systematic review and meta-analysis. *Cancer Med.* **2018**, *7*, 1070–1080. [CrossRef]
26. Stone, J.C.; Furuya-Kanamori, L.; Barendregt, J.J.; Doi, S.A. Was there really any evidence that rosiglitazone increased the risk of myocardial infarction or death from cardiovascular causes? *Pharmacoepidemiol. Drug Saf.* **2015**, *24*, 223–227. [CrossRef]
27. Loke, Y.K.; Kwok, C.S.; Singh, S. Comparative cardiovascular effects of thiazolidinediones: Systematic review and meta-analysis of observational studies. *BMJ* **2011**, *342*, d1309. [CrossRef]
28. Seferovic, P.M.; Petrie, M.C.; Filippatos, G.S.; Anker, S.D.; Rosano, G.; Bauersachs, J.; Paulus, W.J.; Komajda, M.; Cosentino, F.; de Boer, R.A.; et al. Type 2 diabetes mellitus and heart failure: A position statement from the Heart Failure Association of the European Society of Cardiology. *Eur. J. Hear. Fail.* **2018**, *20*, 853–872. [CrossRef]
29. Camara, A.K.; Bienengraeber, M.; Stowe, D.F. Mitochondrial approaches to protect against cardiac ischemia and reperfusion injury. *Front. Physiol.* **2011**, *2*, 13. [CrossRef]
30. Riess, M.L.; Camara, A.K.S.; Chen, Q.; Novalija, E.; Rhodes, S.S.; Stowe, D.F. Altered NADH and improved function by anesthetic and ischemic preconditioning in guinea pig intact hearts. *Am. J. Physiol. Heart Circ. Physiol.* **2002**, *283*, H53–H60. [CrossRef]
31. Riess, M.L.; Kevin, L.G.; Camara, A.K.S.; Heisner, J.S.; Stowe, D.F. Dual exposure to sevoflurane improves anesthetic preconditioning in intact hearts. *Anesthesiology* **2004**, *100*, 569–574. [CrossRef] [PubMed]
32. Nabbi, R.; Gadicherla, A.K.; Kersten, J.R.; Stowe, D.F.; Lazar, J.; Riess, M.L. Genetically determined mitochondrial preservation and cardioprotection against myocardial ischemia-reperfusion injury in a consomic rat model. *Physiol. Genom.* **2014**, *46*, 169–176. [CrossRef] [PubMed]
33. Salzman, M.M.; Cheng, Q.; Deklotz, R.J.; Dulai, G.K.; Douglas, H.F.; Dikalova, A.E.; Weihrauch, D.; Barnes, B.M.; Riess, M.L. Lipid emulsion enhances cardiac performance after ischemia-reperfusion in isolated hearts from summer-active arctic ground squirrels. *J. Comp. Physiol. B* **2017**, *187*, 715–724. [CrossRef] [PubMed]
34. Baker, J.E.; Konorev, E.A.; Gross, G.J.; Chilian, W.M.; Jacob, H.J. Resistance to myocardial ischemia in five rat strains: Is there a genetic component of cardioprotection? *Am. J. Physiol.* **2000**, *278*, H1395–H1400. [CrossRef] [PubMed]

35. Kevin, L.G.; Novalija, E.; Riess, M.L.; Camara, A.K.; Rhodes, S.S.; Stowe, D.F. Sevoflurane exposure generates superoxide but leads to decreased superoxide during ischemia and reperfusion in isolated hearts. *Anesth. Analg.* **2003**, *96*, 949–955. [CrossRef] [PubMed]
36. Kevin, L.G.; Katz, P.; Camara, A.K.; Novalija, E.; Riess, M.L.; Stowe, D.F. Anesthetic preconditioning: Effects on latency to ischemic injury in isolated hearts. *Anesthesiology* **2003**, *99*, 385–391. [CrossRef] [PubMed]
37. Sandhu, R.; Diaz, R.J.; Mao, G.D.; Wilson, G.J. Ischemic preconditioning: Differences in protection and susceptibility to blockade with single-cycle versus multicycle transient ischemia. *Circulation* **1997**, *96*, 984–995. [CrossRef]
38. Altman, F.P. Tetrazolium salts and formazans. *Prog. Histochem. Cytochem.* **1976**, *9*, 1–56. [CrossRef]
39. Riess, M.L.; Rhodes, S.S.; Stowe, D.F.; Aldakkak, M.; Camara, A.K. Comparison of cumulative planimetry versus manual dissection to assess experimental infarct size in isolated hearts. *J. Pharmacol. Toxicol. Methods* **2009**, *60*, 275–280. [CrossRef]
40. Shidham, S.V.; Nabbi, R.; Camara, A.K.S.; Riess, M.L. Development of automated infarct size measurement in TTC stained rat isolated hearts after global ischemia/reperfusion. *FASEB J.* **2011**, *25*, 1130–1132.
41. Peng, X.; Chen, R.; Wu, Y.; Huang, B.; Tang, C.; Chen, J.; Wang, Q.; Wu, Q.; Yang, J.; Qiu, H.; et al. PPARgamma-PI3K/AKT-NO signal pathway is involved in cardiomyocyte hypertrophy induced by high glucose and insulin. *J. Diabetes Complicat.* **2015**, *29*, 755–760. [CrossRef]
42. Peymani, M.; Ghaedi, K.; Irani, S.; Nasr-Esfahani, M.H. Peroxisome Proliferator-Activated Receptor gamma Activity is Required for Appropriate Cardiomyocyte Differentiation. *Cell J.* **2016**, *18*, 221–228. [PubMed]
43. Chance, B.; Williamson, J.R.; Jamieson, D.; Schoenner, B. Properties and kinetics of reduced pyridine nucleotide fluorescence of the isolated and in vivo rat heart. *Biochem. Zeit* **1965**, *341*, 357–377.
44. Camara, A.K.; Aldakkak, M.; Heisner, J.S.; Rhodes, S.S.; Riess, M.L.; An, J.; Heinen, A.; Stowe, D.F. ROS scavenging before 27 degrees C ischemia protects hearts and reduces mitochondrial ROS, Ca^{2+} overload, and changes in redox state. *Am. J. Physiol. Cell Physiol.* **2007**, *292*, C2021–C2031. [CrossRef] [PubMed]
45. Cheng, D.; Gao, H.; Li, W. Long-term risk of rosiglitazone on cardiovascular events—A systematic review and meta-analysis. *Endokrynol. Pol.* **2018**, *69*, 381–394. [PubMed]
46. Varga, Z.V.; Ferdinandy, P.; Liaudet, L.; Pacher, P. Drug-induced mitochondrial dysfunction and cardiotoxicity. *Am. J. Physiol. Heart Circ. Physiol.* **2015**, *309*, H1453–H1467. [CrossRef]
47. Sivarajah, A.; McDonald, M.C.; Thiemermann, C. The cardioprotective effects of preconditioning with endotoxin, but not ischemia, are abolished by a peroxisome proliferator-activated receptor-gamma antagonist. *J. Pharmacol. Exp. Ther.* **2005**, *313*, 896–901. [CrossRef]
48. Morrison, A.; Yan, X.; Tong, C.; Li, J. Acute rosiglitazone treatment is cardioprotective against ischemia-reperfusion injury by modulating AMPK, Akt, and JNK signaling in nondiabetic mice. *Am. J. Physiol. Heart Circ. Physiol.* **2011**, *301*, H895–H902. [CrossRef]
49. Chen, T.; Jin, X.; Crawford, B.H.; Cheng, H.; Saafir, T.B.; Wagner, M.B.; Yuan, Z.; Ding, G. Cardioprotection from oxidative stress in the newborn heart by activation of PPARgamma is mediated by catalase. *Free Radic. Biol. Med.* **2012**, *53*, 208–215. [CrossRef]
50. Nagashima, A.; Watanabe, R.; Ogawa, M.; Suzuki, J.; Masumura, M.; Hishikari, K.; Shimizu, T.; Takayama, K.; Hirata, Y.; Nagai, R.; et al. Different roles of PPAR-gamma activity on physiological and pathological alteration after myocardial ischemia. *J. Cardiovasc. Pharmacol.* **2012**, *60*, 158–164. [CrossRef]
51. Han, J.; Wang, D.; Ye, L.; Li, P.; Hao, W.; Chen, X.; Ma, J.; Wang, B.; Shang, J.; Li, D.; et al. Rosmarinic Acid Protects against Inflammation and Cardiomyocyte Apoptosis during Myocardial Ischemia/Reperfusion Injury by Activating Peroxisome Proliferator-Activated Receptor Gamma. *Front. Pharmacol.* **2017**, *8*, 456. [CrossRef] [PubMed]
52. Ravingerova, T.; Adameova, A.; Carnicka, S.; Nemcekova, M.; Kelly, T.; Matejikova, J.; Galatou, E.; Barlaka, E.; Lazou, A. The role of PPAR in myocardial response to ischemia in normal and diseased heart. *Gen. Physiol. Biophys.* **2011**, *30*, 329–341. [CrossRef] [PubMed]
53. Hoffmann, B.R.; El-Mansy, M.F.; Sem, D.S.; Greene, A.S. Chemical proteomics-based analysis of off-target binding profiles for rosiglitazone and pioglitazone: Clues for assessing potential for cardiotoxicity. *J. Med. Chem.* **2012**, *55*, 8260–8271. [CrossRef] [PubMed]
54. Feinstein, D.L.; Spagnolo, A.; Akar, C.; Weinberg, G.; Murphy, P.; Gavrilyuk, V.; Dello Russo, C. Receptor-independent actions of PPAR thiazolidinedione agonists: Is mitochondrial function the key? *Biochem. Pharmacol.* **2005**, *70*, 177–188. [CrossRef]

55. Gardner, O.S.; Shiau, C.W.; Chen, C.S.; Graves, L.M. Peroxisome proliferator-activated receptor gamma-independent activation of p38 MAPK by thiazolidinediones involves calcium/calmodulin-dependent protein kinase II and protein kinase R: Correlation with endoplasmic reticulum stress. *J. Biol. Chem.* **2005**, *280*, 10109–10118. [CrossRef] [PubMed]
56. Mughal, R.S.; Warburton, P.; O'Regan, D.J.; Ball, S.G.; Turner, N.A.; Porter, K.E. Peroxisome proliferator-activated receptor gamma-independent effects of thiazolidinediones on human cardiac myofibroblast function. *Clin. Exp. Pharmacol. Physiol.* **2009**, *36*, 478–486. [CrossRef]
57. He, H.; Tao, H.; Xiong, H.; Duan, S.Z.; McGowan, F.X., Jr.; Mortensen, R.M.; Balschi, J.A. Rosiglitazone causes cardiotoxicity via peroxisome proliferator-activated receptor gamma-independent mitochondrial oxidative stress in mouse hearts. *Toxicol. Sci.* **2014**, *138*, 468–481. [CrossRef]
58. Chen, Q.; Vazquez, E.J.; Moghaddas, S.; Hoppel, C.L.; Lesnefsky, E.J. Production of reactive oxygen species by mitochondria: Central role of complex III. *J. Biol. Chem.* **2003**, *278*, 36027–36031. [CrossRef]
59. Krenz, M.; Oldenburg, O.; Wimpee, H.; Cohen, M.V.; Garlid, K.D.; Critz, S.D.; Downey, J.M.; Benoit, J.N. Opening of ATP-sensitive potassium channels causes generation of free radicals in vascular smooth muscle cells. *Basic Res. Cardiol.* **2002**, *97*, 365–373. [CrossRef]

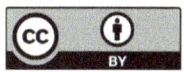

© 2020 by the authors. Licensee MDPI, Basel, Switzerland. This article is an open access article distributed under the terms and conditions of the Creative Commons Attribution (CC BY) license (http://creativecommons.org/licenses/by/4.0/).

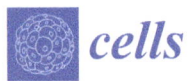

Article

Advanced Age Is Associated with Iron Dyshomeostasis and Mitochondrial DNA Damage in Human Skeletal Muscle

Anna Picca [1,2], Robert T. Mankowski [3], George Kamenov [4], Stephen D. Anton [3], Todd M. Manini [3], Thomas W. Buford [5], Sunil K. Saini [3], Riccardo Calvani [1,2], Francesco Landi [1,2], Roberto Bernabei [1,2], Emanuele Marzetti [1,2,*] and Christiaan Leeuwenburgh [3]

1. Institute of Internal Medicine and Geriatrics, Università Cattolica del Sacro Cuore, 00168 Rome, Italy; anna.picca1@gmail.com (A.P.); riccardo.calvani@gmail.com (R.C.); francesco.landi@unicatt.it (F.L.); roberto.bernabei@unicatt.it (R.B.)
2. Fondazione Policlinico Universitario "Agostino Gemelli" IRCCS, 00168 Rome, Italy
3. Department of Aging and Geriatric Research, Institute on Aging, University of Florida, Gainesville, FL 32611, USA; r.mankowski@ufl.edu (R.T.M.); santon@ufl.edu (S.D.A.); tmanini@ufl.edu (T.M.M.); sunil.saini@ufl.edu (S.K.S.); cleeuwen@ufl.edu (C.L.)
4. Department of Geological Sciences, University of Florida, Gainesville, FL 32605, USA; kamenov@ufl.edu
5. Department of Medicine, University of Alabama at Birmingham, Birmingham, AL 35205, USA; twbuford@uabmc.edu
* Correspondence: emanuele.marzetti@policlinicogemelli.it; Tel.: +39-(06)-3015-5559; Fax: +39-(06)-3051-911

Received: 21 October 2019; Accepted: 25 November 2019; Published: 27 November 2019

Abstract: Whether disruption of iron metabolism is implicated in human muscle aging is presently unclear. We explored the relationship among iron metabolism, muscle mitochondrial homeostasis, inflammation, and physical function in older adults and young controls. Eleven young and 23 older men and women were included. Older adults were classified into high–functioning (HF) and low–functioning (LF) groups according to their Short Physical Performance Battery score. Vastus lateralis muscle biopsies were assayed for total iron content, expression of 8-oxoguanine and DNA glycosylase (OGG1), 3-nitrotyrosine (3-NT) levels, and mitochondrial DNA (mtDNA) content and damage. Circulating ferritin and hepcidin levels were also quantified. Muscle iron levels were greater in the old group. Protein expression of transferrin receptor 1, Zrt-Irt-like protein (ZIP) 8, and ZIP14 were lower in old participants. Circulating levels of ferritin, hepcidin, interleukin 6 (IL6), and C-reactive protein were higher in the old group. Old participants showed lower mtDNA content and greater mtDNA damage. OGG1 protein expression declined with age, whereas 3-NT levels were greater in old participants. Finally, a negative correlation was determined between ZIP14 expression and circulating IL6 levels in LF older adults. None of assayed parameters differed between HF and LF participants. Our findings suggest that muscle iron homeostasis is altered in old age, which might contribute to loss of mtDNA stability. Muscle iron metabolism may therefore represent a target for interventions against muscle aging.

Keywords: iron overload; hepcidin; transferrin; ferritin; ZIP; inflammation; mtDNA; mitochondrial dysfunction; muscle aging; physical performance

1. Introduction

Iron is the most abundant transition metal in living organisms and is involved in multiple biochemical processes including oxygen binding and transport, energy production, regulation of cell growth and differentiation, and a variety of enzyme reactions. Most body iron is incorporated into haem proteins (e.g., haemoglobin, myoglobin, cytochromes, and haem thiolates). Non-haem iron serves instead as an enzyme cofactor (i.e., atomic iron) or iron reserve (e.g., bound to cytosolic ferritin and haemosiderin) and is integral to electron transport chain complexes (i.e., iron-sulphur clusters) and transferrin (Tf) [1,2]. Approximately 5% of cellular iron exists as chelatable non-haem iron, referred to as labile iron pool. This iron fraction consists of both ferrous (Fe^{2+}) and ferric (Fe^{3+}) ions associated with a variety of small molecules, including organic anions, polypeptides, and phospholipids. Fe^{2+} ions can participate in Fenton reactions thereby producing highly destructive radicals, which are thought to be major contributors to the generation of protein and DNA oxidative adducts [3–5]. Hence, a tight coordination encompassing iron absorption, uptake, efflux, and sequestration is crucial to preserve cell homeostasis.

Circulating iron is bound and transported by Tf. However, in the setting of iron overload, the iron-binding capacity of plasma Tf can be exceeded and accumulation of non-Tf-bound iron (NTBI) occurs [6]. As such, NTBI needs to be adequately disposed. Fourteen divalent metal transporters belonging to the Zrt-Irt-like protein (ZIP) family, named ZIP1 to ZIP 14, have been identified [7]. Of them, ZIP8 and ZIP14 have similar amino acid sequences [8] and contribute to the import of several divalent ions, including iron [9]. In particular, Zip14 mediates, at least in part, NTBI uptake by hepatocytes in the context of iron overload [10].

Iron metabolism is modulated by the defensin-like hormone hepcidin [11] via binding and subsequently degrading of the iron exporter ferroportin at the level of key iron sources [i.e., duodenal enterocytes (absorption of dietary iron), splenic and hepatic macrophages (recycling iron from erythrophagocytosis), and hepatocytes (iron stores)] [12]. In particular, circulating iron concentrations decrease as a consequence of intestinal absorption and release of iron from recycling macrophages [11].

Skeletal muscle is a major reservoir of body iron, which is comprised by 60% of non-haem fraction [13]. Studies have shown that non-haem iron accumulates in muscle during ageing possibly causing oxidative damage to biomolecules and organelles, including mitochondria [14–18]. As such, iron dyshomeostasis is advocated as a mechanism involved in the pathogenesis of sarcopaenia of ageing and disuse-induced muscle atrophy [19].

Along with iron imbalance and mitochondrial dysfunction, chronic inflammation is a hallmark of ageing and a factor involved in functional decline [20,21]. A link between mitochondrial damage and chronic low-grade inflammation has recently been hypothesised [21,22]. However, little is known about the relationship among iron dyshomeostasis, inflamm-ageing, mitochondrial dysfunction, and physical performance in older adults. To provide an initial appraisal of the subject, the present study was undertaken to assess total iron content, the expression of selected iron transporters, and indexes of mitochondrial damage in muscle biopsies obtained from healthy young adults and older people with varying levels of physical performance. The relationship between muscle iron content and systemic inflammation was also explored.

2. Materials and Methods

2.1. Participants

Participants were community-dwelling men and women aged 70 years or older. Healthy young adults between the ages of 18 and 35 years were recruited as controls. Participant recruitment was coordinated by the Recruitment Core of the University of Florida Claude D. Pepper Older Americans Independence Center, as detailed elsewhere [23–25].

A set of eligibility criteria was chosen to minimise the possible confounding effect of co-morbid conditions, medications, or lifestyle habits on the relationship among physical performance, iron metabolism, and indexes of muscle mitochondrial damage [26]. Briefly, candidates were not included if presenting with any of the following characteristics: smoking in prior 12 months; engagement in regular physical exercise; history of drug or alcohol abuse; active treatment for cancer or cancer in the past three years; heart failure New York Heart Association class III–IV; stroke with upper and/or lower extremity involvement; Parkinson's disease or other neurological disorders likely to interfere with physical function; major psychiatric illnesses; peripheral vascular disease Lériche–Fontaine stage 3–4; history of life-threatening cardiac arrhythmias; cognitive impairment (i.e., Mini Mental State Examination score ≤ 21); renal disease requiring dialysis; lung disease requiring steroids; chronic viral diseases (e.g., hepatitis B and C, HIV); lower extremity amputation; severe knee or hip osteoarthritis limiting mobility; diabetes with visual, vascular or neuropathic complications; inflammatory diseases (e.g., rheumatoid arthritis, vasculitis, autoimmune disorders, inflammatory bowel disease); taking growth hormone, oestrogen replacement, testosterone, anticoagulants, steroids, or non–steroidal anti–inflammatory drugs on a regular basis; severe obesity [i.e., body mass index (BMI) ≥35]; underweight (i.e., BMI ≤18.5); active weight loss >5 kg in prior three months; life–threatening illnesses with an estimated life expectancy <1 year. Candidates on statin treatment were asked to refrain from drug administration one month prior to blood drawn upon their general practitioner's approval.

Old enrolees were categorised as high–functioning (HF) and low–functioning (LF) based on their Short Physical Performance Battery (SPPB) summary score [27]. Specifically, participants with a SPPB score ≥11 were classified as HF, while those who scored ≤7 were categorised as LF. These cut-offs were selected based on their ability to predict several relevant health outcomes in older adults (e.g., functional limitations, institutionalisation, mortality) [27–31]. Individuals scoring 8–10 on the SPPB were excluded to allow greater discrimination in physical function and possibly biochemical parameters between groups.

Prior to enrolment in the study, all participants provided written informed consent. The study protocol was approved by the University of Florida's Institutional Review Board (IRB201300790).

2.2. Blood Collection and Processing

Blood samples were obtained in the morning by venipuncture of the median cubital vein after overnight fasting, using commercial ethylenediaminetetraacetic acid (EDTA) collection tubes (BD Medical, Franklin Lakes, NJ, USA). Samples were immediately centrifuged at 1000× g for 10 min at 4 °C, aliquots were prepared, and stored at −80 °C until analysis.

2.3. Collection of Muscle Biopsies

Muscle samples were obtained from the vastus lateralis of the dominant lower extremity by percutaneous needle biopsy, under local anaesthesia, as previously described [25]. Muscle specimens were cleaned of any visible blood and fat, snap-frozen in liquid nitrogen, and subsequently stored at −80 °C until analysis.

2.4. Measurement of Circulating Iron Transporters and Inflammatory Biomarkers

Plasma levels of the iron transporter ferritin and the iron regulator hepcidin as well as those of C-reactive protein (CRP) and interleukin (IL) 6 were measured using enzyme-linked immunosorbent assays (ferritin: Human ELISA Kit, Thermo Scientific (Waltham, MA, USA); hepcidin: Intrinsic Hepcidin IDx™ ELISA Kit, Intrinsic LifeSciences (La Jolla, CA, USA); CRP: Human C-Reactive Protein/CRP Quantikine ELISA Kit, R&D Systems (Minneapolis, MN, USA); IL6: Human IL-6 Quantikine HS ELISA Kit, R&D Systems). Plate processing and data collection were carried out according to the manufacturer's instructions. Absorbance was read on a Synergy HT Multi-Detection microplate reader (BioTek, Winooski, VT, USA). Concentrations of ferritin, hepcidin, and CRP are shown as ng/mL, whilst IL6 levels are reported in pg/mL.

2.5. Inductively Coupled Plasma-Mass Spectrometry (ICP-MS) Determination of Total Iron in Muscle Biopsies

Total iron content in muscle samples was determined by ICP-MS as described previously with modifications [32]. Briefly, 15–30 mg of vastus lateralis muscle samples were digested in 1 mL concentrated nitric acid (HNO_3 Optima-grade) in capped Teflon (Savillex Corporation, Eden Prairie, MN, USA) vials for 24 h. Afterwards, 1 mL of 30% hydrogen peroxide (H_2O_2 Optima-grade) was added to each vial and placed opened on a hot plate (100 °C) to let the mixture evaporate. Subsequently,

1 mL of HNO$_3$ and 1 mL of H$_2$O$_2$ were added to the dry residue and incubated on the hot plate (100 °C) overnight to digest any remaining organic material. After this second digestion, samples were evaporated to dryness, followed by addition of 0.8 N HNO$_3$ spiked with 8 parts per billion (ppb) rhenium (Re) and rhodium (Rh). Vials were then incubated at 100 °C overnight to ensure complete dissolution. A fraction of the sample solution was removed and further diluted with 0.8 N HNO$_3$ spiked with 8 ppb Re and Rh to obtain a final dilution of approximately 300×. The exact final dilution for elemental analyses was achieved according to the weight of each sample. Trace element analysis was conducted on a Thermo Finnigan Element2™ high–resolution ICP-MS (Thermo Fisher Scientific, San Jose, CA, USA) in medium resolution using Re and Rh as internal standards. In order to avoid analytical biases, all samples were run in the same day and in the same sequence. Results were quantified by external calibration using a combination of gravimetrically prepared ICP-MS standards obtained from QCD Analysts (www.qcdanalysts.com). Iron concentrations are reported in parts per million (ppm), with an analytical error < ±5%.

2.6. Western Immunoblotting

Protein content of Tf receptor 1 (TFR1), ZIP8, ZIP14, and 8-oxoguanine DNA glycosylase (OGG1), and levels of 3-nitrotyrosine (3-NT) were measured in muscle samples by Western immunoblotting. Whole-tissue extracts were prepared as described elsewhere [24]. Briefly, 50 µg proteins were separated on 12%–15% polyacrylamide gels (Bio-Rad Laboratories, Hercules, CA, USA), transferred onto polyvinylidene difluoride membranes (Bio-Rad Laboratories), and blocked for 1 h in 5% milk in Tris-buffered saline Tween (Bio-Rad Laboratories). Blots were probed with commercially available primary antibodies for OGG1 (1:2500, Abcam, Cambridge, MA, USA; #ab63942), TFR1 (1:1000, Cell Signaling Technology, Beverly, MA, USA; #13113), ZIP14 (1:1000, Sigma–Aldrich, St. Louis, MO, USA; #HPA016508), and 3-NT (1:1000, Cell Signaling Technology; #9691S). A custom-made polyclonal rabbit primary antibody was used for detecting ZIP8 (1:1000). The antibody was raised to a peptide [(NH$_2$) FGNDNFGPQEKT (COOH)] selected from the full-length sequence [33] designed by Dr. Tolunay Beker Aydemir (University of Florida, Gainesville, FL, USA) who also performed the purification [34]. To allow affinity purification, a cysteine residue was added to the N terminus for coupling to the carrier protein and for conjugation to Sulfolink (Pierce, Rockford, IL, USA). The antibody was prepared in rabbit as previously described [35]. Anti-rabbit secondary antibody conjugated with horseradish peroxidase (1:10000, Cell Signaling Technology; #7074) was used to enable subsequent protein detection. Protein bands were visualised with SuperSignal West Femto Maximum Sensitivity Substrate (Thermo Scientific) using a ChemiDoc XRS imager (Bio-Rad Laboratories). Spot density of the target bands was normalised to the amount of protein loaded in each lane, as determined by densitometric analysis of the corresponding Ponceau S-stained membranes [36]. Bands were quantified using Image Lab 6.0 software (Bio-Rad Laboratories) according to the "Total Lane Protein" setting.

2.7. Quantification of Mitochondrial DNA (mtDNA) Content

Genomic DNA was purified from muscle samples using a Wizard Genomic DNA Purification Kit according to the manufacturer's instructions (Promega, Madison, WI, USA). Briefly, 10–20 mg of muscle tissue were homogenised in 1 mL of nuclei cell lysis solution using a hard tissue disposable probe (Omni international, Kennesaw, GA, USA) on a PowerGen 500 homogenator (Thermo Fisher Scientific). Total DNA quantification was carried out on a NanoDrop 1000 spectrophotometer (Thermo Fisher Scientific) and integrity was verified by gel electrophoresis on 0.8% agarose gel in 1× Tris-borate-EDTA (TBE) (90 mM Tris-borate pH 7.4, 90 mM boric acid, 2.5 mM EDTA). Determination of mtDNA content was performed with the Human Mitochondrial DNA Monitoring Primer Kit (Takara Bio, Mountain View, CA, USA) using real-time polymerase chain reaction (RT-PCR). Amplification reactions were run on a CFX96 Touch™ Real-Time PCR Detection System (Bio-Rad Laboratories). Primers included in the kit specifically amplified mitochondrial genes corresponding to mitochondrial NADH dehydrogenase subunit 1 and 5 (ND1, ND5) and nuclear genes corresponding to solute carrier organic anion transporter family, member 2b1 (SLCO2B1), and serpin family A member 1 (SERPINA1) [37]. Melting curve analysis, non-template control reactions, and gel electrophoresis of PCR products were used to check amplification specificity of each experiment. Each sample was analysed in triplicate in 20 µL final volume. The reaction mixture consisted of 1× Terra qPCR Direct SYBR Premix (Takara Bio), 0.2 µM forward and reverse primers, and 10 ng of genomic DNA template. Amplification proceeded for 40 cycles. Quantification of relative mtDNA content was accomplished according to the Pfaffl mathematical model [38]. Differences in threshold cycle values for the ND1/SLCO2B1 pair ($\Delta Ct1$ = Ct for SLCO2B1 − Ct for ND1) and the ND5/SERPINA1 pair ($\Delta Ct2$ = Ct for SERPINA1 − Ct for ND5) were calculated, and the average of $2^{\Delta Ct}$ for the values of $\Delta Ct1$ and $\Delta Ct2$ was used as a measure of relative mtDNA abundance.

2.8. Analysis of mtDNA Damage

Quantitative RT-PCR was used to assess mtDNA damage according to the method described by Furda et al. [39] with minor adjustments. Briefly, 225 ng of purified total DNA was digested with PvuII Restriction enzyme (New England Biolabs, Ipswich, UK). Fifteen ng of digested DNA were used to amplify a 8.9-kb mtDNA fragment (accession number: J01415; 5' sense position: 5999; 5' antisense position: 14841) [39] with a TaKaRa LA Taq® DNA Polymerase with GC Buffer (Takara Bio) and a 221-bp mtDNA fragment (accession number: J01415; 5' sense position: 14620; 5' antisense position: 14841) [39] with a DreamTaq DNA Polymerase (Thermo Fisher Scientific). Amplification was carried out using a CFX96 Touch™ PCR Detection System (Bio-Rad Laboratories) as described by Furda et al. [39]. Each sample was analysed in triplicate in 20 µL final volume. The reaction mixture for the 8.9-kb mtDNA fragment consisted of 1× GC Buffer I, 2U TaKaRa LA Taq® DNA Polymerase (Takara Bio), 0.2 mM dNTPs, and 0.4 µM forward and reverse primers. The reaction mixture for the 221-bp mtDNA fragment included 1× DreamTaq Buffer (Thermo Fisher Scientific), 0.2 mM dNTPs, and 0.4 µM forward and reverse primers. Prior to quantification, amplification products of the 8.9-kb and the 221-bp fragments were electrophoresed on 0.8% agarose and 1.5% agarose gels, respectively, to check for PCR product specificity. Amplicons were quantified by Pico-Green (Thermo Fisher Scientific) using a Synergy HT multidetection microplate reader (BioTek) with excitation and emission wavelengths at 485 and 530 nm, respectively. Data obtained from the 221-bp mtDNA fragment were used to normalise results of the 8.9-kb fragment amplification. The number of mtDNA lesions was calculated using the equation: $D = [1 - 2^{-(\Delta 8.9\text{-kb} - \Delta 221\text{-bp})}] \times 10{,}000 \text{ bp}/8900 \text{ bp}$ [40].

2.9. Statistical Analysis

The normal distribution of data was ascertained through the Kolmogorov–Smirnov test. Comparisons for normally distributed continuous variables were performed by one-way analysis of variance (ANOVA) followed by Tukey's post-hoc test when applicable. The non-parametric tests Mann–Whitney U and Kruskal–Wallis H (with Dunns' post-hoc test as appropriate) were applied to assess differences for non-normally distributed continuous data. Differences in categorical variables among groups were determined via χ^2 statistics. Correlations between variables were explored via Pearson's or Spearman's tests as appropriate. All analyses were performed using the GraphPrism 5.03 software (GraphPad Software, Inc., San Diego, CA, USA), with statistical significance set at $p < 0.05$.

3. Results

3.1. Characteristics of Study Participants

A total of 34 volunteers were enrolled, 11 young (six men and five women; mean age: 24.7 ± 4.4 years) and 23 older persons (14 men and nine women; mean age: 77.5 ± 8.0 years). Participant characteristics according to age groups and physical performance categories are shown in Table 1. No differences were observed among groups for gender distribution, BMI, or number of disease conditions and medications. The two subgroups of older adults did not differ for age. As per the study design, HF participants showed higher SPPB scores than LF older adults ($p = 0.0002$).

Table 1. Participant characteristics according to age groups and physical performance categories.

Characteristic	Young ($n = 11$)	Old ($n = 23$)		p Value
		HF ($n = 16$)	LF ($n = 7$)	
Age (years), mean ± SD	24.7 ± 4.4	76.0 ± 6.0 *	81.0 ± 3.7 *	<0.0001
Gender (female), n (%)	5 (45.5)	4 (25.0)	5 (71.4)	0.1076
BMI (kg/m^2), mean ± SD	24.9 ± 4.2	27.7 ± 3.6	27.8 ± 4.2	0.1604
Number of diseases ¥, mean ± SD	1.0 ± 0.8	1.9 ± 1.4	2.1 ± 1.8	0.1274
Number of medications #, mean ± SD	2.9 ± 2.6	3.7 ± 3.2	1.7 ± 1.4	0.3112
SPPB summary score, mean ± SD	–	11.4 ± 0.5	6.1 ± 1.7 §	0.0002

Abbreviations: BMI, body mass index; HF, high functioning; LF, low functioning; SD, standard deviation; SPPB, Short Physical Performance Battery. * $p < 0.05$ vs. young group. § $p < 0.05$ vs. HF. ¥ includes hypertension, coronary artery disease, prior stroke, peripheral vascular disease, diabetes, chronic obstructive pulmonary disease, and osteoarthritis. # includes prescription and over-the-counter drugs.

3.2. Quantification of Total Iron and Selected Metal Transporters in Vastus Lateralis Muscle Biopsies

To evaluate whether iron levels in muscle were associated with age and physical performance, total iron content was quantified by ICP-MS. Iron levels were significantly greater in muscles of old enrolees compared with the young group ($p < 0.05$), with no differences between SPPB categories (Figure 1).

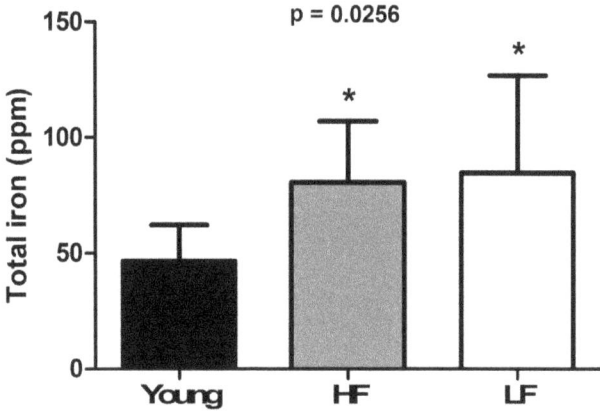

Figure 1. Total content of iron in the vastus lateralis muscle of young and old participants. Bars represent mean values (± standard deviation) in the three experimental groups. Values are expressed in ppm. * $p < 0.05$ vs. young group ($n = 11$). HF: high-functioning ($n = 16$); LF: low-functioning ($n = 7$).

Protein levels of selected iron transporters (TFR1, ZIP8, and ZIP14) were assayed by Western immunoblotting. The expression of TFR1, the primary cellular iron importer, was significantly lower in old LF participants compared with the young group ($p < 0.05$; Figure 2A). Also, lower protein levels of ZIP8 were detected in old enrolees compared with their younger counterparts (Figure 2B). A pattern similar to TFR1 was found for ZIP14 ($p < 0.05$; Figure 2C).

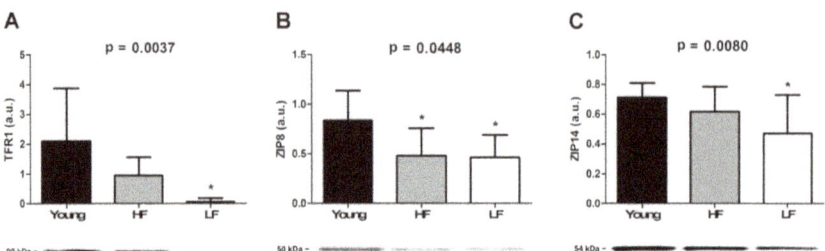

Figure 2. Protein expression of (**A**) transferrin receptor 1 (TFR1), (**B**) Zrt-Irt-like protein (ZIP) 8, and (**C**) ZIP14 in the vastus lateralis muscle of young and old participants. Bars represent mean values (±standard deviation) in the three experimental groups. Values are expressed in arbitrary units (a.u.). Representative blots are shown. * $p < 0.05$ vs. young group ($n = 11$). HF: high-functioning ($n = 16$); LF: low-functioning ($n = 7$).

3.3. Circulating Levels of Ferritin, Hepcidin, and Selected Inflammatory Biomarkers

Perturbations in iron status have been associated with chronic low-grade inflammation during ageing [41]. In turn, inflammation is acknowledged as a major mechanism contributing to functional impairment [42]. We, therefore, verified whether circulating levels of ferritin, hepcidin, and selected inflammatory biomarkers were associated with age and functional status.

An age-dependent increase was observed for plasma ferritin concentrations ($p = 0.0291$; Figure 3A), with no differences between SPPB categories. Circulating levels of the defensin-like hormone hepcidin were also increased with age ($p = 0.0232$; Figure 3B). The post-hoc test revealed significantly higher hepcidin concentrations in LF older adults compared with young enrolees.

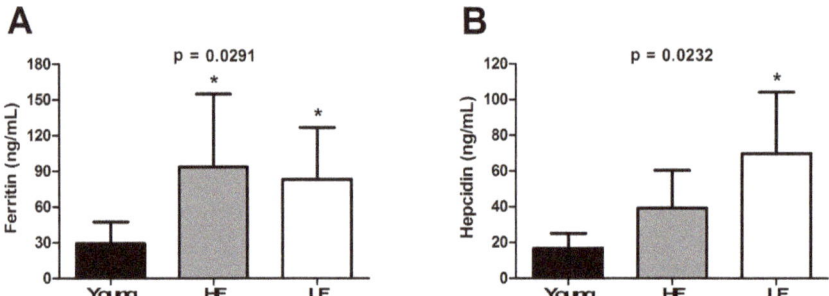

Figure 3. Plasma levels of (**A**) ferritin and (**B**) hepcidin in young and old participants. Bars represent mean values (± standard deviation) in the three experimental groups. * $p < 0.05$ vs. young group ($n = 11$). HF: high-functioning ($n = 16$); LF: low-functioning ($n = 7$).

A similar pattern was described for plasma IL6 ($p = 0.0174$; Figure 4A) and CRP ($p = 0.0488$; Figure 4B).

We performed a correlation analysis to test the hypothesis of an association between inflammation and iron status in LF older adults. As reported in Table 2, ZIP14 was the only iron transporter showing a significant negative correlation with IL6.

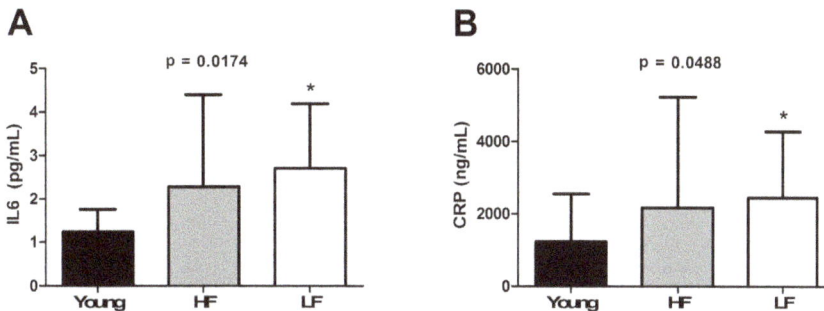

Figure 4. Plasma levels of (**A**) interleukin 6 (IL6) and (**B**) C-reactive protein (CRP) in young and old participants. Bars represent mean values (±standard deviation) in the three experimental groups. * $p < 0.05$ vs. young group ($n = 11$). HF: high-functioning ($n = 16$); LF: low-functioning ($n = 7$).

Table 2. Relationship between plasma concentrations of IL6 and protein expression of iron transporters in muscle in old low-functioning participants.

	TFR1	ZIP14	ZIP8
Pearson r	−0.09161	−0.9976	0.5968
95% confidence interval	−0.8408–0.7779	0.0444	−0.4167–0.9488
R square	0.008392	0.9951	0.3561
p value (two-tailed)	0.863	0.0444	0.2111

Abbreviations: TFR1, transferrin receptor 1, ZIP, Zrt-Irt-like protein.

3.4. Determination of mtDNA Content and Damage

mtDNA homeostasis in muscle becomes impaired during ageing and in the setting of atrophying conditions [43]. However, whether the abundance and integrity of mtDNA in muscle are associated with physical function in old age is still debated [44]. In the attempt to shed light on this relevant research question, we determined the relative content of mtDNA and mtDNA damage load in muscle samples of young and old enrollees. As depicted in Figure 5, older participants showed lower mtDNA content ($p = 0.0012$, Figure 5A) and greater mtDNA damage ($p = 0.0001$, Figure 5B) compared with young controls, with no differences between HF and LF individuals.

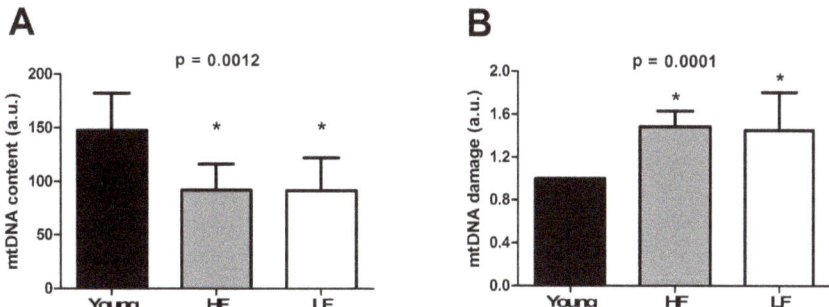

Figure 5. (**A**) mtDNA content and (**B**) mtDNA damage in the vastus lateralis muscle of young and old participants. Bars represent mean values (± standard deviation) in the three experimental groups. * $p < 0.05$ vs. young group ($n = 11$). HF: high-functioning ($n = 16$); LF: low-functioning ($n = 7$).

3.5. Protein Levels of Selected Markers of Oxidative/Nitrosative Damage

Protein expression of the repair enzyme OGG1 and levels of nitrosative stress-associated 3-NT were determined in muscle samples to obtain indications on the extent of oxidative-related molecular damage [45].

OGG1 protein expression declined with ageing ($p = 0.0435$), with no differences among individual groups (Figure 6A). An age-related increase in 3-NT levels was observed ($p = 0.0005$, Figure 6B), without differences between the two old groups.

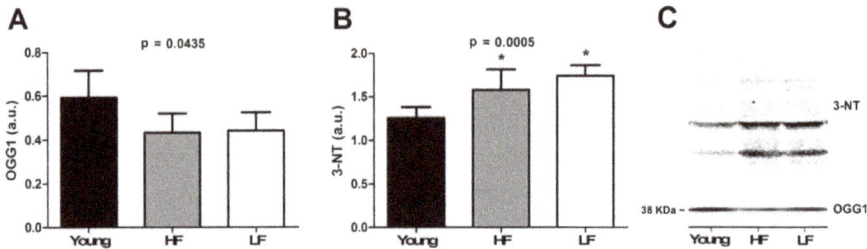

Figure 6. Protein expression of (**A**) 8-oxoguanine DNA glycosylase (OGG1) and (**B**) levels of 3-nitrotyrosine (3-NT) in the vastus lateralis muscle of young and old participants. Bars represent mean values (±standard deviation) in the three experimental groups. Representative blots of OGG1 and 3-NT are shown in panel (**C**) a.u. arbitrary units. * $p < 0.05$ vs. young group ($n = 11$). HF: high functioning ($n = 16$); LF: low functioning ($n = 7$).

4. Discussion

Iron homeostasis is altered in muscle of old rodents, possibly contributing to muscle fibre atrophy and loss via oxidative stress-mediated signalling pathways [18]. A specific form of non-apoptotic cell death, referred to as ferroptosis, seems to occur upon intracellular iron overload, causing oxidative injury which probably involves lipid peroxidation [46]. This iron-driven cell death may operate via mitochondrial and NADPH-dependent oxidases reactive oxygen species burst [46]. However, to the best of our knowledge, the relationship between iron status and physical function in old people was not previously explored.

Studies from our group showed increased levels of muscle non-haem iron, including labile fraction, with age in old rats following hind limb suspension [18]. Such changes were associated with elevated expression of ferritin and decreased TFR1 content [18]. Age-dependent iron accumulation was also reported in muscle subsarcolemmal mitochondria of rats [47]. Notably, mitochondrial iron levels were shown to impact organelle RNA damage as well as the susceptibility to opening of the mitochondrial permeability transition pore [47]. This prompted us to test the hypothesis of a relationship between iron status and age-related functional decline involving muscular mitochondrial damage.

Our finding of an age-dependent accumulation of iron in skeletal muscle (Figure 1) paralleled by decreased expression of two of the three metal importers assayed (i.e., TFR1 and ZIP14) in the LF group (Figure 2A–C) supports the idea of a link between iron dyshomeostasis in muscle and functional status. The analysis of iron-related circulating factors offered further insights into this association. Indeed, ferritin levels, an indicator of stored iron, were found to be higher in both HF and LF older adults (Figure 3A), which might arise from chronic inflammation [48]. This view is consistent with our observation of an age-dependent elevation of plasma IL6 and CRP, the levels of which were both higher in LF relative to HF participants (Figure 4A,B).

Although in apparent contrast to our original hypothesis, the measurement of circulating levels of hepcidin provided interesting information regarding such an association. This defensin-like hormone, produced mainly by the liver, plays a major role in modulating iron metabolism [11]. Indeed, via binding to the iron exporter ferroportin at the level of key iron sources [i.e., duodenal enterocytes (absorption of dietary iron), splenic and hepatic macrophages (recycling iron from erythrophagocytosis), and hepatocytes (iron stores)], hepcidin induces its own endocytosis and lysosomal degradation as well as of ferroportin [12]. As a consequence, decreased intestinal absorption and release of iron from recycling macrophages occur, ultimately resulting in lower circulating iron concentrations [11].

In the present investigation, higher levels of hepcidin were found in older participants, especially in those classified as LF (Figure 3B), with a parallel increase in IL6 and CRP (Figure 4A,B). These results are in line with previous reports pointing to IL6 as a major hepcidin inducer in older adults [49–51], in whom it may be responsible for iron-limited erythropoiesis [52,53]. Whether inflammation reduces iron availability for myoglobin assembly, thereby contributing to impairing muscle function, is presently unknown. Further support to the link among inflammation, iron status, and functional impairment is lent by the strong negative correlation ($r = -0.99$, $p = 0.04$) between circulating IL6 levels and muscle expression of ZIP14 in LF older participants (Table 2). Although our experimental design does not allow inferring about a direct involvement of ZIP14 in muscle iron clearance, a link between ZIP14 expression and IL6 induction has previously been reported and a role for ZIP14 in iron uptake has been hypothesised [54].

A hepcidin-independent regulation of iron status with ageing cannot be excluded. Indeed, studies conducted in older adults with anaemia and chronic inflammation did not detect increased levels of hepcidin in urine or serum [55,56]. In this context, the co-occurrence of multiple age-related conditions may explain changes in the iron status [57,58]. This could be the case for higher circulating ferritin levels in HF participants, which may result, for instance, from the stimulation of ferritin expression by reactive species [59,60].

mtDNA content and damage (Figure 5A,B) as well as the expression of OGG1, one major enzymatic system of mtDNA base excision repair, and 3-NT (Figure 6A,B) showed an age-related association rather than changes dependent on functional status. These findings are in line with previous results in other aged post-mitotic tissues [61].

Taken as a whole, results from the present study suggest that altered iron metabolism during ageing may predispose to oxidant generation and damage to cell components, including mitochondria. In particular, the association of iron dyshomeostasis with systemic inflammation might represent a kingmaker towards functional decline. Disruption of iron metabolism in myocytes might therefore represent a novel target for interventions aimed at preserving muscle health in old age.

5. Limitations of the Study

While reporting novel findings, our work is not devoid of limitations that need to be discussed. First of all, the study is exploratory in nature due to the small sample size and the limited amount of muscle tissue available for analyses. In addition, the cross-sectional design hampers inference about the time course of changes in analysed mediators and the development of functional decline. Also, only total iron levels were measured and no information is available about haem and non-haem iron. Likewise, neither haemoglobin levels nor mean corpuscular haemoglobin concentration in erythrocytes were measured. Furthermore, plasma iron levels, Tf affinity and saturation, and ferritin capacity were not assessed, which impeded a comprehensive appraisal of body iron homeostasis. Finally, the study did not include a group of actively exercising older people. Both categories of old participants were physically inactive and this did not allow appreciating the possible effect of physical activity on iron status in muscle in old age.

Author Contributions: Conceptualization, A.P. and R.T.M.; methodology, A.P. and R.T.M.; formal analysis, A.P., E.M., R.C., T.M.M., and T.W.B.; investigation, A.P., G.K., and S.K.S.; resources, C.L., F.L., and R.B.; data curation, R.T.M.; writing—original draft preparation, A.P., E.M., and S.D.A.; writing—review and editing, C.L. and R.C.; supervision, E.M. and C.L.; funding acquisition, C.L., F.L., and R.B.

Funding: This research was funded by the National Institute on Aging [R01AG17994], Innovative Medicines Initiative-Joint Undertaking [IMI-JU #115621], Intramural Research Grants from the Università Cattolica del Sacro Cuore [D3.2 2013 and D3.2 2015], and the nonprofit research foundation "Centro Studi Achille e Linda Lorenzon".

Acknowledgments: The authors thank Robert J. Cousins (Dept. of Food Sciences and Human Nutrition, University of Florida. Gainesville, FL) for providing insightful scientific inputs on metal transporters.

Conflicts of Interest: The authors declare no conflict of interest.

References

1. Maio, N.; Rouault, T.A. Iron-sulfur cluster biogenesis in mammalian cells: New insights into the molecular mechanisms of cluster delivery. *Biochim. Biophys. Acta* **2015**, *1853*, 1493–1512. [CrossRef]
2. Kohgo, Y.; Ikuta, K.; Ohtake, T.; Torimoto, Y.; Kato, J. Body iron metabolism and pathophysiology of iron overload. *Int. J. Hematol.* **2008**, *88*, 7–15. [CrossRef] [PubMed]
3. Papanikolaou, G.; Pantopoulos, K. Iron metabolism and toxicity. *Toxicol. Appl. Pharmacol.* **2005**, *202*, 199–211. [CrossRef] [PubMed]
4. Bresgen, N.; Eckl, P.M. Oxidative stress and the homeodynamics of iron metabolism. *Biomolecules* **2015**, *5*, 808–847. [CrossRef]
5. Emerit, J.; Beaumont, C.; Trivin, F. Iron metabolism, free radicals, and oxidative injury. *Biomed. Pharmacother.* **2001**, *55*, 333–339. [CrossRef]
6. Hentze, M.W.; Muckenthaler, M.U.; Andrews, N.C. Balancing acts: Molecular control of mammalian iron metabolism. *Cell* **2004**, *117*, 285–297. [CrossRef]
7. Lichten, L.A.; Cousins, R.J. Mammalian zinc transporters: Nutritional and physiologic regulation. *Annu. Rev. Nutr.* **2009**, *29*, 153–176. [CrossRef] [PubMed]
8. Taylor, K.M.; Morgan, H.E.; Johnson, A.; Nicholson, R.I. Structure-function analysis of a novel member of the LIV-1 subfamily of zinc transporters, ZIP14. *FEBS Lett.* **2005**, *579*, 427–432. [CrossRef] [PubMed]
9. Gao, J.; Zhao, N.; Knutson, M.D.; Enns, C.A. The hereditary hemochromatosis protein, HFE, inhibits iron uptake via down-regulation of Zip14 in HepG2 cells. *J. Biol. Chem.* **2008**, *283*, 21462–21468. [CrossRef] [PubMed]
10. Liuzzi, J.P.; Aydemir, F.; Nam, H.; Knutson, M.D.; Cousins, R.J. Zip14 (Slc39a14) mediates non-transferrin-bound iron uptake into cells. *Proc. Natl. Acad. Sci. USA* **2006**, *103*, 13612–13617. [CrossRef]
11. Ganz, T.; Nemeth, E. Hepcidin and disorders of iron metabolism. *Annu. Rev. Med.* **2011**, *62*, 347–360. [CrossRef] [PubMed]
12. Nemeth, E.; Tuttle, M.S.; Powelson, J.; Vaughn, M.B.; Donovan, A.; Ward, D.M.; Ganz, T.; Kaplan, J. Hepcidin regulates cellular iron efflux by binding to ferroportin and inducing its internalization. *Science* **2004**, *306*, 2090–2093. [CrossRef]
13. Chen, L.H.; Thacker, R.R. Effects of dietary vitamin E and high level of ascorbic acid on iron distribution in rat tissues. *Int. J. Vitam. Nutr. Res.* **1986**, *56*, 253–258. [PubMed]
14. Altun, M.; Edström, E.; Spooner, E.; Flores-Moralez, A.; Bergman, E.; Tollet-Egnell, P.; Norstedt, G.; Kessler, B.M.; Ulfhake, B. Iron load and redox stress in skeletal muscle of aged rats. *Muscle Nerve* **2007**, *36*, 223–233. [CrossRef] [PubMed]
15. Hofer, T.; Marzetti, E.; Xu, J.; Seo, A.Y.; Gulec, S.; Knutson, M.D.; Leeuwenburgh, C.; Dupont-Versteegden, E.E. Increased iron content and RNA oxidative damage in skeletal muscle with aging and disuse atrophy. *Exp. Gerontol.* **2008**, *43*, 563–570. [CrossRef]
16. Jung, S.H.; DeRuisseau, L.R.; Kavazis, A.N.; DeRuisseau, K.C. Plantaris muscle of aged rats demonstrates iron accumulation and altered expression of iron regulation proteins. *Exp. Physiol.* **2008**, *93*, 407–414. [CrossRef]
17. Xu, J.; Knutson, M.D.; Carter, C.S.; Leeuwenburgh, C. Iron accumulation with age, oxidative stress and functional decline. *PLoS ONE* **2008**, *3*, e2865. [CrossRef]
18. Xu, J.; Hwang, J.C.Y.; Lees, H.A.; Wohlgemuth, S.E.; Knutson, M.D.; Judge, A.R.; Dupont-Versteegden, E.E.; Marzetti, E.; Leeuwenburgh, C. Long-term perturbation of muscle iron homeostasis following hindlimb suspension in old rats is associated with high levels of oxidative stress and impaired recovery from atrophy. *Exp. Gerontol.* **2012**, *47*, 100–118. [CrossRef]
19. Xu, J.; Marzetti, E.; Seo, A.Y.; Kim, J.-S.; Prolla, T.A.; Leeuwenburgh, C. The emerging role of iron dyshomeostasis in the mitochondrial decay of aging. *Mech. Ageing Dev.* **2010**, *131*, 487–493. [CrossRef]
20. López-Otín, C.; Blasco, M.A.; Partridge, L.; Serrano, M.; Kroemer, G. The hallmarks of aging. *Cell* **2013**, *153*, 1194–1217. [CrossRef]

21. Picca, A.; Lezza, A.M.S.; Leeuwenburgh, C.; Pesce, V.; Calvani, R.; Landi, F.; Bernabei, R.; Marzetti, E. Fueling inflamm-aging through mitochondrial dysfunction: Mechanisms and molecular targets. *Int. J. Mol. Sci.* **2017**, *18*, 933. [CrossRef]
22. Picca, A.; Lezza, A.M.S.; Leeuwenburgh, C.; Pesce, V.; Calvani, R.; Bossola, M.; Manes-Gravina, E.; Landi, F.; Bernabei, R.; Marzetti, E. Circulating mitochondrial DNA at the crossroads of mitochondrial dysfunction and inflammation during aging and muscle wasting disorders. *Rejuvenation Res.* **2018**, *21*, 350–359. [CrossRef] [PubMed]
23. Buford, T.W.; Lott, D.J.; Marzetti, E.; Wohlgemuth, S.E.; Vandenborne, K.; Pahor, M.; Leeuwenburgh, C.; Manini, T.M. Age-related differences in lower extremity tissue compartments and associations with physical function in older adults. *Exp. Gerontol.* **2012**, *47*, 38–44. [CrossRef] [PubMed]
24. Joseph, A.-M.; Adhihetty, P.J.; Buford, T.W.; Wohlgemuth, S.E.; Lees, H.A.; Nguyen, L.M.-D.M.-D.; Aranda, J.M.; Sandesara, B.D.; Pahor, M.; Manini, T.M.; et al. The impact of aging on mitochondrial function and biogenesis pathways in skeletal muscle of sedentary high and low functioning elderly individuals. *Aging Cell* **2012**, *11*, 801–809. [CrossRef] [PubMed]
25. Marzetti, E.; Lees, H.A.; Manini, T.M.; Buford, T.W.; Aranda, J.M.; Calvani, R.; Capuani, G.; Marsiske, M.; Lott, D.J.; Vandenborne, K.; et al. Skeletal muscle apoptotic signaling predicts thigh muscle volume and gait speed in community-dwelling older persons: An exploratory study. *PLoS ONE* **2012**, *7*, e32829. [CrossRef] [PubMed]
26. Marzetti, E.; Landi, F.; Marini, F.; Cesari, M.; Buford, T.W.; Manini, T.M.; Onder, G.; Pahor, M.; Bernabei, R.; Leeuwenburgh, C.; et al. Patterns of circulating inflammatory biomarkers in older persons with varying levels of physical performance: A partial least squares-discriminant analysis approach. *Front. Med.* **2014**, *1*, 27. [CrossRef]
27. Guralnik, J.M.; Simonsick, E.M.; Ferrucci, L.; Glynn, R.J.; Berkman, L.F.; Blazer, D.G.; Scherr, P.A.; Wallace, R.B. A short physical performance battery assessing lower extremity function: Association with self-reported disability and prediction of mortality and nursing home admission. *J. Gerontol.* **1994**, *49*, M85–M94. [CrossRef]
28. Vasunilashorn, S.; Coppin, A.K.; Patel, K.V.; Lauretani, F.; Ferrucci, L.; Bandinelli, S.; Guralnik, J.M. Use of the Short Physical Performance Battery Score to predict loss of ability to walk 400 m: Analysis from the InCHIANTI study. *J. Gerontol. A Biol. Sci. Med. Sci.* **2009**, *64*, 223–229. [CrossRef]
29. Studenski, S.; Perera, S.; Patel, K.; Rosano, C.; Faulkner, K.; Inzitari, M.; Brach, J.; Chandler, J.; Cawthon, P.; Connor, E.B.; et al. Gait speed and survival in older adults. *JAMA* **2011**, *305*, 50–58. [CrossRef]
30. Pahor, M.; Guralnik, J.M.; Ambrosius, W.T.; Blair, S.; Bonds, D.E.; Church, T.S.; Espeland, M.A.; Fielding, R.A.; Gill, T.M.; Groessl, E.J.; et al. LIFE study investigators. Effect of structured physical activity on prevention of major mobility disability in older adults: The LIFE study randomized clinical trial. *JAMA* **2014**, *311*, 2387–2396. [CrossRef]
31. Marzetti, E.; Cesari, M.; Calvani, R.; Msihid, J.; Tosato, M.; Rodriguez-Mañas, L.; Lattanzio, F.; Cherubini, A.; Bejuit, R.; Di Bari, M.; et al. The "Sarcopenia and Physical fRailty IN older people: Multi-componenT Treatment strategies" (SPRINTT) randomized controlled trial: Case finding, screening and characteristics of eligible participants. *Exp. Gerontol.* **2018**, *113*, 48–57. [CrossRef]
32. Li, M.; Zhang, Y.; Liu, Z.; Bharadwaj, U.; Wang, H.; Wang, X.; Zhang, S.; Liuzzi, J.P.; Chang, S.-M.; Cousins, R.J.; et al. Aberrant expression of zinc transporter ZIP4 (SLC39A4) significantly contributes to human pancreatic cancer pathogenesis and progression. *Proc. Natl. Acad. Sci. USA* **2007**, *104*, 18636–18641. [CrossRef] [PubMed]
33. Begum, N.A.; Kobayashi, M.; Moriwaki, Y.; Matsumoto, M.; Toyoshima, K.; Seya, T. Mycobacterium bovis BCG cell wall and lipopolysaccharide induce a novel gene, BIGM103, encoding a 7-TM protein: Identification of a new protein family having Zn-transporter and Zn-metalloprotease signatures. *Genomics* **2002**, *80*, 630–645. [CrossRef] [PubMed]
34. Aydemir, T.B.; Liuzzi, J.P.; McClellan, S.; Cousins, R.J. Zinc transporter ZIP8 (SLC39A8) and zinc influence IFN-gamma expression in activated human T cells. *J. Leukoc. Biol.* **2009**, *86*, 337–348. [CrossRef] [PubMed]
35. Liuzzi, J.P.; Bobo, J.A.; Lichten, L.A.; Samuelson, D.A.; Cousins, R.J. Responsive transporter genes within the murine intestinal-pancreatic axis form a basis of zinc homeostasis. *Proc. Natl. Acad. Sci. USA* **2004**, *101*, 14355–14360. [CrossRef]

36. Marzetti, E.; Carter, C.S.; Wohlgemuth, S.E.; Lees, H.A.; Giovannini, S.; Anderson, B.; Quinn, L.S.; Leeuwenburgh, C. Changes in IL-15 expression and death-receptor apoptotic signaling in rat gastrocnemius muscle with aging and life-long calorie restriction. *Mech. Ageing Dev.* **2009**, *130*, 272–280. [CrossRef]
37. Yu, Y.; Liu, H.; Ikeda, Y.; Amiot, B.P.; Rinaldo, P.; Duncan, S.A.; Nyberg, S.L. Hepatocyte-like cells differentiated from human induced pluripotent stem cells: Relevance to cellular therapies. *Stem Cell Res.* **2012**, *9*, 196–207. [CrossRef]
38. Pfaffl, M.W. A new mathematical model for relative quantification in real-time RT-PCR. *Nucleic Acids Res.* **2001**, *29*, e45. [CrossRef]
39. Furda, A.M.; Bess, A.S.; Meyer, J.N.; Van Houten, B. Analysis of DNA damage and repair in nuclear and mitochondrial DNA of animal cells using quantitative PCR. *Methods Mol. Biol.* **2012**, *920*, 111–132. [CrossRef]
40. Jablonski, R.P.; Kim, S.-J.; Cheresh, P.; Williams, D.B.; Morales-Nebreda, L.; Cheng, Y.; Yeldandi, A.; Bhorade, S.; Pardo, A.; Selman, M.; et al. SIRT3 deficiency promotes lung fibrosis by augmenting alveolar epithelial cell mitochondrial DNA damage and apoptosis. *FASEB J.* **2017**, *31*, 2520–2532. [CrossRef]
41. Broedbaek, K.; Siersma, V.; Andersen, J.T.; Petersen, M.; Afzal, S.; Hjelvang, B.; Weimann, A.; Semba, R.D.; Ferrucci, L.; Poulsen, H.E. The association between low grade inflammation, iron status and nucleic acid oxidation in the elderly. *Free Radic. Res.* **2011**, *45*, 409–416. [CrossRef] [PubMed]
42. Calvani, R.; Marini, F.; Cesari, M.; Buford, T.W.; Manini, T.M.; Pahor, M.; Leeuwenburgh, C.; Bernabei, R.; Landi, F.; Marzetti, E. Systemic inflammation, body composition, and physical performance in old community-dwellers. *J. Cachexia Sarcopenia Muscle* **2017**, *8*, 69–77. [CrossRef] [PubMed]
43. Calvani, R.; Joseph, A.-M.; Adhihetty, P.J.; Miccheli, A.; Bossola, M.; Leeuwenburgh, C.; Bernabei, R.; Marzetti, E. Mitochondrial pathways in sarcopenia of aging and disuse muscle atrophy. *Biol. Chem.* **2013**, *394*, 393–414. [CrossRef] [PubMed]
44. Hepple, R.T. Mitochondrial involvement and impact in aging skeletal muscle. *Front. Aging Neurosci.* **2014**, *6*, 211. [CrossRef] [PubMed]
45. Picca, A.; Pesce, V.; Sirago, G.; Fracasso, F.; Leeuwenburgh, C.; Lezza, A.M.S. "What makes some rats live so long" The mitochondrial contribution to longevity through balance of mitochondrial dynamics and mtDNA content. *Exp. Gerontol.* **2016**, *85*, 33–40. [CrossRef] [PubMed]
46. Dixon, S.J.; Lemberg, K.M.; Lamprecht, M.R.; Skouta, R.; Zaitsev, E.M.; Gleason, C.E.; Patel, D.N.; Bauer, A.J.; Cantley, A.M.; Yang, W.S.; et al. Ferroptosis: An iron-dependent form of nonapoptotic cell death. *Cell* **2012**, *149*, 1060–1072. [CrossRef]
47. Seo, A.Y.; Xu, J.; Servais, S.; Hofer, T.; Marzetti, E.; Wohlgemuth, S.E.; Knutson, M.D.; Chung, H.Y.; Leeuwenburgh, C. Mitochondrial iron accumulation with age and functional consequences. *Aging Cell* **2008**, *7*, 706–716. [CrossRef]
48. Torti, F.M.; Torti, S.V. Regulation of ferritin genes and protein. *Blood* **2002**, *99*, 3505–3516. [CrossRef]
49. Andrews, N.C. Anemia of inflammation: The cytokine-hepcidin link. *J. Clin. Investig.* **2004**, *113*, 1251–1253. [CrossRef]
50. Ferrucci, L.; Corsi, A.; Lauretani, F.; Bandinelli, S.; Bartali, B.; Taub, D.D.; Guralnik, J.M.; Longo, D.L. The origins of age-related proinflammatory state. *Blood* **2005**, *105*, 2294–2299. [CrossRef]
51. Maggio, M.; Guralnik, J.M.; Longo, D.L.; Ferrucci, L. Interleukin-6 in aging and chronic disease: A magnificent pathway. *J. Gerontol. A Biol. Sci. Med. Sci.* **2006**, *61*, 575–584. [CrossRef]
52. Ganz, T. Hepcidin, a key regulator of iron metabolism and mediator of anemia of inflammation. *Blood* **2003**, *102*, 783–788. [CrossRef] [PubMed]
53. McCranor, B.J.; Langdon, J.M.; Prince, O.D.; Femnou, L.K.; Berger, A.E.; Cheadle, C.; Civin, C.I.; Kim, A.; Rivera, S.; Ganz, T.; et al. Investigation of the role of interleukin-6 and hepcidin antimicrobial peptide in the development of anemia with age. *Haematologica* **2013**, *98*, 1633–1640. [CrossRef] [PubMed]
54. Liuzzi, J.P.; Lichten, L.A.; Rivera, S.; Blanchard, R.K.; Aydemir, T.B.; Knutson, M.D.; Ganz, T.; Cousins, R.J. Interleukin-6 regulates the zinc transporter Zip14 in liver and contributes to the hypozincemia of the acute-phase response. *Proc. Natl. Acad. Sci. USA* **2005**, *102*, 6843–6848. [CrossRef] [PubMed]
55. Ferrucci, L.; Semba, R.D.; Guralnik, J.M.; Ershler, W.B.; Bandinelli, S.; Patel, K.V.; Sun, K.; Woodman, R.C.; Andrews, N.C.; Cotter, R.J.; et al. Proinflammatory state, hepcidin, and anemia in older persons. *Blood* **2010**, *115*, 3810–3816. [CrossRef]

56. Waalen, J.; von Löhneysen, K.; Lee, P.; Xu, X.; Friedman, J.S. Erythropoietin, GDF15, IL6, hepcidin and testosterone levels in a large cohort of elderly individuals with anaemia of known and unknown cause. *Eur. J. Haematol.* **2011**, *87*, 107–116. [CrossRef]
57. Guralnik, J.M.; Eisenstaedt, R.S.; Ferrucci, L.; Klein, H.G.; Woodman, R.C. Prevalence of anemia in persons 65 years and older in the United States: Evidence for a high rate of unexplained anemia. *Blood* **2004**, *104*, 2263–2268. [CrossRef]
58. Makipour, S.; Kanapuru, B.; Ershler, W.B. Unexplained anemia in the elderly. *Semin. Hematol.* **2008**, *45*, 250–254. [CrossRef]
59. Tacchini, L.; Recalcati, S.; Bernelli-Zazzera, A.; Cairo, G. Induction of ferritin synthesis in ischemic-reperfused rat liver: Analysis of the molecular mechanisms. *Gastroenterology* **1997**, *113*, 946–953. [CrossRef]
60. Goodall, E.F.; Haque, M.S.; Morrison, K.E. Increased serum ferritin levels in amyotrophic lateral sclerosis (ALS) patients. *J. Neurol.* **2008**, *255*, 1652–1656. [CrossRef]
61. Chimienti, G.; Picca, A.; Sirago, G.; Fracasso, F.; Calvani, R.; Bernabei, R.; Russo, F.; Carter, C.S.; Leeuwenburgh, C.; Pesce, V.; et al. Increased TFAM binding to mtDNA damage hot spots is associated with mtDNA loss in aged rat heart. *Free Radic. Biol. Med.* **2018**, *124*, 447–453. [CrossRef]

© 2019 by the authors. Licensee MDPI, Basel, Switzerland. This article is an open access article distributed under the terms and conditions of the Creative Commons Attribution (CC BY) license (http://creativecommons.org/licenses/by/4.0/).

MDPI
St. Alban-Anlage 66
4052 Basel
Switzerland
Tel. +41 61 683 77 34
Fax +41 61 302 89 18
www.mdpi.com

Cells Editorial Office
E-mail: cells@mdpi.com
www.mdpi.com/journal/cells

Ingram Content Group UK Ltd.
Milton Keynes UK
UKHW021022240523
422268UK00017B/59